ATTENTION AND BRAIN FUNCTION

ATTENTION AND BRAIN FUNCTION

Risto Näätänen

University of Helsinki
and
The Academy of Finland

LEA
1992

LAWRENCE ERLBAUM ASSOCIATES, PUBLISHERS
Hillsdale, New Jersey Hove and London

Lawrence Erlbaum Associates, Inc., Publishers
365 Broadway
Hillsdale, New Jersey 07642

Library of Congress Cataloging in Publication Data

Näätänen, Risto.
Attention and brain function / by Risto Näätänen.
p. cm.
Includes bibliographical references and indexes.
ISBN 0-8058-0984-8
1. Attention. 2. Evoked potentials (Electrophysiology)
3. Neuropsychology. I. Title.
QP405.N33 1992
612.8′13—dc20 92-15395
CIP

Printed in the United States of America
10 9 8 7 6 5 4 3 2

To my wife Marjatta
and my sons
Petri, Marko, and Janne

Contents

Foreword

This book by R. Näätänen, *Attention and Brain Function,* presents original psychophysiological research based on computerized techniques of recording and evaluating event-related brain potentials. The application of multichannel magnetoencephalography greatly contributes to exact localization of corresponding neuronal generators responsible for attention. The book contains a bulk of information concerning data obtained by cognitive psychology in the area of study of attention. These results are closely linked with neurophysiological investigation of attention.

The problem of attention has been studied in classical psychology mainly by using introspection data concerning an enhancement of subjective phenomena, improvement of task performance, and modification of motor responses due to a voluntary set or a given instruction. Thus, the psychological research of attention has focused on the voluntary (active) forms of attention. Two main difficulties arose on this pathway. On the one hand, under a voluntary set or due to a verbal instruction, attention was integrated into a behavioral act requiring a later separation of attentional mechanisms from decision making, response elicitation, and reinforcement. On the other hand, voluntary set and verbal instructions could not be applied for research of involuntary (passive) attention.

Cognitive psychology, however preoccupied with computer metaphor, was separated from the neurophysiological basis of attention. Such terms as *allocation of resources* used in explaining attention were influenced by computer science. No attempts were made to bridge the gap between the concept of resource allocation and its structural implementation into neural networks.

The objection against undifferentiated resources equally available to all tasks has led to a theory of multiple resources, which is still far from neurophysiological foundation.

The stimulus acting as a distractor of voluntary attention invokes a call for involuntary, automatic attention. Involuntary attention disrupts the voluntary attention system with stimuli characterized by intensity and suddenness. The psychological study of involuntary attention was based on its destructive effects on voluntary attention.

The direct investigation of involuntary attention was initiated by I.P. Pavlov's (1927) discovery of the orienting reflex (OR). In the framework of the physiology of the higher nervous activity, OR research was regarded as a logical extension of physiological research strategies which view psychological phenomena as complex brain functions.

Initially the OR was viewed as an interruption of ongoing activity (external inhibition of conditioned reflexes). Later, specific somatic OR components (eye and head movements) were identified, known after J. Konorski (1948) as the *targeting response.* However, the external inhibition of the ongoing activity and targeting responses constitute only a tip of the iceberg of OR components hidden from direct observation. The possibility of looking at this part of the iceberg of OR components was opened by the remarkable discovery of brain waves by H. Berger (1929). It was shown that the alpha-rhythm depression closely corresponds to the OR and involuntary attention. A very important step forward in the study of involuntary attention was the discovery made by Moruzzi and Magoun (1949) of the reticular activating system. It was shown that the alpha-rhythm depression, the OR, and involuntary attention can be integrated within the framework of a control system of arousal.

The study of cardiovascular, humoral, and sensory components of the OR has revealed an even more complex structure of involuntary attention. The main characteristic of the OR is its selective habituation during repeated presentation of a stimulus. It was suggested that in the process of repeated stimulus presentation, a neuronal model of a stimulus in the brain is established. The evocation of an involuntary OR depends on a mismatch signal generated by a disconcordance of the neuronal model and the stimulus presented. The progress in the identification of such a mismatch signal in the brain was based on the application of computerized averaging techniques for the study of the event-related potentials (ERPs). Using ERP shape comparisons on frequently presented standard and infrequent, deviant stimuli, Professor R. Näätänen found a specific brain wave, termed *the mismatch negativity* (MMN), specifically linked with deviation of the test stimulus from the standard stimulus. The mismatch negativity depends on a short-living stimulus trace caused by frequent stimulus of the specific projection area of the neocortex. Such a directly demonstrated mismatch signal differs from the classical OR in two basic aspects: short-living memory trace and modality-specific generation.

Another mismatch signal underlying classical involuntary OR was revealed by a specific computerized technique used to separate single ERPs evoked by stimuli presented with long intervals. M. Verbaten's (Verbaten, Roelofs, Sjouw, & Slangen, 1986) recordings of single skin-conductance responses (SCRs) and N1 peaks of ERPs have demonstrated a parallel habituation of a nonspecific part of the N1 wave of the ERP and the SCR. A novel stimulus results in a reestablishment of the nonspecific part of N1 and SCR. The nonspecific component of N1 has demonstrated a long-living trace, as well as modality-nonspecific effects. It might consequently be suggested that mismatch signals contributing to involuntary OR generation are based on at least two different kinds of traces: short-living modality-specific and long-living modality-nonspecific ones. The separation of two different involuntary OR-related ERPs opens a new perspective on the neuronal interpretation of the OR.

There are two basic concepts relating ERPs to neuronal activity: synaptic and glial. According to the synaptic hypothesis, ERPs are due to overlap of excitatory and inhibitory postsynaptic potentials (EPSPs and IPSPs, respectively). The glial hypothesis suggests that depolarizing–hyperpolarizing events are due to an increase and a subsequent decrease of spike-dependent potassium release affecting surrounding astrocytes. According to the glial hypothesis, spiking of different populations of novelty-responsive cells contribute to the mismatch negativity and the nonspecific component of the N1 peak.

An important step toward the understanding of the neuronal basis of attention was taken by the detector theory of perception suggesting, parallel selective coding of stimulus features within local brain modules. The stimulus features are coded by means of feature-detector maps. Viewing the nonspecific thalamic reticular formation as a spotlight emphasizes particular combinations of feature detectors constituting the focus of attention. The concept of the attentional spotlight can be explained by a local modular organization of feature detectors. Two stimuli within one module are fused, generating a single percept in one spatial locus. The stimuli acting on two different modules produce two different percepts in two spatial loci.

The shift of attention from a particular set of modules to another is due to the contribution of nonspecific local arousal evoked with participation of the thalamic reticular formation. Local arousal also participates in integration of features for object perception. The concept of local feature-detector modules as a basis of parallel information processing should be supplemented by the time-quanta principle. The duration of a time-quantum equals the period of local arousal. Different stimuli occurring during a single time-quantum within a local feature-detector module generate a single sensory event due to the fusion of separate excitations. The genetically prewired feature detectors are complemented by formation of learning-dependent long-term memory units of complex stimuli (gnostic units), which, after being established, are involved in OR elicitation selectively with respect to patterned stimuli. The feature detectors and memory units constitute a preattentional mechanism of input-signal analysis generating the stable part of the N1. The cortical mismatch negativity might depend on modality-specific novelty neurons of reticular thalamic nuclei.

Modality-nonspecific novelty detectors habituated in parallel with the SCR and the nonspecific part of the N1 component were demonstrated in the hippocampus by O. Vinogradova (1975). Thus separate ERPs, the mismatch negativity, and the nonspecific part of the N1 can be interpreted in terms of functioning neuronal circuits (neocortical and hippocampal novelty detectors).

Using a strategy of ERPs, one can initiate the study of voluntary OR as a basis of voluntary attention. The verbal instruction to attend to particular signal stimuli by counting their presentations among nonsignal stimuli results in an enhancement of the SCR and an increase in the N1 amplitude. The question arises whether the effects result from intensification of the involuntary OR or whether, in addition, a voluntary OR is initiated. Professor R. Näätänen has presented evidence that voluntary attention is characterized by a separate brain potential called the processing negativity (PN). The neuronal basis of this attentional ERP is linked with memory units. The memory units are switched to novelty neurons in two different ways: directly, as complex feature detectors for generation of an involuntary novelty effect, and indirectly, through their participation in a voluntarily kept template producing the significance effect of voluntary attention. By repeated presentation of a stimulus, its direct involuntary novelty effect is eliminated, while the significance effect remains operating in voluntary attention. A novel stimulus deviating from the relevant ones increases its novelty effects (the mismatch negativity and the nonspecific N1) and reduces the contribution of its significance (the processing negativity).

The voluntary OR acts together with the involuntary one in the sense that, during voluntary attention to relevant stimuli, irrelevant stimuli are handled in parallel by involuntary attention. A verbal instruction given to the subject to attend to a particular stimulus results in an evocation of the processing negativity when that stimulus is presented. The PN amplitude increases as the correspondence between the presented stimulus and the template constructed from memory units by verbal instruction becomes closer. The maintenance of the template depends on frontal-lobe neurons. According to A.R. Luria (Luria & Homskaya, 1970), in patients with frontal-lobe lesions having intact involuntary OR, verbal instruction does not facilitate the OR. In terms of neuronal populations, the processing negativity is a match signal evoked by a coincidence of the stimulus and the template composed of the neurons recruited from a pool of memory units constituting long-term memory.

Such long-term memory units formed in the process of learning were demonstrated by Y. Miyashita (1988) in the anterior ventral temporal cortex of a monkey. The template is maintained in an operational memory with the participation of frontal-lobe units. The recruitment of memory units into the template and the activation of the frontal-lobe units that keep the template in operational state are determined by reinforcement procedures during conditioning in animals or by semantic units analyzing verbal instruction in humans.

The neuronal basis underlying attentional ERPs can be presented as follows. The verbal instruction via semantic units organizes a template from memory units constituting long-term declarative memory. This template representing a brain copy of a relevant stimulus is kept as an operational memory mechanism with the participation of frontal-lobe voluntary control units. The memory units of the template are switched to novelty detectors at the neocortical and hippocampal levels. The stimulus presented is acting in parallel on feature detectors, gnostic units, and memory units of the template.

The response of the feature detectors and gnostic units generates the specific, nonhabituating N1. The signals are fed to short-living, neocortical short-term memory units generating the mismatch negativity. The pathway reaches hippocampal novelty detectors linked with the activating system. The spiking of activating-system neurons affects neocortical feature detectors and gnostic units by generating a nonspecific, habituating part of N1.

At the same time, the stimulus is matched in parallel against the template. By a coincidence of the stimulus with memory units within the template, spikes are generated constituting the processing negativity. The match signals passing to hippocampal novelty detectors reach the system of activating units and produce the significance effects of the OR and voluntary attention.

In the case of the disconcordance of the stimulus and the template, the match signal is not generated, the processing negativity is lacking, and the significance effect of the OR is not observed. The mismatch negativity is, however, generated by any short-term stimulus change, independently of verbal instruction.

—E.N. Sokolov

Preface

This book was started in early 1986 when I was a fellow in the Neurosciences Institute of the Neurosciences Research Program in New York, based on the initiative of Professor V.B. Mountcastle. I am greatly indebted to the staff of the institute, in particular to Dr. Einar Gall, for support during the initial preparatory phases of this volume. This work was interrupted following my return to Helsinki in April 1986 and remained dormant until my next long stay abroad, this time at the Wissenschaftskolleg zu Berlin (Institute for Advanced Study, Berlin) in West-Berlin from 1988-1989. This stay, based on the initiative of Professor Rudolf Cohen (University of Konstanz, Germany), gave me an opportunity to continue the book as well as prepare some articles. I am grateful to the whole staff of the Wissenschaftskolleg, especially to its Rector, Professor Wolf Lepenies, its Secretary, Dr. Nettel-Geck and Dr. Joachim Nettelbeck, for providing me with excellent conditions and support for this project, and to Mrs. Firooza Kraft for her competent and patient text-editing work.

On my return to Helsinki in August 1989, I believed that the work was almost done but in retrospect, more than 2 years later, it is now clear that I was not even halfway through. I considerably underestimated the amount of revision needed on the earlier draft of this book. In addition, the field was rapidly moving forward, not least because of the extremely fast technological and methodological development, and I kept changing the text as new results emerged. The manuscript was submitted to Lawrence Erlbaum Associates on July 8, 1991 (but even thereafter, several additions and changes were made). I regret that it was not possible to include animal research on attention and psychopathology of attention.

Many of my colleagues and friends have given an essential contribution to this book. In October 1989, I spent several days with Professor Terry Picton (Ottawa General Hospital) in Ottawa, Canada, who managed to greatly clarify my thinking and text with regard to some of the toughest theoretical problems encountered. A year later, in October 1990, I spent some time with Professor Walter Ritter (Albert Einstein College of Medicine, N.Y.) in New York who checked and commented a large portion of the text. In spring 1991, Professor Nelson Cowan from the University of Missouri, a specialist in cognitive psychology, spent a period of 3 months in our laboratory in Helsinki during which time he read most of the manuscript.

Also Professor E.N. Sokolov, from the Moscow State University, spent some time in Helsinki in early 1991 and read a large part of the manuscript. The contact with Professor Sokolov starting from my visit and lecture series in the Moscow University in the fall of 1981 has had a most deep influence on my thinking. As an acknowledgment to this fact, I have asked him to write the Foreword of this book.

Other senior colleagues who have continuously supported my scientific work are Professor Donald B. Lindsley (UCLA) in whose laboratory I got my training in this field and collected data for doctoral-thesis work in 1965-1966, Professor Friedhart Klix (Humboldt University, Berlin) whose help during the 1980s played a very significant role in creating the background conditions for this book work, and Professor Kai von Fieandt, my teacher in the University of Helsinki. Of particular importance have also been long discussions with Professor F. K. Graham (University of Delaware), Dr. N. E. Loveless (University of Dundee, Scotland), and Professor A. Öhman (University of Uppsala, Sweden).

Professor S.A. Hillyard, who has given me inspiration in all these years through his ingenious experimental work, has read an early version of the text on attention effects on visual event-related potentials. Dr. Marie-Helene Giard (INSERM, Lyon) has greatly helped the book project by clarifying some parts of the text and in many other ways.

Several other colleagues have also given helpful comments to previous drafts of the text of this book. They include: Cheryl Aine (Los Alamos National Laboratories, N.M.), Kimmo Alho (University of Helsinki), Deborah Arthur (Los Alamos National Laboratories, N.M.), Valéria Csépe (The Hungarian Academy of Sciences), Steven A. Hackley (University of Missouri), Heikki Hämäläinen (University of Helsinki), Riita Hari (Helsinki University of Technology), Jim Hoffman (University of Delaware), Risto Ilmoniemi (Helsinki University of Technology), Dan Javitt (Albert Einstein College of Medicine, N.Y.), William A. Johnston (University of Utah), Lloyd Kaufman (New York University), Art Kramer (University of Illinois at Urbana-Champaign), Heikki Lang (University of Turku,

Finland), Heikki Lyytinen (University of Jyväskylä, Finland), Jyrki Mäkelä (Helsinki University of Technology), Ronald Mangun (University of Dartmouth), Patricia T. Michie (Macquarie University, Sydney), Gisbertus Mulder (University of Groningen, The Netherlands), Christo Pantev (University of Münster, Germany), Michael I. Posner (University of Oregon), Jarl Risberg (University of Lund, Sweden), Per Roland (Karolinska Hospital, Stockholm), Walton T. Roth (Stanford University and V.A. Hospital, Palo Alto), Michael Rugg (University of St. Andrews, Scotland), Jukka Saarinen (University of Helsinki), Mikko Sams (Helsinki University of Technology), Michael Scherg (Max-Planck Institut für Psychiatrie, München), R. J. Seitz (University of Düsseldorf, Germany), Christopher D. Wickens (University of Illinois at Urbana-Champaign), Veijo Virsu (University of Helsinki), Samuel Williamson (New York University), István Winkler (The Hungarian Academy of Sciences), C.C. Wood (Los Alamos National Laboratories, N.M.), J.M. von Wright (University of Helsinki), and D.L. Woods (University of California, Davis).

I am also indebted to Kenneth Campbell (University of Ottawa), Emanuel Donchin (University of Illinois at Urbana-Champaign), Aki M. Johansson (University of Lund, Sweden), Gregory A. Miller (University of Illinois at Urbana-Champaign), and Peter Ullsperger (Institute of Occupational Health, Berlin) for their help.

This book would not have been possible without the experimental work conducted by my research group: Kimmo Alho, Juha Lavikainen, Teija Nittyvuopio, Petri Paavilainen, Kalevi Reinikainen, Mikko Sams (until 1989), Wolfgang Teder, Mari Tervaniemi, Hannu Tiitinen, and István Winkler. I wish also to acknowledge experimental collaboration with A. Algazi, N. Cowan, N. Donauer, M.-H. Giard, H. Hämäläinen, M. Hämäläinen, R. Hari, R. Ilmoniemi, D. Jiang, S. Karakas, M.-L. Karlsson, E. Kaukoranta, J. Kekoni, R.T. Knight, A. Lähteenmäki, H. Lang, P. Laurinen, N. E. Loveless, H. Lyytinen, G. Nyman, T. Radil, W. Ritter, E. Schröger, M. Simpson, E.N. Sokolov, K. Töttölä, M. Wagner, and D.L. Woods. A.W.K. Gaillard and S. Mäntysalo have had an essential role in the initial findings on which our current research work is based. Theoretical and reviewing work conducted with T.W. Picton, A.W.K. Gaillard, and P.T. Michie in the past has helped me in developing some of the conceptual tools for dealing with the phenomena addressed in the book.

My research group has been of crucial importance also in practical realization of the book. I am especially indebted to Mari Tervaniemi, M.A., who has done most of the text-editing work and to Juha Lavikainen, M.A., who has taken the main responsibility for the preparation of the figures.

From the publisher's side, I wish in particular to thank Dr. Chava Casper, Assistant Editor, for her help, advice, and encouragement and Mr.

Christopher Pecci for his careful and skillful editing work. Of course, I am more than grateful to Lawrence Erlbaum Associates, Inc., for their willingness to publish the book.

Finally, I wish to express my sincerest gratitude to The Academy of Finland, especially to its Council of Social Sciences, and to the University of Helsinki, for their financial support without which our laboratory and research group could not exist. Support has also been received from The Emil Aaltonen Foundation, European Science Foundation, The Finnish Academy of Science and Letters, The Finnish Cultural Foundation, The Gyllenberg Foundation, U.S. Public Health Service (Fogarty International Research Fellowship to K. Alho), and Väinö Tanner Foundation. In addition, Professor O.V. Lounasmaa has kindly provided us with a possibility to conduct magnetoencephalographic studies in his laboratory in The Helsinki University of Technology. The Department of Psychology, University of Helsinki, in particular its Chairman, Professor G. Nyman, has also supported our research group in several important ways.

Last but not least, I wish to express my gratitude to my family for their (almost) never-ending patience and support during this project, which turned out to be tremendously more demanding and time consuming than I initially expected and promised.

—Risto Näätänen

1

Introduction: What Is Attention?

1.1. ON THE HISTORY OF THE CONCEPT

The scope of this book is attention, although as James (1890) said:

> Everyone knows what attention is. It is the taking possession of the mind, in clear and vivid form, of one out of what seem several simultaneously possible objects or trains of thought. Focalization, concentration of consciousness are of its essence. It implies withdrawal from some things in order to deal effectively with others, and is a condition which has a real opposite in the confused, dazed, scatterbrained state . . . (pp. 403–404)

We cannot easily attend to more than one thing at a time, James (1890) maintained:

> . . . unless the processes are very habitual; but then two, or even three, without very much oscillation of the attention. Where, however, the processes are less automatic, as in the story of Julius Caesar dictating four letters whilst he writes a fifth, there must be a rapid oscillation of the mind from one to the next, and no consequent gain of time. Within any one of the systems the parts may be numberless, but we attend to them collectively when we conceive the whole which they form. (p. 409)

It is easy to agree with Horn (1965) that almost everything that is intuitively obvious about attention was stated more than a century ago by William James (James, 1890). Moreover, the respect for James' views has even increased since the mid-1960s when this opinion was expressed—

perhaps prompted by setbacks, blind alleys, and persistent conceptual confusion prevailing in attention research. James' thoughts are now viewed by many as having penetrated the "intuitively obvious," and much beyond that, to a level perhaps superior in several ways to where we are now, a century later, with all our new techniques and methodologies. In their excellent review of the field, Johnston and Dark (1986), bewildered by all these problems, confessed:

> At a time of despair and panic we turned to William James (1890), where we found new hope and inspiration. The reader will understand, therefore, if from time to time we betray a reverential awe of James. We believe that James understood attention better than most contemporary theorists; he articulated many of the same phenomena with which current theories are concerned, but he managed to avoid some of the pitfalls of many current theories. (p. 44)

Attention is one of the most popular constructs in modern cognitive psychology, psychophysiology, and related fields; in fact, it is hard to understand how we could do without it. Nevertheless, it was possible for our respectable predecessors in psychological research in the first half of this century to develop influential theories of human behavior, mind, subjective experience, and the biological basis of all that, without using the concept of attention at all. Also many notable contemporaries of James, such as Wundt, Helmholtz, Hering, Exner, Külpe, Donders, and Cattell, showed marked experimental and theoretical interest in attention, but after these pioneers, the subject of attention was put aside. For example, only six brief items are listed under the heading "Attention" in Stevens' monumental *Handbook of Experimental Psychology* (1951). And in Boring's *Sensation and Perception in the History of Experimental Psychology* (1942), surveying an area of research highly geared to the use of reporting and introspection, "Attention" is a subheading under "Attributes" in the index, and only two brief items are listed.

This reluctance to use the concept of attention strikes many as very strange because this concept refers to something that seems to be absolutely essential in us as perceiving, thinking, and behaving organisms. This reluctance can, however, be understood as an overshooting response to the introspectionistic trends in psychology when it became increasingly clear that the human mind cannot understand itself by trying to observe itself. The behaviorist movement in American psychology, fostered by Watson, Holt, Weiss, and others, rejected the idea of subjective descriptions of experiences and abandoned the use of the concepts of attention and consciousness.

> They substituted description and measurement of overt behavioral responses, including vocal, subvocal and other responses of semiovert nature, detectable

> only by special measuring or recording instruments. From the point of view of objective measurement and the establishment of reliable, though perhaps limited, criteria of response, this was an advance. However, it overlooked the fact that not all stimulation which is capable of excitation of, or influence upon, the central nervous system results in overt behavior of an immediate and measurable nature. (Lindsley, 1960, p. 1554)

Lindsley, a great pioneer of cognitive neuroscience, emphasized that although behavioral criteria of sleep and wakefulness, and even of attention and consciousness, may be established, it has become apparent that one cannot depend solely on these criteria. In his view, the very essence of attention and consciousness seems "to reside in shifting processes and states within the central nervous system, some of which are detectable through changes in electrical potentials recorded indirectly and diffusely from the brain, or directly and focally in certain regions of the brain" (Lindsley, 1960, pp. 1554–1555).

Another important reason for the neglect of attention in psychology is the long dominance of Gestalt psychologists and their great influence on contemporary thinking. Gestalt psychologists emphasized their intrinsic Gestalt laws as central determinants of our percepts, of course, leaving no role to attention in perceptual organization. For example, according to Rubin (1921), one cannot abolish the fundamental differences between the figure and the ground by seeking it through a change in the direction of attention. *"Die . . . Unterschiede zwischen Figur und Grund sind desgleichen ganz konkret, und die Verwendung des Wortes Aufmerksamkeit hat sich als überflüssig erwiesen"* ["The differences between figure and ground are essentially concrete; thus the use of the term attention rendered itself as obsolete."] (Rubin, 1921, p. 101).

Worden (1966) wondered how it is possible to have so much psychology with so little attention and he explained: "The lens of science is difficult to focus on the phenomena termed attention so that one may be tempted to turn it on something else to get a sharper scientific image" (pp. 48–49). According to him, this is due to severe conceptual and methodological problems associated with attention. The essence of the conceptual problem is, in his view, that the selectivity so evident in the performance of organisms results from the operation of selective forces at all psychological levels, from sensation through cognition to response.

However, the rapid technological development during the World War II and immediately thereafter and the consequent change in the demands on human performance soon led to a revival of attention and related concepts (Evarts, Shinoda, & Wise, 1984; Kahneman & Treisman, 1984). A new important field of psychology, human performance research, emerged as a response to different kinds of questions involving the human being as a task performer. Human operators monitoring radar screens, dials, and other information sources became the models of the new research area. Variations in human perception and performance in such situations soon made it clear that perceptual acuity and similar concepts were not sufficient to explain limitations and extensive variations in performance.

> The revival of interest in attention in the 1950s was motivated at least in part by the discovery of surprising limitations in the handling of simultaneous messages by air-traffic controllers and by subjects in dichotic listening tasks. Perceptual overload seemed to be the problem, and the experimental situations of the time were designed to induce overload in order to explore the efficacy with which limited resources could be directed to the most relevant information. (Kahneman & Treisman, 1984, p. 29)

Attention returned to psychology and has made a comeback in a manner compensatory to its long-time absence. The concept is now frequently used and, it seems, often even in inappropriate connections. It appears that it would be best to try to use other, more specific, terms wherever possible and to describe the process involved as accurately as possible. The conceptual problem associated with the term attention will be dealt with later.

1.2. PHENOMENA COMMONLY REFERRED TO AS "ATTENTION"

Situations and phenomena in which the attention concept has been commonly used are briefly described first. Thereafter analogous phenomena in situations where the term has not been generally used are examined. In this way, we may, hopefully, understand attention better and gain some conceptual clarity.

To describe some of the principal uses of the attention concept, we can, for instance, selectively attend to one of the concurrent streams of input such as the voice of a certain speaker in a cocktail party where all the people are speaking at the same time. Or, when only one person is speaking, we can attend to that voice, in order to get the message, as opposed to attending to something else or to nothing. Further, we can well direct our attention to the voice of the speaker but listen to it as an acoustic phenomenon, without caring about the linguistic message that this voice is carrying. Attention can scan or focus on different objects depending on our momentary or permanent interests and goals as well as on the properties of the stimuli involved.

The complexity of objects of attention can vary from simple physical attributes, such as the tonal frequency or the locus of origin of a sound, to complex stimuli and stimulus combinations, even to subtle semantic aspects of the stimuli. Apparently, we can attend to any aspect of stimuli or their combinations, within the limits of discriminability. It is of course easier to attend to stimuli that are very different from other concurrent stimuli than to those that are easily confused with the concurrent stimuli.

Further, selective attention can have a broad or narrow focus, and this does not have to depend merely on physical stimulus properties such as the width (visual angle) of a radar screen monitored. Thus, even in an identical stimulus situation, attention can have a narrower or a broader focus, or be directed to molecular or molar aspects of stimulation (e.g., to individual dots on a visual display or to the pattern formed by them). One popular assumption (Easterbrook, 1959) holds that when we become more aroused the focus of attention gets narrower.

Divided attention occurs when the subject is instructed to monitor simultaneously two or several input sources such as to listen to two dichotically presented stories, that is, one story to one ear and the other story concurrently to the other ear. The interest here has, in general, been in clarifying how well people can perform two simultaneous tasks, for instance, how much, if any, performance decrement in one task occurs due to performing the other task. This decrement has usually been explained in terms of "capacity" limitations (Kahneman, 1973) or of incompatibility of the response patterns required by the two tasks. (For penetrating analyses of the capacity concept, see Allport, 1980; Navon, 1985; Wickens, 1984.) The performance in the secondary task has often been used as a measure of the spare capacity left over by the primary task in which the performance may remain at a steady level, due to compensatory "resource allocation."

On the other hand, "sustained attention" or "vigilance" is studied when interest is in long-term performance decrement, mainly in detecting infrequent and unpredictable weak signals, as a function of the time on task. (For a review, see Parasuraman, 1984.)

All the preceding cases involve active or voluntary attention; we can choose the object of our attention. This can, however, be the other way round also. Abrupt loud sounds, infrequent events, unfamiliar objects, incongruent object combinations, significant stimuli (e.g., our name being mentioned in some unattended conversation), all such events and many others tend to attract our attention away from the task we are performing. This attention switch was named "passive attention" by William James (1890). Stimuli that elicit passive attention also tend to elicit what is called the "orienting reflex" or the "orienting response" (Sokolov, 1963), a complex pattern of overt and covert bodily changes often associated with such an attention switch. This response pattern was called the "what-is-it-reaction" or the "investigatory reaction" by the famous Russian neurophysiologist Ivan Pavlov (1927), who first described it.

This brings us to the issue of *distraction.* When we try to concentrate on some demanding mental task, occasional sounds and other irrelevant stimuli are usually regarded as distracting, causing distraction away from the task. We can often maintain our level of performance irrespective of distraction but this may occur at the cost of increased effort (Kahneman, 1973; Woodworth, 1938; see also Wickens, 1984). The essence of the distracting effect is, evidently, that those irrelevant stimuli tend to attract our attention, at least momentarily, away from the task. Research interest here has been in the effects of different distractors on performance, on physiological responses and states, as well as on various subjective variables.

When attention is caught by a stimulus from a task we are performing, it is usually almost instantaneously pulled back to the task performance (voluntary attention). The duration of passive attention to the stimulus which caused the attention switch usually depends on the time needed for stimulus recognition and evaluation. However, when we start to follow a conversation whose onset initially caught our attention away from the task, it is a case where involuntary attention changes to voluntary attention without a concomitant change of the object of attention.

1.3. ATTENTION TO PAST AND FUTURE STIMULI

Whereas involuntary attention only operates in the present time—only stimuli here and now can elicit it—voluntary attention can be directed to past or future stimuli and events. For instance, we can attend to a sound that occurred 2 seconds ago by attending to its representation in echoic memory (Neisser, 1967), which is discussed in chapter 2. This ability has certainly saved us many times from awkward social situations caused by not listening to a speaker at the moment of his or her speaking. If it suddenly turns out to be very important to know what that person just said—for instance, he or she unexpectedly asks a question related to what he or she had just said—it is possible to internally "listen" to the auditory events of the immediate past just as from a tape recording. But these internal auditory stores decay very rapidly, so that we can maximally get back only a few words or a short sentence. On the other hand, when we perform a long-term memory search for some stimulus or event of the past, this form of backwards-directed attention is not limited by a fast decay of its target.

Future-directed attention is involved when we, say, concentrate on responding as fast as possible to a visual signal to be delivered in the immediate future (simple reaction time) or to a certain one of three visual stimuli delivered in random order (go/no-go or choice reaction time). The form of attention involved could be called "expectant" or "anticipatory attention." In this case, attention is set for detecting the target as soon as possible and releasing a prompt response to it.

This future-oriented, anticipatory attention was extensively investigated by Posner. In his studies of the costs and benefits of expectations (see Posner, 1978), the first stimulus was usually not to be responded to but it delivered to the subject some information with regard to the imperative stimulus, for instance its probable locus of appearance in the visual field. If the imperative stimulus indeed occurred in the expected locus, the reaction time (RT) was shorter than when the warning stimulus contained no spatial information. This RT gain was regarded as the measure of the benefit of the specific expectation. On the other hand, if the imperative stimulus was presented in an unexpected locus, the RT was longer than when the warning stimulus was uninformative with regard to the locus of the imperative stimulus. This RT prolongation served as Posner's measure of cost of a wrong expectancy. This design involves selection only in the sense that the subject is selectively prepared for some future events rather than for others (Kahneman & Treisman, 1984).

1.4. ATTENTION IN THE MOTOR DOMAIN

As already mentioned, the concept of attention is relevant even in the motor domain where phenomena analogous to those referred to by attention in the sensory domain occur. In attention research, however, there has been a very strong emphasis on the sensory side.

> Attention, as a concept covering selective activity, is responsible for the modulation of information processing and has generally been considered, until recently, as mainly acting upon sensory input. This has most often been explicitly stated in the definitions proposed for attentional processes, which emphasize the role of attention in the selection of stimuli. Furthermore, at the end of the 1970s, although several studies addressed the question of the attentional demand of movement in the frame of dual-task paradigm, no more than half a dozen papers were written under titles associating attention with movement. . . . (Requin, 1985, pp. 147–148)

Requin (1985) regarded the linkage of attention and consciousness as an important reason for the long-lasting separation between attention and movement. This is because, according to him, internal signals that determine the biomechanical features of a movement are likely to have no direct access to consciousness. Consequently, the involvement of consciousness in movement is only indirect: "What is most conscious is the stored representation or online perception of the changes that a movement introduces in the outside world . . . and, perhaps, what it feels like during its execution" (Requin, 1985, p. 148).

Evarts, Shinoda, and Wise (1984) provided an excellent discussion of the role of attention and set in motor behavior. A difficult motor performance needs strong concentration of the mind in order to succeed. Such performances are based on motor programs stored in the central nervous system, and their adequate selection and release often require total involvement of the mind in this performance. Requin (1985) observed that "because the concepts both of selective attention and of specific preparation can be viewed as covering internally triggered selective sets, they are closely related and possibly not separable" (p. 149) and, further, referring also to the hypothesis of Sternberg, Monsell, Knoll, and Wright (1978), that "both processes are optional and flexible, either governed by some central processor or automatized. Note that it thus would be legitimate to utilize the notion of perceptual preparation to define selective set acting on input processing, as well as that of motor attention to define selective set acting on output processing" (Requin, 1985, pp. 151–152).

In "ballistic" movements, the performance is so short that once its release has started, there is no chance of correcting the course. Thus, attentional effects determining the performance occur before the actual movement. On the other hand, in the nonballistic performance, the motor program of the performance involved is not fully determined at the onset of the release but can be modified on the basis of the subsequent feedback (which may have internal or external sources, or both). The level of excellence of many performances depends on how the feedback is used. A typical motor control situation critically depending on the adequacy of feedback utilization is manual tracking of a moving visual target or driving along a winding road.

Consequently, motor control may, in fact, involve a complex integration task. In addition to concentrating on selection and release of an optimal motor program, one continually utilizes the sensory feedback from the ongoing motor behavior and from the effects of this behavior on the situation, including the changing spatial relation of our body to the environment.

A complex motor performance can become automatized, of course, as a result of frequent repetition over a long period of time. A man who has just learned the steps of a difficult dance usually is quite a quiet partner. His mind is involved in the release of the appropriate motor program and in coordinating this release to information provided by sensory feedback, there being less time, or capacity, for long-term memory search for suitable topics of conversation and also a reduced sensitivity to situational cues for such topics. After a couple of hours of practice, he gains his talkativeness back, however.

Our musculature obeys central commands within its anatomical and physiological limits. These commands have to be adequately chosen, both qualitatively and quantitatively, as well as correctly timed in order for the desired behavioral pattern to occur (Näätänen, 1973). The crucial importance of this mental concentration in control of difficult motor performance has become increasingly clear to those who aim at top-level athletic performance: In sports, a popular training method nowadays is called "mental training." In it, the athlete just imagines, during motor quiescence, his or her motor performance, the sequence of the motor-activation patterns involved. Some positive effects on motor performance have been reported. (For a review, see Feltz & Landers, 1983.)

In conclusion, selective mental activity or work can be observed as governing motor behavior in a way analogous to the role of selective mental work when we focus our mind on, that is, select, some specific type of sensory information among all concurrent sensory input.

1.5. ATTENTION AND THINKING

The attention concept is relevant even in the analysis of purely central events, that is, when neither sensory nor motor connections of the organism with the external world are involved. Much of the time, however, our thinking may be characterized as associative, one thought, or mental representation, activating the next, one memory calling for another, this sequence reflecting the strength of connections between different items stored in long-term memory. Such associative chains of thought, which psychoanalysts are tracing, typically occur in a perceptually static situation when our mental activity momentarily has no definite goal.

Usually our thinking, however, has a definite goal, and can then be characterized as *directed thinking* or, to use Roland's (1981, 1985) term, *mental work*. This is the case when we try to solve a problem, or to recall urgently the name for some familiar disappointed face, and so forth. The aspect of selection in this mental work is evident here: When the chain of thoughts slips away from the task, due for instance to associations emerging during the purposeful thought process or to environmental distracting stimuli, thinking is usually returned back to the relevant track from the irrelevant track or chain of thoughts. Evidently, the ongoing mental process is monitored with reference to, and guided toward, its goal; there is the memory of the decision of what should be achieved by mental work in progress. The thinking process is *self-corrected* moment by moment until the desired end state is achieved (see also Ingvar, 1985).

Hence we can have a selective mental focus even with no sensory or motor control operation. Again, the ability to concentrate on the activity pursued is a crucial condition of success, that is, the ability to maintain the mental focus and to shift it according to the changing mental environment. Even here selection continuously occurs between numerous alternatives, among them those provided by the irrelevant stimuli or action patterns, potential chains of thought, tempting the mind to sidetrack from the goal-oriented focus or sequence of thought. Goal-directed thinking is, thus, another form of *directed central activity,* in principle very similar to that underlying the aspect of continuous selection in sensory or motor contact with the environment.

2

Attention and Automaticity in Information Processing

2.1. INTRODUCTION

Although the attention construct plays a critical role in scientific analysis of various forms of information processing and behavior, a good deal of these processes run their course independently of attention. Indeed, much of the information processing in our brain occurs without any voluntary effort or experienced mental involvement. Certainly everybody has such experiences of his or her own. One time the motor of my car extinguished while standing in traffic lights when the amber turned green, there typically being a slope backwards and a long queue of impatient drivers. In this anxiety-provoking situation, I observed that my right hand had very quickly moved behind the driver's seat as if searching for something. Afterward, I recalled that the start button of the van that I had had a long time ago when I had a butcher's shop in Helsinki was located in a location compatible to that strange hand movement. Later, I decided to become a psychologist, but from that background, it was possible to become only a psychophysiologist.

Here we come to the distinction between automatic and attentional (nonautomatic, controlled; Shiffrin & Schneider, 1977) processes, a distinction of central importance in current research of human information processing. The so-called automatic processing was indeed a favored topic during the 1970s and 1980s, and the interest mainly involved the borderline between the automatic and attentional processes. Thus the investigators have sought for answers to questions such as what type of sensory processing can occur automatically, in the sense of being free from capacity limitations, to what extent these limits can be pushed farther by extended practice, which tasks can be combined with one another without performance decrement, and how much processing occurs to unattended sensory input.

This chapter first examines some leading views on the nature and extent of automatic processing, and thus on the borderline between automatic and attentive processing. This issue of course is intimately intertwined with that involving the mechanisms of attention itself; these mechanisms, their nature and extent, determine the space left for automaticity in information processing. Therefore, after examining views on automatic processing, theories of attention are discussed.

2.2. DIFFERENT FORMS OF AUTOMATICITY

Criteria of Automaticity. Posner and Snyder (1975), in their highly influential paper, proposed three criteria for a process to be purely automatic: The process occurs (a) without intention, involuntarily, (b) without giving rise to any conscious awareness, and (c) without producing interference with other ongoing mental activity (i.e., not using limited-capacity resources of the organism). The authors maintained that "even with these stringent requirements it is possible to show that many complex but habitual mental processes can operate automatically and thus, in principle, be strategy-independent . . . Many cognitive tasks may be viewed as combining automatic activation and conscious strategies" (Posner & Snyder, 1975, p. 56).

As an example of processing occurring without intention, in fact even against intention, the authors referred to the so-called Stroop effect (Stroop, 1935). This effect provides excellent evidence that the subject cannot always avoid processing of aspects of an input item which he or she desires to ignore. In this task, the subject is presented with a name of a color printed in a different color and is asked to name the color of the ink. This performance is slowed down by the competition between vocal responses to the printed word, involuntarily activating its name code, and the ink color. Consistently with this, words often facilitate the ink-color naming response when the ink and the word share a common color name (Hintzman et al., 1972).

Posner and Snyder concluded from Stroop studies that color naming and reading go on in parallel and without interference until close to the output. "If they result in look-up of the same name, the overall reaction time is speeded; if they produce different names and a vocal output is required, the word tends to compete with the color name and reaction time is increased" (Posner & Snyder, 1975, p. 57).

As a further example of unintentional, and in this sense automatic, mental events, the authors referred to the well-established phenomenon of the spreading of activation in long-term memory. For instance, a word not only activates its representation in long-term memory but also, to some extent, related representations, and this spreading activation is stronger for more closely associated words (Warren, 1972, 1974). This effect occurs without any apparent intention of the subject.

Posner and Snyder's (1975) second criterion for an automatic process was lack of awareness. Here the authors pointed to the Stroop results of Conrad (1974), which they interpreted as showing that the subject may be quite unaware of the activation pattern produced by input words. Subjects were orally presented with sentences that ended with an ambiguous word (e.g., "bank"). In some cases, the word was disambiguated by the context, in others not. The orally presented sentence was followed by a single visual word in colored ink, and the subject's task was to name the color of the ink.

Conrad found that the time to name the color of the ink was longer when this word was related to the last word of the sentence than when the visually presented word was neutral. This result might be interpreted as suggesting spreading of activation to semantically related items in long-term memory (Posner & Snyder, 1975). The finding of particular interest here is that the prolongation of the color-naming response was similar for the two meanings of the ambiguous word even when the sentence context had disambiguated this word.

Thus, a word, which has two meanings when presented alone, activates both meanings even in a sentence context that clearly specifies, disambiguates, the meaning of the word in that sentence. Posner and Snyder (1975) concluded that since a word disambiguated by context is consciously perceived in only one way, the fact that both meanings are nevertheless activated provides evidence that "the activation pattern is not dependent on the subject's conscious percept" (p. 59). Holender (1986), however, regarded it possible that an ambiguous word in a disambiguating context might nevertheless initially cause a short-lasting awareness of both of its meanings (of which the one compatible with the context then remains; Swinney, 1979, 1982). Therefore, he maintained that these studies do not warrant the inference that the initial activation of multiple meanings is unconscious.

As further evidence for the claim that semantic activation can occur without awareness, Posner and Snyder (1975) pointed to results of a number of dichotic-listening studies, concluding that a large amount of automatic semantic processing still occurred for the to-be-ignored input. Holender (1986), however, again denied the value of these kinds of data as evidence for the occurrence of semantic processing without awareness. He concluded that dichotic-listening tasks are "simply ill-suited" for fulfilling his first criterion for the occurrence of semantic activation without conscious identification. This criterion, slightly modified from that proposed by Dixon (1971), was that the data should provide "positive indirect evidence of semantic activation together with negative direct evidence of stimulus identification at the time of presentation" (Holender, 1986, p. 3).

Posner and Snyder's (1975) third criterion for a purely automatic process was that it does not produce interference with other ongoing mental activity. Parallel semantic processing occurring in different kinds of situations was pointed to as evidence for these kinds of processes. Such semantic activation was, according to the authors, caused by to-be-ignored (aspects of) stimulation in the Stroop and dichotic-listening tasks and also when the to-be-ignored stimuli have differed in modality from the to-be-attended stimuli.

As further evidence, the authors referred to RT studies (e.g., LaBerge, 1973) showing that although the response to an unexpected stimulus is considerably delayed, the accuracy of the response, either physical or semantic discrimination, is very high, even higher than for the expected stimulus. While considering also some other possibilities, Posner and Snyder (1975) proposed, as a possible explanation of these results, that "information from the unattended channel is building up in a normal way even though the subject is not attending to it" (p. 63). They admitted, however, that these data by themselves are not totally convincing as evidence for parallel processing but when coupled with the Stroop and dichotic-listening data referred to, "there begins to build a picture of stimulus information automatically activating those internal representations that have been habitually associated with it" (p. 63; see also LaBerge & Samuels, 1974, and Keele, 1973).

Interestingly, Posner and Snyder emphasized that this view makes the automaticity of a perceptual pathway "closely related to the degree of learning or experience that the subject has had to particular associations" (1975, p. 63). In this way the authors anticipated the extensive evidence for parallel processing occurring as a result of extended training in visual search, which was obtained in the latter half of the 1970s and thereafter. It is now time to turn to this evidence, which underlies much of the current theorizing on the nature of automatic processing.

Automaticity Produced by Extended Training. This evidence originates mainly from the studies initiated by Shiffrin and Schneider (1977; Schneider & Shiffrin, 1977), and provides the empirical basis of the popular distinction between automatic and controlled processes proposed by the authors. These studies used a modification of the memory-search paradigm introduced by Sternberg (1966, 1969, 1975) for investigating short-term memory search (the "Sternberg paradigm"). In essence, a small set of items (typically one to six in number), called the memory set, is presented to the subject.

Shortly thereafter a single input item ("probe") is presented, and the subject reacts as rapidly as possible with one response if the input item is in the memory set (a positive response) and with a different response if it is not (a negative response).

The typical finding was that the RT is a linear function of the memory-set size, with the RT increasing by about 40 msec for each additional item in the memory set. This was true for both positive and negative responses. Sternberg proposed that the input item was compared in turn with each memory-set item at a rate of 40 msec per comparison.

Very similar results have been obtained in research on visual search. In a typical study (Atkinson, Holmgren, & Juola, 1969), a single item to be stored in short-term memory was first delivered, followed by a presentation of a visual display containing several items. The task was to decide as quickly as possible whether or not the display contained the memory-set item. Again, there was a linear relationship between the number of items in the visual display and the RT. Further, the RT regularly increased at a rate of about 40 msec per item (both for the positive and negative responses).

In the multiframe visual-search paradigm of Shiffrin and Schneider (1977) and Schneider and Shiffrin (1977), the frames (displays) are presented in immediate succession, and each frame is presented only for a brief period of time. The subject's task is to memorize a set of visually presented items (memory-set items) such as letters of the alphabet and to respond, say, with the left hand if one of these letters (target) appears in a subsequently presented set of visual items (probes), and with the right hand if no target appears in the latter set (i.e., all the probes in the frame are "distractors").

In Shiffrin and Schneider's *consistent-mapping* condition, targets are always selected from one set of items (e.g., letters from A to N) and distractors are selected from another, nonoverlapping set of items (e.g., letters from O to Z). Thus, the mapping of stimuli to responses does not vary over trials. After extensive practice, the target-recognition performance, measured in speed and accuracy, becomes independent or almost independent of the memory-set size and of the frame or display size (the number of visual items in the frame; Schneider & Shiffrin, 1977). For such results, see Fig. 2.1. This type of performance was termed by the authors *automatic*. It was characterized as fast, inflexible, difficult to suppress once learned, and not limited by short-term memory capacity or attention (see Schneider, Dumais, & Shiffrin, 1984).

On the other hand, when targets and distractors are chosen from the same set of items and thus exchange roles over trials, it is not possible for the subject to consistently map stimuli to responses. Under these *varied-mapping* conditions, the increase in the memory-set size or in the frame size considerably increases the RT and the number of errors irrespective of the amount of practice, there being only little improvement with extended

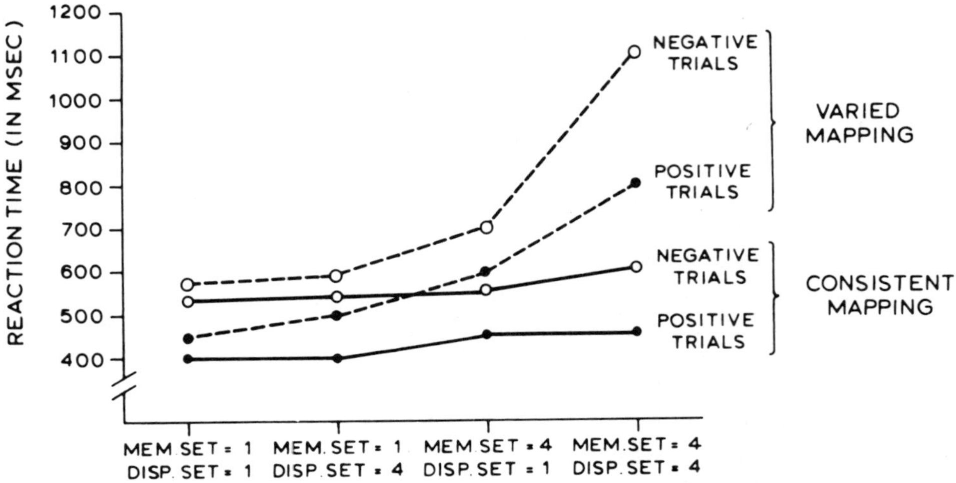

FIG. 2.1 The effects of memory-set size and display-set size on speed of response in a target-detection task separately for varied-mapping and consistent-mapping conditions. (Adapted from Schneider & Shiffrin, 1977, by Eysenck, 1982. Copyright © 1982 by Springer-Verlag. Reprinted with permission.)

practice. This type of processing was called *controlled processing* by Shiffrin and Schneider (1977) and by Schneider and Shiffrin (1977). Controlled (control) processing was characterized by Schneider et al. (1984) as slow, serial, and capacity-limited.

How Automatic is "Automatic" Processing? One is indeed impressed by the magnitude of the training effect under the consistent-mapping conditions, that is, by the large amount of parallel processing that seems to occur as a result of the extended consistent-mapping training. However, this performance is not fully independent of the memory-set and display-set sizes, that is, on the magnitude of parallel processing to be performed. Eysenck (1982) observed that a typical finding was that "increases in memory-set size and visual display size led to increases of approximately 15% in reaction time under consistent mapping conditions" (Eysenck, 1982, p. 23; see also Hoffman & MacMillan, 1985; Hoffman, Nelson, & Houck, 1983). Thus, although coming close to it, completely parallel processing was not achieved with extended consistent-mapping training. These data therefore do not quite fulfill Posner and Snyder's (1975) third criterion of pure automaticity of a mental process, namely that the process occurs without producing interference with other ongoing mental activity.

On the other hand, as to the occurrence of the process without giving rise to any conscious awareness (Criterion 2), the consistent-mapping performance appears to meet this criterion quite well, judging from the multitude of processes that must be occurring simultaneously. Consistently with this, the authors themselves (Schneider et al., 1984) characterized awareness of their automatic processes as "low."

As to unintentionality (Criterion 1), this criterion appears to be perfectly fulfilled (although Schneider et al., 1984, referred to instances in which automatic processing depends on controlled processing). The striking evidence for unintentionality is provided by reversing the roles of the targets and the distractors after consistent-mapping performance is fully developed. After this reversal, the detection accuracy dramatically decreased; in fact, it dropped well below the level obtained at the start of the training when subjects were completely unpracticed, and it took almost 1,000 trials to reach this initial level. It appeared that automatic processes were continuing to detect items that had been targets during the first part of the experiment but were no longer, and these automatic detection processes interfered with the performance of the reversed task. (Notice that the involuntary attention switches caused by processes regarded as automatic do not violate the lack-of-awareness criterion, for the processes leading to attention switch are themselves unconscious; see Schneider et al., 1984, pp. 16–17).

Interestingly, similar involuntary processes appeared to have teased subjects even after returning home from consistent-mapping sessions. Subjects who were exposed to hundreds of trials of consistent mapping with the memory-set items always being drawn from a limited number of consonants reported that these items seemed to "pop out" from the page during normal reading. One subject even found this phenomenon so distracting that he would not attempt to read for an hour or more after the end of the experimental session. Eysenck (1982) described this as a certainly novel excuse for not studying.

Consequently, it is evident, as Schneider et al. (1984) maintained, that after a process has become automatized, it is rigid and inflexible. It is even turned on by the occurrence of appropriate stimuli irrespective of the possible adverse effect on the current behavioral goal of the organism. In considerable contrast, controlled processing is highly flexible. The harmful effects of altering the conditions for subjects exposed to varied mapping were relatively small compared with such effects when consistent-mapping conditions were changed.

This same difference between consistent and varied mapping was also shown by changing the subject's task so that the search for target(s) was to be performed in only one part of the visual display while targets located elsewhere in the display were to be ignored. This ignoring proved to be much harder for subjects who had been performing consistent mapping than for those who had performed varied mapping before the instruction was given to limit the search to only a certain part of the display.

Thus, in conclusion, the automatism developed by Shiffrin and Schneider appears to satisfy some but not all the criteria for purely automatic mental processes proposed by Posner and Snyder (1975). The criterion involving parallel processing, that is, that the concurrent processes should not interfere with each other, was not quite filled (Eysenck, 1982; Hoffman & MacMillan, 1985). The assessment of the degree of fulfillment of this criterion, however, seems to be resting on a somewhat arbitrary basis because this fulfillment depends on the experimenter's choice of the ranges of the memory- and display-set sizes included in the study. If these ranges are progressively increased, even an approximate fulfillment of the zero-slope criterion (the lack of the processing-load effect) in consistent mapping becomes more and more difficult or impossible, and vice versa. Schneider, Dumais, and Shiffrin (1984) stated that "most of the research showing no performance reduction with increasing number of channels have tested in the range of 1 to 9 simultaneous inputs" (p. 17). Also, a further prolongation of the consistent-mapping training might bring the performance even closer to the zero-slope criterion as that now observed. "We know that as the amount of consistent training increases so does the number of stimuli that can be processed simultaneously without interference" (Schneider et al., 1984, p. 17).

Although Shiffrin and Schneider's experiments differed considerably from those on which Posner and Snyder (1975) based their suggestions involving automaticity, the theoretical positions of the two groups resemble one another (Eysenck, 1982). In Schneider and colleagues' (1984, Table 1) characterizations of automaticity, Posner and Snyder's three automaticity criteria are well represented. Schneider et al. (1984) propose some additional characterizations (such as that the modification of automatic processes is difficult and the effort needed by these processes is little if any) but most of them are either implicated or easily accommodated by Posner and Snyder's criteria. Schneider and his colleagues, however, assumed that the storage in long-term memory is little or none for the automatic processes. In contrast, much of Posner and Snyder's automaticity is based on strong connections on the one hand between external stimuli and their representations in long-term memory and, on the other hand, between the different representations in long-term memory (automatic spreading of activation to related representations).

This difference in views with regard to the extent of long-term memory involvement is probably due to the very different data bases on which the two groups drew in their theorizing. Whereas Schneider and Shiffrin developed their automaticity from the very beginning, training it in the course of their experiments, that is, produced arbitrary stimulus–response contingencies (the choice of the targets), Posner and Snyder (1975) utilized the already existing connections produced by a year-long experience.

As to the nature of the Schneider and Shiffrin automaticity, the authors themselves regarded this processing as *qualitatively* different from the processing occurring before the automaticity has developed, or from that occurring under conditions in which automatic processing cannot emerge (varied mapping). Schneider et al. (1984) suggested that:

> human performance is the result of two qualitatively different processes referred to as automatic and control processing . . . Automatic processing is fast, parallel, fairly effortless process that is not limited by short-term memory (STM) capacity, is not under direct subject control, and is responsible for the performance of well-developed skilled behaviors. Automatic processing typically develops when subjects process stimuli consistently over many trials . . . Control processing is characterized as a slow, generally serial, effortful, capacity-limited, subject-regulated processing mode that must be used to deal with novel or inconsistent information. Control processing is expected when the subject's response to the stimulus varies from trial to trial. (Schneider et al., 1984, pp. 1–2)

As already mentioned, consistent mapping performance does not quite fulfill the criterion for parallel, capacity-free processing in the sense of being composed of processes that do not interfere with one another. Shaw interpreted her own results as suggesting that the striking improvement caused by extended consistent-mapping practice is an effect on "the efficiency with which processing resources are used, rather than being explicable as the development of 'automatic' search" (Shaw, 1984, p. 120). Therefore she suggested that limited-capacity processes are not "bypassed" (Shaw, 1984, p. 117). Also Hoffman, Nelson, and Houck (1983) found evidence that a performance thought to be "automatic" by Schneider and Shiffrin (1977) made extensive use of one or more limited-capacity processes. Physiological data, reviewed later in this book (Section 4.5), also suggest that consistent-mapping processes regarded as automatic in fact demand some capacity. Thus, one might choose to talk about *automatized* rather than *automatic* processes as a consequence of extended consistent-mapping practice (Näätänen, 1985).

Automaticity in Basic Sensory Processing. Fully automatic processing can be encountered in the realm of basic, *task-independent processing* (Näätänen, 1985, 1990; Rugg, 1991). This processing is predominantly of inborn nature, and mainly involves certain basic sensory-analysis and storing functions. *Task-dependent processing* in turn refers to processing that is specific to a task and does not occur without it. For instance, certain processes occur in response to two consecutive stimuli when a subject is instructed to compare them with one another, but do not occur when these stimuli are presented with no such instruction (and the subject does not try to compare them).

As to fully automatic processes, they are probably illustrated by the analysis of environmental stimuli, leading to their initial cerebral representations, performed by different feature-detector neurons (task-independent processing). Each stimulus is in parallel analyzed by different feature-detector systems, these processes providing the sensory data base for corresponding percepts. Recently, Livingstone and Hubel (1988) reviewed convincing anatomical and physiological evidence in monkeys that indicates that the primate visual system consists of several separate and independent subdivisions that analyze different aspects of the same retinal image. According to these authors, cells in cortical visual areas 1 and 2, as well as in higher visual areas, are segregated into three subdivisions differing in their selectivity for color, stereopsis, movement, and orientation. Such different systems represent fully parallel channels which can operate without causing interference to the simultaneous operation of the other channels.

The action of such very fast but inflexible, parallel, in part subcortical, systems is not conscious but the stimulus information extracted by these processes may become consciously represented as is discussed later in this book. Consequently, such initial processes have been characterized as preconscious or preattentive (Neisser, 1967). These initial processes are turned on by the occurrence of appropriate stimuli quite irrespective of the state of the organism; such processes tend to occur even in sleep (chapter 4), which provides good evidence for their unconscious nature. Thus, they are turned on even in the absence of attention; whether attention can affect them is an issue of great current interest, as is discussed later in this book.

Evidence for such preattentive processes in visual analysis provides the starting point for Treisman and Gelade's (1980) feature-integration theory of visual attention. In essence, these authors suggested that (a) different basic features of visual stimuli such as color, form, and orientation (but not location) are analyzed in parallel by the preattentive feature-detector systems, and (b) the role of attention is to "glue" the outcomes from these different separate analysis systems together to make possible a perception of an object (in a certain spatial location). It is as if attention were placing the outcomes from the different analysis systems to their appropriate spatial locations of origin where these outcomes (a certain color, form, etc.) overlap one another, thus forming a coherent representation of a visual object with the corresponding spatial location.

This theory appears to be supported by a number of studies. Treisman and Schmidt (1982) reported that simple features were correctly conjoined when the stimuli fell within a narrowly focused "spotlight" of attention (the area of the attentional focus in the visual field; see Johnston & Dark, 1986), but that illusory conjunctions often occurred when attention was widely distributed over the visual field. Further, detection of feature conjunctions, but not of single features, was necessarily accompanied by correct localization of the stimuli (Treisman & Gelade, 1980). In addition, as reviewed by Johnston and Dark (1986), in a multielement display, detection of single features appears to be based on parallel processing, but detection of feature conjunctions seems to be based on serial processing (e.g., Egeth, Virzi, & Garbart, 1984; Hoffman, 1979; Treisman, 1982; Treisman & Gelade, 1980; see, however, Nakayama & Silverman, 1986; Pashler, 1987; for a review, see Treisman, 1988). Moreover, accurate visual processing could occur farther away from the fixation point for simple features than for feature conjunctions (Vaughn, 1984).

Thus, these studies suggest, according to Johnston and Dark (1986), the crucial role of visual attention in creating the spatial organization of the multiple parallel visual impressions or sensations, that is, in object perception. Hence, stimuli outside the attentional spotlight seem to receive less accurate spatial processing in the sense that outcomes of the different parallel processing systems for different features may not be properly localized and conjoined in the subjective visual space.

Impaired processing of physical stimulus features outside the spatial focus of attention has also been demonstrated in studies on identity priming. (Identity priming is usually explained as "the establishment of durable physical codes in memory by the prime presentation that benefits processing of the test presentation"; Johnston & Dark, 1986, p. 47.) Johnston and Dark (1985) found that the identity priming caused by words falling inside the spatial focus of attention was consistently larger than that caused by words falling outside the focus of attention.

Rayner, McConckie, and Ehrlich (1978) also reported evidence that processing of physical stimulus features is attenuated for stimuli outside the attentional spotlight. The authors delivered different strings of letters to the subject's left and right parafoveas. When the eye started to move toward one of the stimuli (a sign of spatial attention being directed to that stimulus), both stimuli were removed and a test stimulus was delivered to the fovea. Only the parafoveal stimulus to which attention had been directed proved to be an effective identity prime for the test word. Johnston and Dark regarded this result as particularly important "because it shows that the stimulus to which spatial attention is directed receives more physical analysis than the other stimulus even though the two stimuli are equidistant from the fovea." (1986, p. 55). The authors concluded that "although some nonsemantic processing may occur for stimuli outside the attentional spotlight, it appears to be much less than that which occurs inside the spotlight." (Johnston & Dark, 1986, p. 55.)

Consequently, it seems that the processing of even physical features of stimuli falling outside visual spatial attention is impaired, and that this impairment involves deficient spatial processing, resulting in impaired object perception.

According to Johnston and Dark's (1986) review, visual stimuli falling outside the spatial focus of attention undergo little or no semantic processing. It is not known, however, how much of this is due to already impaired processing of physical stimulus features (spatial processing). On the other hand, as the Stroop studies reviewed earlier in this chapter clearly show, processing of irrelevant semantic information contained by stimuli falling on the attentional spotlight usually cannot be avoided. Consistently with this, the Stroop effect can be eliminated by introducing a spatial separation between the color and the conflicting color name (12.5° in the study of Kahneman & Henik, 1981).

The Texton Theory of Preattentive Vision. Julesz' (e.g., Julesz & Bergen, 1983) texton theory proposes a preattentive visual analysis system that resembles that suggested in the feature-integration theory but that allows automatic processing of some feature conjunctions. (For a comparison between the theories, see Treisman, 1985.) The preattentive visual system proposed by Julesz cannot process complex forms but can, almost instantaneously, without effort or scrutiny, detect differences in some local conspicuous features, regardless of where they occur. Hence this preattentive system inspects a large portion of the visual field in parallel. These features—"textons"—are often elongated blobs (e.g., rectangles, ellipses, or line segments) with specific properties such as color, angular orientation, width, and length. Other textons are ends-of-lines ("terminators") and crossings of line segments.

Only differences in textons or in their density (or number) can be preattentively detected while this system does not perceive the positional relationship between neighboring textons. For an illustration, see Fig. 2.2. Such positional information was regarded as the essence of form (and object) perception, and can be extracted only by a time-consuming and spatially very restricted process, "focal attention" (Julesz & Bergen, 1983). The aperture of focal attention changes, according to the authors, its spatial scale depending on the situation and task (e.g., on the size of the feature being sought), and can be very narrow, even restricted to a small portion of the fovea, and shifting its locus requires about 50 msec. Consequently, Julesz and Bergen regarded preattentive vision as an "early warning system" that points out loci of texton differences for closer scrutinizing by the attentive visual system.

Thus the function of the large-capacity, parallel, visual preattentive system is to segregate the visual field into figure and ground and in this way to guide the limited-capacity, sequential visual focal-attention system,

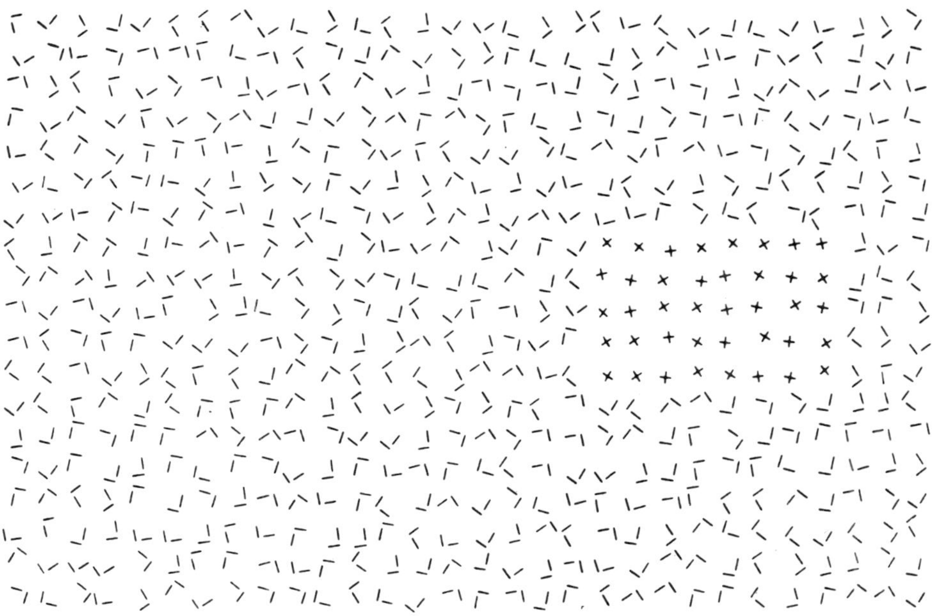

FIG. 2.2 "Preattentive texture discrimination" occurs between areas composed of +s and Ls, while element-by-element scrutiny, called "focal attention", is required to find the Ts embedded in the Ls. (From Julesz & Bergen, 1983. Copyright © 1983, American Telephone & Telegraph Company.)

capable of detailed scrutiny of a small part of the visual field at any one time, to examine the potentially most informative part of the visual field.

> The textons reported here help to discriminate textures, mainly surfaces of objects, without the need of complex familiarity cues. Such an early separation of the visual environment into figure and ground, or objects and their backgrounds, is a fundamental operation of visual perception. Lack of understanding of this process is, as of now, the greatest bottleneck in machine vision, which in turn is necessary in extending the capabilities of robots. . . . It should be stressed that the textons of preattentive vision only draw attention to certain areas, and we do not claim that these same textons are also the building blocks of form vision. (Julesz & Bergen, 1983, pp. 1641–1642)

It is clear that the data base underlying the Treisman and Gelade (1980) and Julesz and Bergen (1983) views of preattentive vision, as well as Livingstone and Hubel's (1988) functional segregation of the visual system, indicate the occurrence of a great number of parallel processes in visual analysis. These processes can be regarded as fully automatic in every possible sense of the concept. They occur irrespective of, and are probably even unaffected by, the direction of attention. As already reviewed, only spatial visual analysis has proved to depend on attention.

Automatic Attention-Control Mechanisms. Because foveal vision and the spotlight of attention usually overlap, the impairment of processing usually involves extrafoveal stimuli. This is, however, compensated by the intimate linkage between the outcome of preattentive visual processing and the visual focal-attention system; this outcome guides the focal-attention system to examine the corresponding part of the visual field. This attention-guiding or "early-warning" function of the preattentive visual system was in particular emphasized by Julesz and Bergen (1983).

It is of course of vital biological significance that pathways of such functions are not inhibited or blocked by withdrawal of attention. That they are not has been demonstrated by a number of studies and also by a multitude of common everyday observations. Hoffman, Nelson, and Houck (1983) reported that the ability of the flickering light to catch spatial attention did not depend on instructions, even though they greatly affected the ability to *report* the location of the flicker. (Hence attention was again shown to be important to the correct perception of visual spatial locus.) Thus, as Hoffman, Nelson, and Houck (1983, p. 405) stated, "it should not be surprising that some stimuli, such as peripheral movement, have a 'built-in' ability to capture attention." Further evidence was provided by Posner, Choate, Rafal, and Vaughn (1985) who found that a peripheral visual event tends to produce an "active orienting of attention" even while the eyes remain fixed. Consistently with this, Jonides (1981) proposed that the subject actively uses central cues in his or her visual field as a basis for orienting attention, whereas the peripheral cues pull attention automatically to their spatial position.

When deeply concentrating on writing this book in the library of the Neurosciences Institute in New York, my attention is frequently caught by something moving on the periphery of my right visual field. Fixating my gaze on this "something moving," it turns out to be somebody walking along a corridor on the next level below, visible through the glass walls. I cannot but feel awe to this automatic perceptual mechanism, which is apparently precisely the same as that which frequently saved our forefathers from their approaching enemies, predators, and other dangers. The physiological work reviewed later in this book reveals some of the cerebral mechanisms of such automatic sensory processing, which underlie attention triggering and switching.

Automatic Processing in Audition. Physical features of auditory stimuli are probably extensively processed even in the absence of attention, as far as sensory information for percepts, that is, creating initial stimulus representations ("basic processing"; Näätänen, 1985, 1990), is involved. For instance, Treisman (1960) found such results in her experiments on auditory shadowing. The subject was required to repeat orally a stream of speech presented to one ear and to report targets occurring in this stream as well as in the concurrent stream of speech presented to the opposite ear. She found that detection of targets in the shadowed ear was far superior to that in the unshadowed ear except when the targets differed from the other stimuli of the two streams of speech in some simple acoustical feature. For instance, the targets were tones. These results demonstrate that simple physical stimulus features were processed in the absence of attention.

These results, corroborated by a number of studies (e.g., Lawson, 1966; Moray & O'Brien, 1967; Treisman & Geffen, 1967; Treisman & Riley, 1969), also point to a possible attention-switch mechanism triggered by deviations in an ongoing acoustic stimulus stream. The neurophysiological basis of such an attention-switch mechanism was revealed by electrophysiological work (reviewed later in this book).

Further evidence that physical features of acoustic stimuli are processed extensively even in the absence of attention is provided by results demonstrating the existence of a short-duration sensory memory, called the sensory register or preattentive store, in audition the "echoic" memory (Neisser, 1967; for a review, see Cowan, 1984, 1988). Even stimuli that were unattended at the moment of their entry are represented in this memory. Thus auditory stimuli are represented there with respect to their pitch, intensity, duration, and so on, as are stimuli in our percepts. This form of memory is characterized as an attention-independent, large-capacity system of rapidly decaying sensory data which usually are outside conscious experience (Kroll, 1975).

Glucksberg and Cowen's study (1970) on selective dichotic listening illustrates the point. Their subjects shadowed (repeated aloud) prose in one ear and attempted to recall single digits that had been embedded in the concurrent prose presented to the to-be-ignored ear. Both the digits from zero to nine and prose words were spoken by the same voice. When the delay between the light onset, signifying the moment at which the subject should report a digit if recalled, and the digit was short, the digit was *correctly* recalled well above the chance level. (No incorrect digits were reported.) The recall performance decreased to zero by a delay of 5 sec in a typical negatively accelerating fashion.

Of course a problem in accepting such results is that subjects might have paid some attention also to the to-be-ignored input because of knowing that the task involves stimuli of this input. However, the rate of the items spoken, and therefore also that of the shadowing, was relatively fast (130/min). Consequently, these results might be taken as providing some additional evidence that physical stimulus features in audition are extensively processed irrespective of the direction of attention.

As to semantic processing occurring to unattended input in audition, it has been repeatedly reported that significant items of this input tend to become consciously perceived. For instance, Moray (1959) found that the subject's own name occurring in the to-be-ignored input in dichotic listening was sometimes detected by the subject. On the other hand, it is clear that semantic processing of the unattended input does not always occur (Johnston & Dark, 1982; for a review, see Kahneman & Treisman, 1984). The safest conclusion at the present moment certainly is that the issue of semantic processing occurring for the unattended auditory input is not yet settled. These studies are further discussed in section 2.3.

Automatic Processing: Summary and Conclusions. This section dealt with different forms of processing claimed to be automatic. Posner and Snyder (1975) put forward three criteria for a mental process to be "purely automatic": the process should occur without intention, it should be accompanied by no conscious awareness, and it should not interfere with the other ongoing processes. These criteria could probably be combined by referring to processes that occur "without attention" (see also Kahneman & Treisman, 1984), but are useful for indicating what we might mean by that. Anyway, these criteria have played an important role in guiding subsequent research in the field. Posner and Snyder themselves, in an attempt to find processes that would meet these criteria, stressed two types of processes as examples of automatic processes: (a) *pathway activation,* which means that stimuli tend automatically to activate their representations in long-term memory (at least if such representations are well-developed); (b) the spreading of activation in long-term memory to related representations. It was suggested in the afore-going that the evidence for automatic pathway activation to semantic meaning is not compelling, that is, semantic activation necessarily caused by unattended items has not been convincingly shown. On the other hand, the spreading of activation from one activated node in long-term memory to related nodes appears to be well-established.

Shiffrin and Schneider developed automatic processing in the course of their experiments (consistent mapping), whereas Posner and Snyder's automaticity (automatic pathway activation) mainly referred to consequences of life-long learning carried by subjects to the experimental situation. Consistent-mapping automaticity seems to fulfill Posner and Snyder's unintentionality and unawareness criteria, whereas the criterion requiring parallel processing without interference between the processes is not satisfactorily fulfilled. Thus it appears that although the consistent-mapping automaticity demonstrates the striking speed and breadth of information processing that the human brain is capable of performing after receiving extended consistent-mapping training, a qualitatively different form of processing, fully automatic search, does not emerge (Shaw, 1984). On the other hand, one might find a reason to reconsider this conclusion on the grounds that this training produced the so-called "pop out" phenomenon: As a result of this training, consistent-mapping targets started to "pop out" from the display, even when this was harmful to the subject's performance (for instance, after the roles of the consistent-mapping targets and distractors had been reversed). This is qualitatively different from the varied mapping which resulted in no pop-out.

However, a fundamentally different, profoundly deeper, form of automatic processes is found in the realm of innate sensory-perceptual processes. In vision, the processing of different stimulus features—except the spatial location—seems to occur fully automatically. In audition, too, physical stimulus features, providing sensory feature-specific information for auditory percepts, appear to receive extensive processing irrespective of the direction of attention. On the other hand, the magnitude of semantic processing of unattended stimuli in audition still appears to be an open question, whereas stimuli falling outside the attentional spotlight in vision have been shown to receive no, or very little, semantic processing.

Thus, there is a multitude of pure or genuine automaticity in sensory processing of physical stimulus features. In addition, the transfer of the stimulus information produced by these automatic processes into sensory memory also is automatic. A further type of fully automatic processes involves the high-priority channels from certain types of input to mechanisms controlling the direction of attention. Some stimuli are inherently attention-catching, irrespective of the direction of attention at the moment of occurrence of such a stimulus. In vision, peripheral movements automatically switch the organism's attention to the stimulus and cause an eye movement to foveate this stimulus. In audition, subjects become aware of the occurrence of a physical stimulus change in the unattended input during dichotic listening. This suggests that there is an auditory attention-switch mechanism that is automatically triggered by stimulus change in an unattended input. Other similar mechanisms are discussed later.

Consequently, we can distinguish three types of fully automatic processes: (a) sensory processes providing sensory feature-specific information for perception; (b) transfer of sensory information to sensory memory; (c) processes leading to an attention switch. The physiological data reviewed later in this book support the existence of each of these three kinds of automatic processes. On the other hand, it is controversial whether stimuli automatically cause semantic activation.

2.3. EARLY- AND LATE-SELECTION THEORIES OF ATTENTION

In the foregoing, the degree of automaticity of different types of mental processes was examined. This also paved the way for discussing different attention theories, for the degree of automaticity proposed by an attention theory is a crucial aspect in any such theory. In fact, the differing stands taken on this issue provide a continuum along which the different selective-attention theories can be meaningfully arranged. The *early-selection theories* allow much less automatic processing than do the *late-selection theories,* with the strong versions of the early-selection theories accepting no semantic processing of the unattended input at all. On the other hand, most early-selection theories hold that even unattended stimuli are extensively processed with regard to their physical features. Thus, on these theories, processing of physical stimulus features would be automatic but processing of semantic features would not.

The late-selection theories in turn propose that even semantic processing is automatic, and that the role of attention is only to select inputs for consciousness, memory, and response. These competing types of theory are examined in more detail in the following text. Thereafter we turn to processing-capacity theories thought by many to represent more modern views on attention, and to have replaced the early- and late-selection theories which both assume a single attentional "bottleneck" of processing. Thereafter the feature-integration theory, the leading theory of visual selective attention, is examined. As already mentioned, this theory proposes a special status for spatial location in visual processing; therefore it appears useful to take a more general look at this issue. Finally, the orienting-response theory, which in essence is a theory of passive attention, is discussed.

Paradigms of Selective-Attention Research. In selective-attention studies, Kahneman and Treisman (1984) distinguished two main types of experimental paradigms, the *filtering* and *selective-set* paradigms. The latter paradigm is most notably represented by Shiffrin and Schneider's visual-search tasks discussed in the preceding section and by Posner's RT studies of costs and benefits of expectations (see Posner, 1978). In selective-set paradigms, stimuli are usually presented at a slow rate, and "the subject chooses which of several possible stimuli to expect or search for rather than which of several actual stimuli to analyze" (Kahneman & Treisman, 1984, p. 31).

On the other hand, the essence of the filtering paradigm is the rapid, often continuous, presentation of "relevant" and "irrelevant" stimuli, usually differing in some physical attribute, for instance, in the locus of spatial origin. The most popular version of the filtering paradigm is dichotic listening. Such tasks of selective, or focused, attention are used to study resistance to distraction from the irrelevant input and to establish the locus beyond which the relevant and irrelevant stimuli are treated differentially, the locus or stage of selection ("the bottleneck"). The resistance to distraction of the relevant processing could be assessed by comparison with a condition in which the relevant input alone is presented (Kahneman & Treisman, 1984). Mechanisms involved and the selective processes emerging in the filtering paradigm might be quite different from those occurring in the selective-set paradigm. "It seems fair to conclude that the subjects in set paradigms resemble automatic processors more than do the subjects in standard filtering paradigms" (Kahneman & Treisman, 1984, p. 34).

Selective Attention in Filtering Paradigm. The differential treatment of relevant and irrelevant input has been the main scope of interest when filtering types of paradigms have been used. The early studies of selective attention, such as the pioneering ones of Cherry (1953) on dichotic listening, typically used complex competing messages, often speech, which constituted a high perceptual load. In these situations, subjects usually performed badly when dividing attention between the two messages, whereas selective attention was very successful both in protecting the relevant message and in screening out the irrelevant message.

Selective attention was viewed as selecting between messages arriving on different "channels" (Kahneman & Treisman, 1984), that is, selecting one "channel" usually defined on the basis of spatial origin or some other distinctive feature. (As Broadbent (1970) remarked, the concept of channel has caused some confusion, due to its obvious connotations for which one should remain alert, but it is handy in referring to a class of input whose items are in some essential physical feature(s) similar or rather similar to one another.) The channels to be ignored appeared to be effectively rejected, providing the empirical basis for the early-selection or filtering theory (Broadbent, 1958, 1970). The most popular illustration was the cocktail-party phenomenon familiar to attendants of scientific conferences. It is evident, even before the very first drink, that only very little information can be extracted or remembered from the messages of the many concurrent speakers, whereas the message chosen stands out from the background formed by the other voices.

Broadbent's Filter Theory. Broadbent's (1958) original version of the filter theory proposed that first, all stimuli are briefly stored and analyzed in parallel for their elementary physical properties (the preattentive level, or the S-system). This stage is, on his theory, followed by a higher-level processing stage (P-system) into which only a subset of stimuli, allowed by the filter, enter.

This later system is of limited capacity and operates serially. According to Broadbent:

> . . . part of the information from the buffer store will fail to pass this stage of serial processing before the time limit on the buffer store expires and those items which are lost in this way will have no further effect on behaviour. Selection of the items in buffer store for further processing was supposed to employ some common characteristics such as location in space, and the class of items possessing such a feature was termed a "channel"; an unfortunate term, as some readers identified it with the stimulation of particular sense organs. (Broadbent, 1970, p. 52)

Broadbent's (1958) theory, which was mainly based on dichotic-listening results, received further support from the pioneering experiments of Sperling and his associates (Averbach & Coriell, 1961; Averbach & Sperling, 1961; Sperling, 1960). Their results suggested the existence of a sensory-buffer type of memory postulated by Broadbent (1958) and, further, that attentional selection could occur within this memory.

Sperling and his colleagues briefly exposed their subjects to a display containing visual letters or similar items, and instructed them to report the items appearing in certain spatial positions in the display. These positions were informed to the subject at various brief time intervals after the display presentation. It was found that the subject was able in this "partial-report" condition to report considerably more items than could be expected on the basis of his or her performance in the "whole-report" condition (report all the items presented).

This advantage of the partial report over the whole report (per location to be reported) seemed to suggest that: (a) there indeed was a preattentive large-capacity visual sensory store; and (b) it was possible by means of the spatial location to choose items within this store, that is, effectively to pay selective attention to a certain subset of items defined on the basis of spatial criteria (stimulus-set attention). The fast disappearance of the partial-report advantage (within approximately 250 msec) indicated that the visual sensory store rapidly decayed after the offset of the visual display.

Subsequent studies showed that stimulus selection, stimulus-set attention, within the visual sensory store, the "iconic" memory (Neisser, 1967), was possible also on the basis of other stimulus attributes. For instance, von Wright (1968, 1970) demonstrated that color belonged to such attributes.

Broadbent (1970) observed, however, that his original filter theory clearly ascribed all selective attention to "stimulus set" and did not consider "response set" at all. Response set is a different mode of selective attention with which Broadbent (1970; Broadbent & Gregory, 1964) later wished to complement his treatment. Broadbent & Gregory explained response set as "a set to make certain responses, rather than a set to react to stimuli from a certain source" (1964, p. 316). According to Broadbent (1970), the relevant and irrelevant stimuli may be distinguished in two ways. First, the vocabulary of responses may determine the selection, because the irrelevant stimuli are not appropriate to any one of the allowable responses. For example, a subject may be asked to report only the digits in a mixed array of letters and digits, and each letter stimulus then has no corresponding member of the allowable class of responses. This illustrates stimulus selection on the basis of response set. In the second type of selection, the relevant and irrelevant stimuli can be separated from one another on the basis of some physical feature. For example, a subject might be asked to report the red digits in a mixed array of red and black digits, where the black stimuli are then irrelevant only by their color. This is stimulus-set selection suggested by the filter theory.

The "Break-Through of the Unattended": The Filter-Attenuation and Late-Selection Theories. In the end of the 1950s and in the 1960s, however, a good deal of data were obtained which were interpreted as indicating that more processing occurs in the unattended "channel" than acceptable to Broadbent's stimulus set. For instance, the subject sometimes responded to the occurrence of his or her own name (Moray, 1959) or to the meaning of some other significant item (Treisman, 1960) in the message to be ignored (see, however, Cowan, 1988).

This "break-through of the unattended" (Broadbent, 1982) resulted in Treisman's (1960) modification of the first version of Broadbent's (1958) filter theory. The filter-attenuation theory assumed that the filter only reduces the information available on a rejected channel and that this reduced information is sometimes sufficient to activate highly primed entries in the "mental dictionary" (Treisman, 1960). The operation of priming was thus assumed to be involuntary and unconscious, features later stressed in theories of selective-set (see, for example, Posner, 1978; Kahneman & Treisman, 1984).

Thus, Treisman (1960) suggested that the meaning of semantic stimuli is analyzed by the system by matching the incoming sensory inputs with a "dictionary store" of known words and, further, that there is a permanent response-set kind of selective facilitation state in this system continuously increasing the probability of certain meanings, such as one's own name, to become activated and hence perceived. Moreover, according to her, the selective facilitation pattern of the dictionary-unit system may also be temporally modified, for instance, by instructions and situational expectancies such as those associated with a specific verbal context. Consistent with this, as discussed previously (section 2.1.), many later studies suggest that a semantic stimulus not only activates the corresponding dictionary unit but also causes a spreading facilitation to the semantically related dictionary units (Warren, 1972, 1974; Posner & Snyder, 1975).

Broadbent (1970) interpreted results suggesting break-through of the unattended as indeed being "less favorable" to his 1958 view by showing that "a strong response set is able to overcome instructions to operate a stimulus set; one will respond to one's own name even if one is listening to speech from a different source. At first sight this seems to imply that all stimuli reaching the senses are fully analyzed for meaning in order that those of importance may receive response. That is, response set is primary. This view is urged by Deutsch & Deutsch (1963) . . ." (Broadbent 1970, p. 53). At second sight, however, things did not appear as gloomy as that to Broadbent (1970) who found good reasons to argue that stimulus set cannot be reduced to a form of response set. He seemed to regard Treisman's (1960) filter-attenuation version of his filter theory as a good compromise which accommodates the new data without sacrificing the principle of the stimulus set (though weakening its power in rejecting the irrelevant channel).

> There is thus something described as an "attenuation" of the signals from some channels; nevertheless, such signals may still convey enough information for their corresponding dictionary state to occur, if there is a strong enough prior tendency in the same direction from the internal factors. Treisman's view thus allows for stimulus set by attenuating some input channels, and for response set by prior biases on certain dictionary units. (Broadbent, 1970, p. 53)

The break-through of the unattended observed in several experiments also resulted in more profound concessions to unattended-channel processing, namely, to the emergence of the late-selection theories of selective attention. Deutsch and Deutsch (1963) proposed that perceptual processing to the semantic level is entirely automatic and independent of selective attention, the role of attention being only to control the access of stimuli to consciousness, memory, and response. This would be the case even in a typical stimulus-set situation, that is, when there is a clear physical difference between the relevant and irrelevant input channels. The authors suggested that "a message will reach the same perceptual and discriminatory mechanisms whether attention is paid to it or not; and such information is then grouped or segregated by these mechanisms. . . . We may suppose that each central structure which is excited by the presentation of a specific quality or attribute to the senses is given a preset weighting of importance" (Deutsch & Deutsch, 1963, p. 83). The emergence of these weightings and the subsequent comparison between different concurrent stimuli were, according to the authors, preconscious, this stage performing selection for conscious experience. "Only the most important signals coming in will be acted on and remembered." (Deutsch & Deutsch, 1963, p. 84). Similar late-selection views have been expressed, among others, by Norman (1968), Shiffrin and Grantham (1974), Shiffrin and Schneider (1977), Moray (1975), and LaBerge (1975).

Early Versus Late Selection: The Current Status. Presently, the controversy between the early- and late-selection theorists still continues, as the case seems to be with regard to most of the key questions in psychology. Broadbent (1982), while admitting that breakthroughs of the unattended message may occur, claimed that this does not mean that the unattended stimuli are fully analyzed before selection. Yet he noted some loss in the memberships of his fan club, giving an estimate that the late-selection theory is in fact supported by "a slight majority of authors" (Broadbent, 1982).

The more recent development in the field, in turn, appears to be more in favor of Broadbent's position. Selective-set studies (e.g., Hoffman, Nelson, & Houck, 1983; Shaw, 1984) demonstrating that the processing believed to be automatic in visual search turned out to be susceptible to attention were already referred to. In addition, the auditory results of Johnston and his associates (Johnston & Heinz, 1978, 1979; Johnston & Wilson, 1980; Johnston & Dark, 1982) with dichotic simulation strongly favor early selection. For instance, Johnston and Dark (1982) showed that attended and unattended auditorily presented words differ considerably in their ability to selectively prime one meaning of an occasional visually presented homonym.

In addition, Kahneman and Treisman (1984) reviewed a good deal of their own data from different paradigms, which they interpreted as surprising within a framework that describes information processing in terms of automatic access to nodes in long-term memory. "We repeatedly found that the impact of an item was affected by the intentional direction of attention or even by the mere presence of other objects in the field. Processing that might be expected to be automatic was thus shown to depend on attention" (Kahneman & Treisman, 1984, p. 54).

Moreover, the authors concluded that the data previously interpreted as favoring late selection provided, in fact, no conclusive evidence (see also Johnston & Dark, 1982). Three major lines of findings have, according to them, substantially contributed to the "growing popularity of generalized late-selection models." These lines of evidence are: (a) semantic processing of unattended material; (b) the "category effect"; and (c) subliminal perception. The authors regarded none of the three as providing compelling support for the view that perceptual processing is completely automatic.

As to semantic processing of unattended material, Kahneman and Treisman concluded:

> the effect is typically a small one: in 12 papers (4 measuring galvanic skin responses, 4 measuring target detection, and 4 measuring biased interpretation of a concurrent attended homonym) reasonable estimates of the proportion of trials showing semantic processing of unattended words ranged from

> about 2% to about 38% and averaged 16%. . . . The evidence suffices to reject the null hypothesis that stimuli on an unattended channel are never processed semantically. It appears quite insufficient to justify the acceptance of the converse null hypothesis, that attention does not affect perception." (Kahneman & Treisman, 1984, pp. 35–36)

The same conclusion is extended to other demonstrated failures of selective attention, including the failure to elicit Stroop-like effects by stimuli presented at some distance from the focus of attention (e.g., Eriksen & Hoffman, 1973; Gatti & Egeth, 1978). The observed effectiveness of the irrelevant stimuli as varying with their distance from the relevant stimuli appears to support "some form of early selection although the observed interference has been cited as evidence for automatic processing" (Kahneman & Treisman, 1984, p. 36).

In the "category effect," it is much easier to find a letter among digits on a visual display than it is to find this letter among different letters (and vice versa). In many of these studies, the target item seems to "pop out" from among the items of a different category, and this effect appears to be independent of the number of the items in the display. The category effect has often been interpreted as implying that the "category label" (e.g., "a letter") is produced automatically and in parallel for all the items presented. The target could then be distinguished from the other items on the display on the basis of its different category code, "just as a red target can be segregated by its color from a field of blue distractors" (Kahneman & Treisman, 1984, p. 37).

The authors, however, questioned this interpretation. They stressed that the categories of both digits and letters are small, and all these stimuli are highly familiar, conditions which usually tend to make pop-out effects possible, and that, as demonstrated by Deutsch (1977), associative connections among the members of a category are exceptionally strong. Because of these connections, the designation of, for instance, a letter as the target probably primes all members of the letter category (Taylor, 1978) and, consequently, when this letter is to be searched for among other letters, these other letters also tend to attract attention, there thus being competition for attention. Further, when an irrelevant stimulus has attracted attention, it can only be rejected by time-consuming further analysis which of course slows down the search. Therefore, the search for a letter among digits is fast because the digits have not been primed, not because they are all simultaneously coded as digits.

For these considerations the authors were able to find a good deal of supportive evidence from the literature and therefore conclude, contrary to many previous discussions, that the category effect does not provide compelling proof that all items presented in an array are automatically encoded to a semantic level.

The third line of evidence often interpreted as supporting the notion of automatic semantic coding involves claimed demonstrations of semantic encoding of subliminally presented material. Kahneman and Treisman (1984) attributed the revival of interest in subliminal perception in large part to some "widely discussed" experiments of Allport (1977) and Marcel (1983; Marcel & Patterson, 1978) which suggested that a stimulus that the subject does not consciously see as a distinct object, let alone recognize, nevertheless primes semantically related stimuli. The occurrence of priming by subliminal words has been demonstrated through speed of lexical decisions (e.g., Balota, 1983; Marcel, 1983), performance in Stroop situations (Marcel, 1983), and picture naming (McCauley, Permelee, Sperber, & Carr, 1980). Consequently, Kahneman and Treisman (1984, p. 38) observed that a new "New Look" is arising "30 years after the first flurry of excitement about subliminal perception in the 1950s" (see Dixon, 1981). They expressed, however, considerable doubt with regard to the significance of these results (if valid) as evidence for automatic semantic encoding.

Holender (1986) provided a penetrating analysis of the data claimed to demonstrate semantic activation without conscious identification, the "central thesis of the controversial research in subliminal perception," from three commonly used paradigms: dichotic listening, parafoveal vision, and visual masking. On the basis of this analysis, Holender concluded that the occurrence of semantic activation without accompanying conscious identification of the stimulus has not yet been unequivocally demonstrated:

> (1) Dichotic listening cannot provide the conditions needed to demonstrate the phenomenon. These conditions are better fulfilled in parafoveal vision and realized ideally in pattern masking. (2) Evidence for the phenomenon is very scanty in parafoveal vision, but several tentative demonstrations have been reported for pattern masking. It can be shown, however, that none of these studies has included the requisite controls to ensure that semantic activation was not accompanied by conscious identification of the stimulus at the time of presentation. (3) On the basis of current evidence it is most likely that these stimuli were indeed consciously identified. (Holender, 1986, p. 1)

In analyzing dichotic-listening results, Holender first discussed studies determining the magnitude of semantic processing of the irrelevant input by requiring the subject to respond to targets presented within this input, if he or she happens to detect any, while performing the task proper involving the input to the opposite ear (usually shadowing, target detection, or both). Holender claimed that there is no valid evidence for semantic activation of *any* of the irrelevant message when attention is stringently focused on the message delivered to the opposite ear in these studies (e.g., Bookbinder & Osman, 1979; Dennis, 1977; Treisman & Geffen, 1967; Treisman & Riley, 1969; Underwood & Moray, 1971). Holender proposed that subjects are basically engaged in dual tasks in which they have to give a higher priority to one task than to the other. The high-priority task consists of shadowing or monitoring the relevant message. The low-priority task, which cannot be neglected completely, is detecting targets in the irrelevant message or recalling some material presented in it. According to Holender, because both tasks are resource-limited, each performance depends on the particular trade-off between the quantity of resources allocated to each task and, further, that it is unlikely that no resources at all are allocated to the low-priority task. The only way to know how resources are allocated is, according to him, to study the performance trade-off by varying the relative emphasis put on each task. In this way, it could be determined, he further proposed, how much semantic processing of the irrelevant message is possible under the most extreme conditions of voluntary resource allocation to the processing of the relevant message. "Unfortunately, no such study is available, so it is impossible to determine whether such a limit in the focusing of attention was indeed reached in the experiments just reviewed" (Holender, 1986, p. 6).

To avoid this trade-off in the allocation of resources between channels, one could eliminate the need to perform any task on the secondary channel. In this case, the secondary-channel processing has to be assessed on the basis of indirect evidence such as possible effects of this processing on (a) the memory or (b) shadowing latencies for relevant items. As to the studies on possible memory effects (Davis & Smith, 1972; Smith & Burrows, 1974; Smith & Groen, 1974; Traub & Geffen, 1979), Holender (1986) concluded that none implied that the to-be-ignored input was scanned together with the to-be-attended input but all implied that some semantic processing of the to-be-ignored input did take place. He pointed, however, to the light load of the tasks used in these studies (monitoring rather than shadowing which demands a much larger amount of resources; for a review, see Holender, 1986), and claimed that such tasks often leave enough spare resources for processing the irrelevant items. Therefore these data cannot, according to him, be interpreted as suggesting some semantic processing of the to-be-ignored stimuli.

The second type of indirect measure used to assess semantic processing of irrelevant input is provided by the effect of this input on the latencies of the shadowing responses to the relevant input. Lewis (1970) found that this latency was prolonged by the simultaneous occurrence of a synonym of this word in the irrelevant input. However, Treisman, Squire, and Green (1974) showed that this effect occurs only at the beginning of a block and vanishes thereafter. They proposed that subjects were unable to focus their attention fully right from the beginning of shadowing, which allowed enough division of attention for irrelevant words occasionally to become processed. Later when the full attentional focus was reached, semantic processing of the irrelevant stimuli apparently no longer occurred. In a somewhat similar study, Underwood (1977) obtained results suggesting that the meaning of individual words but not of the whole sentence in the to-be-ignored input could sometimes be processed.

Another way to study semantic processing in the unattended input without requiring any response to items of that input is to present ambiguous sentences in the attended input and information disambiguating these sentences in the unattended input. This design allows us to measure unattended-channel semantic processing via the magnitude of the disambiguating effect. Two early studies along these lines were conducted by Lackner and Garrett (1972) and MacKay (1973). Both studies reported such disambiguating effects, but Holender (1986) found good reason to claim that the semantic processing of the unattended input implied did not occur without attention. Consistently with this, when attention deployment was better controlled in these types of studies (Johnston & Dark, 1982; Johnston & Wilson, 1980; Newstead & Dennis, 1979), no disambiguating effect was found.

Skin-Conductance Responses (SCR) as Indicants of Automatic Semantic Processing. Irrelevant-channel semantic processing has also been measured in a number of studies by recording the SCR to irrelevant-channel items. These results are frequently referred to as firm evidence for semantic processing of unattended input. The design of these studies has usually closely followed that of Moray's (1969) pioneering study. Moray first administered a conditioning phase in which a word was paired with an unpleasant but harmless electric shock. The subsequent presentation of this word in a list mainly composed of neutral words elicited an SCR in some of the subjects. (This response was resistant to extinction even when the shock was no longer associated with the word.)

During the subsequent experimental phase using the dichotic-listening paradigm, the shock-associated word was embedded in the irrelevant message while the relevant message was shadowed. The question was whether this word still elicits a SCR, and, if so, whether this response generalizes to *semantically related* words which themselves had never been associated with a shock. This generalization would indicate that semantic, rather than physical, properties of the shock-associated word are the ones responsible for the SCR to this word embedded in the irrelevant channel (Holender, 1986).

A number of studies conducted along these lines (e.g., Corteen & Dunn,

1974; Corteen & Wood, 1972; Forster & Govier, 1978; von Wright, Anderson, & Stenman, 1975) reported SCRs to shock-associated words as well as to semantically related words, although Wardlaw and Kroll (1976), using exactly the same design as Corteen, completely failed to replicate these results. This probably occurred because of some problem in conditioning the subjects (see Forster & Govier, 1978); therefore Holender (1986) rejected Wardlaw and Kroll's (1976) results as "completely inconclusive."

The afore-mentioned studies interpreted as supporting semantic processing of the to-be-ignored input were in turn criticized by Holender (1986) for providing no satisfactory independent assessment of attention deployment. In the only study providing such an assessment, that conducted by Dawson and Schell (1982), SCRs were found to be almost always confined to (shock-associated and semantically related) words that had received some attention. This measure of the deployment of attention was obtained by recording shadowing latencies and errors to words of the relevant message. The probability of shadowing errors considerably increased when a shock-related word occurred in the irrelevant channel and, further, almost all SCRs occurred when either an error or an increase in latency of the shadowing response occurred. The SCRs found with no indication of attention switch in shadowing performance were recorded in a slight but significant number from subjects who received the relevant message in the right ear and the irrelevant message in the left ear, whereas the subjects receiving the two messages in the opposite arrangement showed no SCRs in these trials associated with undisturbed shadowing performance. For a discussion on this effect, see Walker and Ceci (1983) and Dawson and Schell (1983).

Holender (1986) concluded that these data are "the only candidate instance of semantic processing without attention in the dichotic literature" (p. 9). These subjects might, however, have been able to shadow with no detectable deterioration in this performance and yet pay minimal attention to the irrelevant channel. It has been demonstrated that well-practiced subjects are able to shadow and to play piano (Allport, Antonis, & Reynolds, 1972), or to shadow and to type (Shaffer, 1975) simultaneously. In general, in trying to determine irrelevant-channel processing, a problem is that the performance does not, at least for the whole time, *fully* load the subject who then has some time and capacity for irrelevant-channel processing (see also Broadbent, 1982; Hartley, 1970; Holender, 1986; Pashler, 1984).

In principle, attention and semantic activation can occur in two orders: (a) semantic processing of the irrelevant input (and disturbance in shadowing) may occur because the subject paid some attention to the irrelevant channel (this may also happen because of some physical event switching attention in the irrelevant channel); (b) semantic processing may occur automatically, that is, without any attention being paid to the irrelevant channel at the moment of stimulus onset, but the outcome of semantic processing causes attention switch to the irrelevant message, accompanied by a disturbance in shadowing performance (see also Holender, 1986).

Only the latter alternative, of course, would make a case for automatic semantic processing. It is not possible, however, to determine which of the two alternatives was involved in shadowing disturbances observed by Dawson and Schell (1982).

Holender (1986) ended his review on dichotic literature by concluding that "in most of the cases, either enough processing resources were available and indirect evidence of semantic activation was present, or resources were scarcer and influences from items in the secondary channel no longer appeared" (p. 9). He admitted however that Dawson and Schell's (1982) afore-mentioned small subset of SCRs elicited by irrelevant words delivered to the left ear might be attention free and thus indicate automatic semantic activation.

Summary and Overview. Early- and late-selection theories of attention were discussed. Both types of theory accept that physical stimulus features are fully processed, whereas the theories differ with regard to how much semantic processing they allow. Strong versions of the early-selection theories such as Broadbent's (1958) original filter theory allow no semantic processing because the rejection of the irrelevant input occurs before the input reaches the mechanisms of semantic analysis. Such an early rejection can occur, in the theory, when relevant and irrelevant inputs clearly differ in some simple physical attribute. Therefore it would be impossible for the items of the irrelevant input to activate their semantic representations.

In contrast, the late-selection theories propose that, irrespective of the possible physical difference (and its magnitude) between the relevant and irrelevant input, both inputs are processed to the point where they contact the semantic analyzers and thus activate the corresponding semantic representations. In this case, the role of attention would only be to select input for conscious awareness, response, and memory.

The strong version of the early-selection theory was quickly complemented by a milder version when the first data signaling the breakthrough of the unattended started to occupy journal pages. This filter-attenuation theory of Treisman (1960) could neatly accommodate these data interpreted as being fatal to Broadbent's (1958) original filter theory. Broadbent (1982) himself also made a concession to these data by admitting that breakthroughs from the unattended do occur; he maintained, however, that this does not mean a full analysis of the unattended: "Getting a few features however is something very different from total analysis of the unattended ear; the latter has not indeed been blocked out altogether, but it is 'attenuated,' in Treisman's term" (Broadbent, 1982, p. 259). Another step in this direction can probably be seen in his distinction between stimulus set and response set (Broadbent, 1970). The response set, or "pigeon-holing," however, was not meant as any milder version of early selection, for this concept addressed a situation in which relevant and irrelevant stimuli differ in no conspicuous physical feature.

In audition, the issue of semantic processing of unattended stimuli during focused attention appears still unsettled. In vision, however, it seems well-established that no, or only very little, semantic analysis occurs outside the attentional spotlight, as indicated by Johnston and Dark's (1986) excellent review. This might be, at least in part, accounted for by the deficient processing of the spatial locations, and thus feature conjunctions giving rise to perceptual objects, of different visual features falling outside the attentional spotlight.

Results from the selective set (Kahneman & Treisman, 1984) and still further paradigms, partially replacing the older dichotic-listening paradigm in attention research, have mainly been interpreted as strongly supporting late-selection theories. These data, however, are not as compelling as they initially appeared to be (Broadbent, 1982). Furthermore, a multitude of still more recent data indicate that there is not as much automaticity in information processing as was initially believed (Kahneman & Treisman, 1984). The physiological results reviewed later in this book shed some more light into the issues raised. These findings reveal the mechanisms of early selection and might, at least in part, explain the data interpreted in terms of the breakthrough of the unattended.

2.4. RESOURCE OR CAPACITY THEORIES OF ATTENTION

The previous section was engaged with the issue of where the attentional bottleneck is located, that is, from what point is processing limited in capacity, so that selection is needed. In other terms, the question was how far, starting from the periphery, the parallel, capacity-unlimited processing occurs. Consequently, both early- and late-selection theorists agree on the presence of an attentional bottleneck beyond which the parallel processing capacity is limited; what is in question is the level of processing at which this bottleneck is located.

On the other hand, many observations are commonly interpreted as contradicting the idea of a single, central bottleneck incorporated by both types of theory, though at very different levels of processing. According to these findings (e.g., Allport et al., 1972; Shaffer, 1975; Treisman & Davies, 1973), interference in "divided attention tasks" is reduced or eliminated when the difference between the concurrent tasks is increased. According to Kahneman and Treisman (1984), this suggests that the brain is organized as a modular system, and that the interference arises chiefly within rather than between the separate, semi-independent subsystems. In this case, they further proposed, the need for early selection should arise only when concurrent activities engage the same processing mechanisms or resources but they added that whether there is in addition some central shared resource or limit (Kahneman, 1973) remains an open question.

The resource theories, regarded as more modern attention theories than the structural theories, are in particular suitable for accounting human performance in dual-task, that is, divided-attention, situations. These resource or capacity theories are examined next, mainly following Wickens (1984).

Time Sharing. It was already mentioned that efficient *time sharing* between two tasks (their simultaneous performance) is possible when the two tasks engage different mechanisms and structures. (Time sharing can be said to be perfect when the two tasks can be performed concurrently as well as each of them can be performed in isolation.) It goes without saying that both tasks must also be well-practiced and easy to the performer. For example, the participation of the car driver in a conversation with his or her passenger is disrupted if the demands posed on the driver are increased by a slippery road, or poor visibility (unless he is a highly experienced driver). Alternatively, driving performance may deteriorate as the conversation becomes very involving. "Tasks are assumed to demand resources for their performance, and these resources are limited in their availability. Therefore, when the joint resource demand of two tasks exceeds the available supply, time-sharing efficiency drops and will be more likely to do so as the difficulty of either component task increases" (Wickens, 1984, p. 63).

Resource Versus Structural Theories. The basic idea of capacity theories might be best illustrated via their contrast to an orthogonal type of attention theory, the structural theories. The early- and late-selection theories were typical structural theories, both proposing that the limited-capacity part of the system is performing only one task at a time. In both theory types, there was a fixed location in the system for the bottleneck beyond which the capacity is limited. However, in Kerr's (1973) bottleneck model, the bottleneck had no fixed location but rather was a single limited-capacity central processor (LCCP), which can operate at different levels but can at any time perform only one task. This processor would be needed, for instance, in selecting a response, performing a mental transformation, or rehearsing material. In general, structural theories tend to explain efficient dual-task performance with rapid switching of attention between the two tasks (and possibly with nonoverlapping, specific performance mechanisms) and also by stressing the remaining difference between performing a given task as the only task and as combined with another task (see Broadbent, 1982). According to Hoffman (1986), the continuous and self-paced nature of many of these tasks "raises the possibility that subjects can 'queue' certain processes and switch attention at critical points in the performance of each task." (Hoffman, 1986, p. 221).

Consequently, whereas the structural theories hold that the attentional limited-capacity mechanisms or structures can perform only one task at a time, the capacity theories in contrast postulate shareability of capacity between two tasks at the same time and, further, that capacity can be allocated in graded quantity between the two tasks. Knowles (1963), concerned with the measurement of human-operator workload, presented a conceptual model of the human operator as possessing a "pool" of limited-capacity resources. As a task (a "primary task") demands more of these resources, fewer resources are available for a concurrent "secondary task," introduced for indirect measuring of the primary-task work load, and the performance of the secondary task deteriorates. An implicit characteristic of capacity in Knowles' (1963) as well as in later conceptions is its shareability (divisibility) and allocatability. A number of later authors (e.g., LaBerge, 1973; Logan, 1979; Schneider & Fisk, 1982), interested in automatization in perceptual and motor tasks, emphasized capacity as a commodity that is needed less as learning proceeds. For example, longer RTs to secondary-task "probe" stimuli in the early rather than in the late part of the session were presumed to indicate greater capacity demands (less automation) of the primary task in the early phase.

Moray (1967), in an influential paper, drew an analogy between human processing resources and the limited capacity of a time-shared computer. In both systems, resources can be allocated, and in different degrees, to any activity, or processing stage, as ordered by a higher-level, executive program. Moray contrasted the ensuing flexibility of locus of the dual-task interference with the fixed locus of interference proposed by the early- and late-selection theories. To him, the locus of interference would merely depend on the capacity demands at any particular stage of processing.

In another important paper, Taylor, Lindsay, and Forbes (1967) outlined a quantitative theory of capacity sharing between different "channels" or sources of perceptual input, thereby highlighting the shareability of attention, as opposed to its dedicated nature, that is, involvement in only one task or performance at a time, as proposed by the structural theories. During the 1970s, the resource metaphor, facilitated by the theoretical treatments of Kahneman (1973), Norman and Bobrow (1975), and Navon and Gopher (1979), underwent an evolution from "a loose concept to a quantitative theory with testable predictions and important implications for the use of capacity assumptions in workload measurement and learning and memory research." (Wickens, 1984, p. 66).

Basic Assumptions of the Resource Theory. The basic assumptions on the relation between resources and performance have been confirmed by a large number of studies on performance in various dual-task situations. When a subject performing a dual task is instructed to allocate more attention to one task than to the other (either explicitly, or implicitly by differential payoff schedules), performance in the favored task improves at the expense of the other task (e.g., Navon & Gopher, 1980; Sperling & Melchner, 1978; Wickens & Gopher, 1977). This suggests, on the resource theory, that there are performance resources that the subject can differentially allocate to the concurrent tasks and, further, that performance in a given task improves with an increased amount of resources allocated to it.

This resource-performance relation was further elaborated by Norman and Bobrow (1975) who introduced the hypothetical construct of the *performance-resource function,* and proposed the important distinction between *data-limited* and *resource-limited* tasks or performances. The hypothetical performance-resource function relates the performance level to the quantity of resources invested in a task (see Fig. 2.3). The maximum single-task performance is assumed to occur when all resources are invested in this task (Point S in Fig. 2.3). Further, when the secondary task is introduced and some resources are shifted to it from the primary task, the primary-task performance deteriorates accordingly.

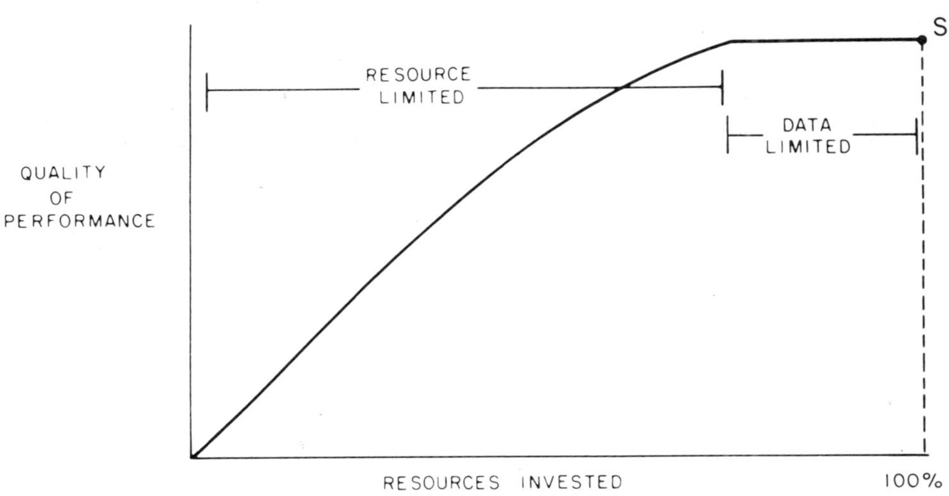

FIG. 2.3 Hypothetical performance-resource function. Single-task performance is at point S. For further explanation, see text. (From Wickens, 1984. Copyright © 1984 by Academic Press, Inc. Reprinted with permission.)

The relation between resources and performance, however, is not necessarily continuous. Norman and Bobrow (1975) proposed that performance initially gains from investment of more resources—the resource-limited portion of the function—but further increase in resource allocation beyond this point results in no further gain in performance level. This is the starting point of the *data-limited* portion of the performance-resource function. This means that performance level, in this portion of the function, is actually not limited by the magnitude of resources—allocation of still further resources would be useless—but by the quality of data. A performance might be data-limited, for instance, because the measurement scale cannot go higher: Perfect performance in an easy task is achieved with few resources—a larger data-limited portion means that maximum-level performance is associated with a larger spare capacity. Performance might also be data limited because the quality of the (perceptual or memory) data is poor. This cannot be compensated with increased resource allocation. In contrast, in the case in which performance would improve if the amount of resources allocated were increased, the performance is resource limited.

When two tasks are performed in parallel under differential resource-allocation instructions which are gradually modified from favoring one task to favoring the other task, the performance in the two tasks may be depicted as two separate performance-resource functions. Performance Operating Characteristic (POC) is obtained by combining this information by using coordinates in which one axis represents performance in one task and the other axis represents performance in the other task. Thus each point of the curve obtained, the POC, indicates the parallel level of performance in both tasks. This is illustrated in Fig. 2.4. The time-sharing efficiency of the two tasks performed in parallel is indicated by the average distance of the curve from the origin. The farther from the origin the curve is, the closer the dual-task performance is to single-task performance. Perfect time-sharing efficiency is represented by the box-like POC: Curve II in Fig. 2.4b. The distance from the origin can be increased by choosing easy tasks, combining only tasks that engage different structures or systems, or by extended practice. The allocation bias is indicated by the proximity of a given point on the POC curve to one axis over the other. Thus movement along the POC curve of Fig. 2.4b indicates a shift in relative resource allocation to the two tasks.

The *degree of linear exchange* between the two variables of the POC function indicates the extent to which resources are shared, or are interchangeable, between the two tasks. A POC curve such as Curve I in Fig. 2.4b indicates that a given amount of resources removed from Task A (thereby deteriorating its performance) can be transferred to, and utilized by, Task B (resulting in improved performance in this task).

A discontinuous, for example, rectangular POC curve, however, suggests that either (a) one of the tasks is in a data-limited region for the range of the

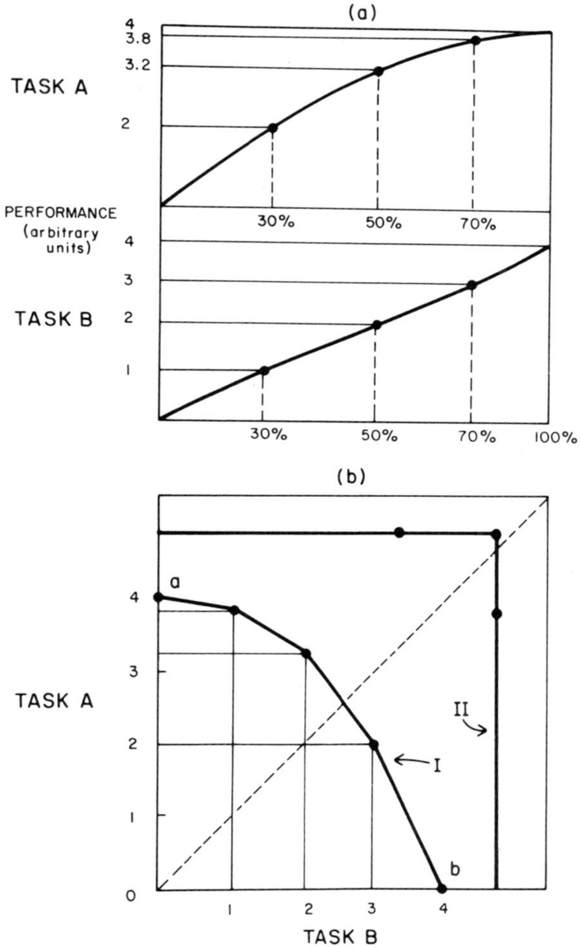

FIG. 2.4 Performance of two tasks under different resource-allocation policies as represented (a) on two performance-resources functions; (b) in The Performance Operating Characteristic (POC; Curve 1). The performance measures 1–4 in arbitrary units in (b) are those derived from the performance-resources functions in (a). Single-task performance indicated by points a and b. Curve II in (b) is a boxlike POC, which illustrates the case of perfect time-sharing efficiency. For further explanation, see text. (From Wickens, 1984. Copyright © 1984 by Academic Press, Inc. Reprinted with permission.)

POC in question, in which case withdrawing resources from the data-limited task will not deteriorate its performance (as long as the performance-resource function remains within its data-limited portion) but can improve performance in Task B; or (b) the resources are not interchangeable between the two tasks, so that resources withdrawn from Task A (thereby possibly deteriorating its performance) cannot be used to benefit Task B performance. In either case, performance change in one task does not occur concurrently with a change in the other performance, and so the POC will be parallel to one of the axes.

It is also noteworthy that points representing single-task performance may often indicate a better performance than the projection of the POC function into the axes signifies. This "cost of concurrence" (Navon & Gopher, 1979) of the two tasks is attributable to the act of time-sharing itself and to peripheral interference (Wickens, 1984).

Problems with Undifferentiated Resources. The afore-examined resource theory assumed a single reservoir of undifferentiated resources only, equally available to all stages of processing or mental operations. This single-resource model, the original resource model, has encountered four different types of difficulties (Wickens, 1984). These four phenomena, listed as follows, each emphasize the importance of *structural* aspects of the tasks to be combined:

1. *Difficulty insensitivity.* This refers to increases in the difficulty or demand of a primary task, which presumably then consume more resources, which fail to deteriorate performance of a secondary task (e.g., North, 1977).

2. *Perfect time sharing.* Examples of this were already referred to. For instance, Allport et al. (1972) showed that well-trained subjects could sight-read music and engage in an auditory shadowing performance concurrently as well as they could perform either task by itself. It is improbable that the findings referred to in 1. and 2. could simply be explained via data-limited nature of the performances involved (Wickens, 1984).

3. *Structural alternation effects.* These are instances in which a change in the processing structure (such as the stimulus modality or the memory code) involved in a performance causes a change in interference with a concurrent task, even when the difficulty of the changed task did not change. Such instances involve the stimulus modality (e.g., Treisman & Davies, 1973), response modality (e.g., McLeod, 1977; Wickens, 1980), and codes of central processing (verbal vs. spatial, e.g., McFarland & Ashton, 1978; Wickens & Sandry, 1982). Such results indicate that the specific structures involved in the two tasks, as related to one another, are of importance, too, and not only the *amount* of resources allocated to each of the two tasks.

Wickens and Liu (1988), however, concluded that separate modalities do not define separate resources. When a cost imposed by visual scanning was eliminated, there did not appear to be better time sharing across modalities than within the visual modality, nor is a performance/difficulty trade-off enhanced under intramodal conditions (Tsang & Wickens, 1988; Wickens, Kramer, Vanasse, & Donchin, 1983).

4. *Uncoupling of difficulty and structure.* This refers to cases in which the more difficult of the two tasks when paired with a third task actually interferes less with the third task than does the easier one of the two tasks when it is paired with the third task. Wickens (1976) paired tracking with an auditory signal-detection task and with an open-loop force-generation task. Subjects assessed the signal-detection task to be more difficult than the force-generation task, and therefore it apparently demanded more resources than the force task. Yet the force task interfered more with tracking than did the signal-detection task. Hence these data also indicate that the specific structures of the two tasks to be combined, as related to one another, are of importance and not just the amount of capacity.

Resources and Structural Factors in Combination. Kahneman (1973), in modifying the original resource theory, which postulated undifferentiated capacity, acknowledged structural factors as potential contributors to interference between tasks. He proposed a model in which the two tasks compete for a general pool of freely allocatable resources and also for more or less dedicated (one performance at a time) satellite structures (e.g., encoding and response modalities).

Multiple Resources. An alternative, though in many ways similar, modification of the undifferentiated resource theory postulates the existence of multiple resources (e.g., Kantowitz & Knight, 1976; Navon & Gopher, 1979; Sanders, 1979; Wickens, 1980). These multiple-resource views hold that there is more than one commodity in the human processing system that may be assigned resource-like properties: shareability, flexibility, allocatability. The implications of the multiple-resource view for time sharing are fourfold (Wickens, 1984):

1. The more separate, rather than common, the resources demanded by the two tasks are, the more efficient the time sharing will be; structural alteration effects on dual-task performance occur when a change in task structure affects the amount of overlap in resource demands of the two tasks.

2. To the extent that the two tasks share common resources, a relatively smooth POC can be obtained between them. Otherwise, the POC will rather assume a box-like form (see Curve II in Fig. 2.4b), as resources freed from one task cannot be used to improve performance in the other task. Nearly perfect time sharing should result when the two tasks demand an entirely nonoverlapping set of resources. The afore-mentioned difficulty-structure uncoupling will result when dual-task performance involving two

tasks placing heavy demands on separate resources is compared with performing two tasks of lesser demands, but imposed on a common resource.

3. If one of the tasks is made more difficult, so that the increasing resource demand involves, at least in part, resources that are also required in a concurrent task, the latter performance will deteriorate. On the other hand, if the increasing resource demand involves resources that are not utilized by the secondary-task performance, then that performance is not affected. Complementarily, in the latter case, a withdrawal of resources from that secondary-task performance to compensate for the increased difficulty of the primary task will not help the primary-task performance.

4. If a primary task is made more difficult so that its demand on resources that are shared with the concurrent task increases, the primary-task performance will become more dependent on the shared resource. The consequence will be a greater effect of priorities, of the resource-allocation policy, on the primary-task performance. The extent to which the two tasks share a common resource determines the degree to which the primary-task performance can be preserved at the same level, despite the increased task difficulty, through resource allocation by sacrificing the secondary task.

If resources in fact are heterogeneous, then it is important to try to establish their identity. Wickens (1980), after analyzing a multitude of dual-task studies which had produced structural alteration effects and difficulty insensitivity, proposed that resources may be defined by a three-dimensional matrix consisting of (a) stages of processing (perceptual–central vs. response), (b) codes used by the perceptual and central processing (verbal vs. spatial); (c) modalities of stimulus input (visual vs. auditory) and of response (manual vs. vocal). For an illustration, see Fig. 2.5.

As to stages of processing, Wickens suggested that perceptual and central processing rely on common resources which in turn are functionally separate from the resources underlying response processes. These stage-defined resources were supported by the afore-mentioned difficulty-structure uncoupling observed by Wickens (1976). In this study, the more demanding signal-detection task caused less deterioration of the tracking performance than the less demanding force task because, presumably, the signal-detection task required primarily perceptual resources, whereas both tracking and force-generation tasks required primarily response-related resources. For further evidence, see Kantowitz and Knight (1976) and Wickens and Kessel (1980).

As to the spatial and verbal processes each drawing on functionally separate resources, support is provided, for instance, by studies of Kinsbourne and his colleagues (for a review, see Kinsbourne & Hicks, 1978) on hemispheric specialization. It appears as an attractive possibility that the

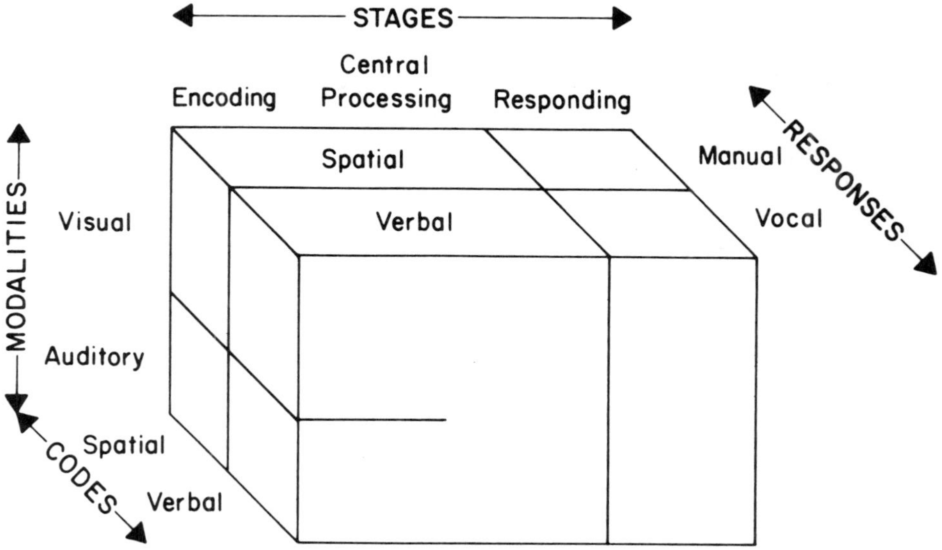

FIG. 2.5 The dimensional structure of human processing resources as proposed in Wickens' (1980) theory of multiple resources. The incomplete separation of auditory and visual resources through the perceptual-central processing stages indicates uncertainty as to whether the benefit of cross-modality presentation is preserved in central processing. For a more detailed explanation, see text. (From Wickens, 1980. Copyright © 1980 by Lawrence Erlbaum Associates. Reprinted by permission.)

resources for spatial and verbal processing are anatomically separated, as these processes occur predominantly in the right and left hemispheres, respectively. Kinsbourne and his colleagues, for example, found that there is a greater interference of a verbal task with dowel balancing when the latter was performed with the right hand (controlled by the left hemisphere engaged in linguistic processing) than when the balancing task was performed with the left hand (controlled by the unused right, "spatial," hemisphere). Further similar evidence was provided by McFarland and Ashton (1978), Brooks (1968), Friedman, Polson, and Dafoe (1988), Friedman, Polson, Dafoe, and Gaskill (1982), and Baddeley and Lieberman (1980). In the perceptual domain, Moscovitch and Klein (1980) found that recognition was more impaired when two spatial targets were simultaneously presented than when a spatial and a verbal target were simultaneously presented.

The third dimension of separable resources proposed by Wickens (1980) involves modalities of input and response. With regard to input modalities, there appears to be some reliable evidence for an advantage of cross-modal over intramodal stimulus presentation. Treisman and Davies (1973) found that detection of both spatial–temporal patterns and semantic targets was better with cross- rather than intramodal stimulus delivery. Further supportive evidence was provided by several studies (e.g., Martin, 1980; see, however, Wickens & Liu, 1988).

Analogous evidence for response modalities was provided by a number of studies (e.g., McLeod, 1977). These studies showed a better time-sharing of tracking when coupled with a discrete task that used vocal as opposed to manual responses.

Thus, Wickens' (1980) theory of multiple resources (see Fig. 2.5) has proposed a set of independent, nonoverlapping resources, each defined by a combination of levels on the three dichotomous dimensions involved. The implications of the model presented, if taken literally, are: (a) two tasks demanding completely nonoverlapping resources will always be perfectly time-shared; and (b) if two tasks demand partially separate resources, the degree of interference between these tasks in a dual-task situation will be unaffected by the "functional distance" (within the model presented in Fig. 2.5) between the nonoverlapping components of these resources (Wickens, 1984). The data, however, do not support the assumption (a) of no interference between two tasks due to simultaneous utilization of nonoverlapping resources as proposed by Wickens (1980). Although many studies have demonstrated that two tasks within a single cell, such as two auditory–verbal tasks, interfere with one another more strongly than two tasks in adjacent cells (e.g., auditory–verbal and visual–verbal or auditory–verbal and auditory–spatial), the data do not suggest perfect time-sharing in the adjacent-cell case. For instance, Treisman and Davies (1973) found considerable cross-modal (auditory-visual) interference between the two tasks performed in two different modalities although less than when the tasks were in the same modality. See also Moscovitch and Klein (1980), Brooks (1968), and Wickens (1989).

Wickens (1984) admitted that although the theory accounts for increasing interference as a function of the increasing proximity in the "resource space," it is not "entirely adequate" in the light of the data available.

Summary. This section reviewed resource or capacity theories of attention. These theories view attention as a commodity that can be shared at a moment between two parallel tasks. This contrasts with the basic assumption of the structural theories, according to which attention can be only in one task or performance at a time (but can be switched back and forth at a very rapid rate). In addition to its shareability, the resource theories propose that attention can be flexibly allocated in different proportions to the two parallel tasks. Attention is characterized by resource theories as shareable, flexible, and allocatable (in different proportions).

Three different main types of resource theories may be distinguished: (a) the undifferentiated-resource theory; (b) Kahneman's (1973) theory proposing undifferentiated highest level resources in conjunction with a set of more or less dedicated (usable only for one task at a time) satellite structures (e.g., modalities of stimulus encoding and response); (c) the multiple-resource theories.

The undifferentiated-resource theory is clearly untenable in light of the multitude of data indicating the important effect of the "structural distance" between two tasks on how well the tasks can be performed in parallel. Attempts to account for these data, which highlight the significance of the structural aspects of tasks in dual-task interference within the framework of resource theory, produced both Kahneman's (1973) theory, limiting the resource notion to the highest level of the processing system, and multiple-resource theories (Wickens, 1980), dividing the processing system into structural compartments each of which was "filled" with a separate resource.

Thus the multiple-resource theories proposed separate specific resources, commodities shareable between two tasks and flexibly allocatable in different proportions to the two tasks. Wickens' (1980) theory postulated three dimensions of separable resources: modalities, codes, and stages of processing. Although data, in general, support separability of resources along these or similar dimensions, the degree of separability, in the light of recent results, seems to be less than that proposed by the theory. In addition to providing some support to the structural views, such findings appear to point to the existence of also undifferentiated resources which would then be located at the highest level, such as those proposed by Kahneman (1973).

2.5. SPATIAL ATTENTION AS THE PRIMARY FORM OF ATTENTION IN VISION: THE FEATURE-INTEGRATION THEORY

The selective-attention theories discussed in Section 2.3. all permitted a completed buildup of a representation of physical features of an unattended stimulus. Even the strong form of the filter theory proposed by Broadbent (1958) held that attention does not affect the buildup of initial sensory stimulus representations. The controversy between different theories involved the magnitude of semantic processing of unattended stimuli. However, Treisman and Gelade's (1980) feature-integration theory of visual attention proposed that the processing of even a physical stimulus feature, namely, the spatial locus, is impaired by lack of attention. According to this theory, attention is needed for spatial processing in vision; without attention, different features of an object are not conjoined, or are often incorrectly conjoined, to feature conjunctions underlying object perception. Hence, this theory gave spatial processing a central integrative role in visual perception. In the following, evidence suggesting the special status of spatial processing in vision is reviewed. Thereafter, the feature-integration theory of visual attention is examined more closely.

There indeed is something primary or basic in the spatial locus in visual attention and perception. Among the sensory cues by which selective attention in vision can be guided, spatial cues seem to be especially effective (Johnston & Dark, 1986; Kahneman, 1973). As already mentioned, perceptual objects primarily depend on the subjective spatial coincidence of different object or stimulus features (Treisman & Gelade, 1980). In the following text, Johnston and Dark's (1986) review of studies demonstrating the fundamental nature of spatial cues in visual perception is followed.

Treisman and Gelade (1980) found that detection of feature conjunctions, but not simple features, was necessarily accompanied by correct localization of the targets (see, however, Sagi & Julesz, 1985). Detection of simple features in a multielement display appears to involve parallel processing, but detection of feature conjunctions probably requires serial processing (e.g., Egeth et al., 1984; Hoffman, 1979; Treisman & Gelade, 1980; Treisman, 1982). When a multi-item visual display is followed by a cue that specifies which items to recall (the Sperling paradigm; see Section 2.3), accuracy of recall is higher when the cue specifies location than when it specifies some other sensory property, for instance, color (von Wright, 1968). Further, studies of Posner and his associates show that spatial cues are particularly effective when they are given in advance of the visual display. For instance, Posner, Snyder, and Davidson (1980) flashed a letter at a particular location in the visual field and found that detection speed was increased by advance cuing of the location of the target but was not increased by advance cuing of the shape and identity of the target. An auditory analog of this result was obtained by Hede (1981). Posner et al. (1980) as well as Eriksen and Schulz (1979) suggested that one of the effects of attending to a certain location is to increase readiness to respond to any event occurring in that location.

Another type of study indicating the fundamental character of spatial cues in relation to other cues was conducted by Nissen (1985). She displayed items of different location, color, and shape, thereafter informing the subject of the dimension on the basis of which to report the remaining two dimensions. The result was that the subject was unable to report the color or the shape of a visual stimulus without knowing its location but could report the color without knowing its shape and vice versa.

Some very interesting data with split-brain patients (the two cerebral hemispheres separated by dissecting the corpus callosum) of Holtzman and his colleagues provide further converging evidence. In these patients, a cue presented to one hemisphere can inform the other hemisphere where, but not what, a stimulus will be in a brief display presented to the other hemisphere (Holtzman, Sidtis, Volpe, Wilson, & Gazziniga, 1984; Holtzman, Volpe, & Gazzaniga, 1984).

All the afore-mentioned studies speak for the fundamental nature of the spatial locus in visual information processing. It appears that the visual attention system first tries to locate the sensory event in subjective spatial coordinates in order to cumulate all the other sensory information to that position (Kahneman & Treisman, 1984; Treisman, 1988). See also Marr (1976) and Fox (1978) for concepts of "place token" or "object token" to denote possible spatial precursors of perceived objects.

The Spotlight Analogy. According to a number of studies, spatial attention in the visual modality can be illustrated via an analogy to a spotlight (for a review, see Johnston & Dark, 1986). The beam of this attentional spotlight can be directed outside the foveal visual field, and this spotlight can assume various sizes and shapes. The adjustable width of the attentional spotlight was demonstrated by LaBerge (1983; see also Hoffman, Nelson, & Houck, 1983). The subject was required to categorize the center letter of a five-letter word displayed on a screen and subtending 1.77 degrees of visual angle. Occasionally, a single probe stimulus was presented in lieu of, or immediately subsequent to, the word, appearing in one of the five letter positions of the word. The RT to the probe stimulus was fastest when the probe appeared in the center position, and slowest for both extreme positions. LaBerge (1983) interpreted this result in terms of the attentional spotlight which was focused on the center position of the letters and facilitated the processing of any stimulus appearing in that position. Consistently with this, when the subject's task was to categorize the whole word, the RT to the probe stimulus did not depend on the position in which the probe appeared. This condition was intended to broaden the beam of the attentional spotlight to cover all the five display positions.

Although the width of the attentional spotlight appears to be adjustable, there is a minimum width to which it can be constricted. This width can be estimated, for example, by determining how far an irrelevant stimulus in the visual field has to be moved away from a relevant stimulus before its disruptive effect on the response to the relevant stimulus ceases.

The dissociability of the attentional spotlight of the fixation point was familiar already to Helmholtz (1896) and James (1890). More recently, Posner and colleagues (1980) and Posner and Cohen (1984) instructed subjects to fixate on the center of a screen and then they presented target stimuli in various positions along the horizontal line on which the fixation point was located. Subjects were either precued with regard to the location of the target or not. Detection of the target was facilitated by spatial precuing. In a minority of trials, however, precuing delivered false spatial information with regard to the target stimulus. The result was that the detection of the target deteriorated and, further, that the degree of this deterioration was proportional to the magnitude of the error in the spatial information.

Although attention can be moved away from the center of the fovea, it becomes less efficient the farther away it is moved, and this decrease of resolution is relatively sharp (e.g., Downing & Pinker, 1985; Egly & Homa, 1984; Inhoff, 1982; Paap & Newsome, 1981; Rayner et al., 1978; Schiepers, 1980; Shulman, Remington, & McLean, 1979). Moreover, the minimum width of the attentional beam increases when attention is shifted from the center of the fovea even slightly off-center (Humphreys, 1981).

Other studies (e.g., Remington & Pierce, 1984; Sperling & Reeves, 1980; Tsal, 1983) suggest that the attentional spotlight can be moved across the visual field independently of eye movements. Some investigations (e.g., Egly & Homa, 1984; Shaw & Shaw, 1977) even suggest that the beam of the attentional spotlight can be split. Although the attentional spotlight may be able to conform to various spatial configurations, some of these configurations are easier than others (Podgorny & Shepard, 1983). "In short, although spatial attention can be directed away from the fovea and assume various shapes, it can do so only at a considerable sacrifice in processing acuity. Processing is most efficient when attention is aligned with the center of the fovea and directed to consolidated regions of space" (Johnston & Dark, 1986, p. 53).

As already mentioned, some data suggest that processing occurring outside the attentional spotlight is rather limited. In these studies, attention was usually aligned with the fovea so that parafoveal stimuli fell outside the so-called attentional spotlight. Semantic processing of these stimuli was measured in terms of both the semantic interference and semantic priming effects that these stimuli have. On the basis of these studies, Johnston and Dark (1986) concluded that "stimuli outside the spatial focus of attention undergo little or no semantic processing" (p. 54).

Even processing of physical stimulus features seems to be deficient outside the attentional focus (e.g., Eich, 1984; Johnston & Dark, 1982; Rayner, McConckie, & Zola, 1980; Treisman & Gelade, 1980). Johnston and Dark (1986) concluded that "stimulus processing outside the attentional spotlight is restricted mainly to simple physical features. Although a sudden and intense event outside the attentional spotlight may receive enough bottom-up processing to draw the spotlight to its location . . ., more detailed physical analysis appears to require that spatial attention be directed to the stimulus" (p. 56). A number of studies (e.g., Treisman & Gelade, 1980; for a review, see Treisman, 1988) have shown, as already mentioned, that object perception depends on attention. These data demonstrate that different simple sensory features, such as color or orientation, of an object need attention to be integrated to a level of perceptual objects. These findings have given rise to Treisman's feature-integration theory, the leading theory of visual attention. This theory is examined in the following.

The Feature-Integration Theory of Visual Attention. Treisman, Sykes, and Gelade (1977; see also Treisman, 1969) proposed a new theory about the role of attention in visual object perception. On this theory, separable features are registered independently and in parallel across the visual field, but focused attention is needed for accurately combining these features of complex objects whenever more than one object is presented in an unpredictable context. Under such conditions, a correct synthesis, underlying correct object perception, can only be achieved by focusing attention on one visual location at a time. Features of a visual object which co-occur in a single fixation of attention in the attentional spotlight combine, and thus form a perceptual object. On the other hand, if attention is diverted or overloaded, the features may be combined incorrectly, forming illusory conjunctions (Prinzmetal, 1981; Treisman & Schmidt, 1982).

The feature-integration theory was tested by Treisman and Gelade (1980) in several experiments. They showed, for instance, that visual search for targets defined by a distinctive feature (e.g., red or horizontal) occurs in parallel across a spatial display, whereas search for a conjunction target (e.g., red and horizontal) occurs as a serial, self-terminating scan through items in the display, suggesting that attention is focused on each item in turn. (It was shown that the serial scan for conjunction targets was not due to the overall level of difficulty.) Treisman and Gelade (1980) further showed that feature targets can be identified without being correctly localized (see, however, Sagi & Julesz, 1985), whereas conjunction targets were correctly identified only if they were correctly localized. This supports the claim of the theory that feature conjunctions are correctly perceived only when attention is focused on their location (Treisman, 1982).

Some predictions about perceptual grouping and segregation, similar to those of Julesz (1975), also follow from the feature-integration theory. One of these predictions, tested and confirmed by Treisman and Gelade (1980), is that if grouping is a very early, preattentive process, it should occur when one region of texture elements is formed by one simple feature and the other by another simple feature, easily separable from the former feature, but not when the two regions differ only in the way in which the same sets of features are combined. The authors showed that elements that differ either in color or shape segregate easily into salient perceptual groups, whereas elements differing only in the conjunction of colors and shapes (for instance red Os mixed with blue Xs in one region, red Xs and blue Os in the other region) do not automatically segregate into perceptual groups. "The boundaries of groups defined only by conjunctions of features are found through slow, perhaps serial, scanning and seem to be inferred rather than directly perceived" (Treisman, 1982, p. 196).

Treisman and Gelade (1980) proposed that preattentive grouping can be mediated by any independent feature-detector population of the visual system. Treisman (1982) regarded it as possible that new, functionally independent feature detectors could be set up through prolonged practice, as might happen, according to her, in Shiffrin and Schneider's (1977) automatization of search with constant mapping of targets and distractors. She further proposed that "any newly acquired feature detectors that allow automatic detection or matching unaffected by expectancy or attention, should then also be capable of mediating perceptual segregation" (Treisman, 1982, p. 196).

The Current State of the Feature-Integration Theory. The initial assumption of the model for feature coding and object perception proposed by Treisman (1988; see also Treisman, 1985, 1986a, 1986b; Treisman & Gormican, 1988; Treisman & Souther, 1985) is that different sensory features, such as colors, sizes, and orientations, are automatically, without focused attention, and in parallel coded in specialized modules. Differences detected by the system at this level of processing can mediate the segregation to figure and ground which sorts the visual field into tentative objects for further perceptual analysis. Further, as illustrated in Fig. 2.6, each module forms different feature maps for the different values on the dimension it codes (for instance, red and blue within the color module; vertical and horizontal within the orientation module).

Treisman (1988) suggested that the feature-detection system organized into different feature maps may be hard-wired into the structure of the visual system, either innately or through early or prolonged experience. In search tasks, these separate maps make it possible to detect targets with a unique sensory feature on the basis of the presence of activity in the separate map for that feature. "My hypothesis is that "pop-out" for a target defined by a single distinctive feature is mediated by the unique activity it generates in the relevant feature map. If activity is detected there, the target must be present; if not, a negative response is made. Note that this criterion requires the relevant features to be unique to the target" (Treisman, 1988, p. 205).

Different features of a visual object must be located and conjoined as the prerequisite of correct perception of this object, and it is here that attention is required. "We inferred that simple, highly discriminable features (whether parts or properties) can be automatically identified with or without focused attention, but that they are accurately located and conjoined only when attention is narrowed to exclude the features of other objects also present in the display" (Treisman, 1988, p. 213). This is spatial

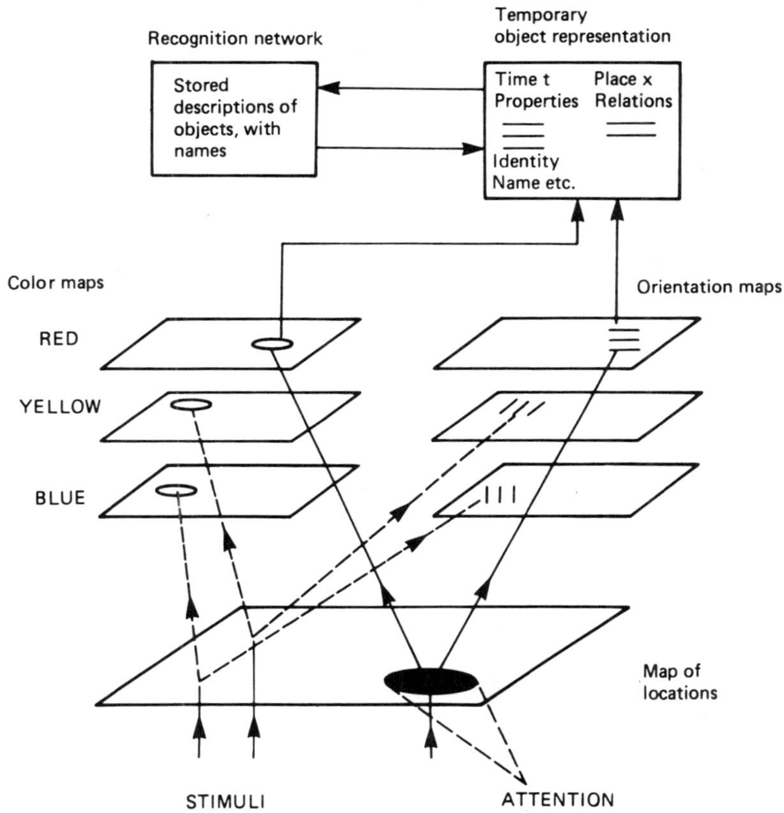

FIG. 2.6 Treisman's model for perceptual processing in object perception. For explanation, see text. (From Treisman, 1988. Copyright © 1988 by the Experimental Psychology Society. Reprinted with permission.)

attention, directed to a certain spot in the visual field. Treisman stressed that the medium of visual attention is a representation of space rather than properties: Conjunctions of properties should, then, be correctly identified as visual objects only when these conjunctions are also correctly localized. (On the other hand, as already mentioned, separate features or properties can be identified without first being accurately localized.)

> Attention selects within a "master map of locations" that shows *where* all feature boundaries are located, but not *which* features are located *where*. Thus it distinguishes "filled" from "empty" locations, where "filled" implies the presence of any discontinuity at the feature level. When attention is focused on a particular location in the master map, it allows automatic retrieval of whatever features are currently active in that location, through links to the corresponding locations in the different modular feature maps.

> My claim is that locations in the feature maps are made available to control responses and conscious experience only through their links to those locations in the master-map that are currently selected by the attentional "spotlight." Attention can be spread over a large or a small area; the narrower the focus, the more precisely located and accurately conjoined the features in that location will be. (Treisman, 1988, p. 203)

In the past, Treisman (1985, 1986a) hesitated where to put the master-map of locations, but more recently (Treisman, 1988; see also Treisman & Gormican, 1988) proposed that different dimensions are initially conjoined in a single representation (master-map of locations) before being separately analyzed, dimension by dimension. As supporting evidence, Treisman (1988) referred to some relatively recent results of Houck and Hoffman (1986) as well as to some single-unit findings.

This suggestion, illustrated in Fig. 2.6, actually holds that object perception is preceded by two different stages of feature integration: (a) an automatic, preperceptual stage leading to the emergence of the master-map of locations; and (b) an attentional stage, wherein attention selects a location within the master-map of locations and conjoins all different features whose locations in their respective feature maps correspond to this location, leading to the emergence of perceptual objects. Treisman (1988) suggested that separate parallel analysis along different dimensions occurs between these two stages, but it appears to the present author that some of this analysis must occur even before the emergence of the master-map of locations to provide the information on feature boundaries or discontinuities represented by this map. These discontinuities can, presumably, be detected only by the feature-detector system specific to the dimension along which the discontinuity occurs.

Thus it might be that (a) a visual stimulus first activates the separate parallel analysis systems for different dimensions; (b) the master-map of locations then emerges on the basis of the first, preliminary results from the operation of these analysis systems; (c) visual perceptual objects can only emerge after that automatic feature-analysis stage has been completed and the attentional spotlight has had time enough, after the emergence of the master-map of locations, to choose a locus in this map if it has not been predirected to a certain locus (e.g., due to precuing).

Treisman (1988) assumed that conscious perception of visual objects, scenes, and events depends on "temporary object representations in which the different features are collected from the dimensional modules and interrelated, then matched to stored descriptions in a long-term visual memory to allow recognition" (p. 204). The model presented in Fig. 2.6 shows long-term memory as interacting only with the object level, after the features have already been conjoined. Treisman and Butler's recent results (reviewed in Treisman, 1988) indeed suggest that features are joined before being compared with stored descriptions for identification. "These temporary assemblies of features with their spatial relations must therefore be distinct from the nodes in semantic memory whose activation mediates perception in many current information-processing models" (Treisman, 1988, p. 218). These temporary assemblies of features, called "object files" by Kahneman and Treisman (1984), are, according to Treisman (1988), "addressed by their spatial and temporal co-ordinates rather than by labels for their identity or for any properties they may contain" (Treisman, 1988, pp. 219–220). Kahneman, Treisman, and Burkell's (1983) results confirm the need to separate the recognition network from the temporary object files, as illustrated by the model presented in Fig. 2.6.

The Feature-Integration Theory: New Findings. As is clear from the aforementioned, the feature-integration theory of visual attention has undergone several steps of modification and elaboration during the last few years to accommodate the most recent data. Due to some new findings (e.g., Houck & Hoffman, 1986; Nakayama & Silverman, 1986; McLeod et al., 1988), it appears to Treisman (1988) that still further modifications might be needed to the theoretical framework she has proposed. Nakayama and Silverman (1986), for instance, have succeeded in developing a display of color and motion that allows the conjunction target to pop out in parallel, and they have also discovered several other instances of pairing of dimensions that produce the same effect. Treisman also referred to some further results of Nakayama along these lines. Some of Treisman and her colleagues' recent results (for a review, see Treisman, 1988) also seem to be somewhat problematic to the present version of the feature-integration theory. At the time of this writing (January, 1989), it is not yet clear how this theory should be modified to account for these new data.

Summary. This section reviewed data interpreted as indicating the special status of spatial processing in visual object perception and selective attention. Visual attention has often been illustrated via a metaphor of a spotlight that can assume different widths and be directed to different locations in the visual field. This spotlight usually moves, but does not have to, with the fixation point of the gaze.

Processing occurring to stimuli falling outside this spotlight is in some aspects seriously limited. According to the feature-integration theory, attention directed to a certain location of the visual field conjoins all the different features (usually of the same object) occurring in this location to form a visual perceptual object. Thus spatial attention would be needed for correct perception of visual objects. On the other hand, processing of separate nonspatial visual features, such as color and orientation, does not require attention.

A later version of the theory explicitly suggests that these different sensory features are automatically coded in respective feature maps of specialized modules (e.g., a color module containing separate feature maps for different colors such as green and yellow). In search tasks, these separate maps allow the detection of a target with a unique sensory feature simply from the presence of activity in the separate map for this feature.

The later version of the theory also proposes that attention selects specific locations within a "master-map of locations." This map, automatically formed in a very early stage of processing, shows where all feature boundaries are located, but not which features are located where. Focusing of attention to a particular location in the master map automatically locates and conjoins all the features currently active in the corresponding locations in all the different feature maps, resulting in the emergence of feature conjunctions, precursors of visual perceptual objects. These feature conjunctions are subsequently compared with long-term memory representations for object identification. Thus, contrary to many modern information-processing models, these temporary feature assemblies with their spatial relations are regarded by the theory as distinct from the nodes in semantic memory.

2.6. PASSIVE ATTENTION AND THE ORIENTING RESPONSE

In the preceding sections, theories of voluntary attention were discussed. Yet attention can also be passively elicited. In introduction, the concept of passive attention was already mentioned several times. Passive attention refers to the phenomenon of attention switch caused by an initially unattended stimulus. "Attention may be either . . . passive, reflex, nonvoluntary, effortless: or . . . active and voluntary" (James, 1890, p. 416). James noted that attention can be drawn automatically to stimuli by virtue of either their sensory ("immediate") characteristics, such as suddenness or high intensity, or their semantic ("derived") characteristics. The latter characteristics were exemplified by James (1890) as follows: A faint tap per se is not an interesting sound: It may well escape being discriminated from the general rumor of the world. But when it is a signal, as that of a lover on the window-pane, it will hardly go unperceived (James, 1890, pp. 417–418).

As already mentioned, Schneider and colleagues (1984) claimed that persistent consistent-mapping training can provide target stimuli with such

valid, conditions is a postural response, including an immediate termination of the ongoing motor behavior and a simultaneous orientation of the appropriate receptor organs so that the sensory input is maximized. This indeed looks like turning attention to the stimulus, that is, passive attention appears to be involved. This is what Pavlov observed to happen in his dogs when he entered the laboratory. The dogs made an orienting response to Pavlov rather than demonstrating the conditioned reflexes which his pupils had succeeded in developing in the dogs and which the pupils were now eager to show to their master.

According to Lynn (1966), in addition to changes in the muscles that direct sense organs, the ongoing motor behavior is temporarily arrested, and there is even a delay in breathing. General muscle tonus increases and the sense organs become more sensitive; the dilation of the pupil is a conspicuous example of such changes. The electroencephalogram (EEG) changes toward faster and lower-amplitude activity which is generally regarded as a sign of increased arousal (Lindsley, 1960, 1961). A number of well-known vegetative responses also occur such as the SCR, heart-rate deceleration, and certain vascular responses. The SCR has served as the most popular index of the occurrence of an orienting response (see also Kimmel, van Olst, & Orlebeke, 1979).

Arousal and Attentional Components of the Orienting Response. Most of the physiological effects occurring in the orienting response can be understood as resulting from a sudden increase in reticular or thalamic nonspecific activation (see Lindsley, 1970), thus suggesting that the principal center of the orienting-response release might be located in the nonspecific activating systems of the brain such as the reticular formation (Sokolov, 1963; see also Rohrbaugh, 1984). These *arousal-related* responses include sensory effects, too, those associated with lowering of sensory thresholds. Consistent with this, such effects can also be induced by electrical stimulation of the reticular formation (see Lynn, 1966).

A number of responses included in the pattern of bodily effects composing the orienting response, can, however, be regarded primarily as *attentional* in nature (Näätänen, 1986a). Such effects include heart-rate deceleration and certain muscular responses, at least those that orient the sensory receptors in the optimal way, a delay in breathing, perhaps even the arrest of the ongoing behavior. Particularly illustrating is the heart-rate deceleration (for reviews, see Graham & Clifton, 1966; Graham, 1979, 1984; Bohlin & Kjellberg, 1979) which is opposite to what could be expected as a result of reticular activation. The heart rate is known to decelerate as a response to attention-provoking stimuli (Lacey, 1967; Graham & Clifton, 1966; Putnam, 1990). Kahneman (1973) regarded heart-rate deceleration as a part of a general somatic inhibitory state that eliminates somatic feedback from interfering with central processing (see also Obrist et al., 1974; Mandler, 1975).

Consequently, Näätänen (1986a) proposed that the pattern of physiological effects known as the orienting response could be viewed as having two components, one controlled by the energetical (arousal), the other by the informational or attentional aspect of brain function:

1. *The arousal component of the orienting response:* This component consists of arousal-related effects, known to facilitate sensory and motor functions as well as their central integration. All these responses can be understood as resulting from a sudden transient increase in reticular (or thalamic nonspecific) activation.
2. *The attentional (informational) component of the orienting response:* This component consists of a reflex-like attention switch to the eliciting stimulus and the accompanying bodily effects specifically associated with an attention switch.

The Repetition–Change Paradigm. The classical, and most commonly used, experimental paradigm to study the orienting response is the so-called repetition–change paradigm. This consists of a sequence of homogeneous stimuli usually presented with rather long interstimulus intervals (ISI), such as 20–30 sec. Such long intervals well permit the recording of slow autonomic responses (chapter 3). A large orienting response, as usually indicated by some autonomic measure, is elicited by the first stimulus in the sequence, but after, say, 5–20 stimulus repetitions, the orienting response is totally extinguished; it has "habituated." However, if some feature of the repetitive stimulus is changed, then the orienting response is re-elicited.

Sokolov's Orienting-Response Theory. To account for this general pattern of data, Sokolov (1960) proposed that the repetitive stimulus results in the development of its cortical "neuronal model," a neuronal representation of the physical features of the repetitive stimulus, and that this development parallels the orienting-response habituation. He explained that the neuronal model inhibits or blocks an input to the reticular formation after a neuronal model corresponding to the repetitive stimulus has developed. On the other hand, when a different stimulus is presented, the afferent input from this stimulus does not encounter the blockage formed by the neuronal model, and the center of the orienting-response release can again be reached.

No direct empirical evidence for the neuronal-model construct was, however, obtained in humans. One important reason, as discussed in chapter 3, is that this research mainly used slow autonomic measures unsuitable for tracing the fast cerebral processes initiating the orienting response (Näätänen, 1979). Another probable reason might be found in the diffuseness or nonspecificity of most of the measures used, making it impossible to clarify the different central processes involved. Therefore Sokolov and his associates have more recently conducted related animal work, recording single-unit responses from different brain structures of unanesthetized rabbits in the repetition–change paradigm (see Vinogradova, 1975).

The responses yielded by hippocampal recordings in these studies seemed to support the neuronal-model concept. Neurons of the dorsal hippocampus were recorded extracellularly by using microelectrodes. The majority of neurons met at certain hippocampal regions responded to any stimulus, and, further, this response decreased with stimulus repetition, vanishing after 10–20 trials. (The constant ISI used was either 2.75 or 5 sec, much shorter than in the classical orienting-response studies). However, any change, even a slight or complex one, in stimulus parameters resulted in the recovery of the initial response. "Thus, the responses of hippocampal pyramids arise as a result of any noncoincidence between the established trace system and the present stimulus . . . ('disconcordance signal')" (Vinogradova, 1975, p. 144).

Consequently, Sokolov (1975) reconsidered the cortical location of the neuronal model and moved it from the cortical feature-detector neurons to the synaptic connections between these detectors and the hippocampal "novelty" neurons. Sokolov's starting point was the assumption that each feature detector is connected to each novelty neuron via interneurons (see also Vinogradova, 1975). Hence, each hippocampal novelty neuron possesses, apparently, numerous synaptic contacts, each representing a certain stimulus property, depending on the corresponding feature detector. When a stimulus is presented for the first time, the feature detectors corresponding to the specific stimulus features activate a large number of hippocampal novelty neurons. These novelty neurons in turn are connected, according to Sokolov (1975), to the center of the orienting-response release in the reticular activating system (and this way to the different orienting-response effectors).

On the other hand, when the same stimulus is repeated, the response of the hippocampal novelty neurons becomes weaker and is finally extinguished, because of the development of "a predominant postactivation potentiation of the responses of the inhibitory interneurons" (Sokolov, 1975, p. 227) in the connections from the feature detectors corresponding to the parameters of the repetitive stimulus to the novelty neurons. The orienting response diminishes and disappears in synchrony with the loss in response of novelty neurons.

When a different stimulus is applied, however, new feature detectors, those with "open" synaptic connections to the novelty neurons, are activated, and the orienting response resumes. The magnitude of the orienting response increases proportionally to the difference (disconcordance signal) between the new stimulus and that corresponding to the neuronal model (Sokolov, 1975).

Thus Sokolov's theory holds that the cerebral initiation of the orienting response occurs similarly to both the beginning of the stimulus sequence and to a stimulus change in this sequence. In both cases, the neuronal model is lacking; therefore the stimulus-initiated process can reach the center of the orienting-response release. O'Gorman (1979), however, proposed an important distinction between the initial orienting response and the change-orienting response, respectively, suggesting that the brain mechanisms of the two are not necessarily identical. This distinction is further discussed and supporting evidence is reviewed in chapter 4.

Criticism of the Orienting-Response Theory. Sokolov's orienting-response theory, the most influential theory in psychophysiology, has also met criticism. It is, for instance, maintained that even though the neuronal-model concept can explain an orienting response to a novel stimulus or stimulus change, it cannot explain the orienting response to a stimulus that is neither novel nor different. Such an orienting response occurs to the second 7 in a sequence 12345677 (Velden, 1978). Moreover, an orienting response can even be elicited in a stimulus sequence in which all the stimuli are physical changes in relation to the previous stimuli, so that there is no such infrequent event that could explain the orienting response. This case is illustrated by an orienting response to 9 in a sequence 12345679, or KAGFBHT9, that is, when expectancy or context is violated (see Unger, 1964). Thus even cognitive mismatches elicit an orienting response.

Moreover, stimulus significance, introduced in the simplest way by instructing the subject to attend to stimuli or to perform a motor response to them (see Lynn, 1966; Sokolov, 1963), enhances the orienting response, makes it much more resistant to habituation, and even brings back an already extinguished orienting response (see Bernstein, 1979; Maltzman, 1979).

None of these cases can be accounted for by the neuronal model and its mismatch process as postulated by Sokolov. However, he did not offer these concepts as the sole account for the initiation of the orienting response kinds of physiological changes (see also Velden, 1978). There are well-established corticoreticular efferent pathways via which the cortex can activate the reticular formation upon detecting an unexpected or otherwise significant stimulus. Such a sudden, strong excitatory influence on the reticular formation could well explain the elicitation of an orienting response type of physiological change (see Lindsley, 1970).

Another criticism, more serious, challenges the basic assumption of the orienting-response theory that a physical stimulus change per se is sufficient to elicit an orienting response. Bernstein (1979) argued that although an orienting response may follow a stimulus change, it is the experienced significance, rather than the change per se as a physical event, that elicits the orienting response. Hence, on the "significance hypothesis," the cortical interpretative and evaluative processes are crucial; if they do not occur, then no orienting response is elicited. This of course means rejecting Sokolov's neuronal-mismatch theory. An orienting response elicited by stimulus change *per se* was described as very disastrous to behavior and performance by significance theorists: We would be continuously orienting to insignificant stimulus changes (Bernstein, 1969). This "significance controversy" was vigorous in the literature some time ago (e.g., Bernstein, 1979, 1981; Maltzman, 1979; O'Gorman, 1979; Siddle, 1979).

One way toward settling this issue, and toward a better understanding of this vital response in general, would be to try to clarify whether any neuronal-mismatch kind of process to a mere physical stimulus change occurs in the human brain. We already examined such a mechanism of the rabbit brain but, as mentioned earlier, a similar mechanism in humans has not been demonstrated. In chapter 4, recent electrophysiological data suggesting the existence of such a mechanism is examined.

Summary. Passive (passively elicited) attention is initiated by stimuli rather than by our own will or choice. Hence this form of attention is involuntary rather than voluntarily controlled. Stimuli can capture our attention for two reasons: for (a) their physical or (b) semantic (derived) properties. Certain physical stimulus events are particularly attention catching; for instance, an abrupt stimulus onset after a period of no abrupt onsets, an offset of a long-duration stimulus, change in a continuous stimulus or in a repetitive sequence of discrete stimuli, stimulus repetition in a continuous change, or regularity in otherwise random change. In addition, peripheral movements in vision are powerful in attracting attention. A stimulus can also catch attention for its meaning or significance, that is, for its derived properties, for instance our name being mentioned in a discussion in the neighboring table. The prerequisite for this type of attention switch is that the input manages to activate its semantic code in long-term memory; whether this can occur in a complete absence of attention is currently a controversial issue.

The orienting-response theory, developed by E.N. Sokolov, is the leading theory of passive attention. This theory proposes a brain mechanism which initiates the orienting-response release. On the present interpretation, the essence of the orienting response is an attention switch to the eliciting stimulus, although research has mainly been engaged with more visible and more easily measurable bodily consequences of this attention switch. The orienting response can, apparently, be divided into two components: (a) attentional (informational) and (b) activational (energetical) responses.

The orienting-response theory primarily addresses the orienting response to physical stimulus events, trying to explain its cerebral initiation and habituation. The theory proposes that a new stimulus, be it the first stimulus in a block or a different stimulus embedded within it, elicits an orienting response, for the sequence of processes initiated by this stimulus has unhindered access to the cerebral center of the orienting-response release. On the other hand, when the stimulus is repeated, the orienting response gets weaker and weaker, and finally habituates completely. This habituation occurs, on the theory, because stimulus repetition leads to a gradual development of the neuronal model, a highly stimulus-specific cerebral inhibition pattern. This theory thus holds that an orienting response is released by a physical stimulus change irrespective of the subjective significance of the change to the organism. This basic claim has elicited much controversy in the literature.

2.7. ATTENTION AND AUTOMATICITY: A SUMMARY

Current research and theories of attention and automaticity in information processing were reviewed and discussed. Since the mid-1970s, there has been a rapidly growing interest in the brain's automatic processing, that is, what the processing system seemed to be able to do without intention, awareness, and capacity limitations, to follow Posner and Snyder's (1975) criteria.

Studies on dual-task (divided-attention) performance of highly skilled individuals and Shiffrin and Schneider's work on automatic search have been particularly illuminating. These authors demonstrated an amazing increase in the subject's ability to perform multielement visual search as a result of extended training under conditions in which target and distractor sets were kept constant, leading to what the authors called automatic search.

The authors regarded their automatic search as a processing mode that is qualitatively different from "controlled" (Shiffrin & Schneider, 1977) or "control" processing (Schneider et al., 1984). This processing, although amazing in its speed and capacity for parallel performance, however, does not seem to be automatic in the same profound sense as are, for instance, innate sensory–perceptual processes. Both in audition and vision, physical stimulus features providing sensory information for percepts appear to be extensively processed automatically (although in vision, processing of spatial information makes an exception).

In general, at least three types of automatic processes may be proposed as far as sensory processing is involved: (a) most sensory processes providing sensory-specific information for perception; (b) transfer of this sensory information to sensory memory; (c) sensory processes leading to attention switch, initiated by certain kinds of physical stimulus events.

The issue of automaticity of information processing has been central also in research on selective attention. Although the main interest has been in the nature, and basic mechanisms, of stimulus selection, automatic processing has been inherently involved. This is because theories of selective processing must, by necessity, also define the processing that occurs automatically. In fact, the position taken by the different theories of selective attention on the nature and magnitude of automatic processing provides a dimension along which these theories can be conveniently arranged. Strong versions of the early-selection theories maintain that, when the to-be-attended and to-be-ignored stimuli clearly differ from one another physically, only the physical, but not semantic, features of completely unattended stimuli are processed. In contrast, the late-selection theories hold that even semantic processing occurs without attention. The latter theories were developed when data interpreted in terms of the breakthrough of the unattended started to accumulate. For instance, it was found that the subject often became aware of the appearance of his or her own name in the to-be-ignored input.

Semantic processing of unattended stimuli may currently still be regarded as an unresolved issue, at least in the auditory modality. On the other hand, in vision, very little or no semantic processing seems to occur to stimuli falling outside the attentional spotlight. This might be attributed, at least in part, to deficient spatial processing of these stimuli.

Although the controversy between the early- and late-selection theorists is thus doomed to continue, a shift of interest from these theories to resource theories has to some extent taken place during the last decade or so. The resource theories, originating from research on dual-task performance, expressed quite a different view of the nature of attention. These theories stressed the flexibility of attention. According to these theories, attention can be allocated to processing occurring at different levels, or attention can be shared between two parallel tasks at the same moment, and allocated in different proportions to them.

Within this framework, the early- and late-selection theories were characterized as structural theories that both assumed (a) the existence of a fixed bottleneck in the processing system above which the attentional capacity is limited (selection could be efficiently made), and (b) that attention could be directed only to one activity at a time (dedicated processing). These structural theories try to account for efficient dual-task performance by rapid attention switching between the two parallel tasks and by stressing the remaining difference to a perfect time sharing. It is of course very difficult to decide experimentally between a very rapid attention switching and a simultaneous sharing of attention between two tasks.

It appears that resource theories cannot replace the early- and late-selection theories. Resource and structural types of theory are mutually complementary. So, the question could be as follows: Given that all resources are allocated to processing of one of two dichotically presented input streams, is the ensuing stimulus selection early or late. Secondly, resource theories try to account mainly for divided-attention performance, whereas the early- and late-selection theories address selective-attention performance.

Whereas even the strong forms of the early-selection theory admitted that physical stimulus features are fully processed in the absence of attention, more recent data indicate even this not to be true in vision. It appeared that although processing of other physical stimulus features is completed without attention, spatial processing of stimuli falling outside the attentional spotlight is deficient; therefore features are often not correctly joined into feature conjunctions, which is a prerequisite of correct perception of visual objects. These data form the central empirical basis for Treisman's feature-integration theory which might, in a way, be regarded as an even more extreme form of early-selection theory than the strong form of filter theory. On the latter theory, physical stimulus features are processed to completion even in the absence of attention, whereas the feature-integration theory makes, with good reason, even this processing depend, in part, on attention.

The feature-integration theory holds that focused attention is needed for accurate localization of the different features processed by the attention-independent, modularly organized parallel-processing systems for these different features. Correct localization of different features results in correctly joined feature conjunctions, precursors for perceptual objects in vision. These objects emerge when feature conjunctions activate corresponding object representations of long-term memory.

The aforementioned theories of attention all are theories of voluntary, active, or controlled attention. The feature-integration theory, however, has some elements of passive attention, namely, involuntary control of the direction of attention by the preattentive texture and figure–ground segregation provided by very early processing (see also Julesz & Bergen, 1983). The control over the direction of attention is, in general, continuously competed for by voluntary and involuntary factors. Involuntary switches of attention, for instance, are caused by abrupt onsets in stimulus energy, especially after a period with no abrupt energy onsets, and changes in some continuous or repetitive stimulus element.

The control of these types of environmental stimulus events over the mechanism directing attention is so powerful that attention is, at least for a short time, captured by such an event irrespective of our voluntary effort to keep attention directed to certain stimuli or performance. Here we are facing a biologically vital mechanism which forcefully provides us environmental information when its potential significance is at its highest (onset, offset, change, regularity in irregularity or noise). The orienting-response theory proposes a brain mechanism to explain attention switch caused by physical stimulus events. Electrophysiological work reviewed later in this book describes these mechanisms in humans in considerably more detail than has been previously possible.

3

Measurement of Brain Activity Underlying Information Processing

3.1. BEHAVIORAL AND PHYSIOLOGICAL RESEARCH

So far this book has focused primarily on behavioral research and theory on human information processing. Despite the ingenious experimental set-ups and brilliant theoretizing of cognitive psychologists, there is an obvious gap between stimulus and response, often called the *black box*. A stimulus triggers a sequence of physiological processes which lead to a required response. These physiological processes provide a potential source for understanding the information processing that occurs between stimulus and response. Psychophysiological research methods can evaluate these physiological processes. These methods can also examine physiological processes that occur before the S–R (stimulus–response) period and determine those occurring during that period. A promising example was provided by Lyytinen (1984) who, using a large set of mainly autonomic measures, was able to demonstrate that each type of selective set, discussed in chapter 2, is associated with, or based on, a highly differentiated physiological anticipatory and preparatory pattern expressing the characteristics of the response or performance required. These methods can also examine physiological processes that underlie self-initiated performance.

3.2. PROBLEMS WITH TRADITIONAL PSYCHOPHYSIOLOGICAL METHODS

The methods of traditional psychophysiology are, however, generally unsuitable for clarifying cerebral mechanisms of attentive and automatic processing. These methods mainly involve sluggish (relative to the speed of cognitive processes) autonomic measures such as the skin-conductance response (SCR), whose onset latency from stimulus onset usually is on the order of 1–2 sec or more (Venables & Martin, 1967). Such long-latency physiological measures—electrodermal, vascular, cardiac—do not usually permit a phase-by-phase analytic mapping of information-processing sequences but rather yield a delayed sum response of the physiological events associated with separate information-processing stages (Näätänen, 1979, 1986a).

Many of these measures also lack a specific pattern. One conspicuous exception to the lack of pattern is the patterning of EMG activity as indicated by simultaneous EMG (electromyogram) recordings from different muscles. For instance, patterning of facial EMG activity is related to emotional states (e.g., Dimberg, 1990). A highly differentiated patterning of EMG activity precedes a motor response and reflects motor systems involved in performance. Such a preparatory patterning can also be obtained by measuring changes in amplitudes of certain monosynaptic reflexes (for a review, see Brunia & Boelhouwer, 1988). But how can, for instance, the heart rate show such a spatial response patterning if we have only one heart? On the other hand, the heart rate can show highly informative temporal patterning.

Response Specificity. In general, the specificity of these measures is low. This means that very different kinds of stimuli or situations, apparently causing very different cerebral processes, can elicit similar responses when measures of traditional psychophysiology are used. The SCR of a suspected murderer to a revealing question may be similar to that of the man on the street excited by the appearance of a sexy female. Hulbert (1957) investigated cab drivers' subjective risk (Näätänen & Summala, 1976) in road traffic by measuring their SCRs to different environmental events. A response was elicited, for instance, when a big truck came threateningly close to the subject's car or when he noticed the presence of a police car, but a similar response was even elicited by an appearance of an attractive female pedestrian. Even steering movements were associated with an SCR. (On the other hand, the low specificity is a problem of many other psychophysiological measures also, including many brain measures of cognitive psychophysiology.)

However, when several autonomic measures are used in combination, some situation-specific autonomic response patterns can be recorded, as in Lyytinen's (1984) aforementioned study (see also Lacey, 1967). Such patterns have given rise to the concept of situational stereotypy of the response pattern (Sternbach, 1966). Certain kinds of experimental situations, such as those that elicit an attention switch, tend to produce an SCR and a heart rate deceleration, whereas others elicit an SCR and heart rate acceleration. As mentioned in the preceding chapter, the orienting response is associated with heart rate deceleration, a "deactivational" change, occurring together with a number of "activational" changes. This deceleration was proposed by Graham and Clifton (1966; see also Graham, 1979; Putnam, 1990) to provide an important defining criterion for distinguishing the orienting response from the defensive response in which the heart rate accelerates. Sokolov (1963) had initially proposed another defining difference between the two response types, namely, that the orienting response is associated with a frontal vasodilation, whereas the defensive response is characterized by a frontal vasoconstriction.

There is also individual stereotypy in autonomic responsiveness; some persons tend to respond to a particular situation with a particular patterning of autonomic changes whereas others respond with a different pattern (Sternbach, 1966).

What is Measured by Traditional Measures of Psychophysiology? It appears that most of the measures of the traditional psychophysiology are only indirect measures of information processing. These measures are primarily sensitive to bodily changes which are of activational or energetical as well as of emotional nature (Duffy, 1962; Hockey, Coles, & Gaillard, 1986; Lindsley, 1960, 1961; Malmo, 1959). These changes can be triggered by certain outcomes of informational transactions; therefore the measures discussed can indirectly serve as measures of information processing and in an important manner complement information provided by more direct measures. It is important to realize that the traditional measures of psychophysiology are not slow when related to the aspects of the organismic processes that they most closely reflect, the activational and emotional processes. Furthermore, autonomic measures played a central role especially in the early research on the orienting response, and thus passive attention (Section 2.6).

In sum, most of the measures of traditional psychophysiological research are suitable for clarifying cerebral mechanisms of attentive and automatic information processing only quite indirectly. For this purpose, the responses recorded usually are:

1. too slow or late;
2. too remote from the processes that are of primary interest;
3. too stimulus- and task-nonspecific, at least when a single measure is concerned (although in combination interesting response patterns may emerge);
4. too nonspecific with regard to different processing stages (Näätänen, 1979);

5. too closely associated with activational or energetical (energy mobilization) bodily events and emotions.

However, these autonomic measures continue to be of great importance in many other fields of psychophysiological research. Perhaps surprising to many brain researchers, the autonomic measures can be very sensitive, such as the SCR and the heart rate, probably to an extent surpassed by no direct measure of cerebral activity available to date. For instance, as reviewed in Section 2.3, SCRs are often elicited by significant items of the to-be-ignored input during dichotic stimulation (but taking this as objective evidence for semantic processing of unattended input is risky). Corresponding ERP data probably do not exist (Näätänen, 1988a). Furthermore, due to its high emotional sensitivity, the SCR has also been the central measure of the polygraph. (There are, however, serious methodological problems here; see Lykken, 1981.) Recent studies recording event-related potentials of the brain (ERP) have, however, shown that some brain measures display a similar sensitivity (Farwell & Donchin, 1986; Farwell & Donchin, 1991).

Electroencephalogram (EEG). Traditional psychophysiology has, however, also measured the EEG which is, of course, generated in the brain. This ongoing rhythmic activity can be recorded simultaneously from very many sites on the scalp; consequently it has been possible to reveal some task-specific patterning in this activity (see, however, Gevins, 1986). This research has often been considered less fruitful in revealing cognitive processing than initially believed (for critical reviews, see Beaumont, 1983; Gevins, 1986; Gevins & Schaffer, 1980). "Despite a number of studies dealing with EEG correlates of higher cortical functions, little fundamental knowledge has been uncovered" (Gevins & Schaffer, 1980, p. 154). Beaumont (1983) agreed but remained optimistic:

> Nevertheless, this area of research still seems well worth pursuing. Given a more rigorous approach to methodological problems, it is still possible that studies of the EEG will form an important bridge between psychological and physiological studies of human behaviour, and enable us to perform direct studies of the cortical activity associated with the cognitive function, validating and extending current models of neuropsychological function. (Beaumont, 1983, p. 406)

Some recent developments in the field, for example those involving event-related desynchronization patterns of the EEG rhythms on the scalp (e.g., Klimesch, Pfurtscheller, & Mohl, 1988; Pfurtscheller & Klimesch, 1991; Pfurtscheller, Steffan, & Maresch, 1988), indeed indicate that the ongoing EEG may serve as an important tool for cognitive brain research (see also Başar, 1980, 1988; Petsche, Lindner, Rappelsberger, & Gruber, 1988; Petsche, Pockberger, & Rappelsberger, 1986, 1988).

3.3. EVENT-RELATED POTENTIALS IN COGNITIVE BRAIN RESEARCH

In view of the limitations of traditional methods, the noninvasive evoked-potential (EP) or event-related potential (ERP) techniques raised great expectations. These new techniques made it possible to study stimulus-evoked brain responses in normal human subjects. It is, of course, this kind of physiological activity which, if any, might interest a cognitive psychologist.

EEG Averaging. After Dawson's (1951) finding that photographic superimposition of EEG traces immediately following a somesthetic stimulus brought out the time-locked, evoked cerebral activity, which was otherwise impossible to see in the "background" activity of higher amplitude, very rapid technical progress took place. Computers were developed to automatically average EEG traces following stimuli. By repeating a stimulus a sufficient number of times, it was possible to record electrical activity evoked by that stimulus, a sequence of positive and negative waves usually lasting a few hundred msec. The background activity not time-locked to the presentation of the stimulus cancels itself out during averaging, revealing the underlying response.

Figure 3.1 illustrates how a useful record was effectively produced by averaging over only 16 consecutive trials. In particular, the pre-S1 trace (the trace before the first stimulus in the figure) shows how the background noise is reduced by averaging. The basic assumptions underlying the averaging procedure are as follows:

> The electrical activity recorded from the scalp after an auditory stimulus contains the response to the stimulus (the "signal") and other unrelated potentials (the "noise"). . . . There are three basic assumptions to the averaging process . . .: the signal and the noise should linearly sum together to produce the recorded activity; the signal should remain constant for each repetition of the stimulus; and the noise should be sufficiently irregular that it can be considered random. With averaging, the signal remains the same, since the average of a constant waveform is that waveform. The background noise, however, since it has a different waveform with each repetition of the stimulus, decreases in amplitude as the averaging progresses. (Picton, Linden, Hamel, & Maru, 1983, pp. 327–328)

A reasonable measure of the background noise is provided by its standard deviation or root mean square value. The standard deviation of the average decreases as the square root of the number of samples in the average (Picton et al., 1983).

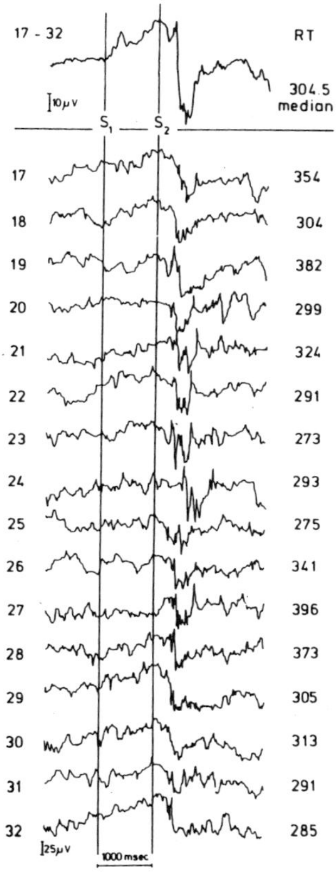

FIG. 3.1. *Top trace:* Vertex (Cz) potential of one subject averaged over trials 17–32 in a visual choice-RT task in which S1 denotes a warning signal and S2 an imperative signal, either an H requiring a left-hand press or an X requiring a right-hand press. The S1–S2 interval was 1 sec. *Lower traces:* Single vertex records resulting in the averaged potential presented by the upper trace. Negativity at the vertex relative to a reference electrode at the left ear is represented by an upward deflection. (From Gaillard & Näätänen, 1973. Copyright © 1973 by the North-Holland Publishing Company. Reprinted with permission.)

Although averaging is almost a rule in ERP research, it is not always a necessity. In certain instances, the evoked activity is so large that the investigator feels confident in measuring this activity even on a single-trial basis. For instance, the response to the first auditory stimulus after a long silence may produce this type of very large response. (See also the slow positivity at a latency of some 300–400 msec in response to S2 in Fig. 3.1.) Moreover, special techniques for analyzing single-trial data with considerably lower signal-to-noise ratios are available (e.g., Glaser & Ruchkin, 1976; Heinze, Künkel, & Scholtz, 1988; Möcks, Gasser, & Pham Dinh, 1984; Ruchkin & Glaser, 1978).

Problems and Limitations Imposed by Overlapping. One of the major limitations of the averaging process is that it necessitates the repetition of the same stimulus numerous times during an experiment. This, of course, imposes limits to the range of experimental paradigms that can be used, making some aspects of information processing very difficult, or at least time-consuming, to study. For instance, it may be difficult to investigate cerebral processes occurring on a trial-by-trial basis during learning, whereas the subsequent steady phase or level of performance can, of course, be evaluated much more easily (Donald, 1979). The same applies to the study of the effects of novel stimuli; each novel stimulus is novel to a subject only once.

Depending on the stimulus paradigm and the aspect of the ERP of interest, the stimulus usually has to be repeated from ten to several thousands of times. The number of repetitions required is particularly large in studying the very small, early responses of the auditory system, the "brainstem responses" (chapter 4). On the other hand, these data accumulate rapidly, because of the very short ISIs that can be used in those recordings. In a long-lasting stimulus block, there is always the danger of seriously violating the constancy assumption, because the signal evoked by the stimulus may considerably change during the course of averaging.

EEG Artifacts. A further difficulty of ERP experiments results from eye blinks and eye movements, because changes in the position of the eyeball induce changes in electrical potentials recorded from the scalp, in particular contaminating data obtained from anterior electrode positions. (The necessity to maintain a steady fixation, of course, involves only the periods over which the EEG is averaged). In long experimental sessions in particular, it may be hard to maintain eye fixation: This then is, in fact, a dual task (Section 2.4), that is, performing the task proper and maintaining eye-fixation (Näätänen & Gaillard, 1974; Weerts & Lang, 1973). This is the case at least when maintaining eye fixation serves no role in task performance, such as during dichotic listening; the subject may even have to counteract a "natural" tendency of eye movement, in this case a shift of the fixation of the gaze to the direction of the attended input.

Ocular potentials are ordinarily handled by using procedures that automatically reject trials on which excessive artifact occurs. However, the procedure is inefficient when using subject populations who cannot adequately control ocular activity (e.g., children), because too many trials would have to be rejected. Consequently, several technologies are now available to subtract the ocular artifacts from the EEG recording (see Brunia et al., 1989). In ERP experiments, it is also important to avoid "unnecessary" body movements during averaging epochs, for these, too, can cause electrical artifacts in scalp recordings.

Moreover, the subject must be in a rather relaxed state. Elevated muscle tension, in particular in the head and neck areas, produces contaminating electrical activity and muscle-reflex artifacts to the records (Bickford, Jacobson, & Cody, 1964; Picton, Stuss, Champagne, & Nelson, 1974), whereas in behavioral research, muscle tension is of no concern. In fact, such an elevated muscle tension belongs to the subject's normal behavior when experimental tasks tap the limits of maximal performance capacity. When we require the subject to perform such a task with relaxed muscles, without biting the teeth firmly together, or without constricting the frontal muscles, we are, in fact, interfering with the normal overlearned behavioral pattern in demanding performance situations.

Why Use ERPs? Despite these limitations, by recording ERPs in appropriate circumstances, it is, in principle, possible to obtain a spatio-temporal picture on the flow of processing events in the brain before, during, and after the critical stimulus or performance. Thus, from ERP data, one can try to infer which regions of the brain are activated and when the activation occurs during stimulus processing and task performance. The sequence of physiological events of the brain reconstructed in this way can then be related to the presumed "psychological" stages or steps of information processing, subjective reports, and objective measures of performance. In addition, the ERPs, like other physiological measures, can provide a measure of information processing without requiring a behavioral response from the subject. For this reason, ERPs provide a relatively unobtrusive measure of the processing of unattended stimuli.

Regan (1981) regarded ERP data as complementing the information provided by the use of the measures of the classical visual psychophysics in several important ways:

> Where EP recordings do not correlate with visual perception, the technique can be used to study those neural activities that do not directly reveal themselves in perception, though they are essential for perception. For example, the transient EPs produced by pattern stimulation include at least four different waves or components, each of which possibly reflect a process necessary for normal form perception. The EP measure is, therefore, richer in information than a simple psychophysical measure of discrimination between a pattern and a blank field. A second example is the use of EPs to study peripheral physiological activities whose effect on perception may be overshadowed by more central properties. (Regan, 1981, pp. 104–105)

It is important, however, not to forget that ERPs provide only a view of those cerebral events that are sufficiently synchronized and organized (in a geometric sense) to create fields at the scalp. A good deal of cerebral activity occurs without generating electrical activity recordable at the scalp (see Donald, 1976; Vaughan & Arezzo, 1988).

3.4. INFERRING FROM EVENT-RELATED POTENTIALS TO BRAIN EVENTS

As already stated, the customary measures of the traditional psychophysiology are, of course, remote from the cerebral processes that are the ultimate objects of interest; with ERPs, we are very close, often only with the skull, the scalp, and the dura separating us from the ultimate target process or mechanism. Now the problem is, however, to be able to study the process(es) of interest separately. The brain is an enormously complex, densely packed collection of structurally and functionally different systems, each having a somewhat different role in various aspects of information processing and behavioral control.

Consequently, what we, in fact, record at any instant as a voltage (potential difference) between the active and inactive electrode sites is usually a composite of temporally overlapping effects from several sources or "generators." At any point in time, multiple cerebral processes may contribute to the ERP waveform. A further problem here is the relatively imprecise spatial resolution of the ERP methodology—however, see following text.

ERP Components. By simultaneously recording from a large number of electrodes attached to different scalp locations, "maps" of electrical activity at consecutive time points are obtained. This is a starting point for an attempt at disentangling various overlapping processes which, rather than the positive and negative waves or peaks of the ERP per se, should be called ERP components (Näätänen & Picton, 1987). "We define an EP 'component' as the contribution to the recorded waveform of a particular generator process, such as the activation of a localized area of cerebral cortex by a specific pattern of input. . . . Whereas the peaks and deflections of an EP can be directly measured from the average waveform, the components contributing to these peaks can usually be inferred only from the results of the experimental manipulation" (Näätänen & Picton, 1987, p. 376) and/or from the "compound source-activity waveforms" (Scherg, 1990). These are obtained by applying certain newly developed data-analysis methods which estimate and separate the overlapping components ("source components") from the scalp-potential distribution over time (Scherg, 1990; Scherg & von Cramon, 1985a; Scherg & Picton, 1991).

Donchin, Ritter, and McCallum (1978) defined an ERP component as "a source of controlled, observable variability." This definition is similar to that of Näätänen and Picton (1987) with respect to how the components are determined, but Näätänen & Picton limited the component by referring it back to a localized physiological activity, to the *generator process* of the component: An ERP component is the contribution of this process to the ERP waveform (see also Jeffreys, 1971; Jeffreys & Axford, 1972a, 1972b; Näätänen, 1975; Scherg & von Cramon, 1985a; Vaughan, Ritter, & Simson, 1983).

Thus, according to this definition, the negative and positive waves visible in the averaged trace should not be called components but rather deflections, waves, peaks, or troughs. The latter do not generally represent any unitary brain event but are usually composed of different components arithmetically summating at the recording electrode. If temporally overlapping components are of opposite polarities, they of course cancel one another either partially or totally.

Determining the ERP Component Structure. As already mentioned, these components can be disentangled by means of experimental manipulations, if they are differentially sensitive in amplitude or latency to different manipulations (Donchin et al., 1978). Subtraction methods (subtracting an ERP waveform elicited in one condition from that of another condition) have often been successfully used in this connection to reveal the underlying component structure of the ERPs elicited. In addition, certain statistical methods, such as the principal-components analysis (Donchin & Heffley, 1978; Glaser & Ruchkin, 1976) have also been used to disentangle components of the recorded ERP waveform, although there are problems with this method (Wood & McCarthy, 1984). A component of the experimental variance may or may not represent a physiological component, an ERP component in the previously defined sense (Näätänen & Picton, 1987).

Further sources of data used for understanding the component structure of the scalp-recorded potentials include intracranial recordings in animals (and in human patients), studies of brain lesions, and comparisons between ERP and magnetoencephalographic (MEG) data. Different generator-modeling techniques have been developed to approximate the loci of cerebral processes generating an ERP with a certain scalp distribution (Darcey, Ary, & Fender, 1980; Scherg, 1990; Scherg & von Cramon, 1985a, 1986; Sidman, Giambalvo, Allison, & Bergey, 1978; Wood, 1982; Wood et al., 1984).

The "Inverse Problem." So, one of the major concerns in the field currently is how to derive from the scalp-recorded data the separate underlying brain processes. As is clear from the preceding, it involves disentangling the different temporally overlapping components and localizing their generator processes. This is the "inverse problem," indeed a problem, because without additional assumptions or information, there is no unique solution to it (Wood et al., 1984; Ilmoniemi, 1991). This is because the potential fields of different sources in a volume-conducting space (such as that inside the skull) sum linearly with each other (Helmholtz's principle of superposition) to give a scalp-recorded potential field which could be produced by any number of source configurations.

The Dipole Assumption. Modeling efforts are largely based on the assumption that the generator source can be approximated by a current dipole, because many empirical ERP phenomena have potential fields on the scalp that closely approximate fields generated by dipole sources. The dipole is used as "an approximation of physiological sources that is mathematically tractable and yet is sufficiently realistic to be useful. The concept of an 'equivalent' or 'resultant' dipole . . . refers to the dipole whose potential field best approximates the summated fields generated by a number of current sources and sinks. For example, the potential field produced by a horizontal layer or sheet of dipoles can be approximated by the field of a single dipole located near the center of the sheet; the latter is said to be the equivalent or resultant dipole of the former" (Wood, 1982, p. 140).

Scherg's Spatiotemporal Dipole Model. This well-known version of the source-fitting or localization techniques was quite recently developed by Scherg and von Cramon (1985a, 1986; see also Scherg, 1990; Scherg & Picton, 1991). The authors expressed the basic assumptions and principles of their "spatio-temporal dipole model" as follows:

> (1) The neural substrate generating the surface EP can be defined as consisting of a limited number of neural subsets (generators), such that each is localized within a small volume as compared to head size.
>
> (2) The external far field of each neural subset adds linearly to the scalp potential according to the laws of electrostatics (spatiotemporal superposition).
>
> (3) The spatial properties, i.e., the scalp potential distribution associated with each generator, can be approximated by the field of an equivalent dipole located within or in close proximity to the neural substrate . . .
>
> (4) The temporal properties of each generator are reflected in the magnitude of the equivalent dipole, which is assumed to be a continuous function of time described by an onset latency and several peaks following. The temporal course of dipole magnitude is thought to depict the compound discharge processes of the underlying structure.
>
> The inverse problem: given a set of potential wave forms measured at different scalp electrodes, location, orientation and wave form parameters of the equivalent dipoles are determined by a least squares fitting procedure minimizing the difference between measured and model-predicted wave forms for all derivations simultaneously. A mathematically unique solution can be found only for a small number of dipoles, limited by the degrees of freedom and the accuracy of the measured signals. (Scherg & von Cramon, 1985a, p. 33–34)

This spatiotemporal dipole model was based on the notion that each activated neural element constitutes a microscopic dipole with respect to the scalp potentials. Taking all the microscopic dipoles of a neural substrate that performs a specific functional process and grouping them together into an equivalent macroscopic dipole results in the component waveshape that is contributed from this brain area, thereby presenting a very accurate approximation of the compound electrophysiological processes underlying an ERP. Using adequate inverse procedures, the component waveshapes of these multiple equivalent dipoles can be estimated from multichannel ERP recordings (Scherg, 1990; Scherg & von Cramon, 1985a).

ERP Components and Scientific Progress. Trying to isolate the components of a response is the direction of progress: In scientific research, decomposing processes of interest represents a central line toward explanation and understanding. Of course a deflection of the ERP waveform is a product of cerebral generator activity, but it is a modified and mixed result of that activity. This is not a satisfying level of data sophistication; major progress from now on requires a strong emphasis on pure measures of brain activity (see also Vaughan, Ritter, & Simson, 1983).

By eliminating a huge source of artificial and misleading variation from our data base through successful component analysis, we might also be in a better position to contribute to a solution of problems raised in cognitive psychology and, in general, become more capable of fruitful interaction with other research fields.

The significance of cognitive ERP research, however, should by no means be evaluated solely in terms of how well this research can decide between different theories of cognitive psychology. Any field or methodology providing data on some aspects of brain function in information processing and behavioral control is important in its own right; in fact, such fields could propose theories of their own, using their own data base as the primary empirical source. Possibilities along these lines are explored later in this book. In ERP research, this will probably be possible only when the relevant data base is organized according to "real" ERP components.

All genuine levels of organization of functional systems are of importance in understanding brain–behavior relationships. Possibly processes generating ERP components belong to the most macroscopic of those levels. It is likely that the information carried by these components is not reducible to microscopic levels such as that represented by single-unit data. Even if it were in theory, in scientific practice it is not, at least in humans: The ERP component as a reflection of some common aspect of activity of a large amount of neurons probably continues to provide an important, in many ways unique, window to the cerebral physiology of information processing. It is also probable that the ERP components, as they appear today, will later be divided into subcomponents as improved methodology provides a better resolution, that is, as the focus of our scientific lens becomes sharper, making it possible to disentangle and reconstruct the processes of interest in considerably more detail. We will certainly be in a better position to understand the mind–body relationships when we know the body better.

3.5. THE MAGNETOENCEPHALOGRAM (MEG)

The advent of the magnetoencephalographic (MEG) methods of brain research has signified a major step forward in attempts at locating electrical activity of the brain. This locating accuracy is often obtained better by recording the magnetic fields (or event-related fields, ERF) caused by and surrounding this activity than by recording the electric fields. In addition, the combined use of both MEG and ERP methodologies has in particular proved useful because of their differential sensitivity to different aspects of cerebral processes. The MEG can therefore complement the information yielded by the ERP techniques (Hari & Lounasmaa, 1989; Kaufman & Williamson, 1982, 1986; Williamson, Hoke, Stroink, & Kotani, 1989; Williamson, Romani, Kaufman, & Modena, 1983).

Magnetic Fields and the Human Body. The first detection of magnetic fields associated with the human body was achieved as recently as 1963, when Baule and McFee (1963) published their study reporting the magnetic field of the human heart. The magnetic counterpart of the human alpha rhythm was reported in 1968 (Cohen, 1968). However, the notion that the human body is associated with magnetic fields traces back at least 200 years: The origin of mesmerism, a concept vaguely familiar to most of us, was vividly described by Williamson and Kaufman (1986) as follows:

> The first association between magnetism and humans to gain prominence was advanced by a charlatan, not a scientist. . . . when a Viennese physician Franz Anton Mesmer arrived in Paris in February 1778 to proclaim an amazing "discovery" his ideas found a receptive audience. . . . Mesmer claimed that an invisible fluid permeates the universe, and in its continual motion it passes through all objects, including the human body. He went on to claim that the body contains poles not unlike those of a magnet, and if they become improperly aligned they impede the flow of this fluid: the result is illness. . . .
>
> In response to scientific and medical criticism a royal commission was established. . . . After extensive studies with the most sensitive electrical instruments and magnetic compasses, this commission issued its conclusion, stating that no evidence was found of a physical manifestation of magnetism to support Mesmer's claims. . . .
>
> We know now, with the benefit of considerably more sensitive instruments, that magnetic fields are indeed associated with the human body—but their origin is of quite a different nature than supposed by Mesmer. (Williamson & Kaufman, 1986, pp. 471–472)

The delay of the more scientific advent of the MEG methodology has to do with the weakness of the body-generated magnetic fields, particularly in relation to the steady magnetic field of the earth and the fields generated by various environmental events (see Williamson, Kaufman, & Brenner, 1977). The magnetic fields emanating from the brain and surrounding the head are much weaker than the fields generated by other organs such as the heart or skeletal muscles, and the magnetic-field changes caused by sensory stimuli are particularly weak. The fields generated by the brain are typically only a few billionths of the strength of the earth's steady field (Kaufman & Williamson, 1982). Therefore, requirements imposed on the recording devices and conditions are extremely stringent.

Development of the MEG Recording Methodology (the "SQUID"). After Cohen (1968) succeeded in recording the human alpha rhythm magnetically, a rapid development in recording devices took place. A highly sensitive magnetic sensor based on a superconducting quantum interference device (SQUID) was developed by Zimmerman and his colleagues in the late 1960s (Zimmerman, 1972; Zimmerman, Thiene, & Harding, 1970). Changes in a magnetic field cause a current flow in the superconducting detection coil of the SQUID magnetometer. By choosing a suitable configuration of coils, a magnetometer can be made relatively immune to fields that arise from distant sources and selectively sensitive to fields arising from nearby sources. This makes it possible to record, with considerable resolution, very weak changes occurring in the magnetic field in the immediate vicinity of the human head, even in magnetically unshielded spaces (Kaufman & Williamson, 1982). However, measurements in magnetically shielded rooms are nowadays preferred. Detailed introductions to biomagnetic measurements of brain activity can be found elsewhere (e.g., Kaufman, Okada, Tripp, & Weinberg, 1984).

The Equivalent Dipole. In order to calculate an equivalent cerebral-source estimate (the equivalent dipole) for an MEG response, the response has to be measured from a number of adjacent locations. In a typical recording session, the detector, or preferably a set of detectors, is sequentially positioned through a matrix of closely spaced points thought to encompass, at the level of scalp surface, the entire extracranial magnetic field produced by a given neural event. The data make it possible to determine the scalp loci of the maxima of the outcoming and reentering magnetic field lines and to reproduce a topographical map representing the spatial distribution of the amplitude and polarity of the magnetic fields at a certain latency (chapter 5). A magnetic field map over the scalp is considered dipolar when it displays symmetrical field extrema of opposite polarity where the flux emerges from and reenters the head and when the strength of the field approaches zero at all borders of the map (Beatty, Barth, Richer, & Johnson, 1986; see chapter 5).

If the field map is dipolar, the equivalent dipole is beneath the midpoint between the maxima, and the depth is proportional to the distance between the two maxima (see Cuffin & Cohen, 1977; Williamson & Kaufman, 1981). The MEG technique makes it possible to locate sources of evoked fields with an accuracy of a few millimeters (Kaufman & Williamson, 1982; Yamamoto, Williamson, Kaufman, Nicholson, & Llinas, 1988). Comparison of MEG localization of brain activity with neuroanatomical information provided by MRI (magnetic resonance imaging) in the same subject provides a very useful test of the validity of the MEG localization (Arthur, Lewis, Medvick, & Flynn, 1991; Pantev, Hoke, et al., 1990; Pantev, Gallen, Hampson, Buchanan, & Sobel, in press; Papanicolaou et al., 1990; Papanicolaou, Rogers, Baumann, Saudjari, & Eisenberg, 1990; Reite, Teale, Zimmerman, Davis, & Whalen, 1988; Yamamoto et al., 1988).

Multi-SQUID Devices. The mapping work has until quite recently been very time-consuming, for only one detector was in use, making it necessary to repeat the same block of stimuli dozens of times. A four-channel SQUID magnetometer was developed in O. V. Lounasmaa's Low Temperature Laboratory in the Helsinki University of Technology in 1983. In 1984, this development was reported (Ilmoniemi, Hari, & Reinikainen, 1984), and the first study (Hari et al., 1984) performed with a multi-SQUID device was published. Presently, many MEG laboratories use seven-channel SQUID magnetometers, and devices with a considerably larger number of channels are already in use (Carelli et al., 1989; Kajola et al., 1989; Pantev, Gallen, Hampson, Buchanan, & Sobel, in press; Schneider et al., 1989). For an illustration of such a device, see Fig. 3.2.

Comparison of ERP and MEG Data. The principal properties of the MEG data may be summarized as follows (Beatty et al., 1986; Hari & Ilmoniemi, 1986; Kaufman & Williamson, 1982; Williamson, Romani, Kaufman, & Modena, 1983, Williamson, Hoke, Stroink, & Kotani, 1989):

1. The generators whose activity can be recorded by the MEG are usually only cortical, because the signal rapidly attenuates with an increasing distance between the generator and the detector (Beatty et al., 1986; Kaufman & Williamson, 1982). This attenuation is much less for ERPs, and therefore subcortical generators contribute to the scalp-recorded ERP. This large (deep) receptive field of the EEG electrodes, though an advantage when the interest is in subcortical events (chapter 4), of course greatly increases the previously discussed overlap problem of the ERP recordings.

2. A generator (electrical current) that is radially oriented to the skull surface gives no MEG response (if a spherical geometry of the head is

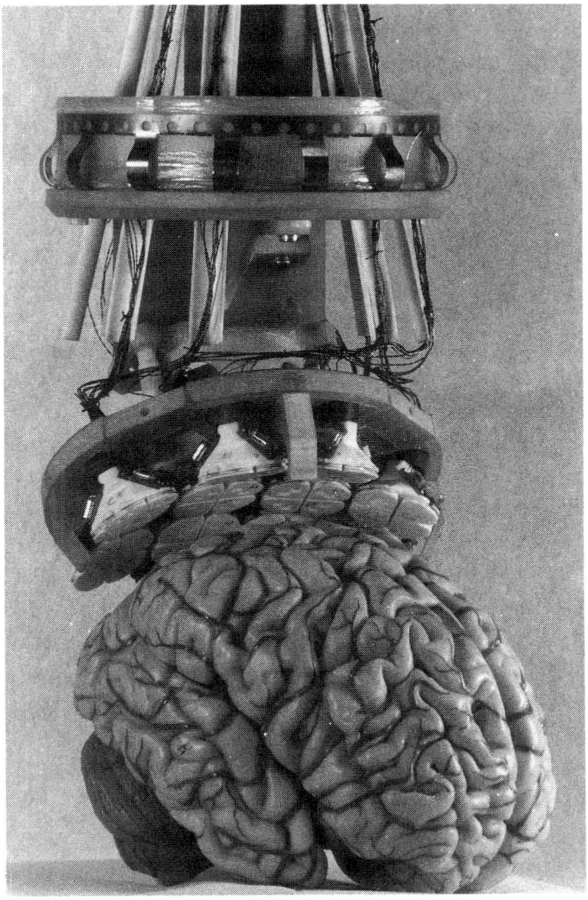

FIG. 3.2. The 24-channel SQUID magnetometer constructed for brain research in the Low Temperature Laboratory of the Helsinki University of Technology in 1989, placed above a brain model at a typical measuring distance. During experiments the device is installed in liquid helium inside a thermos container (a dewar) in a temperature of −269°C. The device enables one to locate current sources generating magnetic fields within a couple of millimeters. (Courtesy of Neuromag Ltd. photo: Jukka Knuutila. Reprinted with permission.)

assumed), whereas a tangentially oriented generator gives the maximal response. This, as well as the relationship of the MEG to the scalp-recorded ERP, is illustrated in Fig. 3.3. When a dipole is tilted from the tangential orientation, but not to the radial orientation, this dipole can be thought of as being equivalent to two weaker dipoles, one parallel to the radius and the

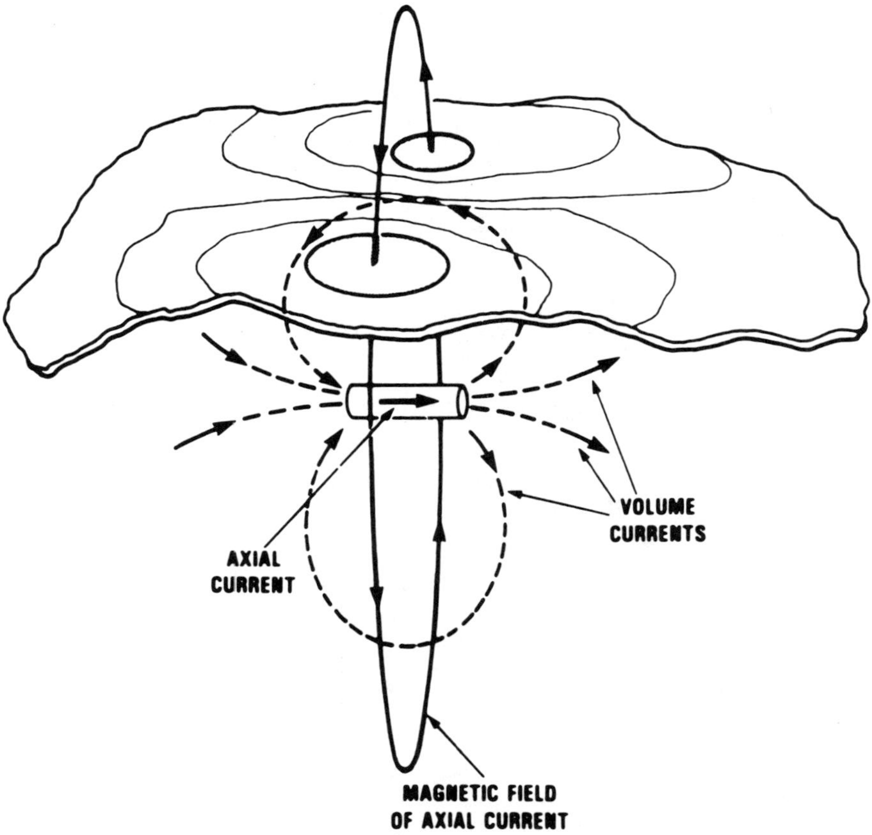

FIG. 3.3. Theoretical distributions of electrical and magnetic fields produced on a surface by a current dipole lying tangentially in a conducting medium below the surface. Dotted lines represent the volume currents resulting from the electric field. The continuous line is the magnetic field produced by the dipole. (Adapted from Kaufman, Okada, Brenner, & Williamson, 1981 by Beatty, Barth, Richer, & Johnson, 1986. Copyright © 1981 by Gordon & Breach Science Publishers. Reprinted with permission.)

other tangential to the outer surface. The external magnetic field is related only to the tangential component, and both the radial and tangential components contribute to the scalp-recorded ERPs (Kaufman & Williamson, 1982). Thus, in a spherical model, the external pattern of the normal field remains constant in shape and position as a current dipole is tilted about its center from the tangential orientation but the field strength diminishes (Williamson & Kaufman, 1981). Field-strength zero represents the case where the dipole is radial in orientation.

Because of its differential sensitivity to tangential current sources, the MEG should be optimal for detecting the activity of dipoles in the cortical fissures (Hari & Ilmoniemi, 1986). "However, the folding of a real brain is quite complex and the cortical surface is not perfectly parallel to the idealized model sphere. Because of the close proximity of the outer cortical layers to the magnetic sensors, complex patterns of overlap from multiple sources may also be present in the MEG" (M. Scherg, personal communication, August 1990).

3. The extracerebral tissues have no significant effects on the magnetic fields, whereas they "smear" the scalp potentials generated by cortical current sources (Hari & Ilmoniemi, 1986). Normal biological tissue is essentially transparent to low-frequency magnetic fields; therefore, a field produced by a source inside the head emerges without much distortion (Kaufman & Williamson, 1982). The determination of the location of a cerebral source is, consequently, often more accurate with the MEG than with the ERP methodology.

4. The aspect of neuronal activity reflected by the MEG is often assumed to be different from that reflected by ERPs. According to these views, the MEG is relatively unaffected by the extracellular volume currents that underlie the ERP, whereas the MEG is generated by the (relatively high-density) intracellular currents flowing in active neural tissue (Cuffin & Cohen, 1977; Hari, Aittoniemi, Järvinen, Katila, & Varpula, 1980; Kaufman & Williamson, 1982). The importance of intracellular currents in the generation of the MEG was proposed on theoretical grounds by Cohen and Cuffin (1977) and on the basis of experimental evidence by Hari et al. (1980).

Ilmoniemi maintained, however, that there is a widely spread misunderstanding in the literature about the generation of MEG and EEG:

> It is often incorrectly claimed that EEG voltage would be due to extracellular currents while MEG would reflect intracellular currents. Electric fields are not produced by volume currents; on the contrary, volume currents are driven by the electric field. It is true that the magnetic field can be directly calculated from the primary current in the infinite homogeneous conductor model, but so can the electric field. Also in the case of the actual head, both electric and magnetic fields can be calculated from the primary current, provided that the conductivity distribution in the different tissues is taken into account. A practical difference between MEG and EEG is that proper interpretation of EEG will require a more detailed knowledge about the shape and conductivity of the skull and the scalp, MEG being relatively insensitive to variations in skull thickness and conductivity. (R. Ilmoniemi, personal communication, September, 1990)

Scherg presented a similar view: "The volume currents generating the EEG derive from the same primary currents responsible for the MEG. Therefore, a more precise localization could also be obtained for ERPs, if more adequate realistic models of the conductivity and geometry of the various head tissues were used." (M. Scherg, personal communication, August, 1990);

5. Whereas the ERP measurement usually requires the use of some "inactive" electrode (whose real inactivity has sometimes been a matter of a major dispute; see chapter 4), the MEG is reference-free (Hari & Ilmoniemi, 1986);

6. Both EEG and MEG methods have a considerable signal-to-noise ratio problem; therefore averaging is necessary also in MEG work.

7. The magnetic field circling a dipole source is measured at the scalp as magnetic flux emerging from the head on one side of the source and reentering the head on the other side of the source (Fig. 3.3). The field obeys the "right-hand rule": If a current source is oriented in the direction of the right-hand thumb, the resulting magnetic field will circulate in the direction of the curled fingers. The electrical field ideally is of opposite polarities at the two ends of the source. The recorded electrical field rarely has such a simple configuration, whereas the magnetic fields are often found to approximate this pattern (Beatty et al., 1986). This is related to a limited view of the MEG, which predominantly looks at superficial tangential dipoles in fissural cortex.

8. Although MEG data also have the component-overlap problem, due to this limited view, the problem is less severe than with ERPs. However, there may still be multiple components even in the MEG waveform (see Achim et al., 1988; Ilmoniemi, 1991; Scherg & Picton, 1991). At present, the dipole-analysis technique used in most MEG work assumes that there is only one spatially limited source area, however (the "one-dipole model"). In general, if two nearby sources are activated in parallel, this analysis technique yields a "point of gravity" that is located midway between the two. Thus the center of activation pointed out by the analysis may even fall on a totally inactive area. Even in the case of a single activated area, the modeling of this area by means of equivalent current dipoles, "point-like currents with strength and orientation" (Mäkelä & Hari, 1990, p. 178), may be seriously misleading (Hari, Joutsiniemi, & Sarvas, 1988; Mäkelä & Hari, 1990; Okada, 1985).

The Import of the MEG. From the preceding, it appears that the main import of MEG methodology to current neurophysiological research on human information processing is: (a) accurately locating, with limitations discussed previously, the cerebral processes that generate recordable MEG responses; (b) complementing and disambiguating ERP information, thereby making it more useful and valuable. This is the case, for instance, when an ERP deflection is an unknown mixture of two components, one of which can be estimated with the MEG (chapter 5). The advantages provided by a combined use of electric and magnetic methods were recently discussed by Ilmoniemi (1991). Achievements of MEG research of human information processing are examined in chapters 5 and 7.

3.6. REGIONAL CEREBRAL BLOOD FLOW (rCBF) AND METABOLISM (rCMR)

Nontomographic rCBF Techniques

Neural activity can be indirectly measured via increases in cerebral metabolic rate and blood flow, which accompany increased neural activity. These changes follow increased neural activity at a relatively short latency and are spatially limited to the region of increased neural activity. The regional cerebral metabolic rate (rCMR) is usually clearly reflected by the amount of blood flow per unit time in this locus: The regional cerebral blood flow (rCBF) is high where the metabolism is fast and low where the metabolism is low. Greenberg, Hand, Sylvestro, and Reivich (1979) showed that the rCBF increases are localized to the active columns of the cortex and hence do not spread around the activated cerebral area or space. Different activities, even in the absence of overt behavior, are associated with notably different rCBF patterns (chapter 8), which therefore reveal the participating cerebral structures.

The rCBF as an Indicator of the Regional Metabolic Rate. The sensitivity of the blood flow distribution to different spatial activation patterns of cerebral tissue is due to the fact that the neural tissue, having no energy reserves, is crucially dependent on immediate supply of oxygen and glucose from blood circulation. The amount of local blood flow is therefore under normal steady-state conditions intimately coupled to local oxygen ($CMRO_2$; cerebral metabolic rate of O_2) and glucose consumption (CMRgl; cerebral metabolic rate for glucose) (Raichle, Grubb, Gado, Eichling, & Ter-Pogossian, 1976; Roland, Eriksson, Stone-Elander, & Widen, 1987; Sokoloff et al., 1977). It is now quite generally accepted that in normal brain under normal conditions rCBF reflects local neural activity (see Roland, 1987; Roland & Widen, 1988). Yet the postulated biochemical mechanism that couples the rCBF to the rCMR has not been identified (Roland & Widen, 1988).

Under some clinical conditions such as acute stroke or encephalitis, however, "uncoupling" of the rCMR and rCBF may occur, so that the rCBF does not always indicate the local metabolism (Fox & Raichle, 1986; Lassen, 1966).

rCBF Measurement: The Intracarotid Method. The basic theory underlying the rCBF methodology was developed by Kety and Schmidt (1948), who also introduced a method for measuring global CBF. Measurements of rCBF became possible during the early 1960s by the development of the intra-arterial, or intracarotid, 133Xenon (Xe) injection method, the Lassen–Ingvar method (see Lassen & Ingvar, 1961). This method reached its full maturity, the ability to describe regional cortical blood-flow patterns in a detailed manner, during the 1970s.

After the injection of the radioactive tracer substance, the clearance of the isotope from the hemisphere is monitored with a multichannel dynamic gamma camera. In Roland's studies (e.g., Roland, 1981, 1982; Roland & Larsen, 1976), this camera monitored the blood flow of the superficial part of the cortex of one hemisphere with 254 detectors, with the distance between the centers of each two adjacent detectors being only 10 mm. The measurement of the isotope clearance began in a few sec after the start of the injection and lasted some 40–50 sec. The flow values determined by the computer from these "wash-out curves," separately for each of the 254 regions, were then displayed on a color-TV screen with colors corresponding to the flow values (chapter 8).

Thus the arrival of the tracer in the brain and its clearance reflect the local blood flow. In general, the higher the blood flow, the faster the tracer concentration will first increase and then decrease and disappear. These tracer-concentration changes observed as a function of time form the data basis from which the flow values, the rCBF, are derived by means of certain computerized procedures (Obrist et al., 1975).

Because blood flow from only superficial parts of the cerebral cortex can be measured with the intra-arterial Xenon-133 method—because of the low energy level of the gamma rays emitted—this is characterized as a two-dimensional (nontomographic) rCBF method. Moreover, the method can only yield unilateral hemispheric information (the side of the intra-arterial injection), and there is the further limitation to the cortical regions supplied by the carotid artery. This method also has the disadvantage of having to puncture the internal carotid artery.

The Noninvasive Method. Therefore, another method was developed, one that is noninvasive and bilateral but nevertheless has a high degree of spatial resolution (Risberg, 1987). In this method, often called the noninvasive two-dimensional rCBF technique (Obrist, Thompson, Wang, & Wilkinson, 1975; Risberg, Ali, Wilson, Wills, & Halsey, 1975), the subject inhales very small amounts of 133-Xenon, usually during a time period of one minute. This physiologically passive tracer thus enters the blood stream via the lungs, and part of the tracer substance diffuses into the brain. After the inhalation minute, the subject again breathes normal air, and the tracer leaves the brain tissue, returns to the lungs with venous blood, and is exhaled. A large set of external detectors (up to 254) again continuously monitor, each recording its own small area, the arrival and disappearance of the tracer in the cerebral cortex.

Advantages of the rCBF Methodology: Good Spatial Resolution. With the previously-described rCBF techniques, one can measure cortical activity with very good spatial resolution. In relation to the MEG methodology, which localizes cerebral activity (that of it eliciting MEG response) better than ERPs do, the rCBF measurements have the advantage of being able to indicate the whole activated region, its size and shape, and even the activation gradients within this focus. The MEG only yields (when the one-dipole model is used) the equivalent (theoretical) dipole that is roughly the center of gravity of the activated area. Therefore different source configurations can yield equivalent dipoles of the MEG that are identical in location, orientation, and strength (see also Stok, 1987), whereas these activated regions are discriminable with the rCBF. The latter does not only show the activation foci but also yields an activity indicator for each single small area (pixel) covered. Thus, even areas with a decreased metabolic rate, and the magnitude of decrease, are indicated.

Disadvantages of the rCBF Methodology: Poor Temporal Resolution. On the other hand, the temporal resolution of the rCBF is very poor in comparison with the msec time scale on which both the ERP and MEG methodologies operate. Although rCBF measurements can yield a distinct response pattern to a sequence of individual stimuli, and thus indicate cortical areas involved in the response, the long measurement period results in the loss of the temporal information. For instance, rCBF measurements cannot determine the order in which the cerebral structures involved are activated. In comparing ERP and rCBF studies of selective attention, Näätänen (1988b) concluded that the two sets of data complement one another in a very important way. "Their mutual usefulness stems from the fact that whereas the ERP methodology, because of its excellent temporal resolution, is primarily aimed at investigating phasic responses . . ., the rCBF techniques monitor, and provide detailed distributional information of, tonic changes and the background state of the cerebral activity which in part determine the phasic responses . . ." (Näätänen, 1988b, p. 152).

Emission Computerized Tomography (PET and SPECT)

One of the weaknesses of the traditional, two-dimensional rCBF methodology was that the blood flow of only the superficial cortex could be monitored. In the intra-arterial method, there was the further limitation to only one hemisphere and there only to the cortical regions supplied by the carotid artery. The most recent technology, however, makes it possible to measure the rCBF everywhere in the brain. These methodologies are PET (Positron Emission Tomography) and SPECT (Single Photon Emission Computed Tomography). Recent reviews of the PET methodology are provided by Raichle (1983, 1987) and Roland and Widen (1988).

With the advent of PET in the late 1970s, it became possible to perform direct, quantitative measurements of blood flow and metabolism everywhere in the human brain. The measurements can be performed regionally from everywhere in the brain simultaneously and with a spatial resolution that permits distinction of most of the anatomical substructures of the cerebrum and even a few major brainstem structures. As Roland and Widen commented, "Obviously this is a breakthrough in brain research" (Roland & Widen, 1988, p. 213).

As discussed in the preceding section, although the rCBF strongly correlates with cerebral metabolism under normal conditions, it does not directly measure this metabolism and, further, the methods examined only "see" a limited part of this blood flow. The introduction of cyclotron-produced, positron-emitting pharmaceuticals for the measurement of brain metabolism and blood flow in the end of the 1960s and in the early 1970s signified, therefore, a major step forward. Techniques based on these radiopharmaceuticals were developed for the three-dimensional measurement of regional blood flow as well as glucose and oxygen utilization. These methods, however, received only limited application, for they required intracarotid injection of radiopharmaceuticals as well as an immediate access to a cyclotron. Moreover, the assessment of cerebral blood flow made possible by these techniques was only quasi-regional, and the metabolic information yielded was rather limited (Raichle, 1983).

These initial steps were followed by a number of further developments on the way toward an adequate three-dimensional regional measurement of blood flow and metabolism (Raichle, 1983). First, cyclotrons and accelerators, devices for producing positrons by nuclear bombardment, became available for use in brain research, coupled with ingenious techniques for rapid synthesis of radiopharmaceuticals suitable for regional metabolic and hemodynamic studies in humans. Second, the parallel development of appropriate mathematical models provided practical algorithms that allow physiological parameters to be estimated from the data. Third, the positron emission tomography (PET) was developed which permits the detection of these radiopharmaceuticals in a truly regional and quantitative manner from everywhere in the living human brain.

Radionuclides Used in PET. A small number of radionuclides, especially oxygen-15 (^{15}O), nitrogen-13 (^{13}N), carbon-11 (^{11}C), and fluorine-18

(^{18}F), possess the following physical and chemical properties which make them uniquely suitable for PET studies:

> 1. These nuclides decay by positron emission. Positrons are emitted from the nucleus of these radionuclides which have too few neutrons to be stable. Emitted positrons lose their kinetic energy in the tissue after travelling a short distance (1–6 mm) and then they interact with an electron. The positron and electron annihilate, giving rise to two photons travelling in opposite directions. . . . It is these annihilation photons that are detected by radiation detectors in the PET. The high energy of the photons gives them excellent tissue penetration and thus good detectability with radiation detectors. The fact that the two photons travel in opposite directions allows tomography algorithms to be applied.
>
> 2. The chemical nature of several radionuclides resembles the normal constituents of molecules of living matter so closely that these radionuclides can be incorporated in substances (such as glucose, water, carbon monoxide and dioxide, various amino acids, nitrous oxide) which are involved in most metabolic processes.
>
> 3. The short half-life of these radionuclides significantly reduces the dose of radiation received by the subject or patient, as well as by those handling the radionuclides.
>
> 4. Because of this short half-life, it is also possible to perform repeated measurements with the same subject, not only because of the low radiation dose but also because of the minimal background activity left from the previous measurements. (Raichle, 1983)

Principles of PET Imaging. As already mentioned, it is the annihilation radiation that is detected by the radiation detectors used in PET. These detectors operate on the principle of coincidence detection. The external detection and localization of a positron emitter inside the brain take advantage not only of the fact that the two annihilation photons travel in opposite directions, but also of the fact that they emerge simultaneously: A coincidence circuit between pairs of opposite detectors arrayed about the imaged object records an event only if both detectors record an event simultaneously (Fig. 3.4). In fact, these coincidence circuits are constructed so that the signal from each detector is compared with signals from many detectors on the opposite side of the object in order to expand the "field of vision" of a detector and hence to increase the effectiveness of the imaging device (Fig. 3.5).

On the basis of the number of coincidence counts between each pair of detectors, images of the distribution of radioactivity in slices of the brain are processed, applying certain corrections (Hoffman & Phelps, 1986). The different concentrations of radioactivity in these images are represented by means of different colors or different shades of gray (chapter 8). The actual

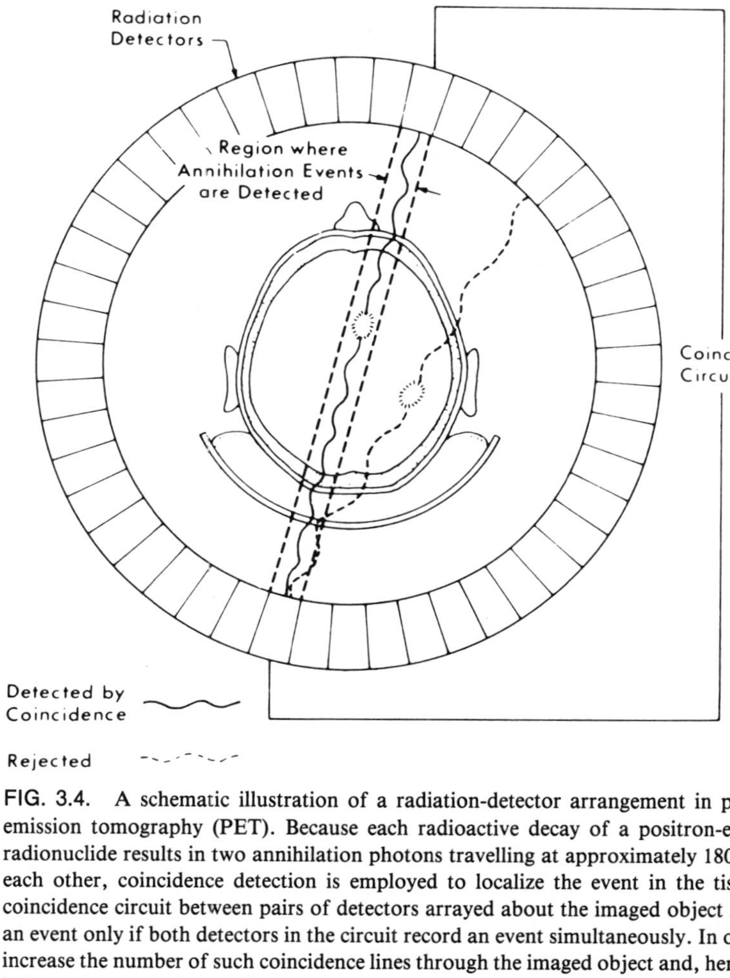

FIG. 3.4. A schematic illustration of a radiation-detector arrangement in positron emission tomography (PET). Because each radioactive decay of a positron-emitting radionuclide results in two annihilation photons travelling at approximately 180° from each other, coincidence detection is employed to localize the event in the tissue. A coincidence circuit between pairs of detectors arrayed about the imaged object records an event only if both detectors in the circuit record an event simultaneously. In order to increase the number of such coincidence lines through the imaged object and, hence, the information-gathering ability of the imaging device, each radiation detector is in coincidence with many opposing radiation detectors (see also Fig. 3.5). (From Raichle, 1983. Copyright © 1983 by Annual Reviews, Inc. Reprinted with permission.)

construction of a PET image of the distribution of a radionuclide in the brain from the corrected count data is a multistep, computerized procedure involving certain specific mathematical methods.

The proper imaging of the brain obviously requires a number of tomographic sections. Modern detection systems of PET are capable of obtaining multiple tomographic sections simultaneously. This makes it possible to reconstruct the data in sagittal and coronal slices in addition to the standard horizontal ones (Raichle, 1983).

The resolution of the PET methodology has steadily improved. The

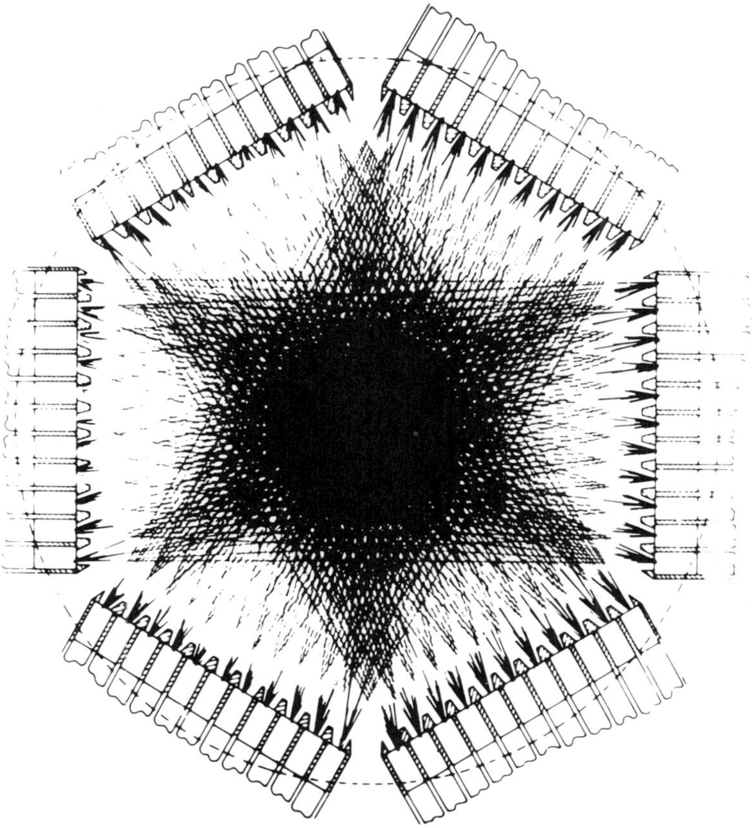

FIG. 3.5. A diagram of a ring of detectors surrounding the body and defining a transaxial field of view in positron emission tomography (PET). The numerous lines of coincidence allow accurate sampling of radioactivity. (From Leenders, 1988. Copyright © 1988 by Hans Huber Publishers. Reprinted with permission.)

resolution of most PET systems currently in use is approximately 8 mm but some have a resolution even below 3 mm (P. Roland, personal communication, February, 1991). Attempts to measure quantitative metabolic rates in structures smaller than permitted by the resolution of PET will lead to serious errors, however (Raichle, 1983; Roland & Widen, 1988).

Measurement of the Metabolic Rate with PET. One of the uses of PET is to measure the regional metabolic rate (rCMR) of the brain. This can be done by measuring the rCMR either for glucose (rCMRgl) or oxygen ($rCMRO_2$). In the glucose measurements, ^{11}C-deoxyglucose or ^{18}F-deoxyglucose is mainly used (Roland & Widen, 1988). Unfortunately, these deoxyglucose methods require a measurement time of about 40 min, which is very long in comparison with performance times of most behavioral tasks given to subjects. Therefore it is not possible to determine whether a given brain structure shows increased rCMRgl because it was active throughout this 40-min measurement period or because it was strongly activated only during certain phases of that period (Roland & Widen, 1988). Also, because of this long measurement time, a behavioral task has to be repeated again and again to determine the participating brain structures. There are also other complications in the rCMRgl determination (Roland & Widen, 1988).

The regional cerebral oxidative metabolism can also be measured with two methods (Roland & Widen, 1988). In contrast to the deoxyglucose methods requiring only a single PET measurement, both methods to determine oxidative metabolism require additional measurements of rCBF and rCBV (regional cerebral blood volume). Thus, three separate consecutive PET measurements are needed to determine the regional cerebral oxidative metabolism of a single behavioral state. In the steady-state method, the subject inhales $^{15}O_2$ for 10–15 min until the radioactivity in brain tissue reaches a steady state. In dynamic method, the subject inhales $^{15}O_2$ only once, and a measurement time of only about 40 sec is required (Roland & Widen, 1988).

rCBF Measurements with PET. The rCBF can be measured with PET in less than one minute. The majority of these PET experiments have used $H_2{}^{15}O$ as the flow tracer. Roland and Widen (1988), however, stated that the results obtained can be considered only semiquantitative, for H_2O is not freely diffusible in the brain.

In addition to the aforementioned metabolic and hemodynamic aspects of brain function, it is possible with PET to measure, for example, amino acid metabolism, membrane transport, certain drug activity, and receptor density of these drugs in the brain.

Although attractive, PET is a very expensive tool and requires an on-site cyclotron to produce the radionuclides. This has limited PET research to a few major medical centers worldwide. The availability of a cyclotron will continue to be a requirement for this type of research in the future, but the number of medical cyclotrons is gradually increasing and their operation is becoming simplified (Raichle, 1983).

Single Photon Emission Computed Tomography (SPECT). There is now another method that has some of the advantages of PET but is much less expensive. This is SPECT. Unlike in PET, substances not normally metabolized are introduced into the brain in the SPECT technique. A gamma-emitting single-photon nuclide, for example, Xenon^{133} (Xe^{133}) or Technetium^{99} (Te^{99}), is administered, and images of slices of the brain are constructed from the gamma counts emitted by the tracer substance. A major requirement is that the detector must be sensitive only to directly incident radiation—otherwise tomography algorithms do not work.

SPECT has so far been used for three-dimensional imaging of the rCBF but the potential exists for some other uses, too (Gordon, Kraiuhin, & Meares, 1986). The principal advantage of SPECT over PET is that long half-life radiopharmaceuticals used in SPECT do not necessitate an on-site cyclotron; the main piece of equipment is usually a rotating gamma camera. On the other hand, because of this long half-life, repeated studies cannot be done with the same subject within short intervals.

DiChiro (1987) listed the principal advantages of PET over SPECT as follows:

> (1) The coincidence detection of the two back-to-back gamma rays emitted following positron annihilation represents an effective and powerful collimation which is difficult to match for SPECT; (2) coincidence techniques permit reasonably accurate compensation for attenuation of the high-energy protons in PET, while accurate attenuation correction has yet to be achieved with SPECT imaging; (3) the radioactive isotopes of some of the biologically most important elements happen to be positron emitters (^{15}O, ^{13}N, ^{11}C). Future advances in attenuation correction and development of newer radiopharmaceuticals for SPECT may alter the situation. (DiChiro, 1987, p. 797)

Thermoencephaloscopy

A new method for noninvasive brain imaging was developed in the Institute of Higher Nervous Activity and Neurophysiology in Moscow by I.A. Shevelev and his colleagues in the beginning of the 1980s. This method, called thermoencephaloscopy (TES), produces dynamic infrared images of the cortical activity and makes use of the fact that changes in cortical activity produce local temperature changes. Like any other body part, the brain produces heat and emits thermal radiation. The heat produced, especially in cortical regions, can reach the cranial bones and the scalp surface by thermal conduction and is then radiated in the infrared range. These temperature changes are based on changes in: (a) the activity of cortical neurons and glia cells, (b) the local metabolism of units, (c) the local cerebral blood flow, and (d) thermo-conductivity in the activated zones, due to changes in the rCBF (Shevelev, Tsicalov, & Gorbach, 1988).

The radiated heat can be detected in the 3–5 or 8–14 μm wavelength range by a thermovision scanner camera from outside the head. This camera produces a thermomap of the surface of the brain over a 40-msec perod and feeds it to a computer at a rate of up to 25 consecutive thermomaps per second for averaging across consecutive maps in time, subtracting the background-state map to focus on the change due to experimental manipulation (Shevelev et al., 1988). Temperature changes are indicated by different colors. This method thus makes it possible to completely noninvasively detect "the activation of small and precisely located cortical zones, and to measure their dynamics before, during and after different forms of sensory stimulation, motor functions and conditioning (associative learning and memory) . . ." (Shevelev et al., 1988, p. 8)

The method has a relatively good spatial resolution, although this resolution is lowered by the diffusing influence of the skull and the scalp and, to some extent, also by scalp circulation, whereas muscle artifacts are not essential (I. Shevelev, personal communication, October, 1990). Thus, for example, changing the position of skin stimulation in the rat leads to a change in location and configuration of the resulting thermal pattern in somatosensory cortex.

Interestingly, the temporal resolution of the technique is far superior to the available techniques of measuring blood flow and metabolism discussed. For example, stimulation of the central retina of a rat with a light flash evokes a clear and local temperature increase in the striate cortex of the amplitude of 0.06–0.014 C° and with an onset latency of 160 msec to 3 sec, and growth time lasting 2–35 sec (Shevelev et al., 1988). Gorbach, Tsicalov, Kuznetsova, and Shevelev (1989) reported such a very early onset latency of the TES response of the primary sensory cortex to electrical stimulation of the skin of the vibrissae of the rat.

Presently, there exists unfortunately no good human data with TES. One problem, although of course not quite insurmountable, is that the surface of the head region monitored should be bald or be covered by hair no longer than 2–3 mm (I. Shevelev, personal communication, October, 1990).

Functional Mapping by Magnetic Resonance Imaging (MRI)

Magnetic resonance imaging (MRI; previously called nuclear magnetic resonance: NMR) is mainly known as a method which provides high-resolution *structural* information (but has also been used to get some functional information: NMR spectroscopy; for a review, see Prichard & Shulman, 1986). Very recent methodological developments have, however, yielded MRI techniques for quantitative imaging of regional cerebral blood volume (rCBV) (see Belliveau, Kennedy, McKinstry, Buchbinder, Weisskoff, Cohen, Vevea, Brady, & Rosen, 1991). In this method, dynamic MRI imaging, based on certain specific techniques, of an intravenously administered paramagnetic contrast agent is used to produce rCBV maps. These maps can then be correlated directly to structural high-resolution MRI images of the underlying anatomy for precise determination of activated areas. The method was successfully used by Belliveau et al. (1991) to determine regions of the human visual cortex that were activated by photic stimulation. These maps had a considerably better spatial resolution than those obtained with PET (Belliveau et al., 1991). In addition, the functional MRI might reach in future also a good temporal resolution: "The sensitivity of our NMR technique to changes in blood volume, as distinguished from changes in blood flow in previous radionuclide studies, offers the possibility of performing continuous serial imaging of cortical function with subsecond temporal resolution using intravascular contrast agents at equilibrium within the vascular space . . . (Belliveau et al., 1991, p. 718).

4

Event-Related Potentials and Automatic Information Processing

4.1. EXOGENOUS AND ENDOGENOUS ERP COMPONENTS

In chapter 2, research and theory of automatic information processing were examined. As might be recalled, according to Posner and Snyder (1975), an automatic process occurs (a) involuntarily, (b) without any conscious awareness, and (c) without competing for resources with other parallel activity. In light of these criteria, a good deal of sensory processing of physical stimulus features, as well as transfer of this sensory information to sensory memory (chapter 2), is automatic. Further, some of the processing that leads to the switch of attention to an eliciting stimulus, as discussed in Section 2.2, also seems to be automatic.

As to the automaticity of sensory processing, ERPs appear, at first glance, to provide an excellent means for investigating this issue, because many ERP components are generated by sensory processes. In fact, the predominant classification divides ERP components into exogenous and endogenous components (see Donchin et al., 1978). The exogenous components are mainly determined by the external stimulus characteristics, whereas endogenous components mostly depend on the subject's intentions and actions.

The exogenous components not only need a sensory stimulus but are, within a wide range of organismic states, obligatorily elicited by the occurrence of an appropriate stimulus. Therefore, these components are also called obligatory ERP components (Näätänen, 1987). Given a certain stimulus situation, exogenous components are, therefore, relatively stable, whereas endogenous components show a great variability and flexibility, usually in accordance with the subject's varying internal state and behavior. The endogenous components:

> are often elicited in the absence of external stimulation. Their characteristics may be related only partially to the physical parameters of the evoking stimulus. A variety of experimental paradigms have shown that these components are associated with such matters as the subject's prior experience, his intentions, and decisions, modulated by task parameters and experimental instructions. . . . Several criteria can be used to identify endogenous components: (1) The components must be nonobligatory responses to stimuli. The same physical stimulus, presented to the same subjects, sometimes will and sometimes will not elicit the component. Moreover, the component could be elicited by the absence of a stimulus, if such absence has the appropriate role in the subject's task. (2) The amplitude, latency, and scalp distribution of the potential are often invariant to changes in the physical parameters of the eliciting stimulus. Quite disparate stimuli, even stimuli in different modalities, elicit the same component if their task-roles are equivalent. (3) The variance of endogenous components is normally accounted for by variation in the tasks assigned to the subject. (Donchin et al., 1978, p. 355)

The exogenous components in the auditory modality are examined in more detail next. For exogenous components in vision, see Halliday (1982) and Regan (1988), and in somesthesis, Desmedt (1988), Desmedt and Cheron (1981), Hämäläinen et al. (1990), Mauguière and Desmedt (1988), and Tomberg, Desmedt, Ozaki, Nguyen, and Chalkin (1989).

4.2. THE EARLY EXOGENOUS ERP COMPONENTS IN AUDITION

The Auditory Brainstem Responses (ABR)

Appearance and Generators of Auditory Brainstem Responses

A discrete sound, such as a brief click stimulus, first elicits cochlear and brainstem potentials recordable from the scalp. These deflections are very small, however, and must therefore be averaged over thousands of stimuli in order to be resolved clearly. It is remarkable that by means of scalp recordings, it is possible to monitor events of the auditory pathways occurring as deep down inside the head as in the brainstem. The "auditory brainstem response" (ABR) or the "brainstem auditory evoked potential" (BAEP) (Jewett & Williston, 1971), as this response is called, is illustrated in Fig. 4.1 (top panel). The ABR consists of seven small deflections, all occurring within the first 10–12 msec from stimulus onset (Legatt, Arezzo, & Vaughan, 1988; Picton, Stapells, & Campbell, 1981; Starr & Don, 1988).

These very short-latency auditory potentials are generated in structures from the auditory (8th) nerve through the thalamus (Vaughan & Arezzo, 1988). Most of these deflections are composed of multiple components, that is, they are generated by multiple sources (Achor & Starr, 1980; Scherg & von Cramon, 1985b; Vaughan & Arezzo, 1988).

Wave I of the ABR is generated by synchronous activity of the 8th nerve (Starr & Don, 1988). Wave II is controversial; possible generators include the distal eighth nerve, the proximal eighth nerve, and the cochlear nucleus and/or its outflow (Legatt et al., 1988). Wave III originates from the pons (Starr & Achor, 1975). The principal generators of Waves IV and V, the latter of which is the largest and most stable ABR component, are probably

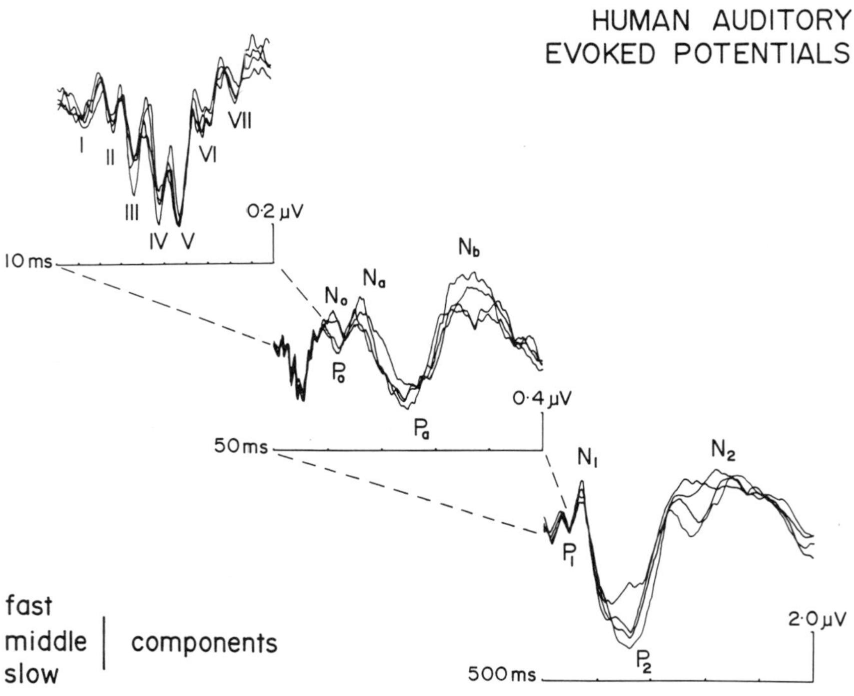

FIG. 4.1 The brainstem (top), middle-latency (middle), and long-latency (bottom) deflections of the auditory ERP (recorded between the vertex and the right mastoid) to a 60-dB SL (sensation level) click stimulus presented to the right ear at a rate of one per second. Relative negativity at the vertex is represented by an upward deflection. Note the different time scales and amplitude calibrations. Each tracing represents the average of 1,024 individual responses. (From Picton, 1980. Copyright © 1980 by Wiley. Reprinted with permission.)

located in the vicinity of the inferior colliculus and in the region of the tegmentum of the midbrain (Starr & Don, 1988; Vaughan & Arezzo, 1988).

Although Waves VI and VII are labelled as part of the ABR, it is uncertain whether brainstem structures are the only main contributors of these highly variable waves (Starr & Don, 1988). According to Vaughan and Arezzo (1988), activity within the thalamocortical radiations is reflected in these two waves which are riding upon a slower negativity preceding the initial cortical response (see Fig. 4.1).

Determinants of the Auditory Brainstem Responses

In general, the latency and amplitude of ABRs strongly depend on the characteristics of stimulation and are relatively insensitive to the conditions of stimulus delivery and to the task performed (for reviews, see Näätänen, 1987; Picton et al., 1981; Starr & Don, 1988). The frequency of tone stimuli has to be rather high for a well-defined response to emerge. Between 2000 and 4000 Hz, all the waves of the response are usually seen, whereas when the tone frequency is below 2000 Hz, only a slow, broad Wave V can be observed (Picton et al., 1981). Click stimuli also elicit good responses; this is mainly due to the shorter-latency waves being mediated through the 2000–4000 Hz region of the cochlea (in the case of a 60–70 dB nHL click; Picton et al., 1981).

Changing the stimulus intensity alters the ABR latency, amplitude, and morphology. All waves increase in latency and decrease in amplitude with a decreased intensity, but the intensity effect on the amplitude is not as reliable and systematic as the effect on the latency (Picton et al., 1981). Therefore, it is primarily the latency rather than the amplitude that is measured in ABR audiometry. At low intensities, ABR amplitudes become very small. In adults, the response, mainly Wave V, to 10/sec clicks is recognizable on the average down to 6 dB above the behavioral threshold for clicks (Pratt & Sohmer, 1978).

Increasing the rate of stimulus presentation increases the latencies and decreases the ABR amplitudes (Picton et al., 1981). However, there are no significant latency changes until the ISI becomes shorter than 100 msec. The amplitude of Wave V remains relatively stable with increasing stimulus rate until the ISI is shortened below 30 msec (Fig. 4.2).

Many studies have reported that a decrease in body temperature can increase ABR latencies. Marshall and Donchin (1981) studied these responses during circadian variation in body temperature. They found that the latencies of Peaks I, III, and V were all negatively correlated with body temperature. Wave V showed an average of a 0.2 msec increase in latency with a decrease of temperature of 1°C.

ABRs do not appear to manifest any overall decrement over time; their

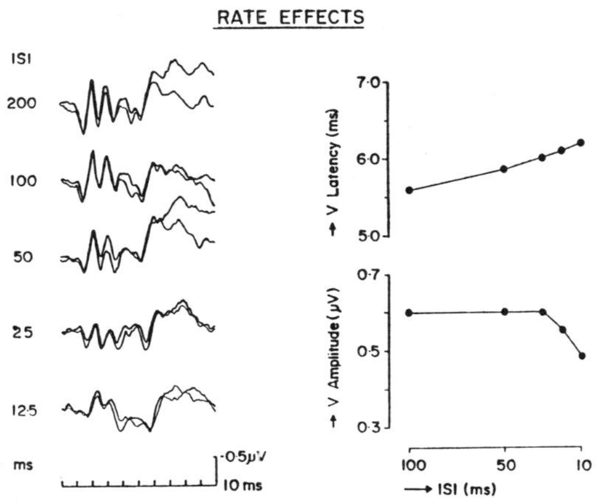

FIG. 4.2 The effect of the interstimulus interval (ISI) on the brainstem responses to click stimuli. *Left:* the responses of one subject to 70 dB nHL clicks presented with alternating polarity at different ISIs. *Right:* the latency and amplitude of wave V as a function of the ISI. The data plotted are diagrammatic and were obtained by combining the published results from many laboratories. (From Picton, Stapells, & Campbell, 1981. Copyright © 1981 by the Canadian Society of Otolaryngology. Reprinted with permission.)

amplitudes are not reduced in the course of a stimulus sequence with a very long duration such as 1 hour (Salamy & McKean, 1977). These responses are even immune to sleep when the temperature drop is taken into account (Amadeo & Shagass, 1973; Campbell & Bartoli, 1986) and probably even to anesthesia (Goff, Matsumiya, Allison, & Goff, 1977).

Auditory Brainstem Responses and Perceptual Experience

Although brainstem responses correlate with stimulus intensity, and in this way with subjective loudness (and are therefore useful in determining hearing thresholds), several studies have dissociated the ABR amplitudes from loudness. For instance, Pratt and Sohmer (1977) concluded that the neural activity recorded as the ABR does not give rise to the subjective loudness estimate, which they suggested is determined by some mechanism more central than the neuronal activity generating the ABR. A particularly striking dissociation between loudness and ABRs was found by Hecox, Squires, and Galambos (1976):

> The correlations between subjective loudness or threshold and the physiological responses observed in this study were poor. Thus no important threshold or loudness changes accompanied the striking shifts in latency observed with altered rise time. In addition, the impressive increase in loudness and improvement in threshold associated with increasing signal duration actually produced little if any change in the physiological responses. One must conclude from these facts either that the "psychological processing" of the acoustic parameters varied in this study occurs above the brainstem level of the auditory pathway, or that it is mediated by brainstem cell population not involved in the production of the brainstem-evoked response. (Hecox et al., 1976, p. 1191)

Further data suggesting a dissociation of the ABR from perception have been reported in several other papers (e.g., Howe & Decker, 1984). Moreover, some patients (for example, those with multiple sclerosis or acoustic neuromas) can have normal perceptual thresholds but almost no ABRs, apparently due to time asynchrony (D. Woods, personal communication, March, 1991).

The Middle-Latency Responses (MLR)

Appearance and Generators of the Middle-Latency Responses

Celesia and Puletti's (1969, 1971; Celesia, 1976) intracortical recordings during surgery have shown that the earliest response of human auditory cortex, a small surface-negative wave, occurs at approximately 9 msec from stimulus onset, followed by two more prominent waves, a positivity at 15 msec and a further negativity at 19 msec (Vaughan & Arezzo, 1988). These waves, recorded with intracranial electrodes in the immediate vicinity of Heschl's gyrus, and thus primary auditory cortex, correspond in their timing to the scalp-recorded deflections No, Po, and Na, the earliest waves of the wave complex called the auditory middle-latency responses (MLR) (Picton, Hillyard, Krausz, & Galambos, 1974; Starr & Don, 1988). For an illustration, see the middle panel of Fig. 4.1.

The primary auditory-cortex origin of the scalp-recorded Po and Na waves was suggested by their polarity reversal across primary auditory cortex. A similar polarity reversal also occurred with a positivity peaking at 32 msec in Celesia's (1976) study, apparently corresponding to the Pa wave of the scalp-recorded MLR (Picton et al., 1974).

These results were corroborated by Cohen (1982), who reported a polarity reversal of Pa across the Sylvian fissure in scalp recordings. Scherg and von Cramon's (1986) dipolar modeling of MLR also supports the hypothesis that auditory cortex in the superior temporal plane is the principal MLR generator. Pa is followed by Nb, usually peaking at 35–40 msec, regarded as the last wave of the auditory MLR.

The very small size of MLRs, as well as their relative lability in comparison with ABR, have often led to difficulties in trying to reliably identify them and to map their scalp topography (Vaughan & Arezzo, 1988). A further problem is an overlap by myogenic potentials (see Bickford et al., 1964) generated especially by post-auricular musculature (Picton et al., 1974; Vaughan & Arezzo, 1988).

Determinants of the Middle-Latency Responses

These problems certainly contribute to the fact that relatively little is known of the determinants of MLR. Regan (1988), however, concluded that these responses are virtually unaffected by arousal and "seem to be essentially exogenous" (p. 270).

When stimulus intensity is decreased, MLR decreases in amplitude and increases in latency (McFarland, Vivion, & Goldstein, 1977; Thornton, Mendel, & Anderson, 1977). In a waking subject, the mean threshold for a recognizable MLR is 18.5 dB nHL (range 10–40 dB) for 1000-Hz tones (Mendel et al., 1975), and the response amplitude rises steeply when threshold-level intensity is increased (Thornton et al., 1977). This, together with the fact that MLR is elicited by tone frequencies within the speech range (too low for most ABRs), makes this response promising in view of evoked-response audiometry (see Thornton et al., 1977).

The influence of the spatial origin of a sound on MLR was investigated by Woods and Clayworth (1985; see also Dobie & Norton, 1980). The results were interpreted as suggesting that functionally distinct generator mechanisms underlie the different MLR waves.

Makeig (1990), in a recent study, found that MLR amplitudes strongly depended on the ISI, being with an ISI of 10 sec about 10 times that with a 100-msec ISI.

The results on sleep effects on MLR are not, unfortunately, consistent (for a review, see Linden, Campbell, Hamel, & Picton, 1985), but the majority of the most recent studies suggest that sleep attenuates the MLR amplitudes (T.W. Picton, personal communication, November, 1989).

Goff et al. (1977) demonstrated that a wave apparently corresponding to Pa was abolished by surgical levels of barbiturate anesthesia. Thornton, Heneghan, James, and Jones (1984) also showed that MLR is very sensitive to anesthesia (see also Galambos, Makeig, & Talmachoff, 1981), and they proposed that MLR could be used in monitoring anesthetic depth. Currently, it is unclear whether selective attention can exert an influence on these components (see Section 6.2.).

Very recent studies suggest that MLR is in fact the early phase of a circa 40-Hz (gamma-band) low-amplitude, transient oscillatory response to the onset of an auditory stimulus (Makeig, 1990; Makeig & Galambos, 1989a; Pantev, Makeig, et al., 1991; for a review of related animal research, see Bressler, 1990). This response is illustrated in Fig. 4.3.

According to Makeig and Galambos (1989a), the transient oscillatory gamma-band response lasts at least 150 msec, and is highly sensitive to stimulus rate (cf. Makeig, 1990). The authors concluded that "a major consequence of each acoustic stimulus is to evoke a rhythmic response consisting of several near-40 Hz oscillations, and that both the conventional 10/sec MLR and the 40/sec steady-state response (SSR) represent partial superimpositions of this 40 Hz-band evoked rhythmicity" (Makeig & Galambos, 1989a, p. 113). Next, SSR is examined.

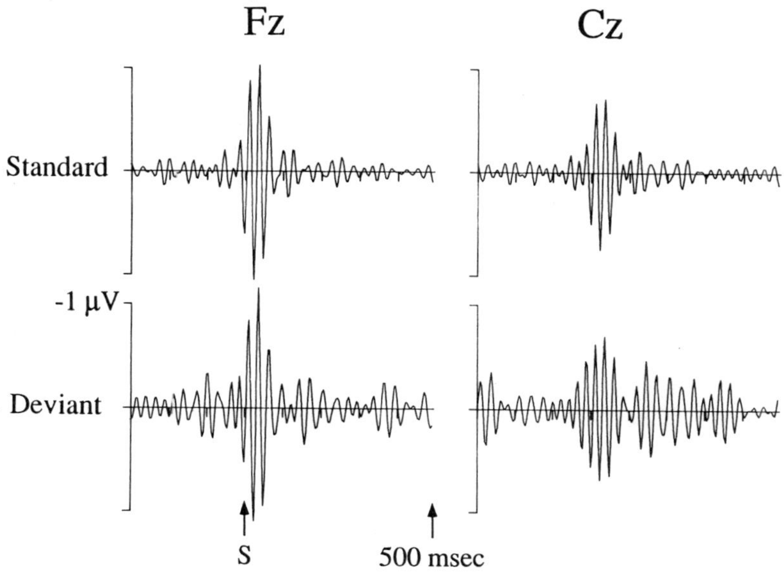

FIG. 4.3 40-Hz responses to auditory stimuli delivered to the left ear of a reading subject. The upper row shows frontal (Fz) and vertex (Cz) responses to standard stimuli (1,000 Hz, 80 dB SPL, 60 msec, $p = 90\%$) and the lower row those to deviant stimuli (1,100 Hz, 80 dB SPL, 60 msec, $p = 10\%$). The reference was at the left mastoid. ISI was 1,000–1,400 msec pseudorandom. Note the temporal spreading of the 40-Hz response caused by the filter. (From Tiitinen et al., in preparation).

The Auditory Steady-State or 40-Hz Response (SSR)

Steady-state responses (as opposed to transient responses) are evoked when stimuli are presented at a rate sufficiently high to cause such an overlapping of the responses to successive stimuli that a periodic response that has a constant phase relation to the repeating stimulus emerges (Picton et al., 1984). Until quite recently, the auditory steady-state responses (SSR) were not widely studied (Linden, Campbell, Hamel, & Picton, 1985) although the response had been known since 1977, when Fergus Campbell, better known for his work on vision, and his colleagues (Campbell, Atkinson, Francis, & Green, 1977), described auditory SSRs to tones presented at rates up to 32 Hz. In addition, Cohen (1977) demonstrated a "following response" to tones presented at rates between 20/sec and 100/sec.

In 1981, Galambos and colleagues (1981; see also Galambos, 1982) reported that the MLR amplitude is considerably larger when auditory stimuli are delivered at a rate of about 40/sec than at lower or faster rates

(Fig. 4.4)—such a phenomenon does not occur with ABRs (see Fig. 4.2). This result reawakened interest in auditory SSRs and in their possible use in objective audiometry. When the stimulus rate is increased to 40/sec, each 25-msec ISI contains a single negative–positive deflection, which resembles the two consecutive deflections occurring during the 50-msec period after stimulus onset when the rate is either 20/sec or 10/sec (Fig. 4.4). Galambos et al. (1981) suggested that the 40-Hz response does indeed result from the superimposition of the MLR components. Stapells, Linden, Suffield, Hamel, and Picton (1984), however, concluded that the relationship between the SSR and the transient MLR is not clear.

The SSR amplitude decreases with decreasing intensity. In response to

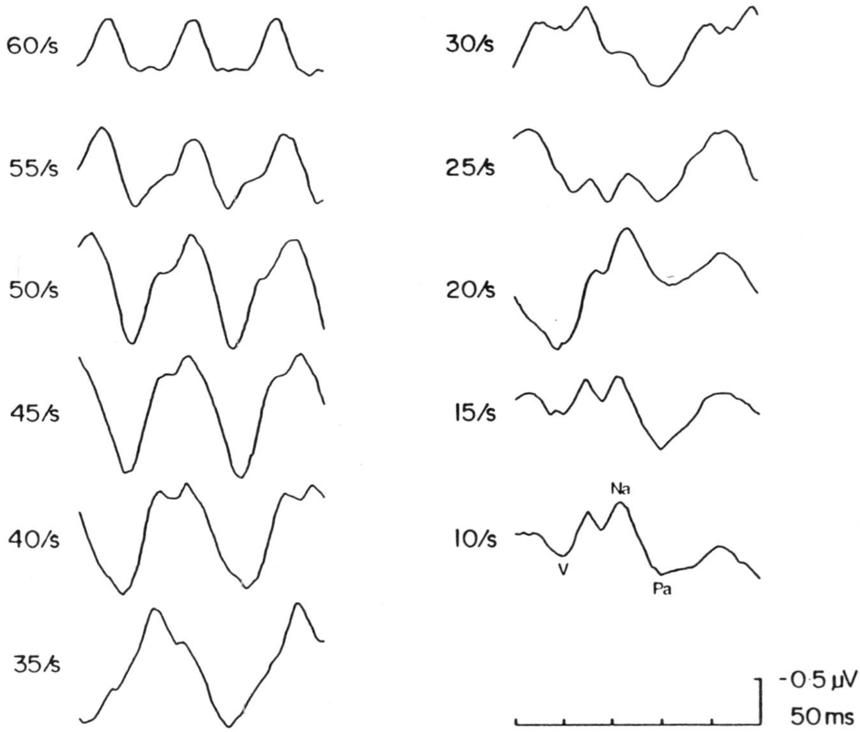

FIG. 4.4 The effect of the rate of stimulus presentation on the middle-latency responses to 500-Hz tones presented at 60 dB nHL (re: a 10/sec presentation rate). The waveforms are the grand averages from 16 subjects. The recordings were taken from the vertex to the mastoid ipsilateral to the ear stimulated. Negativity at the vertex is plotted as an upward deflection. Wave V of the brainstem response and waves Na and Pa of the transient middle-latency response are clearly visible in the 10/sec response. Around 40 to 45/sec, a large-amplitude sinusoidal wave, the 40-Hz ERP, of the same frequency is recorded. (From Stapells D.R. et al., 1984). Copyright © 1984 by Williams and Wilkins. Reprinted with permission.)

500-Hz tones, the 40-Hz response amplitude decreases linearly from about 1.6 μV at 90 dB nHL to about 0.3 μV at 20 dB nHL (Stapells et al., 1984). These larger SSR amplitudes with regard to those of the transient MLR make SSR more easily detectable at intensities near the subjective threshold (Rodriguez et al., 1986). In fact, Galambos et al. (1981) had already predicted the value of the method in evoked-response audiometry, stressing also that this method can even cover the speech-frequency range left uncovered by the ABR audiometry.

A large number of studies have subsequently clarified the relation of SSR to subjective thresholds in both normal subjects and in hearing-impaired patients. On the basis of these studies, Rodriguez, Picton, Linden, Hamel, and Laframboise (1986) concluded that auditory SSRs can provide a reliable and objective assessment of auditory function in waking adults but stressed caution in generalizing these results to sleeping subjects or children.

Quite recently, Makeig and Galambos (1989b) described event-related amplitude and latency perturbations in SSR that lasted several hundreds of msec, which they called "complex event-related potentials" (CERP). This SSR perturbation occurred when the background tone pip, presented to the subject at the rate of 40/sec, changed in frequency from 1000 Hz to 1200 Hz, and when it changed back to the original frequency a couple of seconds later. This response is illustrated in Fig. 4.5. The left side of the figure shows that the SSR amplitude is considerably reduced soon after the occurrence of the frequency change and, further, that the transient amplitude dampening is followed by a period of SSR-amplitude enhancement. This enhancement usually peaked at 300 msec from stimulus (change) onset (Makeig & Galambos, 1989b).

The amplitude-modulation response is paralleled by a latency-shortening response, which peaks at about 200 msec from stimulus onset (see the right side of Fig. 4.5). Makeig and Galambos (1989b), however, concluded that the amplitude and latency perturbations do not have a common cause because their time courses somewhat differed from one another. Moreover, the latency perturbation was often a one-phasic response (only latency shortening), whereas the amplitude perturbation showed two consecutive phases (amplitude reduction followed by amplitude enhancement).

Similar responses occurred when the intensity of the 40-Hz background stimulus was reduced or increased for a period of a couple of seconds and also when the original intensity returned back to the initial level. In addition, an omission of just one of the stimuli of the background sequence elicited a similar response. Interestingly, a subsequent stimulus omission following the initial omission at an interval of only about 0.5 seconds caused a perturbation that was not at all attenuated relative to the perturbation caused by the initial omission.

In a further condition, Makeig and Galambos (1989b) presented parallel

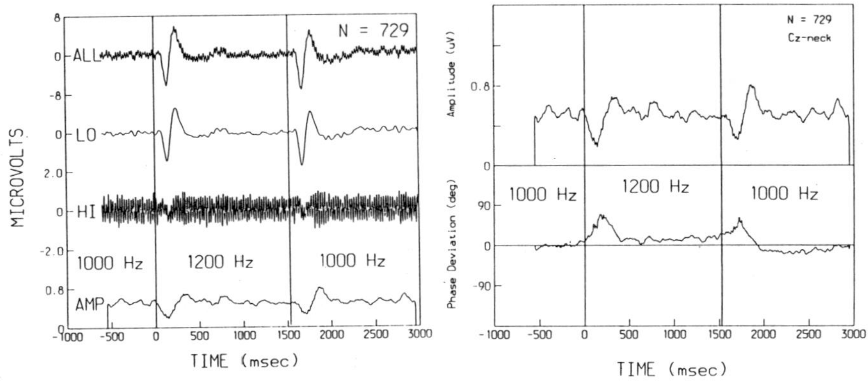

FIG. 4.5 *Left:* Extraction of ERPs (event-related potentials) and CERPs (complex event-related potentials) from the EEG of a subject presented with short tone bursts at a rate of 40/s, which were shifted up and down in pitch every few seconds. The *top trace* contains both the rapid sinusoidal potentials evoked by the individual tone pips (the 40-Hz SSR) and the conventional ERPs produced by the pitch changes. Filtering the EEG at exactly the repetition rate of the tone bursts (40 Hz) extracts the sinusoidal SSR (steady-state response) shown in the *third trace* and leaves behind the ERPs shown in the *second trace.* The *bottom trace* plots the amplitude fluctuations visible in the *third trace* and represents one of two components of the CERP. *Right:* The SSR amplitude fluctuations shown in the bottom trace of the figure on the left are reproduced in the *top line* for comparison with the SSR phase deviations *(bottom line)* that accompany the shifts in pitch of the tones to which the subject was listening. (From Makeig & Galambos, 1989b. Copyright © 1989 by Springer-Verlag. Reprinted with permission.)

sequences of auditory and visual background stimuli (with slightly differing rates). Occasional intensity changes in the auditory background stimulation caused perturbations in the auditory SSR similar to those just described but did not affect the parallel visual SSR. Conversely, intensity changes in the visual background stimulation caused perturbations in the visual SSR resembling those in the auditory SSR but did not affect the parallel auditory SSR. These data consequently suggest modality-specific mechanisms of SSR generation.

Makeig and Galambos (1989b) concluded that although SSR can be explained with a summation of consecutive MLRs elicited by consecutive stimuli of the 40-Hz sequence, SSR perturbations observed cannot be simply accounted for by an effect on any single MLR. This is because of the relatively long duration of the event-related perturbations observed, which suggests that the MLR mechanism is modulated for a much longer time, so that many consecutive MLRs generated by the mechanism are affected. The origin of the modulating, apparently modality-specific, effect remained unclear but it appeared that rather than one, two or several mechanisms were involved.

Rohrbaugh and his colleagues have also studied event-related SSR perturbations but, in contrast to Makeig and Galambos (1989b), they used separate "foreground" stimuli rather than inserting changes in the 40-Hz stimulation itself. In one of these studies, Rohrbaugh, Varner, Paige, Eckardt, and Ellingson (1989) found that the latency of the SSR to a weak, background 40-Hz stimulus was shortened by some 4–5 msec by a foreground stimulus presented with a mean ISI of 10 sec. (On the other hand, the SSR-amplitude response was quite inconsistent.) This effect, illustrated in Fig. 4.6, reached its maximum at 150–200 msec from the onset of the foreground stimulus and lasted several hundred msec. The magnitude of the effect was proportional to the amplitude of the simultaneous slow-wave responses to the foreground stimulus and, to a lesser extent, to the magnitude of heart-rate deceleration caused by this stimulus. Also, the latency-reduction response was larger when the foreground stimuli required a discrimination than when they were only passively observed. The authors proposed that the latency-reduction response may reflect "a transient period of sensitization during orienting" (Rohrbaugh et al., 1989, p. 247).

These results were corroborated by Rohrbaugh, Varner, Paige, Eckardt, and Ellingson (1991). They found that the latency-reduction response was larger for intense than weak foreground stimuli. Further, response was larger to infrequent ($p = 0.3$), counted than to frequent ($p = 0.7$), uncounted foreground stimuli differing in pitch, and was considerably smaller during Session 2 than during Session 1.

In another study, Rohrbaugh, Varner, Paige, Eckardt, & Ellingson (1990) found that the latency-reduction response of the auditory SSR can also be produced with visual foreground stimuli. This response was much smaller in magnitude than that obtained with auditory foreground stimuli, however. The authors related this intermodal difference to the generally smaller alerting effects of visual stimuli as compared to auditory stimuli (e.g., Posner, Nissen, & Klein, 1976).

4.3. THE LATE EXOGENOUS ERP COMPONENTS

The Late Transient Responses: N1 and P2

The auditory middle-latency responses are followed by large N1 and P2 waves; N1 denotes a negativity that usually peaks at about 100 msec from stimulus onset and P2 indicates a positivity that peaks at around 180–200 msec in the auditory modality (Fig. 4.1). N1 is preceded by a small positivity, P1, which peaks at about 50 msec. (In the visual and somatosensory modalities, the latencies of corresponding responses are somewhat longer.) The N1 and P2 waves do not represent a single cerebral event

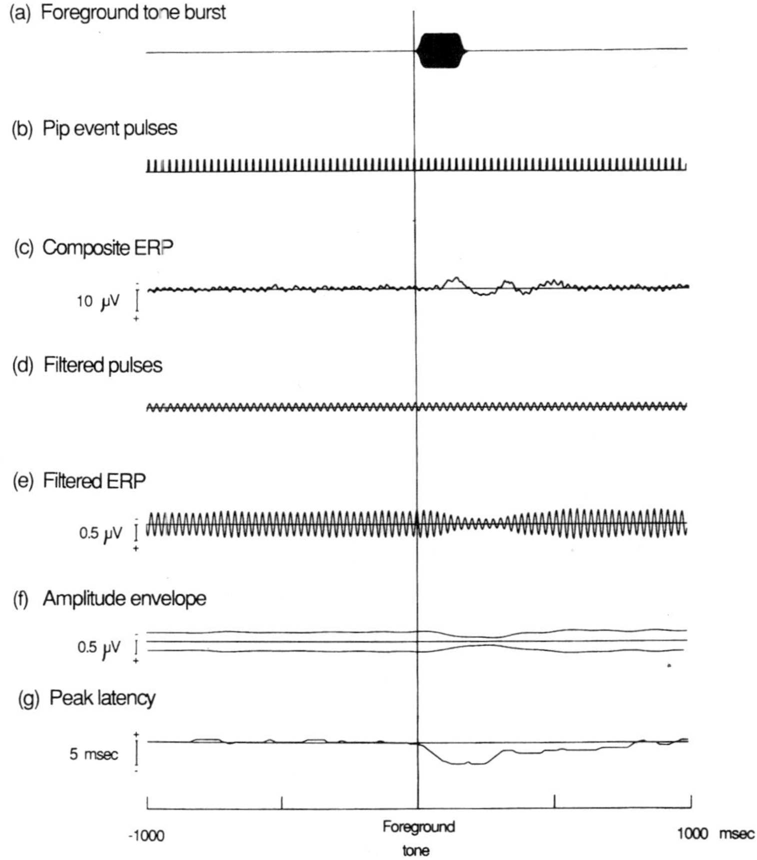

FIG. 4.6 An illustration of the analysis procedure and representative results for event-related perturbations in the 40-Hz steady-state response (SSR). (a) envelope of a 200-msec foreground tone stimulus; (b) pulses, 5 msec in duration, synchronous with the train of background pips at 41 Hz; (c) ERP complex elicited by foreground tone and background pips, averaged over trials; (d) filtered record of synchronous pips, used as temporal referent for computing latency values of individual peaks in filtered 40-Hz SSR record; (e) ERP complex after narrow-band digital filtering to extract 40 Hz SSR; (f) amplitude envelope of filtered 40-Hz SSR; (g) function describing the peak-by-peak latency of the filtered 40-Hz SSR. A decrease in peak latency is plotted as a downward deflection. This decrease reaches its maximum at about 155 msec after the onset of the foreground tone stimulus. (From Rohrbaugh, Varner, Paige, Eckardt, & Ellingson, 1990. Copyright © 1990 by Elsevier Science Publishers BV, Ireland. Reprinted with permission.)

because they respond differently to experimental manipulation and differ in scalp distribution (Knight, Hillyard, Woods, & Neville, 1980; Näätänen & Picton, 1987).

Auditory Cortex as a Possible Generator of the Auditory N1. Vaughan and Ritter (1970) found that N1 to brief 1000-Hz tones presented every 2 sec, recorded along a coronal chain of electrodes using the nose as a reference, reversed its polarity over the Sylvian fissure. The authors therefore proposed that the auditory N1 is generated in primary auditory cortex on the superior aspect of the temporal lobe. A dipole located in primary auditory cortex would be oriented vertically. The surface potentials generated by such a dipole would be of one polarity at the vertex or frontal regions of the scalp and of the opposite polarity below the level of auditory cortex.

This interpretation was soon questioned by Kooi, Tipton, and Marshall (1971). They suggested that the nose was not an inactive reference but could pick up activity from the frontal pole. If this activity were similar in morphology, even though smaller in amplitude than that picked up from the vertex, an apparent polarity inversion would result when this activity was subtracted (by the differential amplifier) from the little or no activity picked up in the temporal and mastoid regions. Lehtonen and Koivikko (1971) and Wood and Wolpaw (1982), however, succeeded, in contrast to Kooi et al. (1971), in recording some degree of polarity reversal across the Sylvian fissure even with a sternovertebral reference. See also Peronnet, Michel, Echallier, and Girod (1974).

Depth-electrode recordings in alert rhesus monkeys (Arezzo, Pickoff, & Vaughan, 1975) showed that the late responses (N70 and P110) recorded epidurally over the frontal and central cortex were mainly volume-conducted from the supratemporal plane. These findings support Vaughan and Ritter's (1970) interpretation of the human scalp recordings, provided that the responses are truly homologous and the intracranial geometries are similar (Näätänen & Picton, 1987).

Subcortical Correlates of N1. Velasco, Velasco, and Olvera (1985; Velasco & Velasco, 1986) have reported subcortical correlates for N1. These authors presented auditory, visual, and somatosensory stimuli randomly at an ISI of 4 sec to patients during stereotactic operations and recorded responses with depth electrodes. Bipolar recordings (Velasco et al., 1985) of the auditory responses indicated rapid changes in potential over very short distances in several subcortical areas: the mesencephalic reticular formation, the medial and dorsal thalamus, the striatum, and the limbic system. These findings suggest that the sources are close to the recording electrodes. No late responses were found in the specific sensory nuclei of the thalamus, which showed only early modality-specific waves.

Velasco and colleagues (1985) postulated that there is a nonspecific sensory system "located in the center of the human brain involving a series of structures with a caudal–rostral arrangement, which extends from the rostral mesencephalon to the striatum and limbic structures of the frontal and temporal lobes" (p. 527). The existence of such a nonspecific generator for N1 was hypothesized in early studies in order to explain such findings as the interactions between sensory modalities (Davis, Osterhammel, Wier, & Gjerdingen, 1972; Walter, 1964), the sensitivity to changes in arousal (Fruhstorfer & Bergström, 1969; Larsson, 1956, 1960a, 1960b; Näätänen, 1967), and very long refractory periods (Allison, 1962; Fruhstorfer, Soveri, & Järvilehto 1970).

Multiple N1 Generators. The idea that multiple generators contribute to the scalp-recorded auditory N1 was first clearly stated by Wolpaw and Penry (1975). They recorded auditory ERPs from Cz, T3, and T4 in response to click stimuli. They found that a temporal "T-complex," with a positive peak at 105 msec (Ta) and a negative peak at 155 msec (Tb), overlapped a separately generated vertex N1–P2 response. They suggested that the T-complex was generated in secondary auditory cortex on the lateral aspect of the temporal lobe, and that N1–P2 was generated in widespread areas of cortex, particularly frontal.

Support was provided by Celesia's (1976) intraoperative recordings from the lateral surface of the temporal lobe. He found waves that were of similar polarity and latency to Wolpaw and Penry's (1975) Ta and Tb waves. Several other papers have demonstrated a temporal N140 wave that is apparently equivalent to the Tb wave (Hackley, Woldorff, & Hillyard, 1990; McCallum & Curry, 1979, 1980; Picton, Woods, & Proulx, 1978a; Woldorff & Hillyard, 1991; Wolpaw & Penry, 1977, 1978; Wood & Wolpaw, 1982). Most papers have suggested that the temporal N140 results from a laterally oriented dipole in the temporal lobe. A concomitant positive wave recorded from the nasopharynx may represent the other side of such a dipole (Perrault & Picton, 1984).

Scherg and von Cramon (1985a, 1986; see also Scherg, 1990) recently developed a technique to model the generator sources for scalp-recorded ERPs (Section 3.3). As already explained, their technique posits dipole sources that generate a waveform over time and contribute to the scalp recordings on the basis of the location and orientation of the source and the conductivity of the head, modeled as a three-layered sphere. Using reasonable restrictions (triphasic dipole waveforms, four sources, spatial accuracy to within 2 cm), they were able to model the scalp-recorded field in response to brief tones presented every 1.5–2.5 sec with two dipole sources in each temporal lobe. One source was oriented vertically (tangentially to the lateral surface of the skull) and the other horizontally (radially). The tangential source gave a negative component at 100 msec and positive at 180 msec; the radial source gave a positive component at 100 msec and negative at 150 msec. These findings are illustrated in Fig. 4.7.

Consequently, the auditory N1 wave is probably generated in at least two different locations in auditory cortex. In addition, there may be a generation locus, responsible for the nonspecific component, outside the auditory cortices. The first N1 component, according to Näätänen and Picton's (1987) classification, is a frontocentral negativity generated by bilateral, vertically oriented dipoles in the auditory cortices on the supratemporal plane. This component, originally proposed by Vaughan and Ritter (1970), is strongly supported by the MEG results (Section 5.1) and by the tangential dipole-source potentials derived by Scherg and von Cramon (1985a) in normal subjects and patients with cerebral lesions.

Näätänen and Picton (1987) estimated that the supratemporal component is about 10% larger to contralaterally than ipsilaterally presented stimuli. This asymmetry probably results from the asymmetry of input to the auditory cortices, each ear sending a larger number of fibers to the contralateral than ipsilateral cortex (Rosenzweig, 1951).

Component 2 is the T-complex with a positive subcomponent at 100 msec and a negative subcomponent at 150 msec, as originally described by

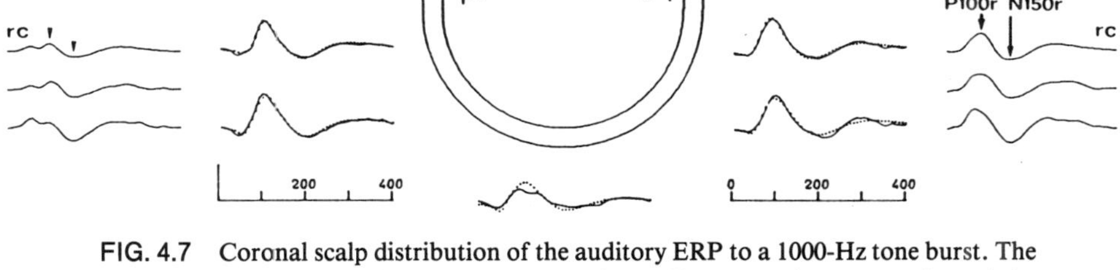

FIG. 4.7 Coronal scalp distribution of the auditory ERP to a 1000-Hz tone burst. The recorded potentials (continuous traces around the diagrammatic cross section of the head) were obtained by using an average reference. The superimposed dotted traces are the best-fit waveforms from the spatio-temporal dipole analyses. Within the cross section are shown the location (dot), orientation (direction of line), and relative strength (length of line) of the tangential (t) and radial (r) dipole-source components in both temporal lobes. On the extreme left and right, tangential (top – tc) and radial (bottom – rc) dipole-source potentials from three different mathematical analyses (a, b, c) are depicted for the left (LH) and right (RH) hemispheres. (From Scherg & von Cramon, 1986. Copyright © 1986 by Elsevier Science Publishers, Ireland. Reprinted with permission.)

Wolpaw and Penry (1975). This complex probably originates in auditory association cortex in the superior temporal gyrus. This complex has received support from intracerebral recordings (Celesia, 1976; McCallum & Curry, 1979, 1980), and it has been convincingly modeled by Scherg and von Cramon (1986). Due to the approximately radial orientation of the underlying current dipole, this component is not picked up with MEG recordings (chapters 3 and 5).

The third component, the one best corresponding to the early notion of the vertex potential, is the nonspecific one that peaks at a latency of about 100 msec and reaches its maximum at the vertex. The location of its generator is not known. The field of this component is widespread, with a maximum that is somewhat posterior to that of Component 1, with which it strongly overlaps. Näätänen and Picton (1987) suggested that the nonspecific component is generated in the frontal motor and premotor cortex under the influence of the reticular formation and the ventral lateral (VL) nucleus of the thalamus.

The justification for this component derives from the studies of Velasco and his colleagues (Velasco et al., 1985; Velasco & Velasco, 1986) who found the reticular formation and the VL nucleus of the thalamus to be very active during the scalp-recorded auditory N1. Furthermore, Arezzo et al. (1975) observed that some areas of the monkey frontal cortex were active during the scalp-recorded N1. In addition, Hari, Kaila, Katila, Tuomisto, and Varpula (1982) found that at long ISIs the vertex-recorded N1 is enhanced independently of the frontally recorded N1 (composed mainly of the supratemporal component) as well as of the magnetic counterpart of the supratemporal N1 component (Section 5.1). These data suggest that at long ISIs, a different, probably nonspecific, source is activated, shifting the scalp distribution of the N1 wave in the posterior direction (Fig. 4.8).

Some recent results point to the possible existence of two further subcomponents of the N1 wave. One of these is the early part of the sustained potential (Scherg, Vajsar, & Picton, 1989) and the other is a frontally generated N1 subcomponent (Giard, Perrin, & Echallier, submitted). Both findings are discussed later.

The P2 Wave. This wave may also have specific and nonspecific components (Vaughan, Ritter, & Simson, 1980). The specific component is generated from a locus in the supratemporal auditory cortex which by means of MEG recordings can be separated from that of the supratemporal N1 component (Section 5.1). Moreover, although the N1 and P2 waves vary quite similarly in most conditions, they can be dissociated from one another (e.g., Knight et al., 1980). In addition, the N1 and P2 scalp distributions differ from one another (Paavilainen et al., 1991).

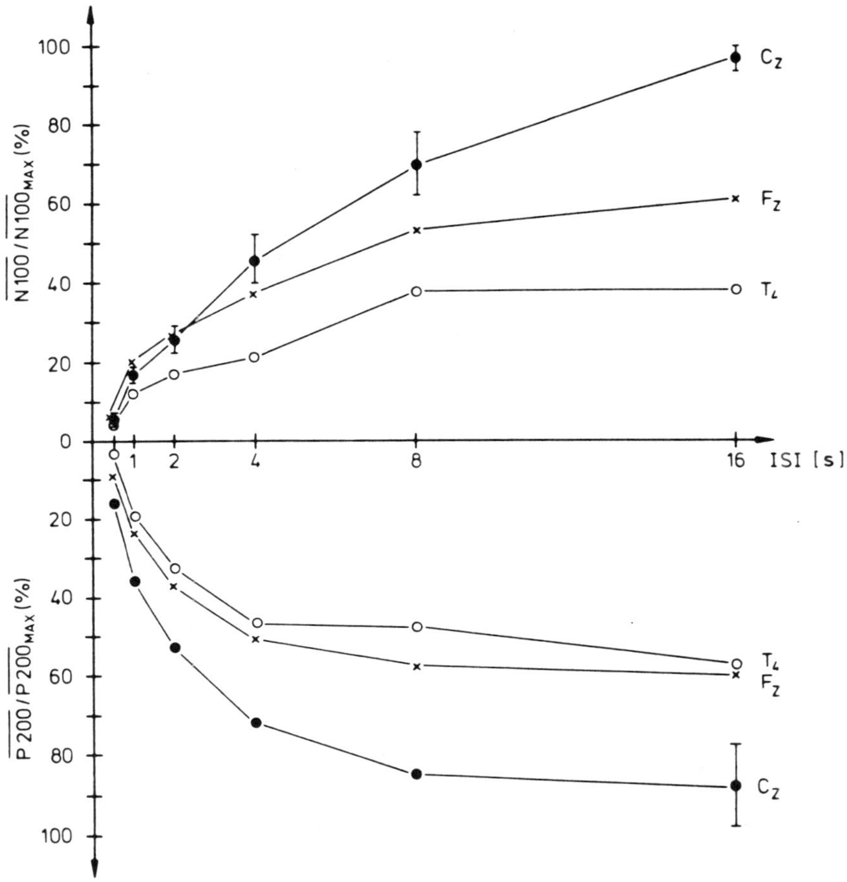

FIG. 4.8 Relative amplitudes of the N1 (N100) and P2 (P200) peaks with different ISIs. Mean of 4 subjects; the amplitudes were normalized separately for each subject. Derivations Cz, Fz, and T4 referred to the right mastoid. (From Hari, Kaila, Katila, Tuomisto, & Varpula, 1982. Copyright © 1982 by Elsevier Science Publishers, Ireland. Reprinted with permission.)

Determinants of the Late Transient Responses

Energy Onset and Offset

The N1 potential is evoked by a relatively abrupt change in the level of energy impinging on the sensory receptors. Stimuli with very slow onsets do not elicit this response (Clynes, 1969). Sustained stimuli elicit the N1 potential only at their onset, with prolongation of the stimulus increasing the N1 amplitude only up to durations of 50 msec (Kodera, Hink, Yamada, & Suzuki, 1979; Onishi & Davis, 1968). Because the majority of cortical neurons, unlike the auditory nerve fibers, respond to the onset and not to the continuation of sensory stimuli (Goldstein, Hall, & Butterfield, 1968), N1 probably represents a true onset response rather than some artifact of synchronization (Näätänen & Picton, 1987).

The N1 response can also be elicited by the offset of a stimulus (Davis, P.A., 1939; Davis, H. & Zerlin, 1966). An offset response is clearly recognizable usually only if the stimulus has been on at least 0.5 sec, and the response increases in amplitude as the stimulus duration is prolonged (Davis & Zerlin, 1966; Hillyard & Picton, 1978; Pfefferbaum, Buchsbaum, & Gips, 1971). For equal on–off cycles, the offset response is smaller than the onset response and its latency is 10–20 msec shorter (Onishi & Davis, 1968).

The N1 latency and amplitude are determined by the slope of the energy change—the rise time or the fall time (Loveless & Brunia, 1990). Several papers have reported that the N1–P2 amplitude decreases as the rise time or fall time of the stimulus exceeds 50 msec (for a review, see Loveless & Brunia, 1990).

N1 to Change in a Continuous Stimulus

N1 can also be elicited by a change in the tonal frequency or intensity of a continuous auditory stimulus (Clynes, 1969; Spoor, Timmer, & Odenthal, 1969). Such a response to a change of a continuous 600-Hz tone to 625 Hz for a duration of 50 msec is shown in Fig. 4.9.

If a continuous stimulus is already changing, even quite slowly, a further change may not elicit a response. Clynes (1969) found that when the amplitude or frequency of a continuous tone changed from one value to another over a steady ramp, the ramp onset elicited an N1–P2 response, but

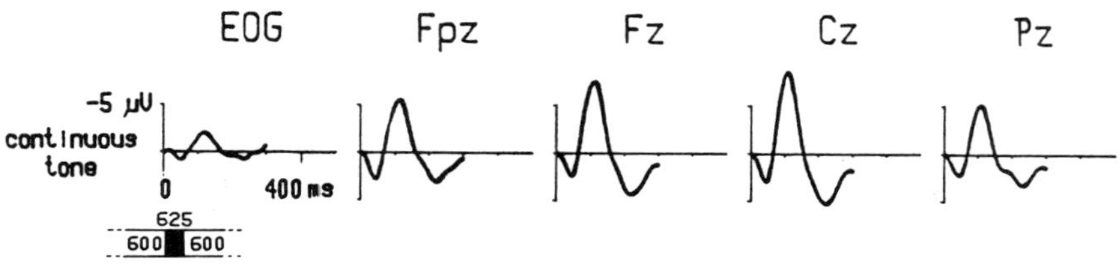

FIG. 4.9 Grand-average (averaged across subjects) ERPs from frontal-pole (Fpz), frontal (Fz), vertex (Cz), and parietal (Pz) electrode positions to a transitory frequency modulation (at 0) from a continuous 600-Hz tone to 625 Hz for a duration of 50 msec. The mean interval between successive frequency modulations was 3.1 sec. (Adapted from Näätänen, Paavilainen, Alho, Reinikainen, & Sams, 1987a. Copyright © 1987 by Butterworths. Reprinted with permission.)

the ramp offset, when the tone became constant again, did not elicit the response (Fig. 4.10, top panel).

Furthermore, the response to a ramp onset could be markedly reduced or eliminated by preceding the ramp by another ramp in the same or different direction (Fig. 4.10, bottom panel). In addition, a ramp change in one attribute attenuated the response to a subsequent change in another attribute. Such interactions occurred between the pitch and intensity of a continuous auditory stimulus. However, these interactions did not cross modality boundaries. An ongoing pitch modulation did not affect the visual response, although there were similar basic rest-motion findings in the visual and also in the somatosensory modality. Clynes (1969) concluded that the N1–P2 response is initiated by a change from sensory "rest" (a

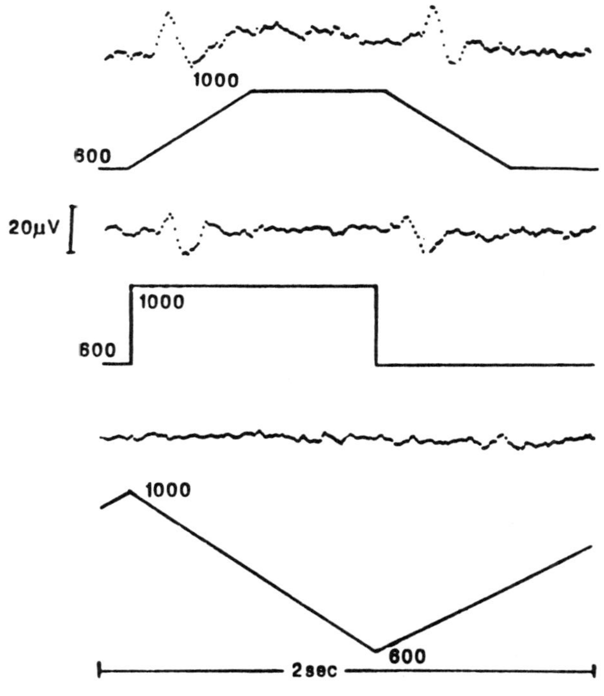

FIG. 4.10 Vertex ERPs to changes in the pitch of a sound with a constant intensity. The pitch of the sound is shown below each of the three paired recordings. The recordings shown at the top are in response to ramp changes in pitch. Note the absence of any response at the end of the ramp. The middle tracings show the responses to abrupt changes in pitch. The bottom recordings show no clear response when the direction of ramp change of pitch is changed. (From Clynes, 1969. Copyright © 1969 by U.S. Government Printing Office. Reprinted with permission.)

steady stimulus or silence) to sensory "motion" (from one level of a stimulus parameter to another).

Because of the similarity of the factors determining this response and the event-related perturbations of the SSR discussed previously, these two phenomena might be expressions of the same or related mechanisms.

Stimulus Intensity

With decreasing stimulus intensity, the N1 response elicited by stimulus onset decreases in amplitude and increases in latency (Beagley & Knight, 1967; Picton, Goodman, & Bryce, 1970; Rapin, Schimmel, Tourk, Krasnegor, & Pollack, 1966). The change in amplitude is more variable than the change in latency.

At high intensities the N1 amplitude often levels off or even reduces (Buchsbaum, 1976). This is particularly true when stimuli are presented at intervals of 2.5 sec or less and the intensity is held constant within blocks (Picton et al., 1970). The saturation of the N1 amplitude occurs well below any saturation of subjective loudness, and thus indicates a clear dissociation between the experienced sensory magnitude and the N1 amplitude. When the ISI is long or if stimuli of different intensity are delivered in the same block, the N1 increases in amplitude with increasing intensity even at high intensities (Gille, Böttcher, & Ullsperger, 1986; see Fig. 4.11).

In some subjects, the N1 amplitude continues to increase with increasing intensity at all levels, whereas in others N1 saturates or becomes smaller at high intensities. This has led to dividing subjects into "augmenters" and "reducers," a classification supposedly reflecting an individual's characteristic response to stimulation (Buchsbaum, 1976). There are, however, several methodological problems in this research. Consequently, a review has concluded that the results of augmenting/reducing research have often been "inconclusive or equivocal" (Prescott, Connolly, & Gruzelier, 1984, p. 32).

Stimulus Rate

The N1 wave is exceptionally sensitive to the stimulus rate. This sensitivity contrasts with the relative resistance to rate shown by earlier auditory ERPs (Picton et al., 1981; see however Makeig, 1990) and later auditory ERPs (Woods, Hillyard, Courchesne, & Galambos, 1980). On the basis of their results, Davis, Mast, Yoshie, and Zerlin (1966) estimated that the N1–P2 amplitude would continue to increase up to ISIs of about 10 sec. Picton and colleagues (1970) and Nelson and Lassman (1973) showed that the N1–P2 amplitude reaches a maximum value at shorter intervals when the stimulus is less intense. These data suggest that for intense stimuli, the recovery period of the N1–P2 amplitude must be very long. More recently,

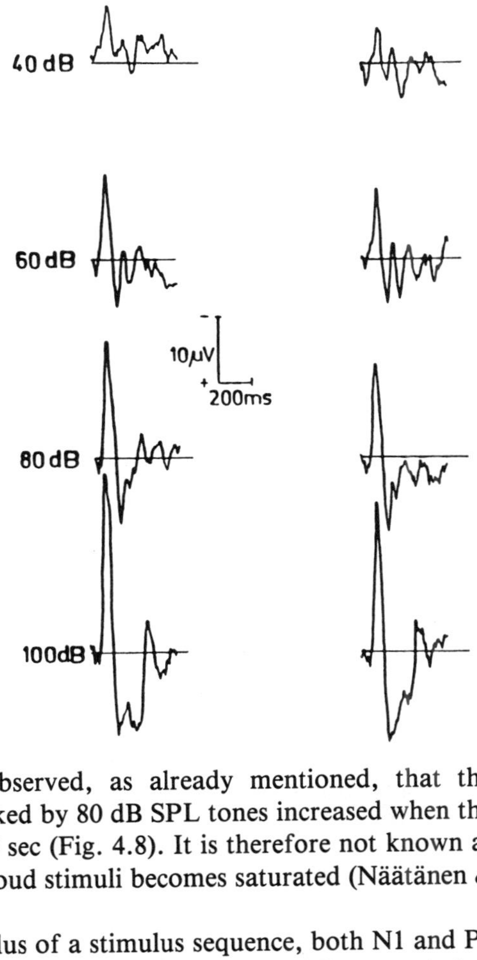

FIG. 4.11 ERPs of a typical subject to 40, 60, 80, and 100 dB stimuli, presented in a pseudo-random order at constant 4-sec ISIs while the subject was reading a book. The left side shows data from the first session, the right from the second session. (Unpublished figure from the study by Gille, Böttcher, & Ullsperger, 1986. Reprinted with permission.)

Hari and colleagues (1982) observed, as already mentioned, that the amplitude of the vertex N1 evoked by 80 dB SPL tones increased when the ISI was prolonged from 8 to 16 sec (Fig. 4.8). It is therefore not known at what interval the vertex N1 to loud stimuli becomes saturated (Näätänen & Picton, 1987).

In response to the first stimulus of a stimulus sequence, both N1 and P2 are much larger than those to subsequent stimuli, provided that a period of silence of several seconds has preceded the first stimulus (Ritter, Vaughan, & Costa, 1968; Roth & Kopell, 1969). Fruhstorfer and colleagues (1970) presented trains of 8 clicks using ISIs of 1 or 3 sec and intertrain intervals of 100 sec. The N1 deflection to the first stimulus of a train was very large in amplitude, about 10 times that elicited by the second stimulus for trains with the 1-sec intervals, and more than 2 times for the trains with the 3-sec intervals (Fig. 4.12). The amplitude decreased further until the third or fourth stimulus and then stabilized.

Fruhstorfer (1971) found that a somatosensory stimulus inserted into a train of clicks evoked an N1 wave that was larger than that evoked by the preceding click, and larger than the N1 wave that would have been evoked if this somatosensory stimulus had been preceded by a train of similar

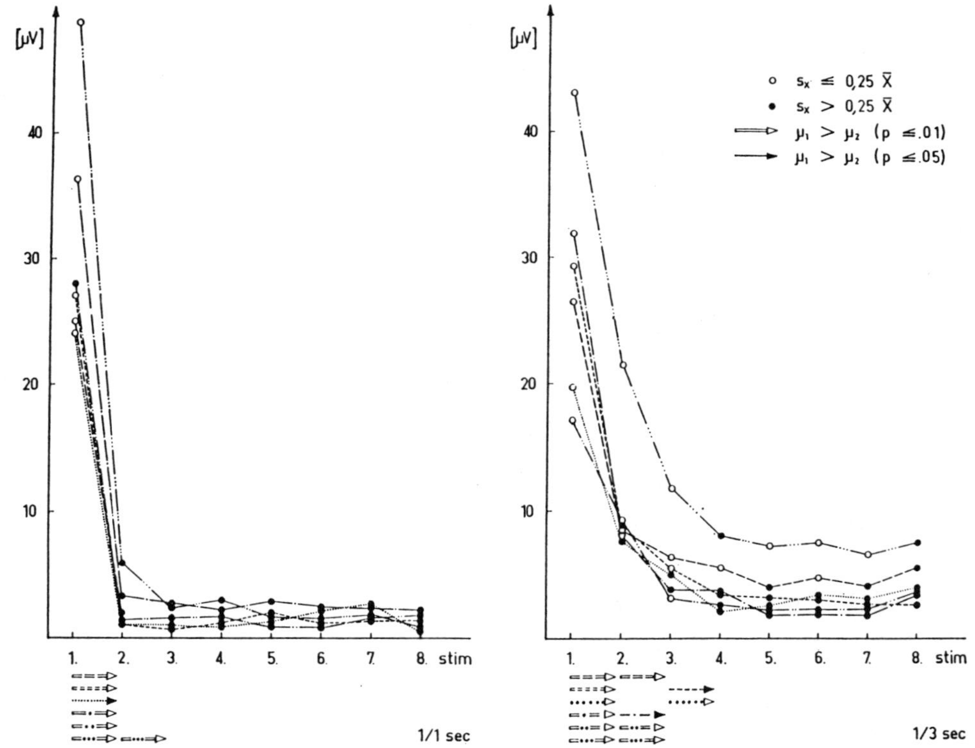

FIG. 4.12 The N1 amplitude as a function of the position of the stimulus in a block separately for each subject. The subject was in an inattentive state when the first stimulus was presented. (Open circles indicate that the value of the standard deviation is equal to or smaller than a quarter of the mean.) Arrows below the diagrams indicate the cases in which the amplitude reduction reaches a significant level (one-tailed rank-sum test). (From Fruhstorfer, Soveri, & Järvilehto, 1970. Copyright © 1970 by Elsevier Science Publishers, Ireland. Reprinted with permission.)

stimuli (Fig. 4.13). The next click after the somatosensory stimulus elicited N1 that was similar in size to the N1 elicited by the click preceding the somatosensory stimulus. Thus the N1 amplitude showed no dishabituation. Analogous results were obtained when an auditory stimulus was inserted into a train of somatosensory stimuli (Fig. 4.13, right).

The P2 response to the modality-deviant stimulus was also enhanced relative to the P2 to the preceding standard (Fig. 4.13). When the deviant stimulus was a somatosensory stimulus in a sequence of clicks, the amplitude of P2 elicited by the somatosensory stimulus even exceeded that for the first stimulus in the somatosensory train. This might, however, be due to some P3 overlap. Like the N1 amplitude, the P2 amplitude showed

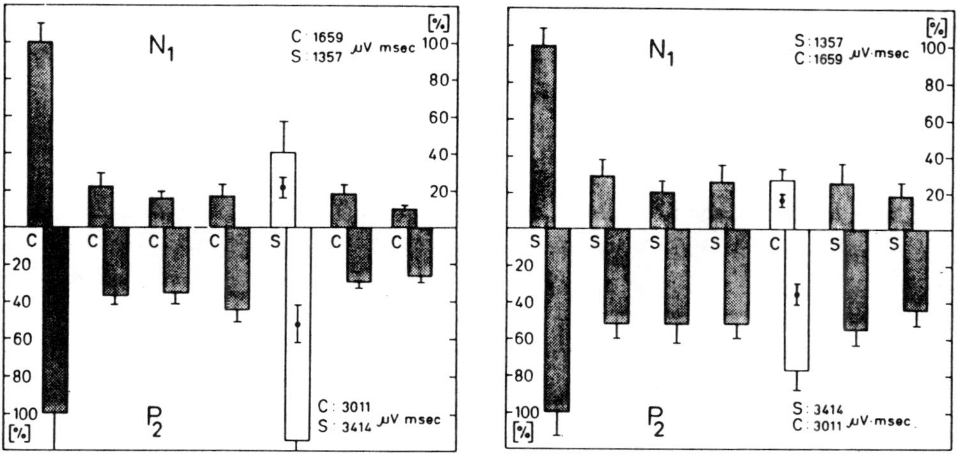

FIG. 4.13 LEFT: Mean changes in the voltage integral of N1 and P2 (in % of the size of the first-stimulus response) during a CCCCSCC train. (C denotes a click stimulus, S a somatosensory stimulus.). The bars indicate the standard error to one side. RIGHT: Mean changes in the voltage integral of N1 and P2 during an SSSSCSS train. (From Fruhstorfer, 1971. Copyright © 1971 by Elsevier Science Publishers, Ireland. Reprinted with permission.)

no amplitude recovery (dishabituation) in response to the standard following the modality-deviant stimulus.

Habituation Versus Refractoriness. The N1-amplitude attenuation with stimulus repetition should be interpreted in terms of refractoriness, as originally proposed by Ritter et al. (1968), rather than of habituation, for no dishabituation was demonstrated (Näätänen & Picton, 1987). Habituation is the progressive decrease in a response with repetition of the stimulus; it differs specifically from other causes of reduced responsiveness by being susceptible to "dishabituation" (Thompson & Spencer, 1966; Thompson, Groves, Teyler, & Roemer, 1973). Dishabituation is the recovery or partial recovery that occurs in a response with no change in the stimulus eliciting the response or in the ISI. Dishabituation can be caused experimentally by inserting a dishabituating stimulus into the train of habituating stimuli, but this has not resulted in N1-amplitude recovery (Fruhstorfer, 1971; Roth, 1973; Woods & Elmasian, 1986). Thus, the recovery of the response with a change in some characteristic (for example, pitch) of the stimulus eliciting the response does not qualify as a demonstration of habituation (Graham, 1973; Loveless, 1983; Öhman & Lader, 1977).

The physiological mechanisms underlying these short-term decrements are not known. "It is unlikely that they are caused by actual refractory periods in simple cellular mechanisms. Synapses do not usually get tired that quickly or recover that slowly. Complex neuronal circuits are probably responsible for these effects" (Näätänen & Picton, 1987, p. 400).

Figure 4.14 schematically illustrates the N1 deflection as a function of the position of the stimulus in a stimulus block (top row). This figure suggests that the exceptionally large response to the first stimulus is mainly due to a very large nonspecific N1 component which is not elicited by the subsequent stimuli. This is supported by the vertex-maximum scalp topography of N1 to the first stimulus (cf. Hari et al., 1982) and by the greatly reduced

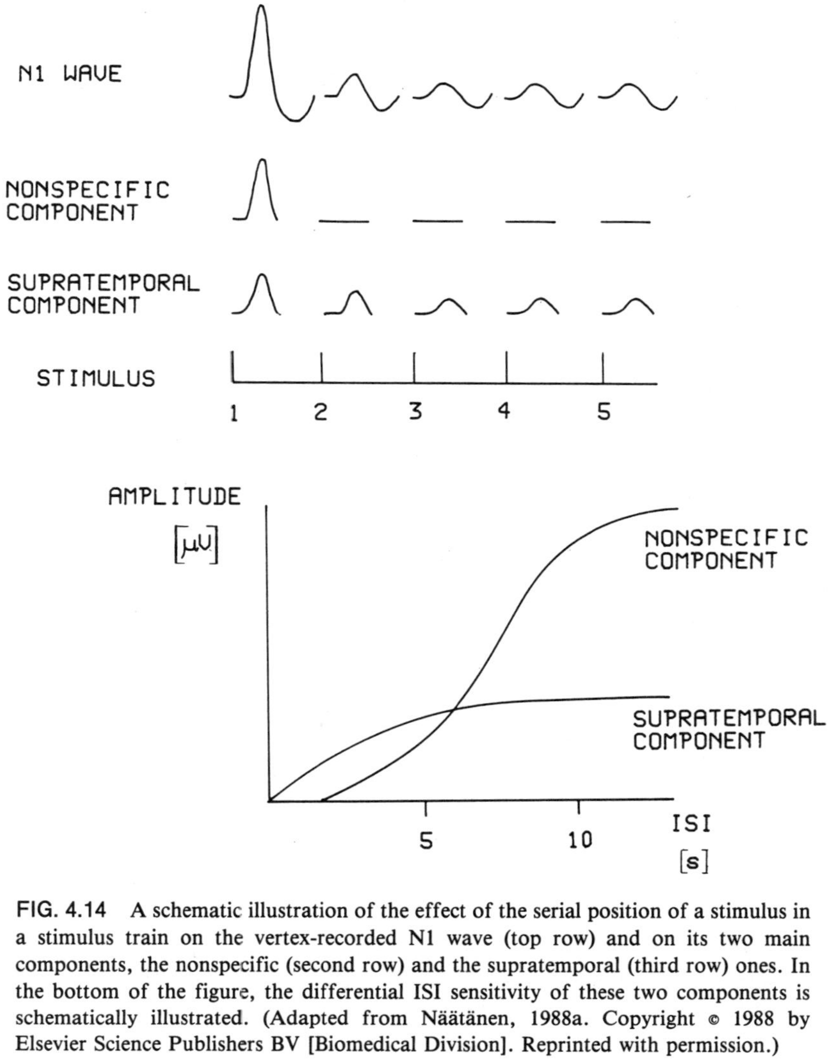

FIG. 4.14 A schematic illustration of the effect of the serial position of a stimulus in a stimulus train on the vertex-recorded N1 wave (top row) and on its two main components, the nonspecific (second row) and the supratemporal (third row) ones. In the bottom of the figure, the differential ISI sensitivity of these two components is schematically illustrated. (Adapted from Näätänen, 1988a. Copyright © 1988 by Elsevier Science Publishers BV [Biomedical Division]. Reprinted with permission.)

amplitude of this N1 when the first stimulus is preceded by a visual stimulus (MacLean, Öhman, & Lader, 1975; Öhman & Lader, 1972). The supratemporal component, too, is larger to the first than to the subsequent stimuli, but this effect is much less dramatic than that on the nonspecific component. (The T-complex is not illustrated because it contributes to the midline-recorded N1 quite little; the attenuation of the T-complex with stimulus repetition probably resembles that of the supratemporal component; see Woods & Elmasian, 1986).

Most of the amplitude reduction caused by stimulus repetition might indeed be accounted for in terms of the refractoriness of the generator. This refractoriness is, at least to some extent, stimulus-specific, because a different stimulus replacing one of the repeating stimuli often enhances N1 (e.g., Woods & Elmasian, 1986) and, apparently, this enhancement is proportional to the magnitude of stimulus change (see Butler, 1968; Näätänen et al., 1988; Picton, Woods, & Proulx, 1978b; see also Bertrand, Perrin, Echallier, & Pernier, 1988). This effect in three different studies is shown in Fig. 4.15.

Such effects could be interpreted in terms of the magnitude of overlap between the neuronal populations activated by the two stimuli (Butler, 1968). It is likely that the stimulus-specific refractoriness develops in the supratemporal N1 generator, whereas the refractoriness of the nonspecific N1 generator is not stimulus-specific. This feature of the nonspecific N1 generator, as well as a very wide receptive field of a large proportion of the supratemporal N1 neurons, might together explain why N1 even to a widely deviant stimulus in a block is much smaller than N1 to the first stimulus of the block (e.g., Fruhstorfer, 1971; see Fig. 4.13).

Time Uncertainty. Wastell (1980) and Wastell, Kleinman, and MacLean (1982) interpreted their attenuated N1–P2 waves at short ISIs (for a review, see Näätänen & Picton, 1987) in terms of reduced time uncertainty (Klemmer, 1956) rather than refractoriness. The idea is that it is much more difficult to predict the moment of stimulus occurrence with long than short ISIs. Näätänen, Muranen, and Merisalo (1974) evaluated the ability of subjects to predict time intervals of different lengths by requesting them to press a button after an estimated duration of 0.25, 0.5, 1, 2, or 4 sec (in separate blocks). With short durations, the timing of the button presses was quite accurate, but for the 4-sec duration, highly variable (Fig. 4.16). With long ISIs the subject probably seldom experiences "peaks of expectancy" that coincide with the stimulus presentation. Time uncertainty is large when the first stimulus of a train occurs after a long intertrain interval and, according to Wastell, this could explain the very large N1 to the first stimulus of a sequence—the "first-stimulus effect." (See also Loveless, 1983.)

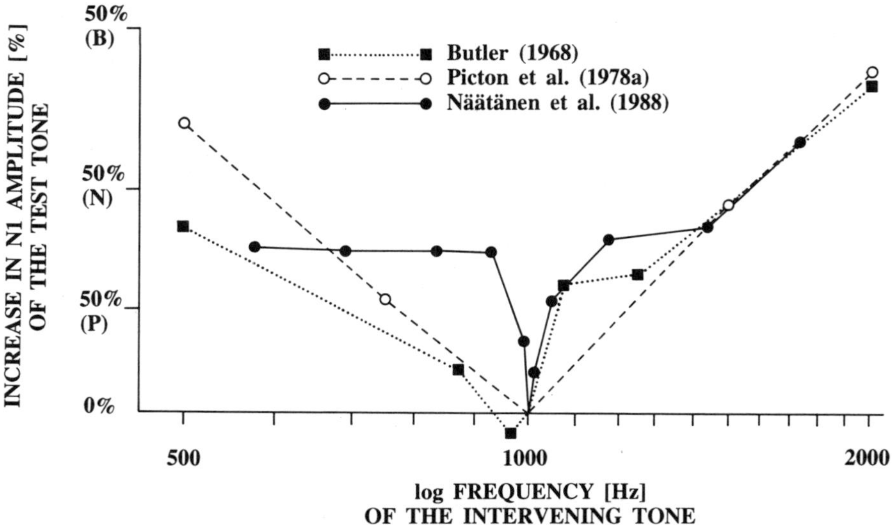

FIG. 4.15 A comparison of the relative frequency specificity of N1 obtained by Butler (1968), Picton, et al. (1978a), and Näätänen et al. (1988). The figure shows the relative increase in amplitude of the response to the test tone of 1000 Hz as a function of the frequency of the intervening tone which was different in different blocks. The increase was calculated in relation to the test-tone N1 amplitude in a condition in which also the intervening stimuli were 1000 Hz. Three different types of measurement were performed in these studies (N1-P2 by Butler, baseline-N1 by Picton et al., P1-N1 by Näätänen et al.). In order to facilitate comparison, three different scales are used [as shown on the vertical axis by B (Butler), N (Näätänen et al., 1988), and P (Picton et al., 1978a)]. (Adapted from Näätänen et al., 1988. Copyright © 1988 by Elsevier Science Publishers, Ireland. Reprinted with permission.)

If the effects of the ISI on the auditory N1 wave are due to the concomitant changes in the subject's uncertainty about the timing of a stimulus, then the response should be larger to irregularly than regularly presented stimuli. Unfortunately, the data reported in the literature are equivocal on this point (Nelson, Lassman, & Hoel, 1969; Nelson & Lassman, 1977; Rothman, Davis, & Hay, 1970; Öhman, Kaye, & Lader, 1972).

Näätänen and Picton (1987) concluded that neural-refractoriness and time-uncertainty factors jointly account for the stimulus-repetition effects on N1. The authors stressed that neural refractoriness should be understood as a temporary decrement in neural responsiveness caused by previous activation of the response mechanism which dissipates only with time, there being no way to expedite the time course of recovery of excitability. Further, the effects of refractoriness on response are maximal when an identical stimulus is repeated but the effects extend to the responses elicited by different stimuli in proportion to the similarity of these stimuli to the

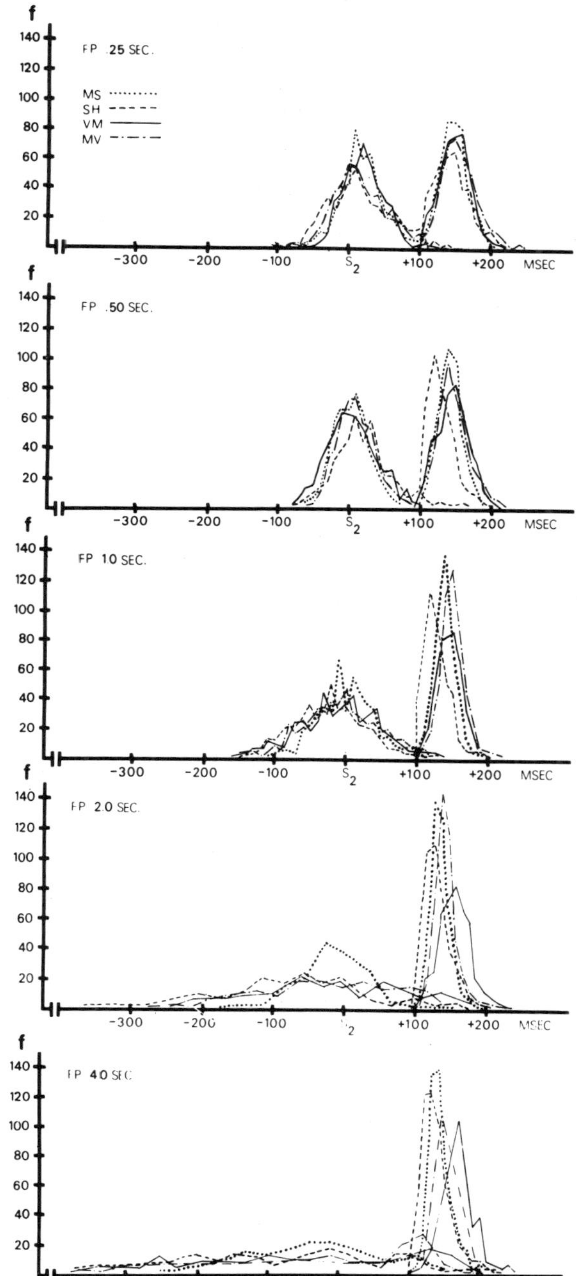

FIG. 4.16 *Left side:* Distributions of anticipation moments (button presses) as a function of the time to be estimated (FP) separately for each subject. S2 indicates the moment of the correct response. Responses to the left of this moment are too early, those to the right are too late responses. *Right side:* RTs at S1–S2 intervals equalling to the durations to be estimated as indicated in the figure. (From Näätänen, Muranen, & Merisalo, 1974. Copyright © 1974 by the North-Holland Publishing Company. Reprinted with permission.)

initial stimulus. Näätänen and Picton (1987) further suggested that neural refractoriness is the major factor in repetition-caused attenuation of the supratemporal and T-complex components of the N1 wave, whereas the amplitude of the nonspecific component is jointly determined by neural refractoriness and temporal uncertainty. According to these authors, reduced temporal uncertainty attenuates the general cerebral excitability (see also Näätänen, 1975).

The suggestion that time uncertainty affects especially the nonspecific N1 component is supported by the results of Schafer and Marcus (1973). These authors reported that the ERP to an auditory or visual stimulus that was triggered by the subject pressing a button was smaller than the ERP evoked by a stimulus presented by a machine. They attributed this effect to temporal uncertainty because "the subjects possessed complete foreknowledge of stimulus timing when they stimulated themselves" and "no foreknowledge when the machine delivered the stimuli randomly in time" (p. 176).

This N1 reduction with decreasing time uncertainty probably stems from the dampening of the nonspecific component. This can be judged from their further results showing that N1 to temporally unpredictable stimuli, but not to predictable stimuli, was attenuated by ethanol and other state factors which are known to attenuate the nonspecific component to a much greater extent than they attenuate the supratemporal component. Moreover, the visual ERP showed the time-uncertainty effect when recorded over the vertex but not when recorded over the occiput. This too suggests that the nonspecific component of N1 was involved in this effect, because the relative contribution of this component is strong in vertex recordings but much smaller in occipital recordings (Lehtonen, 1973).

Reduced time uncertainty also decreases other physiological responses (Lykken & Tellegen, 1974). The SCR (Grings, 1973) and the cardiac acceleration (Lykken, Macindoe, & Tellegen, 1972) elicited by an electric shock are smaller with more predictable timing. Further, Epstein (1973) found a smaller SCR to a "punishing sound" when the timing of the sound was predictable than when it was not predictable. Although subjects rated the loudness of the sound as the same in both conditions, they rated their reactivity as having been higher under time uncertainty.

State Factors

Alertness and Arousal. Several studies have clarified the dependence of the N1 amplitude on various general state factors. N1 evoked by unattended auditory stimuli is larger at higher levels of alertness, as estimated on the basis of the prestimulus EEG (Fruhstorfer & Bergström, 1969). Because the mean ISI used was 12 sec (and the response was recorded between the vertex and the forehead, cancelling most of the supratemporal component), the nonspecific N1 component was probably mainly responsible for this relationship.

Arousal may not always enhance N1, however. Schafer (1978) found no difference in the N1 amplitude to a probe stimulus, a momentary slight increase in the brightness of a TV picture, when subjects watched a dull TV program (Dick and Jane Talk) and when they watched a program they regarded as considerably more interesting (Dick and Jane Make Love).

Sleep. The late ERP components are dramatically affected by sleep (Fruhstorfer & Bergström, 1969; Osterhammel, Davis, Wier, & Hirsh, 1973; Picton et al., 1974; Weitzman & Kremen, 1965; Williams, Tepas, & Morlock, 1962). One of the most striking effects is the emergence of a large negative wave with a peak latency of around 300 msec. This wave is often visible in the unaveraged EEG as the "vertex sharp wave" or "sleep N2" (Fig. 4.17). The nature of this N2 wave is not known.

The waveform at the N1 latency shows complex changes during sleep. Most reports have indicated a decrease in N1 amplitude with sleep (Anch, 1977; Kevanishvili & Specht, 1979; Paavilainen et al., 1987). In Bell and

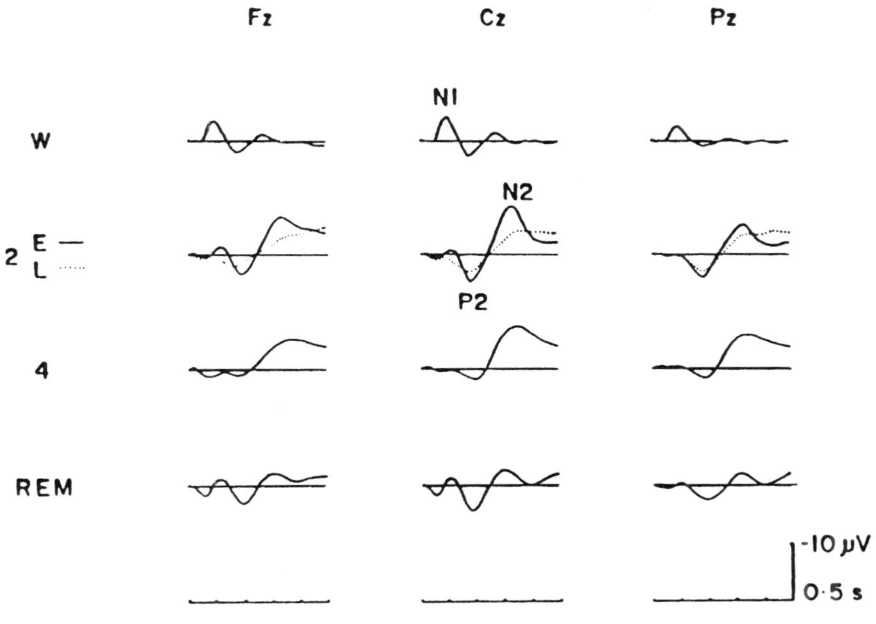

FIG. 4.17 Grand-average frontal (Fz), vertex (Cz), and parietal (Pz) ERPs from 10 young adults recorded before and during overnight sleep to 80-dB SPL, 1,000-Hz tonebursts presented once every 1.1 sec. Recordings were made during wakefulness (W), and during stages 2, 4, and REM sleep. The recordings during Stage 2 are separated into those recorded early (E) and those recorded late (L) in the night. (Unpublished data of Ian Bell and Kenneth Campbell. Reprinted with permission.)

Campbell (Fig. 4.17) and Paavilainen and colleagues' (1987) data, sleep appears to add a positive component that lasts through the latencies of the waking N1 and P2 waves, or to remove a negative component of similar duration.

Drugs. Sedative drugs that bring on sleep cause changes in the auditory ERP that are characteristic for sleep. When the subject is under the influence of a sedative medication but remains awake, N1 is often attenuated. This reduction in amplitude might vary with a drug-related decrease in alertness (Born, Brüninger et al., 1987).

The effect of ethanol has been extensively evaluated since Gross, Begleiter, Tobin, and Kissin (1966) found that ethanol reduces the amplitudes of the auditory N1 and P2 deflections. Ethanol has a much greater effect on N1 evoked by the first stimulus in a brief train than on the later responses (Fruhstorfer & Soveri, 1968; see also Järvilehto, Laakso, & Virsu, 1975). This result supports the suggestion that the N1 wave to the first stimulus of the block is to a great extent composed of the nonspecific component that is not elicited, or is elicited at a much lower amplitude, by subsequent stimuli. Furthermore, Wolpaw and Penry (1978) reported that ethanol attenuated the vertex N1–P2 waves but did not affect the Ta–Tb complex recorded from temporal electrodes (although there were some latency changes). These studies thus indicate that the nonspecific N1 component is the most sensitive of the three N1 components to ethanol.

Task Performance

Several studies, but not all, suggest that the N1 amplitude correlates with task performance, and that it is larger when the level of performance is higher. Näätänen and Picton (1987) concluded that there is some evidence for task- or attention-induced *stimulus-nonspecific* increase in the excitability of some neuronal population contributing to the N1 wave. This increase causes the N1 amplitude to any input, relevant or irrelevant, to be larger when the subject is engaged in a task rather than relaxing, and larger when performing a more rather than less involving task (Näätänen, 1967, 1970, 1975). Similarly, if the subject can predict the order of delivery of relevant and irrelevant stimuli above the chance level, then relevant stimuli tend to be preceded and coincided by an excitability increase enhancing the N1 amplitude selectively to the relevant stimuli (Näätänen 1967, 1970). Possibly this nonspecific excitability increase is not exclusively due to increased arousal but also to a general increase in sensory sensitivity which might also vary independently of arousal:

> It is therefore possible that the brain possesses a general gain control over its own sensory input. This is proposed, for instance, in the orienting-response

theory . . . and there is strong evidence for that proposal (for a review, see Lynn, 1966). When an unpleasant stimulus is anticipated, the sensory sensitivity is decreased ("negative preception"; Lykken & Tellegen, 1974) whereas, when a pleasant, important or interesting stimulus is expected, sensitivity is increased ("positive preception"). A similar basic assumption underlies the "directional-fractionation" hypothesis (Lacey, 1967) which proposes that the heart rate changes differentially depending on whether the subject prepares for stimulus intake (heart rate deceleration) or for stimulus rejection (acceleration). (Näätänen & Picton, 1987, pp. 407–408)

Late Transient Responses and Perception

Studies trying to relate N1 to perceptual experience have revealed no clear perceptual correlate of this wave. N1 can be dissociated from loudness in many ways: At short ISIs, N1 is considerably reduced (Figs. 4.12, 4.13, and 4.14) although loudness remains the same; loudness summation occurs over a much longer stimulus duration than that affecting the N1 amplitude; N1 may saturate at high intensities but loudness does not (Näätänen & Picton, 1987). Similar evidence exists also for P2 (Picton et al., 1978a; for similar evidence for the somatosensory P2, see Donald, 1976).

The relationship of N1 to auditory pitch perception is no closer. Parasuraman, Richer, and Beatty (1982) reported that the N1 amplitude correlated with the detection of a threshold-level tonal stimulus but not with the recognition of its pitch. Butler (1972) found that a 1000-Hz tone amplitude-modulated at 200 Hz, with a perceived pitch similar to that of a 200-Hz pure tone, affected N1 evoked by a subsequent 1000-Hz tone much more than it affected N1 to a subsequent 200-Hz tone. This suggests that the N1-generator activation does not underlie pitch perception.

Sustained Potential

Sustained potentials elicited by long-duration acoustic stimuli were first recognized by Köhler and his associates (Köhler, Held & O'Connell, 1952, Köhler & Wegener, 1955). In contrast to the transient response occurring to stimulus onset, the sustained potential found in direct-coupled (DC) recordings of the human EEG lasted throughout the duration of the stimulus (Fig. 4.18). The sustained potential followed the transient N1–P2 response and reached its maximum amplitude in the fronto-central scalp regions, which was explained by the authors with the orientation of human primary auditory cortex on the supratemporal plane. A similar sustained potential was also recorded from the corresponding modality-specific cortices of the cat as a response to an auditory or a visual stimulus (Köhler, Neff, & Wegener, 1955; Köhler & O'Connell, 1957).

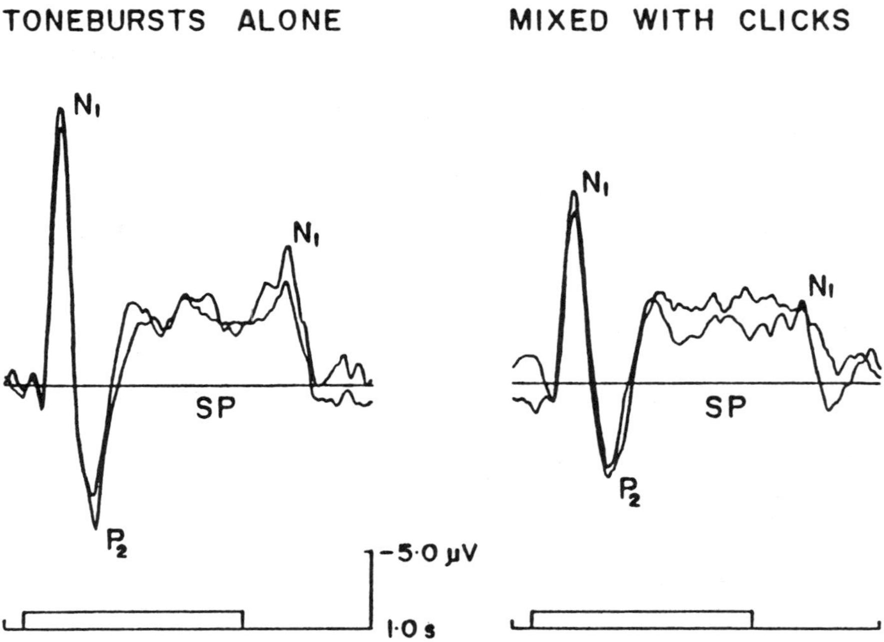

FIG. 4.18 Vertex ERPs of one subject to tonebursts of 600 msec duration with an intensity of 70 dB HL and a frequency of 1,000 Hz presented every 4 sec to the left ear. *Left:* tonebursts alone; *right:* mixed with 0.1 msec click stimuli of 75 dB HL presented with a random ISI of 200–500 msec. (From Picton, Woods, and Proulx, 1978b. Copyright © 1978 by Elsevier Science Publishers, Ireland. Reprinted with permission.)

Keidel and his colleagues (David, Finkenzeller, Kallert, & Keidel, 1969; Keidel, 1971, 1976) have described the relationship of the human auditory sustained potential to various acoustic stimulus parameters. David and colleagues (1969), varying the stimulus duration between 0.6 and 3.5 sec, found that the negative shift lasted for the whole duration of the auditory stimulus and, further, that the amplitude of this slow negative shift increased with stimulus intensity. The authors proposed that this potential was generated by neural processing of the stimulus in the specific auditory projection area (see also Lickey & Fox, 1966). Keidel (1971) even suggested that the sustained potential represents "an objective correlate of the stimulus." Keidel and his colleagues therefore regarded the sustained potential as distinct from the contingent negative variation (CNV), which is rather nonspecific, independent of the physical stimulus features, and tends to grow in amplitude toward the end of the S1–S2 interval (Fig. 6.6).

Picton and colleagues (1978a, 1978b) provided convincing evidence for a distinction of the sustained potential from the transient N1 and P2 responses. Figure 4.18 shows the ERP to a 600-msec toneburst when tonebursts were presented (a) alone every 4 sec, (b) every 4 sec with multiple intervening click stimuli. The introduction of the clicks considerably attenuated the transient N1 and P2 responses but did not affect the sustained potential. This result clearly indicates that the generator mechanisms of these transient responses and the sustained potential are at least in part separate. This is also supported by the difference found in the midline scalp distribution between N1 (both to tone onsets and offsets) and the more frontal sustained potential.

Furthermore, Picton and colleagues (1978b) found that stimulus repetition attenuated N1 and P2 much more than it attenuated the sustained potential. In addition, the amplitude of the sustained potential was more closely related to stimulus intensity than were the N1 and P2 amplitudes and, in contrast to the N1 amplitude, was larger to binaural than monaural stimulation and showed no hemispheric asymmetry as a function of the ear stimulated. Moreover, the frequency dependence was somewhat different for the sustained potential and N1.

Separability of the sustained potential from the CNV types of slow endogenous negativities was demonstrated by Picton and colleagues (1978b), who found that the sustained potential is generated even in sleep. Furthermore, this potential recorded during sleep was of at least the same amplitude as during wakefulness. Attention directed to stimulus duration increased the amplitude of the long-duration negativity, but this effect might be due to a superimposition of a CNV type of wave rather than to a stronger activation of the generator mechanism of the sustained potential. This possibility is supported by Järvilehto, Hari, and Sams' (1978) data suggesting that the sustained potential elicited by a long-duration stimulus may in some conditions be overlapped by a CNV. See also Keidel (1976).

The onset latency of the sustained potential is only some 150 msec (Picton et al., 1978b) or even shorter (Scherg, Vajsar, & Picton, 1989), another feature dissociating it from the CNV (see Tecce, 1972).

Even brief stimuli may elicit the sustained potential. Scherg et al. (1989), by using Scherg's (1990) dipole-modeling techniques, have in fact demonstrated this component in response to brief stimuli, although one with a comparably short duration. This negative component might summate with, and thereby attenuate, the P2 wave.

As already mentioned, the sustained potential is much more closely related to stimulus intensity, and thus to loudness, than the N1 and P2 waves (Picton et al., 1978a). The sustained potential can nevertheless be dissociated from perception. For instance, the sustained potential attenuates toward the end of longer-duration tones, although loudness is not affected (Picton et al., 1978a). Furthermore, stimulus repetition attenuates the sustained potential, although much less than N1 and P2 amplitudes, whereas loudness is not affected (Picton et al., 1978a).

4.4. THE MISMATCH NEGATIVITY (MMN)

MMN: A Change-Detector Response

In contrast to the previously reviewed exogeneous components, an ERP component called the *mismatch negativity* (MMN) appears to provide a physiological measure, although an indirect one, of the actual sensory information processed by the brain. This component was isolated from the auditory N2 wave by Näätänen and his colleagues (Näätänen, 1979; Näätänen & Gaillard, 1983; Näätänen, Gaillard, & Mäntysalo 1978, 1980; Näätänen & Michie, 1979a, 1979b; Näätänen, Sams, & Alho, 1986; Näätänen, Sams, Järvilehto, & Soininen, 1983; Näätänen, Simpson & Loveless, 1982; Sams, Paavilainen, Alho, & Näätänen, 1985). These authors divided the auditory "N2" reported in previous studies (Ford, Roth, Dirks, & Kopell, 1973; Ford, Roth, & Kopell, 1976a, 1976b; Ritter, Simson, & Vaughan, 1972; Ritter, Simson, Vaughan, & Friedman, 1979; Simson, Vaughan, & Ritter, 1976, 1977a, 1977b; K. Squires, Donchin, Herning, & McCarthy, 1977; N. Squires, Squires, & Hillyard, 1975) in response to deviant, usually target, stimuli into two components: an earlier-latency MMN and a later N2b. An N2 kind of wave was first described by Klinke, Fruhstorfer, and Finkenzeller (1968). This was elicited by an infrequent, too early stimulus in a sequence of somatosensory stimuli presented with constant ISIs.

MMN is illustrated in Fig. 4.19. In that study, Sams, Paavilainen, Alho, & Näätänen (1985) presented their subjects with blocks of auditory stimuli consisting of standard stimuli of 1000 Hz (80%) and deviant stimuli (20%) of a slightly higher frequency. This frequency was, in different blocks, either 1004, 1008, 1016, or 1032 Hz. The order of the standard and deviant stimuli was randomized, and the ISI was constant at 1 sec. Subjects were reading a book during the recordings.

The N1 wave in response to the various deviant stimuli is similar to the one evoked by the standard stimulus because the two stimuli were quite similar. As shown by the difference waveforms in the bottom of Fig. 4.19 obtained by subtracting the ERP to the standard stimulus from that to the corresponding deviant stimulus, a clear MMN is elicited by deviant stimuli with frequencies higher than 1008 Hz. MMN appears as a negativity that commences at about 100 msec from stimulus onset and lasts until about 250 msec post-stimulus. Even the 1008-Hz stimuli, which in a separate discrimination task were found to be at about the discrimination threshold, elicited MMN, although a very small one. In a control experiment, MMN was elicited even when the subject, instead of reading, performed a difficult visual discrimination task.

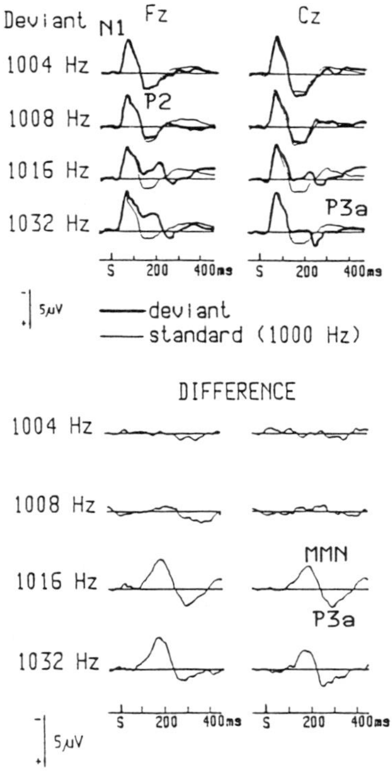

FIG. 4.19 *Top:* Grand-average ERPs to standard stimuli of 1,000 Hz (thin line) and deviant stimuli (thick line) of 1,004, 1,008, 1,016, and 1,032 Hz. In each block, 80% of stimuli were standard stimuli and 20% were deviant stimuli in a random order (one type in a block). *Bottom:* The corresponding difference waveforms obtained by subtracting the standard-stimulus ERP from the deviant-stimulus ERP. (From Sams, Paavilainen, Alho, & Näätänen, 1985. Copyright © 1985 by Elsevier Science Publishers, Ireland. Reprinted with permission.)

When the magnitude of deviation is further increased, the decreased MMN latency results in increasing temporal overlap between the MMN and N1 components (Duncan & Kaye, 1987; Näätänen & Gaillard, 1983; Näätänen et al., 1982; Novak, Ritter, Vaughan, & Wiznitzer, 1990; Scherg, Vajsar, & Picton, 1989; Winkler, Paavilainen, & Näätänen, in press), and the amplitude of the deviance-related difference wave may increase (Scherg et al., 1989; Winkler et al., in press). Näätänen and Gaillard (1983) concluded that the MMN latency is a more reliable correlate of the magnitude of frequency difference than the MMN amplitude, which may saturate at a moderate magnitude of stimulus deviation (Fig. 4.19; see also Novak et al., 1990; Sams, Paavilainen, et al., 1985).

Some data (see Näätänen & Gaillard, 1983) from Loveless' laboratory in Dundee, Scotland, hint at the possible existence of a subliminal MMN. In this study, the standard stimulus was of 1000 Hz and the deviant stimulus around 1010 Hz, individually determined for each subject according to his or her discrimination accuracy. When the subject was certain that a deviant stimulus was presented, the response was to be given with one hand and when he or she was not certain, the other hand was to be used.

It was found that even undetected deviant stimuli elicited MMN and, further, that this MMN was of about the same magnitude as that for (correct) detections (Fig. 4.20) and "not-sure" responses. In contrast, the late positivity was only elicited by detected deviants (see Pz in Fig. 4.20) and "not-sures". This suggests that MMN is generated by an automatic cerebral process that is a necessary, but not sufficient condition, for the conscious perception of a stimulus change (Näätänen et al., 1978).

In the aforementioned studies, the ISI was of the order of 1 sec. Had a shorter ISI been used, MMN of a larger amplitude, longer duration, and lower threshold of elicitation would probably have been obtained.

It has been established that MMN is elicited only when a change in a stimulus sequence occurs. Thus MMN is not elicited when a stimulus sequence begins or, similarly, when stimuli are presented with very long ISIs (Sams, Hämäläinen, et al. 1985; Lounasmaa, Hari, Joutsiniemi, & Hämäläinen, 1989; Näätänen, Paavilainen, Alho, Reinikainen, & Sams, 1989; see also Snyder & Hillyard, 1976). Consequently, no stimulus per se is an adequate stimulus for the MMN-generator mechanism, as the system responds to a *difference* between the consecutive stimuli. This response pattern is orthogonal to that shown by N1. The N1 wave is largest in response to the first stimulus of a series; it attenuates strongly thereafter

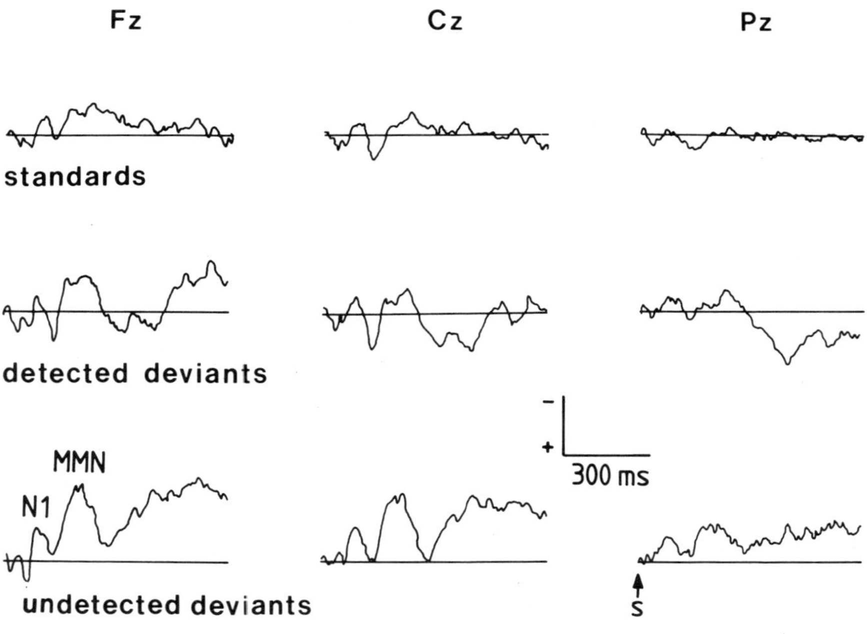

FIG. 4.20 Frontal (Fz), vertex (Cz), and parietal (Pz) ERPs of one subject to standard stimuli of 1,000 Hz as well as to detected and undetected deviant stimuli of 1,010 Hz. (Unpublished data of Loveless, Simpson, & Näätänen, 1979.)

and shows only a partial recovery to a subsequent different stimulus (Section 4.3.).

Thus, MMN is a response to a difference between sequentially presented stimuli. In principle, this type of response, for example to frequency change, can be explained in two ways:

1. *New afferent elements:* MMN is generated by new afferent elements, those corresponding to the frequency of the deviant rather than standard stimulus (see Thompson, Berry, Rinaldi, & Berger, 1979). In the course of the block, these neurons will remain responsive, because of long ISIs between consecutive deviant stimuli. In contrast, neurons responsive to the standard-stimulus frequency, as well as those responsive to both frequencies, will become strongly refractory because of the fast rate of the effective stimuli.
2. *Memory trace:* Rather than by mere activation of "fresh" afferent elements, MMN is generated by a process that registers, that is, is a neural code of, the stimulus difference or change. This would implicate the existence of a memory representation of the standard stimulus (Näätänen, Paavilainen, Alho, et al., 1989; Näätänen, Paavilainen, & Reinikainen, 1989). Studies reviewed below strongly support this interpretation.

Type of Stimulus Change Eliciting MMN

MMN in audition has thus far been found for changes in frequency (see Fig. 4.19), intensity (Näätänen et al., 1978; Näätänen et al., 1987b, 1989; Paavilainen, Alho, Reinikainen, Sams, & Näätänen, 1991; Woldorff, Hackley, & Hillyard, 1991), spatial locus of origin (Paavilainen, Karlsson, Reinikainen, & Näätänen, 1989), rise time (Lyytinen, Blomberg, & Näätänen, in press), duration (Näätänen, Paavilainen, & Reinikainen, 1989; Paavilainen et al., 1991), and phonetic structure (Aaltonen, Niemi, Nyrke, & Tuhkanen, 1987; Aaltonen, Tuomainen, Laine, & Niemi, in press; Sams, Aulanko, Aaltonen, & Näätänen, 1990) of an auditory stimulus. MMN can even be elicited with occasional decrements of a short, constant ISI in the stimulus block (Ford & Hillyard, 1981; Nordby, Roth, & Pfefferbaum, 1988a) or with a partial omission of a compound stimulus (Nordby, Hammerborg, Roth, & Hugdahl, 1991; Winkler & Näätänen, in press).

MMN to Intensity Change. MMN to an intensity reduction in reading subjects is illustrated in Fig. 4.21. The standard stimulus was of 80 dB SPL and, in different blocks, the deviant stimulus was either of 77, 70, 57

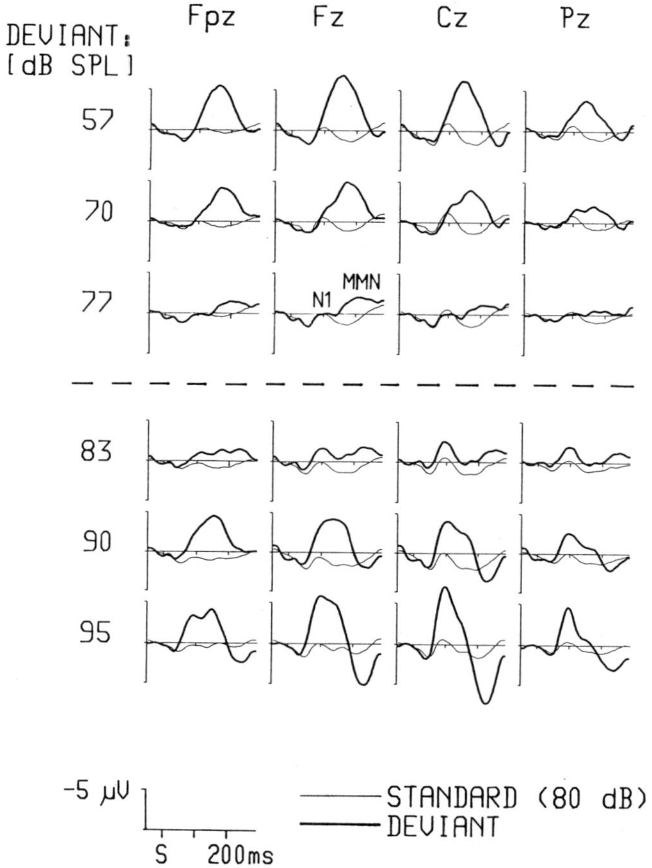

FIG. 4.21 Grand-average frontal-pole (Fpz), frontal (Fz), vertex (Cz), and parietal (Pz) ERPs to standard stimuli of 80 dB (thin lines) and to deviant stimuli of different intensity (thick lines) as indicated on the left side of the figure. (From Näätänen, Paavilainen, Lavikainen, Alho, Reinikainen, Teder, Sams, Strelets, & Rosenfeld, in preparation.)

(intensity decrements), 83, 90, or 95 dB (intensity increments). MMNs are large in amplitude due to the short ISI of 460 msec.

Let us first examine the vertex (Cz) responses to the 77-dB deviants (Fig. 4.21). N1 is attenuated in response to these slight intensity decrements in comparison with the response to the standard stimulus. This results from the intensity dependence of N1 (Section 4.3). N1 to deviants is followed by MMN, not seen in response to standards. When the deviant-stimulus intensity is further reduced, the MMN component becomes larger and earlier, making it impossible to measure N1 and MMN separately. The extreme end of intensity reduction, of course, is stimulus omission, but the results of omission, in the previous studies, have not been clear, as some subjects disclosed a small MMN type of wave, whereas the others did not (Näätänen et al., 1987b; see also Ford et al., 1976a).

Paradoxically, it appears that the weaker the stimulus intensity (down to a certain limit), the larger is the response elicited. This suggests that the generator mechanism in fact responds to the difference between consecutive stimuli, not to the eliciting stimulus per se. Consistently with this, when presented without the intervening, loud standard stimuli, the soft 57-dB stimuli elicited no MMN but rather a large N1 (Fig. 4.22). Therefore it is unlikely that intensity-specific neurons (Brugge & Reale, 1985) could explain MMN elicited by intensity decrements.

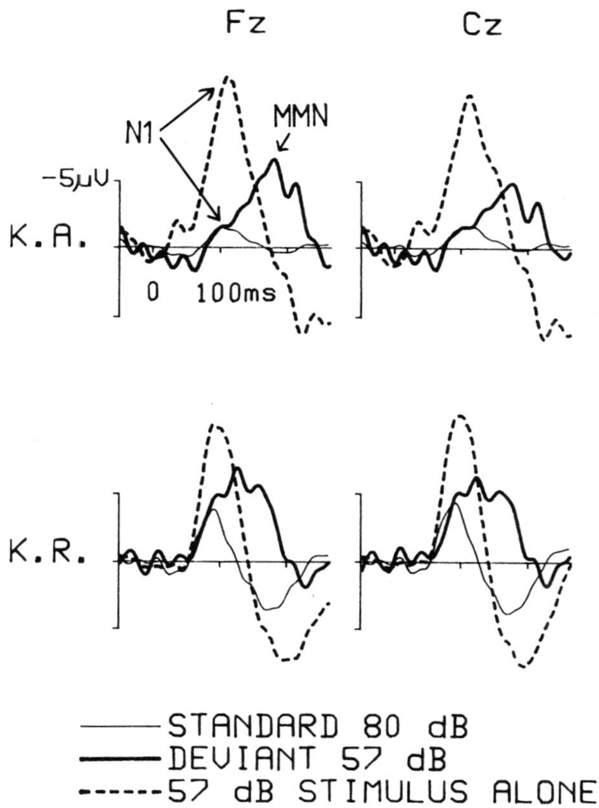

FIG. 4.22 Frontal (Fz) and vertex (Cz) ERPs of two subjects to 80-dB standard stimuli (thin lines), 57-dB deviant stimuli (thick lines), and to identical 57-dB stimuli (dashed lines) when presented with no standards (without changing the ISIs between the 57-dB stimuli). (From Näätänen, Paavilainen, Alho, Reinikainen, & Sams, 1989. Copyright © 1989 by Elsevier Science Publishers, Ireland. Reprinted with permission.)

When deviant stimuli are intensity increments rather than decrements, MMN is again elicited. Moreover, the amplitude of this MMN is increased with the increasing intensity of the deviant stimulus. In addition, the N1 component is enhanced in response to these deviants, and this enhancement, too, is proportional to the intensity increment (Fig. 4.21). This is in keeping with the known intensity dependence of the N1 amplitude (Fig. 4.11).

ERP effects of intensity change can perhaps be better understood by looking down the column for the Fpz recording in Fig. 4.23 showing the deviant-standard difference waves. It can be seen that N1 to the deviant stimulus, with a peak latency of about 100 msec, becomes larger than that to the standard stimulus as the deviant stimulus becomes more intense than the standard stimulus and, further, the N1 enhancement increases with

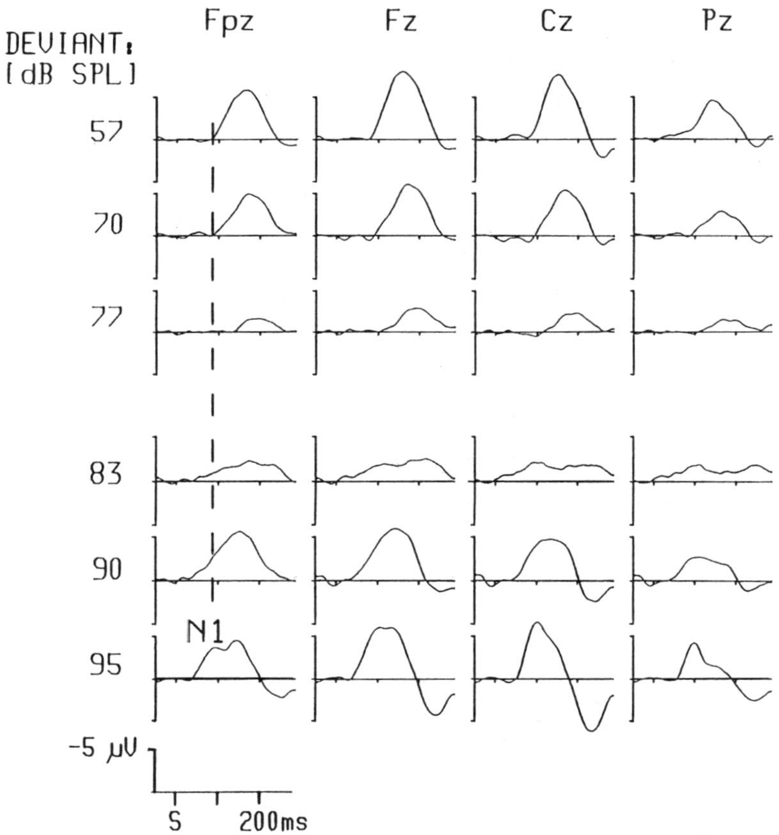

FIG. 4.23 Difference curves for the data presented in Fig. 4.21 obtained by subtracting ERPs to standards from those to the corresponding deviants. (From Näätänen et al., in preparation.)

increasing intensity. By contrast, looking down the column from the top, MMN (with a peak latency between 150–200 msec) gradually *decreases* in amplitude and increases in latency as the deviant stimulus becomes more intense (and therefore becomes closer in intensity to the 80-dB standard stimulus). Then, after the standard-stimulus intensity is passed, MMN becomes gradually larger in amplitude and shorter in latency again as the deviant stimulus becomes yet more intense (and therefore becomes further away in intensity from the 80-dB standard). In other words, the N1 amplitude is a linear function of intensity, whereas the MMN amplitude is a curvilinear function of intensity, with the zero point matching the intensity of the standard stimulus.

Thus, the MMN generator responded to intensity deviation irrespective of whether intensity decreased or increased. The N1 generator, in contrast, responded to stimulus intensity regardless of the relation of this intensity to that of the standard stimuli: N1 was largest for intensity increments and larger for standards than intensity decrements. Thus, whereas stimulus deviation was necessary for MMN elicitation, N1 was also elicited by standards, that is, by stimulus repetitions. The insensitivity of N1 to the relation between the stimuli in the block was also evidenced by the N1 latency which, in contrast to the MMN latency, did not vary as a function of stimulus deviation. So, N1 is a response to individual stimuli, whereas MMN responds to the relation (difference) between consecutive stimuli.

MMN to Temporal Changes. MMN to change in stimulus duration was demonstrated by Näätänen, Paavilainen, and Reinikainen (1989). The standard and deviant stimuli were similar tone bursts except that the deviant stimulus lasted only half of the duration of the standard. The stimuli were presented in random order and at a constant ISI (from onset to onset) of 510 msec while the subject was reading.

As shown in Fig. 4.24, a clear MMN was elicited by duration decrements, even by the 200-msec deviant stimuli. At least the latter MMN is a genuine duration MMN rather than one resulting from a diminished input to the temporal-summation mechanism of loudness, for this temporal summation only continues up to 200 msec from stimulus onset (Scharf & Houtsma, 1986). MMN was also elicited by duration increments (Fig. 4.24).

Thus, even temporal stimulus changes elicit MMN. This is also supported by Ford and Hillyard's (1981) finding that an MMN kind of response is elicited when a stimulus is presented too early in a block with otherwise constant ISIs. Nordby et al. (1988a) obtained a similar result by using a constant ISI of 800 msec and occasionally shortening it to 400 msec.

Nordby, Roth, and Pfefferbaum (1988b) found MMN with even more complex temporal changes. In one of their conditions, the deviant event that elicited an MMN kind of effect was an occasional stimulus repetition

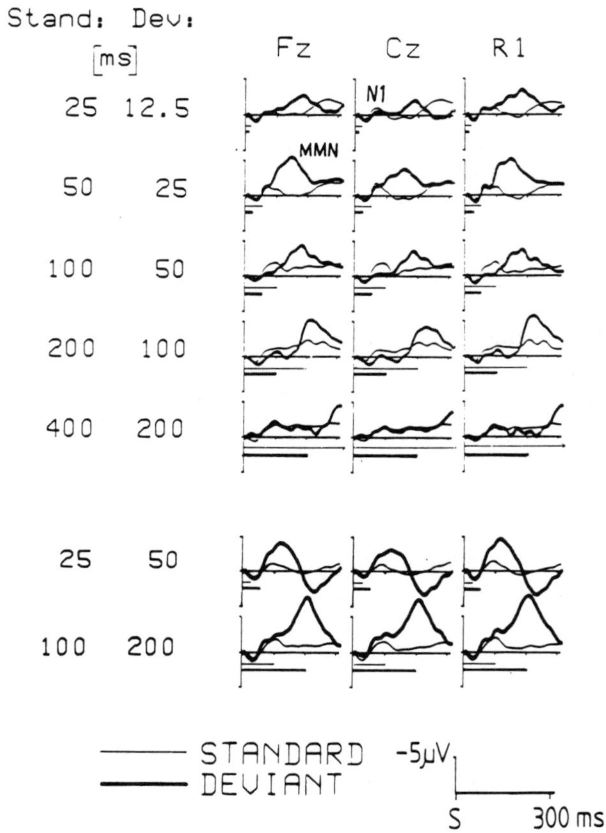

FIG. 4.24 Grand-average frontal (Fz), vertex (Cz), and right-hemispheric (R1 = ⅓ of the Fz- right-mastoid distance) ERPs to standard (thin line) and deviant (thick line) stimuli differing in duration as indicated on the left. In separate blocks, the standard stimulus (probability 90%) was either 25, 50, 100, 200, or 400 msec. In duration–decrement blocks (5 top rows), the duration of the deviant stimulus (probability 10%) was a half of that of the standard stimulus. In duration–increment blocks (2 bottom rows), the deviant stimulus was two-fold the standard stimulus in duration. (Otherwise the two stimuli were identical.) The horizontal lines under the traces illustrate the corresponding stimulus durations. (Adapted from Näätänen, Paavilainen, & Reinikainen, 1989. Copyright © 1989 by Elsevier Science Publishers, Ireland. Reprinted with permission.)

in a sequence of two alternating tones. The authors suggested that the neuronal model underlying MMN generation "could contain two pitches in succession as a single unit" (Nordby et al., 1988b, p. 267).

An occasional stimulus repetition against a changing background does not always elicit MMN, however. Ritter, Paavilainen, Lavikainen, Reinikainen, Alho, Sams, and Näätänen (1991) found no MMN when a repetition (20% of the stimuli) occurred against an irregular background of

5 equiprobable tones. Thus some regularity, even one formed by regular change, in a stimulus block is necessary for MMN elicitation. Apparently, the neural trace underlying MMN generation—if this interpretation is correct—requires some form of regularity in stimulation.

Nordby et al. (1988b) also had a condition with alternating short (400 msec) and long (800 msec) ISIs. A small, MMN type of negativity was elicited by infrequent repetitions of the short ISI but was not statistically significant. In a very recent study with paired tones (60-msec tones of 660 Hz and 740 Hz separated by 40 msec; the inter-pair silent interval 640 msec), Tervaniemi, Saarinen, Paavilainen, and Näätänen (in preparation) obtained an MMN to an infrequent reversal of the order of the stimuli composing the pair. MMN was also obtained when the second member of the pair was occasionally identical to the first member or was omitted.

MMN to Change in Locus of Spatial Origin. Paavilainen et al. (1989) demonstrated MMN to a change in sound location. In their free-field conditions, one loudspeaker was positioned straight in front of the subject for standards and the other speaker was either 10°, 45°, or 90° to its right for deviants. In the conditions that employed earphones, the apparent change in stimulus location was created by manipulating either the inter-aural phase (for low tones) or intensity (for high tones) difference. This was done so that the apparent angle differences between the standards and deviants matched with those of the free-field conditions.

Figure 4.25 illustrates low-tone (600-Hz) data. Whereas the MMN amplitude grows as a function of the (apparent) angle when earphones were used (left), the free-field MMN seems to be quite large even with the smallest angle difference (right). This increased sensitivity to change in stimulus location may result from the larger number of spatial cues operational in the free-field conditions (Paavilainen et al., 1989).

MMN to Phonetic Change. MMN is elicited by changes even in complex stimulus aspects such as those underlying phonetic stimulus properties. Aaltonen et al.'s (1987) standard stimulus was a synthetic vowel /y/ (F2 = 2500 Hz) and the deviant stimulus an /i/ (F2 = 1800 Hz), or vice versa, both representing the end points of the Finnish /i/–/y/ continuum. The other formants were the same for the two stimuli. A distinct MMN was elicited by this phonetic deviation (Fig. 4.26; bottom). A smaller and later MMN was elicited when either the standard or deviant was a boundary stimulus equiprobably identified as an /i/ or a /y/ (Fig. 4.26; top).

The phonetic MMN was confirmed and extended to synthetic consonant–vowel (CV) syllables by Sams et al. (1990). Their standard stimulus was a syllable /bae/ and the deviant stimulus was given different values on the /bae/–/gae/ continuum. Hence the difference between standards and

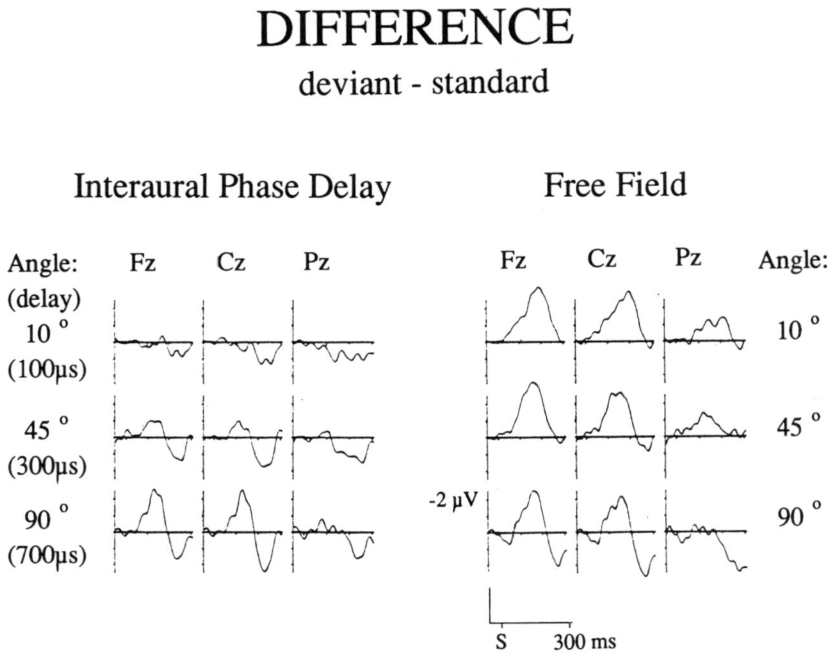

FIG. 4.25 Grand-average frontal (Fz), vertex (Cz), and parietal (Pz) difference waveforms (obtained by subtracting ERPs to standards from those to the corresponding deviants) showing the effect of spatial stimulus deviation. Stimuli were tones of 600 Hz. Spatial deviation was produced either by introducing a phase delay between the inputs to the two ears when earphones were used (left) or, in free-field conditions (right), by presenting a stimulus via a loudspeaker positioned to the right of the standard-stimulus loudspeaker located directly in front of the subject. Three levels of (real or apparent) spatial separation were used in both conditions: 10°, 45°, and 90°. (Adapted from Paavilainen, Karlsson, Reinikainen, & Näätänen, 1989. Copyright © 1989 by Elsevier Science Publishers, Ireland. Reprinted with permission.)

deviants was introduced only by changing the starting frequency of the second-formant (F2) transition.

It was found that a clear MMN was elicited even by a deviant stimulus sharing the phonetic category with the standard stimulus. Also, the N1 amplitude was enhanced by stimulus deviation. The MMNs elicited in this study were of a considerably longer duration than those for simple stimulus features.

The MMN amplitude did not systematically increase with the magnitude of stimulus difference, however, as the intermediate differences were associated with the largest amplitudes. In addition, it appeared that there might be a step-like increase in MMN amplitude as the deviant stimulus moves from the phonetic category of the standard stimulus to a different, adjacent category.

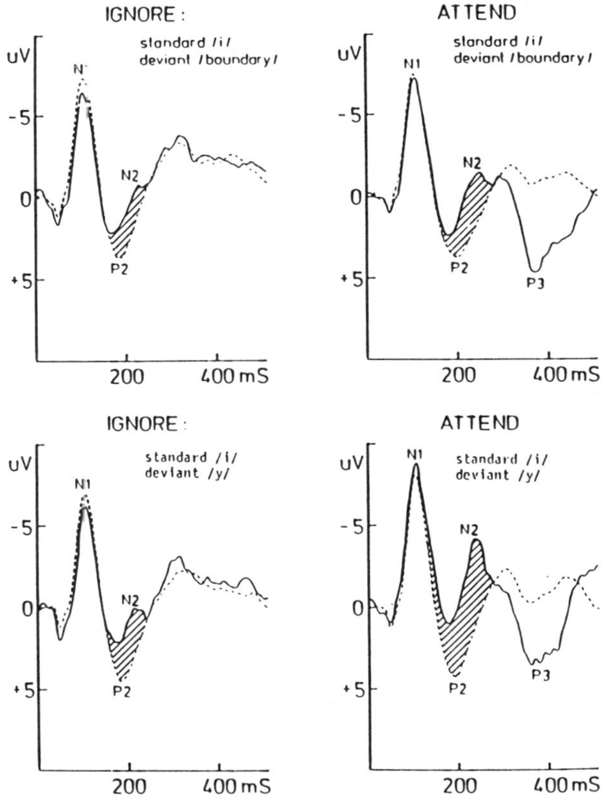

FIG. 4.26 Grand-average vertex (Cz) ERPs when the standard stimulus was an /i/ and the deviant stimulus an /y/ (bottom) or a boundary (top) between the two vowels in ignore (left) and attend (right) conditions. Dashed line = standard, solid line = deviant. (From Aaltonen, Niemi, Nyrke, & Tuhkanen, 1987. Copyright © 1987 by Elsevier Science Publishers BV [Biomedical Division]. Reprinted with permission.)

MMN to Partial Omission. Winkler and Näätänen (in press) and Nordby, Hammerborg, Roth, and Hugdahl (1991) demonstrated MMN to a partial stimulus omission. Nordby et al.'s standard stimulus was a combined tone and noise burst; the deviant stimulus was one element of the standard stimulus alone. The tone presented alone as a deviant event elicited a distinct MMN, which is difficult to explain in terms of new afferent elements. This is because MMN was then elicited by a deviant stimulus that was an element of the standard stimulus, and hence contained no features that were not present in the standard stimulus also. On the other hand, the noise burst presented alone as a deviant event elicited no MMN.

Winkler and Näätänen (in press) found MMN to a partial stimulus

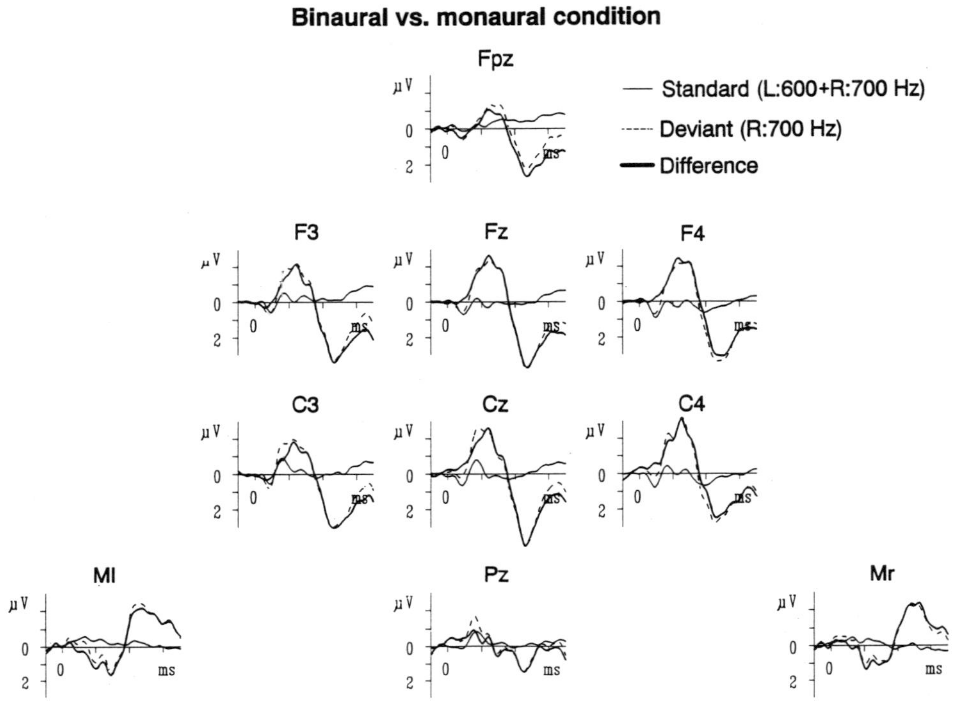

FIG. 4.27 Grand-average ERPs from different electrode locations when the standard stimulus (thin line) consisted of a left-ear tone of 600 Hz and a simultaneous right-ear tone of 700 Hz and the deviant stimulus only the right-ear tone of 700 Hz (dashed line). (Electrode locations Ml and Mr refer to the left and right mastoids, respectively.) The difference wave obtained by subtracting the standard-stimulus ERP from the corresponding deviant-stimulus ERP is indicated by the thick line. (From Winkler & Näätänen, in press. Copyright © in press Birkhäuser, Verlag, Basel. Reprinted with permission.)

omission with standard stimuli composed of concurrent 600- and 700-Hz tones. The deviant stimulus was one of the two tones presented alone. This MMN occurred when the two tones forming the standard stimulus were presented to the same ear or opposite ears and, further, when the weaker intensity of the deviant event was compensated or was not compensated. Some of these data are illustrated in Fig. 4.27.

Determinants of MMN

Magnitude of Stimulus Deviation

The results with simple stimulus changes just reviewed show that, in general, with an increasing magnitude of stimulus deviation, MMN gets larger and earlier and its duration may be shortened. However, the growth of the MMN amplitude, at least for stimulus frequency, may reach a plateau quite soon when the magnitude of stimulus deviation is further increased (Novak et al., 1990; Sams, Paavilainen, et al., 1985; see also Näätänen & Gaillard, 1983). The Sams, Paavilainen, et al. (1985) results suggested that the MMN peak latency for frequency change is more systematically related to the magnitude of stimulus deviance than is the MMN amplitude.

The saturation of the amplitude, however, was not observed with regard to intensity MMN, by Näätänen, Paavilainen, Alho, et al. (1989). Similarly, Paavilainen et al.'s (1989) MMN to change in apparent stimulus location increased in amplitude in proportion to the width of the location change.

With changes in more complex stimuli such as phonetic ones, the magnitude functions appear, in the light of the meager data available, discontinuous and more complex in nature.

Probability of Stimulus Deviation and Sequential Effects

Näätänen and colleagues (1983) found a much larger MMN when the probability of deviant stimuli was 2% than when it was 10% (Fig. 4.28). This effect could of course be due to a change in the temporal probability of the deviant stimulus, that is, in the probability of the deviant stimulus for a given period of time. Näätänen, Paavilainen, Alho, Reinikainen, and Sams (1987a) suggested that both event and temporal probabilities (see Fitzgerald & Picton, 1981) affect MMN. This is discussed later.

A low probability of the deviant stimulus is not necessary for MMN elicitation, however. This was shown by Sams et al. (1983) who found MMN in a stimulus block consisting of two equiprobable stimuli. A sequential ERP analysis, following the pioneering one conducted by Squires, Wickens, Squires, and Donchin (1976) for P3, revealed that this MMN was elicited when one stimulus followed several exemplars of the other stimulus. Furthermore, MMN was larger, the more exemplars of the other stimulus had preceded the eliciting stimulus (Fig. 4.29, left). Although this effect was not significant, it has recently been confirmed and statistically verified by Giese-Davis, Miller, and Knight (1991) (Fig. 4.29, right).

Thus, the MMN amplitude strongly depends on the local probability of the immediately preceding sequence of stimuli. Therefore the effects of the global probability on MMN seem to be, at least to a great extent, mediated by the distribution of the different types of local probabilities in the block.

These findings also illustrate a limitation of simple data averaging: When only two averages are obtained in the oddball paradigm, one for the standard and one for the deviant, the incorrect conclusion can be drawn

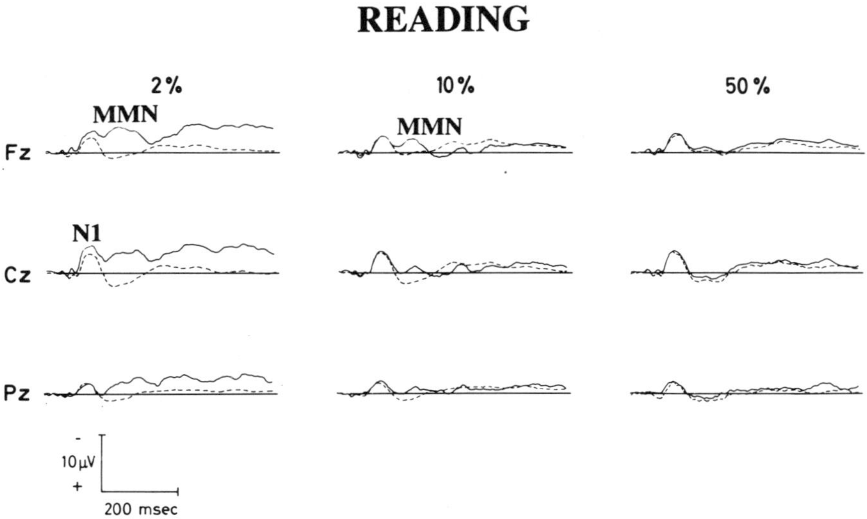

FIG. 4.28 Grand-average frontal (Fz), vertex (Cz), and parietal (Pz) ERPs to standard (dotted line) and to deviant (solid line) stimuli as a function of the probability of the deviant stimuli (2, 10, or 50%) while subjects are reading a book. Stimulus onset is at 30 msec from the beginning of the trace. The horizontal line is drawn along the average level of this 30-msec period. (Adapted from Näätänen, Sams, Järvilehto, & Soininen, 1983. Copyright © 1983 by Elsevier Science Publishers BV [Biomedical Division]. Reprinted with permission.)

that only the deviant elicits MMN, or other components, such as N2b and P3 (see Section 6.1), that are inversely related in amplitude to stimulus probability. Actually, both stimuli elicit these components, but because in the local sequences deviants are much more often preceded by a series of standards than vice versa, in the overall averages it appears that only the deviants elicit these components.

In their subsequent study, Sams, Alho, and Näätänen (1984) investigated sequential effects in the oddball paradigm, using the typical stimulus probabilities of 90% and 10%. MMN was elicited by the deviants; a small MMN was even elicited by the "second deviant," that is, the deviant that happened immediately following another deviant (Fig. 4.30). These stimulus events were of course very infrequent ($p = .01$). On the other hand, when the first deviant was followed by a standard, even that standard elicited MMN, though a small one. The authors (Sams et al., 1984) interpreted these data as suggesting that two neural stimulus representations can exist in parallel:

> Because some MMN was still seen to the second deviant, we infer that the neuronal model (see Sokolov, 1975) formed by the standard was not immediately replaced by a new one formed by the deviant. On the other hand,

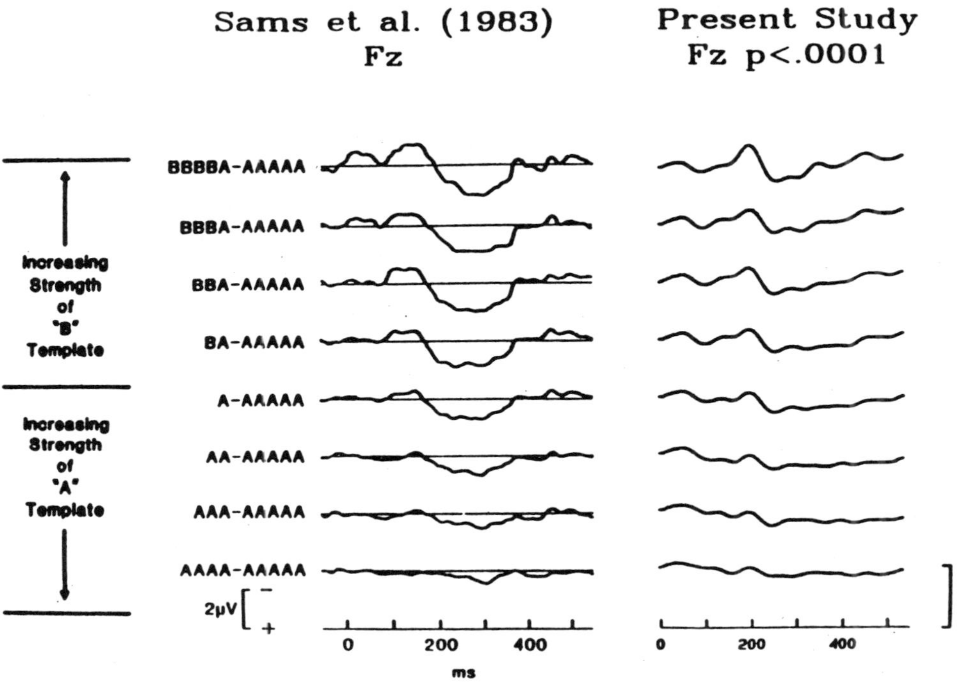

FIG. 4.29 Difference waves of the frontal (Fz) grand-average ERPs elicited by an A stimulus (the last in the letter sequences on the left) in the reading condition as a function of the preceding stimuli when two equiprobable stimuli differing in pitch were presented in a random order. The ERP to the category AAAAA stimulus (an A preceded by 4 As) is subtracted from the other A-stimulus categories. For example, BBBBA-AAAAA compares ERPs elicited by a stimulus change after an uninterrupted occurrence of the other stimulus at least 4 times (A after 4 Bs) with the ERP elicited by an identical stimulus (A) when preceded by itself at least by 4 times. On the left, data of Sams et al. (1983), on the right, data of Giese-Davis et al. (1991). (From Giese-Davis, Miller, & Knight, 1991. Reprinted with permission.)

when a standard was delivered after the first deviant . . . some MMN was elicited also. . . . Consequently, a deviant stimulus, in addition to causing a mismatch process with the neuronal model of the standard, also produces a neuronal model of its own. These findings suggest that the neuronal mechanism preserving the physical features of the auditory stimulus is not a limited-capacity system able to store just one stimulus-feature combination at a time. This is because a MMN was obtained to either stimulus delivered after the first deviant. This can be explained only by assuming the existence of neuronal models both for the standard and for the deviant at the moment of the stimulus following the first deviant. (p. 440)

In conclusion, local sequences of stimuli preceding a deviant stimulus are important determinants of MMN elicited by the deviant stimulus. Conse-

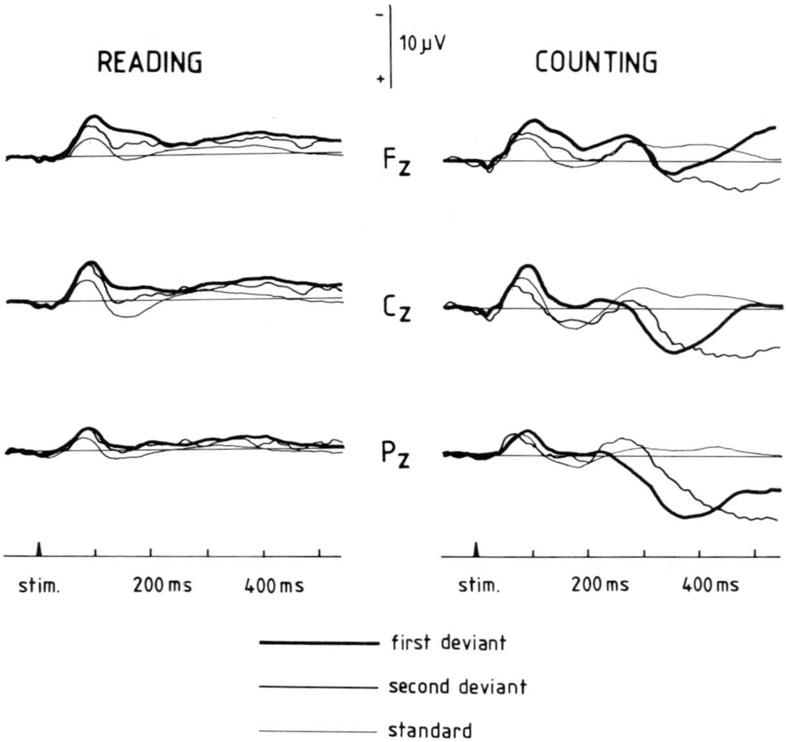

FIG. 4.30 Grand-average frontal (Fz), vertex (Cz), and parietal (Pz) ERPs to the standard stimulus preceding the deviant stimulus, to the deviant stimulus (first deviant), and to the deviant stimulus immediately after the first deviant (second deviant) in reading (left) and counting (right) conditions. Standard stimuli (90%) were tones of 1,000 Hz, deviant stimuli (10%) tones of 1,250 Hz. (Copyright © 1984 The Society for Psychophysiological Research. Reprinted with permission of the publisher from 'Short-term habituation and dishabituation of the mismatch negativity of the ERP,' by Sams, Alho, & Näätänen, 1984).

quently, it appears that the neural stimulus representations involved in MMN generation are most strongly affected by stimulus events occurring during the last few seconds. This suggests that these neural representations might decay at a quite rapid rate (Näätänen, 1985). To determine this decay function has been the principal goal in the studies of ISI effects on MMN that are examined in the next section.

Interstimulus Interval (ISI)

The logic underlying the design of these studies is that by prolonging the ISI of a stimulus block composed of standard and deviant stimuli, MMN is no longer elicited by deviants when the decay of the neural representation of the standard stimulus reaches some limit. Similarly, the gradual reduction in the MMN amplitude as the ISI is prolonged might reflect the gradual decay of this trace in time. In one of these studies, Mäntysalo and Näätänen (1987) found a clear MMN when the constant ISI in a block was either 1 or 2 sec but did not with ISIs of 4 or 8 sec. A small MMN might have been present in the 4-sec stimulus blocks, however. In a subsequent study, Näätänen and colleagues (1987a) found MMN with the 4-sec ISI but unfortunately did not use longer ISIs.

The more recent data of Böttcher-Gandor and Ullsperger (in press) considerably extend the estimate for the duration of neural representations (or of their active phase) involved in MMN generation (see also Cowan, Winkler, Teder, & Näätänen, 1991, to be reviewed later). The ISI in their stimulus blocks was randomly either 1, 6, or 10 sec. The data obtained, illustrated in Fig. 4.31, suggest that MMN was elicited even with ISIs of 6 and 10 sec. These authors used a considerably larger stimulus deviation and longer stimulus duration than did Mäntysalo and Näätänen (1987), which might explain the different results between the two studies. Some of Böttcher-Gandor and Ullsperger's (in press) long-ISI deviance-related negativity might be due to the N2b component, however, judging from the longer latency and (slightly) more posterior midline topography of this long-ISI negativity in comparison with the 1-sec negativity.

Näätänen and colleagues (1987a), in their aforementioned study, tried to determine the shortest ISI at which MMN can still be elicited. They found MMN even with an ISI of 101 msec (onset to onset), possibly even with an ISI of 51 msec, but in the latter case, the effect could also have resulted from an N1 enhancement. With the 101-msec ISI, on the average, 9 standards and one deviant were delivered in one second. In a later study, Näätänen, Teder, Alho, and Lavikainen (1992) found a clear MMN with a constant onset-to-onset ISI of 60 msec.

The MMN amplitude became larger with a decreased probability of the deviant stimulus when the stimulus rate in a block was held constant. It was also found that when the temporal probability of the deviant stimulus was held constant, these stimuli elicited a larger MMN with faster rates of standard stimuli. This supports the assumption of MMN generation being based on neural representations of standard stimuli because a more rapid repetition of standard stimuli should result in the development of a stronger trace.

Consequently, the rate of both standard and deviant stimuli is of importance in ISI effects on MMN. The ISI between deviant stimuli might be important because it determines whether a trace of a previous similar deviant stimulus is still present in the system at the arrival of the sensory input from the next deviant stimulus: The MMN process elicited by a

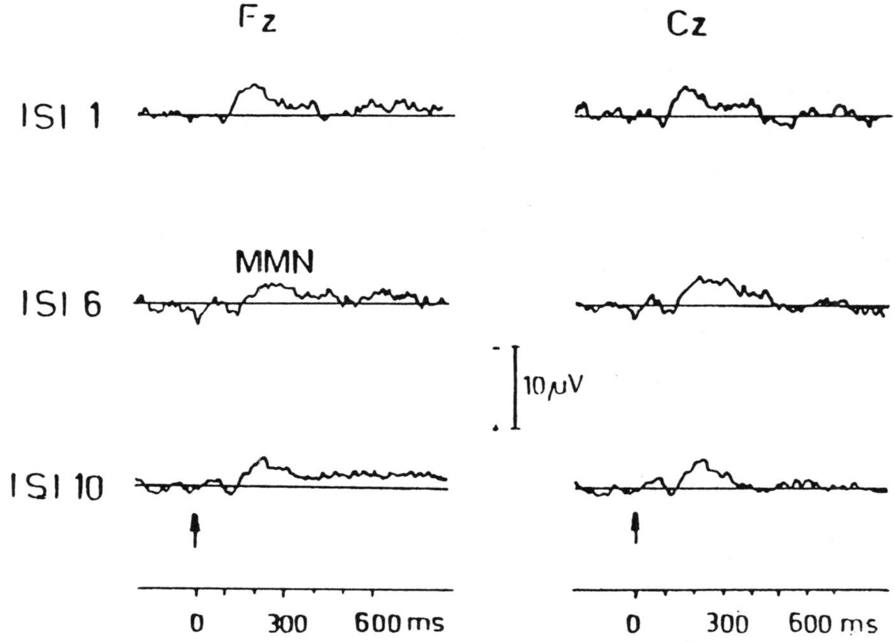

FIG. 4.31 Grand-average frontal (Fz) and vertex (Cz) ERP difference waves (obtained by subtracting the standard-stimulus ERP from the corresponding deviant-stimulus ERP) separately for blocks with ISIs of 1, 6, and 10 sec. The standard stimulus was a tone of 1,000 Hz, the deviant stimulus a tone of 1,500 Hz. (Copyright © in press The Society for Psychophysiological Research. Reprinted with permission of the publisher from "Mismatch negativity in ERPs to auditory stimuli as a function of varying interstimulus interval," by C. Böttcher-Gandor and P. Ullsperger.)

deviant stimulus might be weakened by a simultaneous match process between this input and the trace of the previous deviant stimuli (Ritter et al., 1991; Sams et al., 1984; Winkler et al., 1990, Winkler, Paavilainen, & Näätänen, in press).

Predictability

If the MMN process is indeed an automatic, preconscious brain event, as originally proposed by Näätänen et al. (1978), then it should not be affected by whether or not the subject can predict when deviant stimuli will be presented in a block. This was studied by Scherg, Vajsar, and Picton (1989). In their regular mode of stimulus presentation, a deviant stimulus always occurred after four intervening standard stimuli. In the irregular mode, the deviant stimulus occurred randomly at the same mean rate. The subject was reading during the recordings. Predictability was found to have no significant effect on MMN.

Stimulus Significance

Näätänen and colleagues (1978) suggested that MMN is not affected by stimulus significance. In testing this prediction, attention paid to the stimulus sequence should be controlled in order not to confuse effects of attention and stimulus significance. This can be done best by presenting significant (e.g., target) and insignificant (nontarget) deviants in a random order in the same attended stimulus block.

This design was used by Näätänen et al. (1982; see also Nordby et al., 1988a). One of the deviant tones was slightly higher and the other slightly lower in frequency than the standard. In some of the blocks, the high proximate was designated as the target to be counted; in others, the target was the low proximate. It was found that MMN elicited by the two proximates was very similar in amplitude irrespective of which of them was designated as the target. Furthermore, these MMNs were similar in amplitude to those elicited by the same proximates when neither of them was a target (the reading condition) or when both were targets. These results therefore suggest that stimulus significance has no effect on MMN.

Sleep Effects

Paavilainen and colleagues (1987) failed to record MMN to a frequency change in sleeping adults. They suggested that the use of a relatively small stimulus deviation (5%), as well as the large slow-wave activity, might have prevented the researchers from seeing MMN which they thought might occur even during sleep but at a reduced amplitude and with a longer latency. In a subsequent study, Campbell, Bell, and Bastien (1991) indeed found evidence for sleep MMN. This appeared to occur during the late stage 2 and REM (rapid-eye-movement) sleep in the second half of the night and was described as quite small in amplitude and "unusually early". It is very difficult, according to the authors, to record MMN in the early portion of the night and does not always succeed even in the second half of the night. In addition, Alho, Sainio, Sajaniemi, Reinikainen, and Näätänen (1990) found a large negativity resembling the adult MMN in sleeping human newborns in response to frequency deviants.

Converging evidence for sleep MMN was provided by intracranial MMN recordings in the cat conducted by Csépe, Karmos, and Molnár (1987, 1988a, 1988b; Csépe, Molnár, Karmos, & Winkler, 1989). The sleep MMN had a longer latency and was less widespread in its cortical area than the waking MMN. Csépe, Molnár, Karmos, and Winkler (1989) observed

MMN, though at a small amplitude and only from a very limited cortical area, even during anesthesia.

Drug Effects

MMN seems to be enhanced by drugs that have a general activating effect on the central nervous system and attenuated by drugs with deactivating effects. Born, Bother et al. (1987) and Born, Fehm-Wolfsdorf, Lutzenberger, Voigt, and Fehm (1986) found that the MMN amplitude for frequency deviation was enhanced by lysine-vasopressin (LVP), which belongs to a group of pituitary–hypothalamic hormones known to enhance cortical arousal (Timsit-Berthier, Mantanus, & Legros, 1983). In another study, hydrocortisone substantially reduced the MMN amplitude for frequency deviants (Born, Brüninger, et al., 1987). Hydrocortisone-induced plasma cortisol levels remained within physiological ranges, that is, ranges that may occur under natural conditions. The N1 amplitude, too, was reduced by hydrocortisone.

These amplitude reductions led the authors to suggest that glucocorticoids not only lower stimulus-induced arousal (N1) but also diminish sensitivity to stimulus change (MMN), attributing these effects to "a reduced sensitivity of the nonspecific sensory system" (Born, Brüninger, et al., 1987, p. 291). The authors further proposed that internally produced cortisol release, induced, for example, by stressful stimuli, may lead to ERP changes similar to those observed in their study.

Using a similar paradigm, Born, Kern, Fehm-Wolfsdorf, and Fehm (1987) found that ACTH (adrenocorticotropic hormone) 4–10 did not affect the MMN amplitude but considerably attenuated certain attention-related waves, discussed later (for corroborating results, see Born, Kern, Pietrowsky, Sittig, & Fehm, 1989; Pietrowsky Fehm, & Born, 1990). Similarly, Duncan and Kaye (1987) found no effect of clonidine on MMN, whereas a certain later, positive wave, P3, which is generally regarded as reflecting controlled processing (Section 6.1), was affected.

Very recently, Javitt, Schroeder, Steinschneider, Arezzo, and Vaughan (in press) found a human analogue of intensity-decrement MMN in the monkey, which was abolished by administration of MK-801, an NMDA (N-methyl-D-aspartate) receptor antagonist (Javitt, Schroeder, Arezzo, & Vaughan, 1991), whereas the exogenous components were present. This important finding is discussed later.

In conclusion, the state of the organism affects MMN, so that changes toward increased cortical activation increase, and those in the direction of decreased activation attenuate, the MMN amplitude. The normal variation of the state does not, presumably, totally eliminate MMN at any point, however.

Long-Term Response Decrement

MMN-amplitude decrement in the course of a long experimental session is negligible (Lyytinen et al., in press; Näätänen & Gaillard, 1983; Paavilainen et al., 1987). Paavilainen et al. (1987) found that MMN was very similar during the different phases of an experiment lasting 2 hours. The small amplitude reduction sometimes observed in the course of a long session might be fully accounted for by a slow state change associated with decreased cortical excitability.

The importance of the state (vigilance) to MMN was also demonstrated by Mikola, Lang, and Eerola (in preparation) who found a correlation between reading speed and the MMN amplitude in their overnight recordings (Fig. 4.32). (Subjects were not allowed to take any naps during the

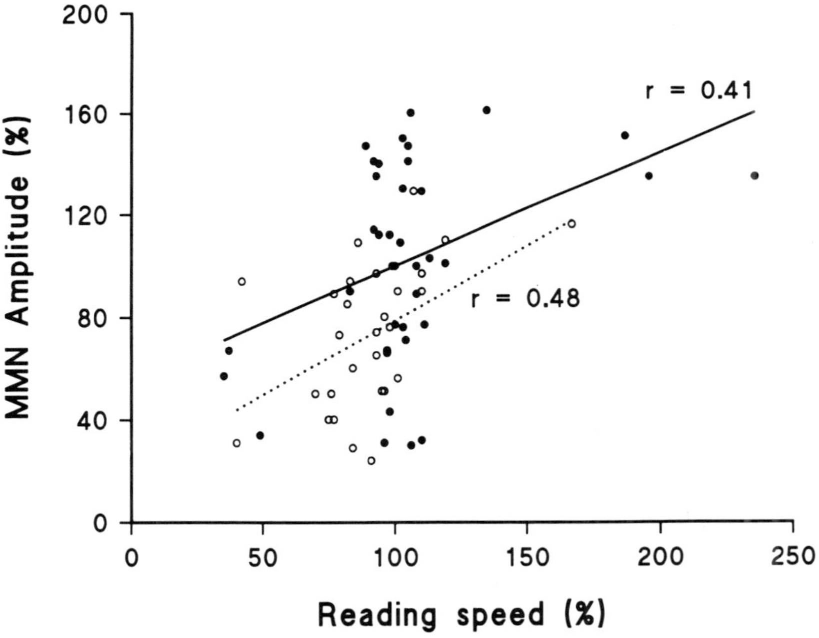

FIG. 4.32 Correlation between reading speed and the MMN peak amplitude in 6 young healthy subjects when trials with slow eye movements were (solid line) and were not (dotted line) eliminated. Open circles represent data from blocks at which slow eye movements were not eliminated, solid circles data from blocks where slow eye movements were eliminated. The tests were made between 17:05 and 07:15, and the subjects were not allowed to fall asleep during the night. The reading speed and the MMN peak amplitude of the first session were set to 100% for each subject. (From Mikola, Lang, & Eerola, in preparation.)

night.) This correlation was stronger when slow eye movements, indicating increased drowsiness, were present than when they were absent in the block, providing further evidence for MMN sensitivity to vigilance.

Constancy of the Standard Stimulus

In all the previously discussed MMN studies, the standard stimulus was constant. In more ecologically valid conditions, however, the (proximal) standard stimulus does not necessarily remain identical over the successive repetitions. The actual acoustic input is affected, for example, by changes in head position relative to stimulus source. Winkler et al. (1990) accordingly studied the tolerance of MMN generation to slight variations in the intensity of the standard stimulus (mean 80 dB SPL). The range of the intensity variation (occurring through 9 equiprobable, equidistant intensity values: "substandards") was different in different blocks, maximally ±6.4 dB. In each block, the intensity of the deviant stimulus was 70 dB.

It was found that MMN occurred when the standard stimulus was varied, but at a reduced amplitude, and, further, that the MMN attenuation was proportional to the range of variation. Similar results were obtained when stimulus deviation involved frequency (Fig. 4.33) rather than intensity. Winkler and colleagues (1990), considering the following two alternatives, interpreted these results in terms of a weakened trace of the standard stimulus:

> (1) The incoming stimulus starts a process whose effect melts into a common trace left by the previous stimuli, i.e., into a "thinner" or "shallower" trace covering a range along the intensity continuum rather than any discrete point on this continuum. (The strength of this distributed trace as a function of intensity might assume the Gaussian form.) If the new stimulus differs from the focal point (strength maximum corresponding to the mean intensity) of the trace a mismatch process occurs. On the other hand, the reinforcing effect of the new stimulus on the common trace decreases with the distance between the stimulus intensity and that represented by the focal point of the trace. (2) Distinctly different substandards are discretely stored, and comparisons are performed in parallel between the current stimulus and each of the existing traces. Thus each of these processes contributes to the mismatch negativity elicited. Further, the incoming stimulus reinforces only the trace left by the previous stimuli with the same parameters. This results in a set of discrete but weak traces because the probability of any substandard is only a fraction of the overall probability of the standard (the whole set of the substandards). (p. 233)

In this study, the number of the different standard stimuli—substandards—was 9, each occurring at a probability of 0.1. In a subsequent study, Winkler et al. (in press) wished to determine whether MMN can be elicited by a deviant stimulus when there are two frequent standards in a block. One

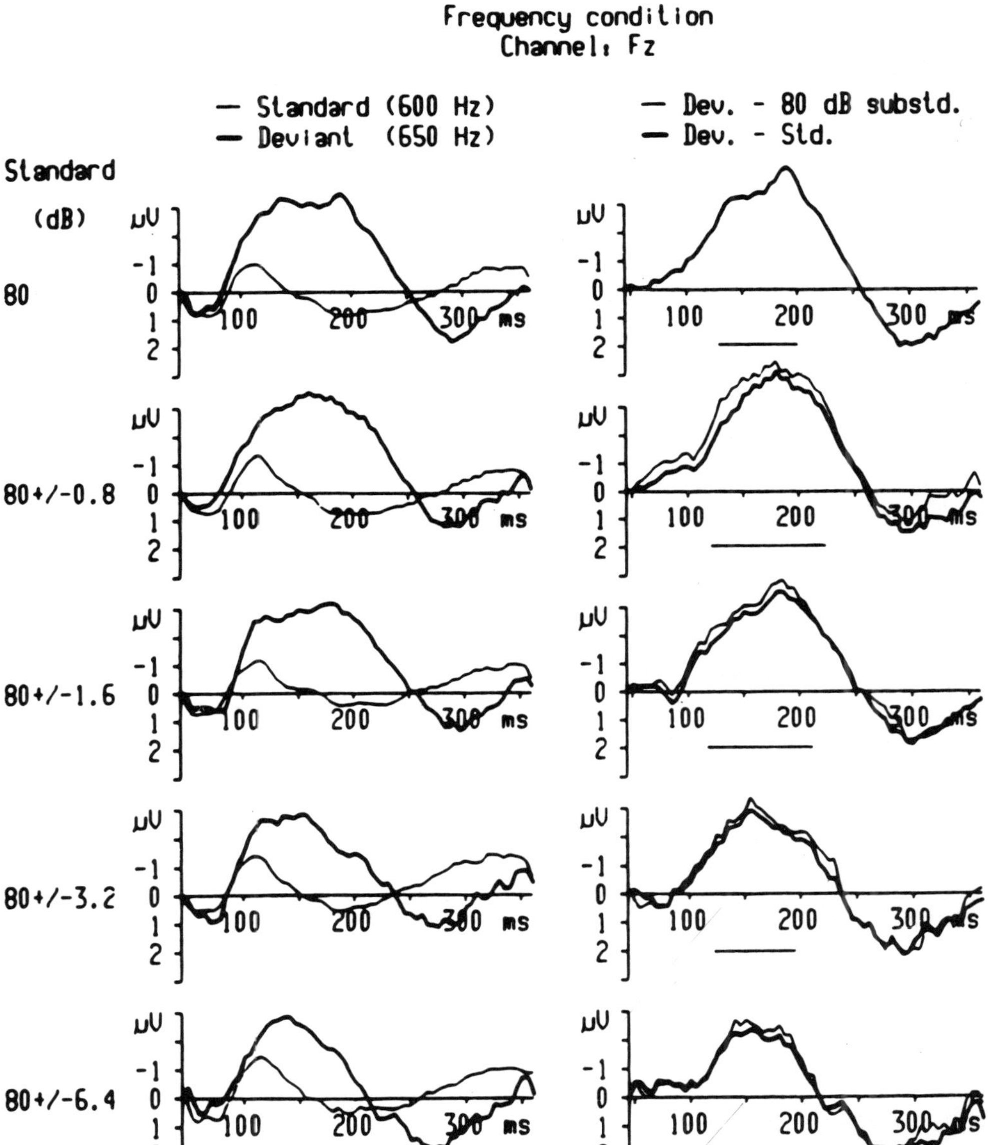

FIG. 4.33 *LEFT:* Grand-average frontal (Fz) ERPs to standard stimuli of 600 Hz (80 dB) (averaged across the different substandards slightly varying in intensity around 80 dB; thin line) and deviant stimuli of 650 Hz (thick line) for the different ranges of the standard-stimulus intensity variability as indicated on the left. *RIGHT:* The corresponding difference waves (*thick line:* deviant-stimulus ERP minus standard-stimulus ERP averaged across the different substandards: *thin line:* deviant-stimulus ERP minus ERP to 80-dB substandards). Intervals with significant ($p < .01$ in point-to-point *t*-tests) differences between ERPs to deviants and standards are underlined. (From Winkler, Paavilainen, Alho, Reinikainen, Sams, & Näätänen, 1990. Copyright © 1990 by The Society for Psychophysiological Research. Reprinted with permission.)

standard was a tone of 600 Hz, the other of 700 Hz; each occurred at a probability of 0.45. In different blocks, a deviant tone ($p = .1$) was either of 625, 650, 675 Hz, or a combined tone including both standards (matched in loudness with the other stimuli).

It was found that all these different deviants elicited MMN. This MMN, however, was much smaller than when there was only one standard ($p = 0.9$) in the stimulus block. Sequential analyses of MMNs in the two-standards conditions suggested a parallel existence of separate traces for the two standards. In addition, in these blocks, MMN was elicited by standards also, apparently due to mismatch processes with the traces of one another. This was also observed in the previous study with 9 equiprobable substandards: Those located at the ends of the range of variation elicited a small MMN (Winkler et al., 1990).

MMN and Masking Effects

One critical test for the memory-trace interpretation of MMN is whether MMN can be eliminated with appropriate masking arrangements. It is known from the behavioral literature that a masking stimulus following a test stimulus at a short interval may erase or deteriorate the memory of the test stimulus. This occurs, for example, when a stimulus of 700 Hz is followed by a louder stimulus of 1000 Hz with an offset–onset interval of 0–150 msec (Hawkins & Presson, 1986).

In an analogous MMN experiment, Winkler, Reinikainen, & Näätänen (1991) found that MMN to a deviant stimulus was indeed eliminated in blocks in which the aforementioned interval was short enough to seriously impair recognition memory but was "normally" elicited in blocks with longer intervals (≥ 150 msec) (Figs. 4.34 and 4.35).

These backward-masking results were complemented by analogous data from forward masking (Fig. 4.35). These masking results belong to the strongest evidence to date for the involvement of memory traces in MMN generation.

Generators of MMN

The early MMN data, usually recorded with only a few electrodes, indicated a midline distribution with an amplitude maximum over frontal areas. In addition, recordings over temporal cortices yielded large MMNs. Näätänen and Michie (1979a) therefore proposed that MMN is actually composed of two subcomponents: (a) a sensory-specific one, generated in the auditory cortices, and (b) a frontal one. They further suggested that the sensory-specific mechanism involves preconscious detection of stimulus deviation which then activates frontal mechanisms related to conscious discrimination of stimulus deviation and to the orienting response.

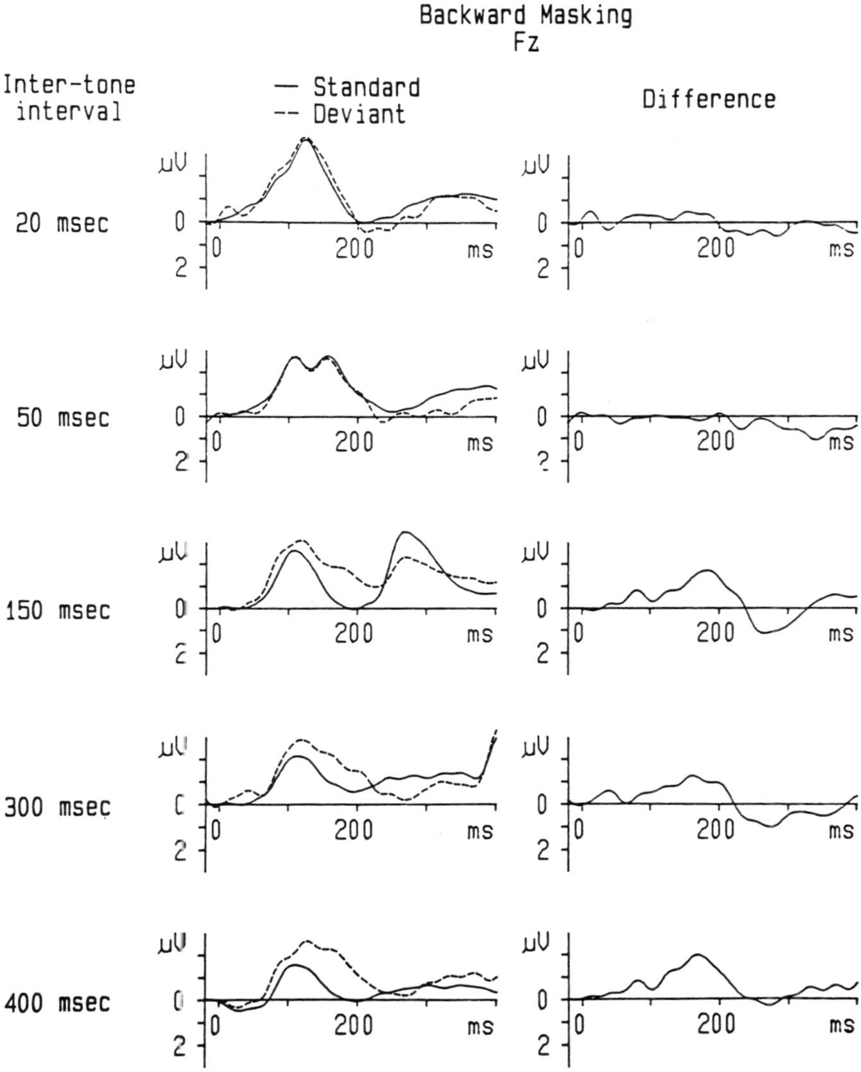

FIG. 4.34 *Left:* Grand-average frontal (Fz) ERPs to standard (600 Hz; solid line) and deviant (700 Hz; dashed line) tones of 25 msec for different intervals, as indicated on the left, from stimulus offset until the onset of a masking stimulus (backward masking) in a reading condition. Each stimulus of the MMN paradigm was followed by a masking stimulus (1,000 Hz, duration 55 msec) with an offset-to-onset interval that differed in different blocks. *Right:* The corresponding difference waves. (From Winkler, Reinikainen, & Näätänen, 1991)

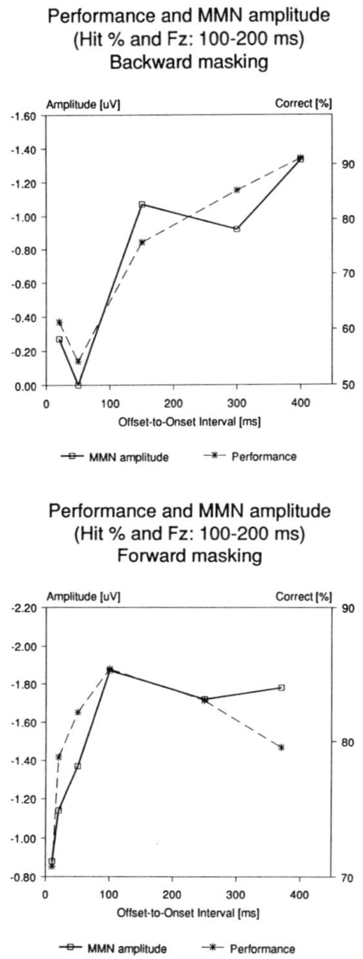

FIG. 4.35 *Backward Masking* (top). Mean frontal (Fz) MMN amplitude (in μV) in a reading condition and the percentage of correctly detected deviant stimuli (dashed line) in a discrimination condition as a function of the interval between the offset of the stimulus of the MMN paradigm (standards 600 Hz, deviants 700 Hz; duration 25 msec) and the onset of the masking stimulus (1,000 Hz; duration 55 msec). Both standards and deviants were followed by a masking stimulus with an offset-to-onset interval which was different in different blocks. *Forward Masking* (bottom). Frontal (Fz) MMN amplitude (μV) in a reading condition (solid line) and the percentage of correctly detected deviant stimuli in a discrimination condition (dashed line) as a function of the interval between the offset of the masking stimulus (600 + 700 Hz; intensity 86 dB SPL; duration 55 msec) and the onset of the stimulus of the MMN paradigm (standards 600 Hz, deviants 700 Hz; intensity 80 dB SPL; duration 25 msec). Both standards and deviants were preceded by a masking stimulus with an offset-to-onset interval which was different in different blocks. (From Winkler, Reinikainen, & Näätänen, 1991.)

These two MMN subcomponents were confirmed by Giard, Perrin, Pernier, and Bouchet (1990) who applied scalp current density analysis (Perrin, Bertrand, Giard, & Echallier, 1987) to their topographical maps for the frequency MMN (Fig. 4.36). Because scalp-current density maps are not sensitive to deep intracranial generator sources, these maps provide a much better basis than ERP maps for inferences concerning cortical ERP generators (Perrin et al., 1987). The results of this analysis suggested that the frequency MMN has two subcomponents: (a) a contralaterally larger component (or pair of components) over the temporal scalp and (b) a frontal component that is larger over the right than the left hemisphere irrespective of ear of stimulation (Fig. 4.36). A separate, frontal subcom-

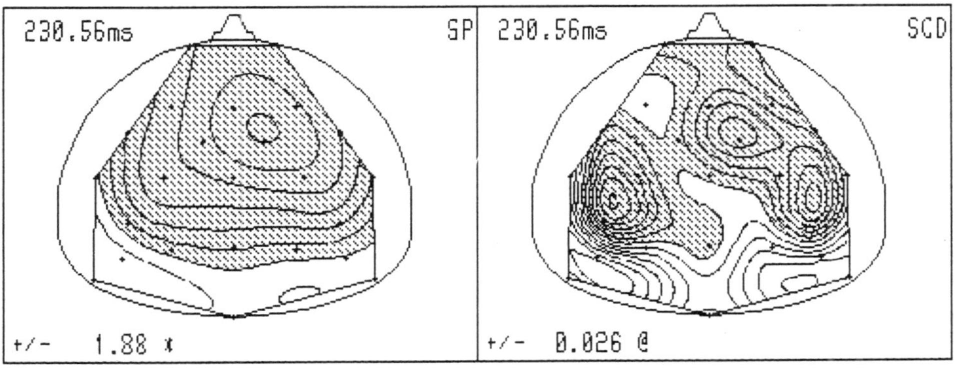

FIG. 4.36 *Ignore condition:* Isopotential (SP) grand-average difference (deviant-standard) map (left) and the corresponding scalp current density (SCD) map (right) at the latency of 230 msec. Standard tones were of 1,000 Hz (low-pitch condition) or 2,000 Hz (high-pitch condition), deviant stimuli of 1,040 or 2,080 Hz, respectively. Data for the two conditions were pooled. (Adapted from Giard, Perrin, Pernier, & Bouchet, 1990. Copyright © 1990 by The Society for Psychophysiological Research. Reprinted with permission.)

ponent of MMN can also be seen in Winkler and Näätänen's (in press) data shown in Fig. 4.27.

The temporal component was explained by Giard et al. (1990) with a bilateral pair of vertically oriented dipole-like generators located in the vicinity of auditory cortex on the supratemporal plane. (MEG evidence for these supratemporal MMN generators for different types of acoustic deviations is reviewed in chapter 5.) Previously, Alho, Sams, Paavilainen, and Näätänen (1986), by using a nose reference, had observed an MMN polarity inversion between recording sites above and below the Sylvian fissure, thus providing some, but not conclusive (because of the possibly active reference electrode), evidence for a supratemporal MMN generator. An MMN-polarity inversion, in another study, is illustrated in Fig. 4.37 and 4.38.

Giard and colleagues (1990) attributed their frontocentral MMN subcomponent to frontal generators, which would be mainly located in the right hemisphere. There is also some evidence for a left-hemisphere frontal MMN generator, however. This is probably located anteriorly to the right-side generator (H. Lang, personal communication, November, 1990). Very recently, Alho, Woods, Algazi, Knight, and Näätänen (1991) found reduced MMN amplitudes in their frontal-lobe patients, supporting a generator in the frontal lobes. The reduction was more marked over the lesioned hemisphere. In contrast, the N1 and P2 amplitudes were similar in patients and controls. In addition, Woods, Knight, Scabini, and Clayworth (1991)

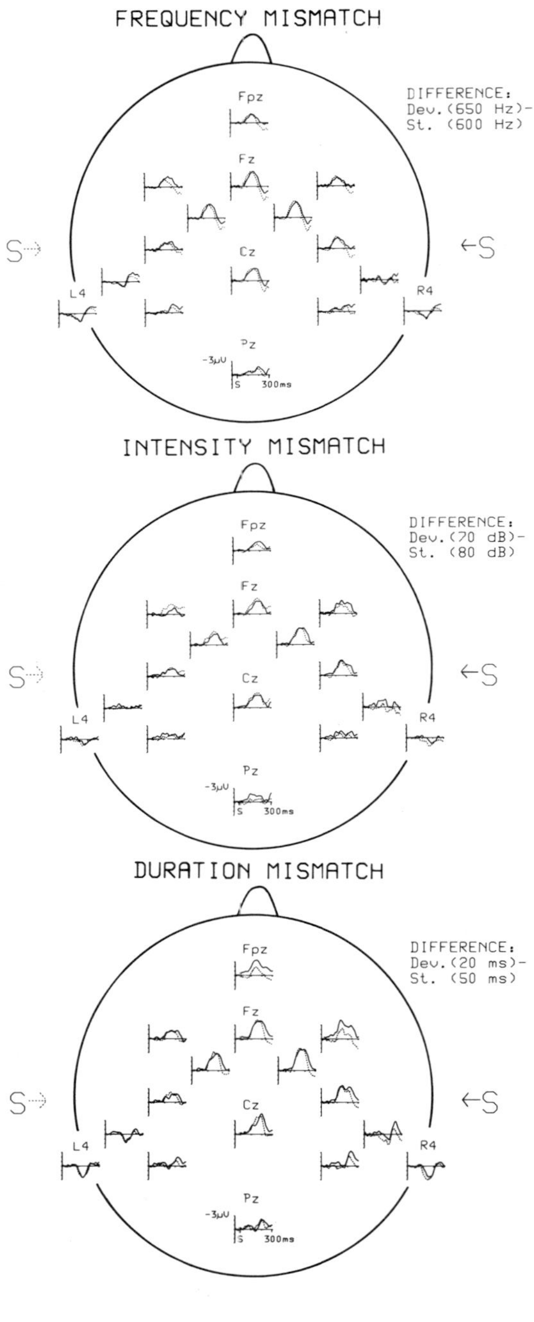

FIG. 4.37 Grand-average ERP difference waves (deviant-stimulus ERPs *minus* standard-stimulus ERPs) for frequency (top), intensity (middle), and duration (bottom) deviation. Continuous lines show results from blocks with right-ear stimulation, dashed lines results from blocks with left-ear stimulation. (From Paavilainen, Alho, Reinikainen, Sams, & Näätänen 1991. Copyright © 1991 by Elsevier Science Publishers, Ireland. Reprinted with permission.)

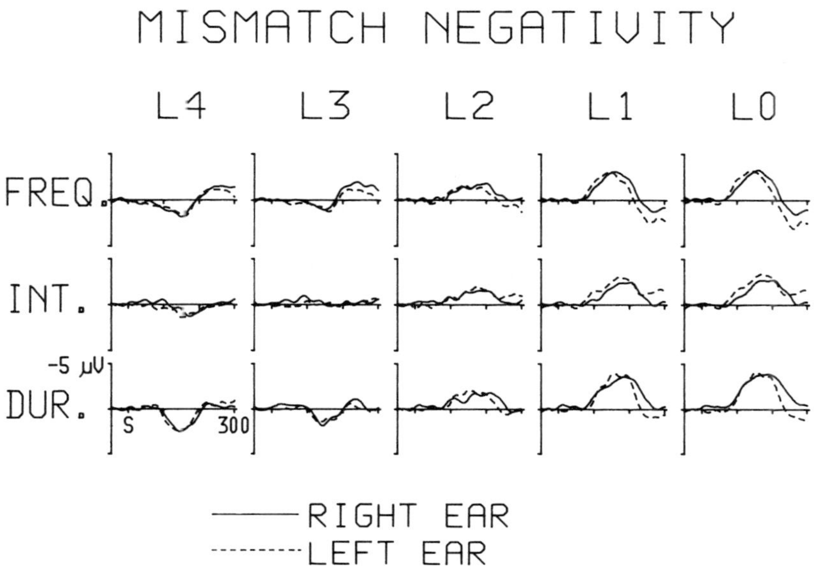

FIG. 4.38 Grand-average ERP difference waves (deviant-stimulus ERPs *minus* standard-stimulus ERPs) for frequency (top), intensity (middle), and duration (bottom) deviations at different electrodes equidistantly located along the left-hemisphere line connecting the midfrontal (Fz) site (= L0) to the mastoid (L4). Continuous lines show results from blocks with right-ear stimulation, dashed lines those from blocks with left-ear stimulation. (From Paavilainen, Alho, Reinikainen, Sams, & Näätänen, 1991. Copyright © 1991 by Elsevier Science Publishers, Ireland. Reprinted with permission.)

found that large temporal/parietal lesions that included auditory cortex reduced the N1 amplitude, particularly to stimuli contralateral to the lesion, whereas MMN was unaffected.

In explaining the right-hemispheric preponderance of their frontal MMN subcomponent, Giard et al. (1990) referred to Luria and Simernitskaya's (1977) observations suggesting a stronger involvement of the "nondominant" hemisphere in automatic information-processing tasks. In addition, patients with unilateral neglect mainly suffer from deficient automatic switching of attention, and this syndrome is more common and severe in patients with right-hemisphere than left-hemisphere lesions (see, e.g., Mesulam, 1981).

Paavilainen et al. (1991) investigated the scalp distribution of frequency, intensity, and duration MMNs. One half of the stimulus blocks were delivered to the left ear, the other half to the right ear. In agreement with Giard et al. (1990), the frequency MMN was larger over the right than left hemisphere irrespective of the ear stimulated (Fig. 4.37). The intensity and duration MMNs were also larger over the right than left hemisphere, and this asymmetry was stronger than that for the frequency MMN. In contrast,

N1 was larger over the contra- than ipsilateral hemisphere throughout the experiment.

A clear polarity inversion was found for each type of MMN (Fig. 4.37). Interestingly, this polarity inversion was strongest for the duration MMN, and stronger for the frequency than intensity MMN. Figure 4.38 shows that at site L3 along the lateral line extending from the midline (LO = Fz) to the mastoid (L4) over the left hemisphere, the duration and frequency MMNs already show some polarity reversal, whereas the intensity MMN does not. Furthermore, at L4, the polarity-reversed "MMN" for intensity is relatively much smaller than that for frequency or duration. The same pattern of data was replicated over the right hemisphere. These data might be taken as tentatively suggesting that MMNs for different auditory attributes are generated in different loci in auditory cortex.

Different generator locations for different MMNs were also suggested by Aaltonen et al.'s (in press) results with aphasic patients with a posterior lesion on the left hemisphere. These patients had a normal frequency MMN but no phonetic MMN (Fig. 4.49). These data are examined later in more detail.

Using Scherg's (1990) dipole-source analysis, Scherg, Vajsar, and Picton (1989; see also Scherg & Picton, 1990) found that their frequency-deviation difference wave was composed of two sequential but partially overlapping components, both originating from the supratemporal plane. The source of the later component was anterior, and oriented laterally, to that of the earlier component. Both components were present for a large (100%) frequency deviation, whereas a much smaller (10%) deviation elicited only the later component.

The early component, elicited only by the wide frequency deviation, was interpreted in terms of an enhancement of the supratemporal N1 generator process. The early part of the negative difference wave for the wide deviation was thus attributed to nonrefractory neurons in the N1 generator that correspond to the frequency of the deviant but not of the standard stimulus. Confirming data were obtained by Novak et al. (1990) and Lang, Nyrke, Ek, Aaltonen, Raimo, and Näätänen (1990).

Consequently, it appears that with wide frequency deviations, the response of the exogenous N1 generator is considerably enhanced, explaining a large portion of the difference wave, at least of its early part (Lang et al., 1990; Novak et al., 1990; Scherg, Vajsar, & Picton, 1989). This N1 enhancement is partially overlapped by a "genuine" MMN component which is also generated on the supratemporal plane. In addition, there is a second genuine MMN component, that generated by a frontal mechanism that is situated predominantly in the right hemisphere, explaining the MMN preponderance over the right hemisphere (Giard et al., 1990; Paavilainen et al., 1991).

When a small frequency change is used, the enhancement of the N1 component is negligible; therefore the negativity of the deviance-related difference wave is probably mainly composed of the previously mentioned "genuine" MMN components. The supratemporal component is earlier (Scherg, Vajsar, & Picton, 1989; Scherg & Picton, 1990) and larger (Giard et al., 1990; Maiste & Picton, 1987; Scherg & Picton, 1990; Scherg, Vajsar, & Picton, 1989) contralateral to stimulation, and is earlier for wider than for smaller stimulus deviations (Lang et al., 1990; Novak et al., 1990; Scherg & Picton, 1990; Scherg, Vajsar, & Picton, 1989).

MMN and ANS Responses

Lyytinen and colleagues (in press) recorded several ANS measures, such as the SCR and the heart rate, in parallel with ERPs. Subjects concentrated on solving difficult Raven-matrix problems while auditory standards and proximate deviants were presented. A good deal of these deviants, especially those at the beginning of the session or of individual stimulus blocks, elicited ANS responses in addition to MMN. Selective averaging of MMN according to whether an ANS response was elicited on a trial or not showed, however, that MMN occurs even without a concomitant SCR or heart-rate response. Furthermore, the MMN amplitude did not, in fact, depend on whether a heart-rate response was also elicited at the trial or not. These data are illustrated in Figs. 4.39 and 4.40.

Studies that try to correlate physiological responses with very different time scales are, of course, methodologically very problematic when short ISIs are used. Because of the long onset latency of an SCR, generally between 1 and 2 sec (Venables & Martin, 1967), it is often not easy to tell which stimulus elicited the response. Also, it is difficult to separate ANS responses elicited by auditory deviants from those associated with primary-task stimuli (Lyytinen et al., in press; Lyytinen & Näätänen, 1987).

Attention and MMN

As already mentioned, there exist several lines of converging evidence for the attentional independence of MMN. These lines of evidence are summarized as follows:

1. *The oddball paradigm.* MMN is even elicited by slight, threshold-level deviations in an auditory stimulus block, while the subject is intensely concentrating on reading. These deviations are hard to discriminate even when the subject is specifically asked to do this (Sams, Paavilainen, et al., 1985).

The value of such results as evidence for automatic processing can of

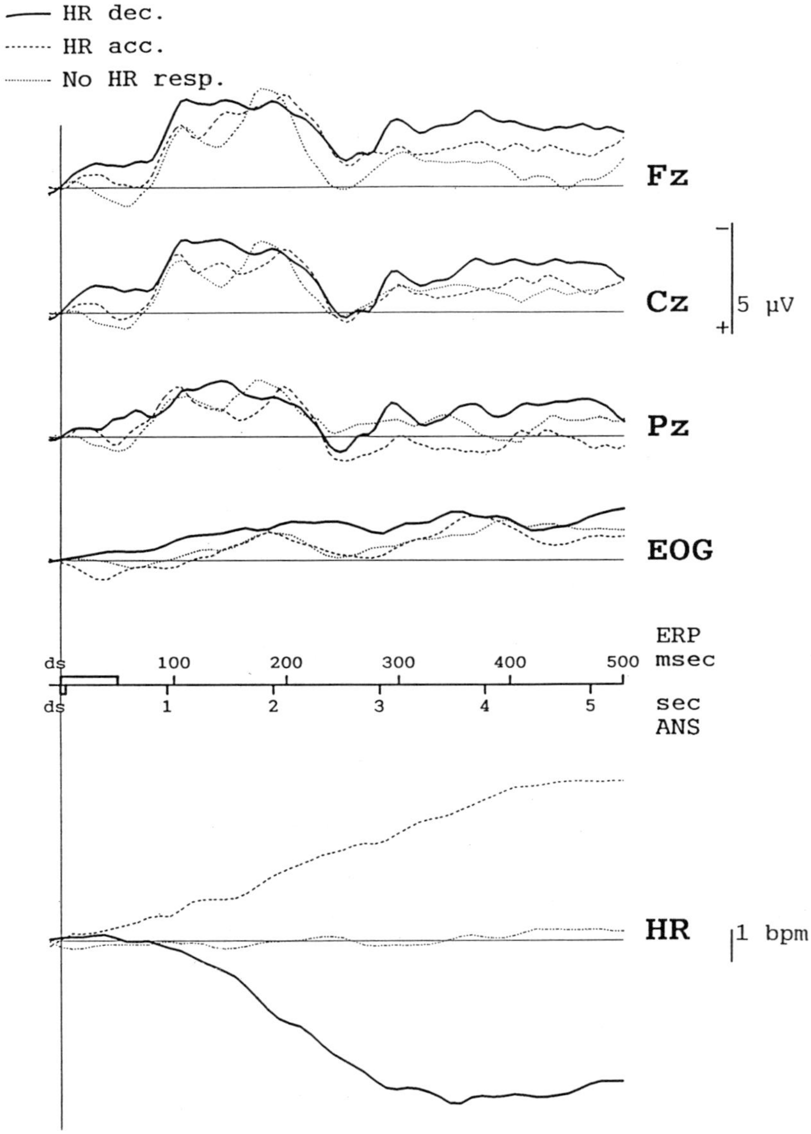

FIG. 4.39 Grand-average ERP, EOG, and heart-rate (HR) curves for pitch-deviant tones for trials classified according to the occurrence of HR deceleration (HR dec., thick line), HR acceleration (HR acc., dashed line), and no-HR response (no-HR resp., dotted line). bpm = beats per minute. Observe the different time scales of the ERP and ANS (autonomic nervous system) responses. (From Lyytinen, Blomberg, & Näätänen (in press). Copyright © in press by The Society for Psychophysiological Research. Reprinted with permission.)

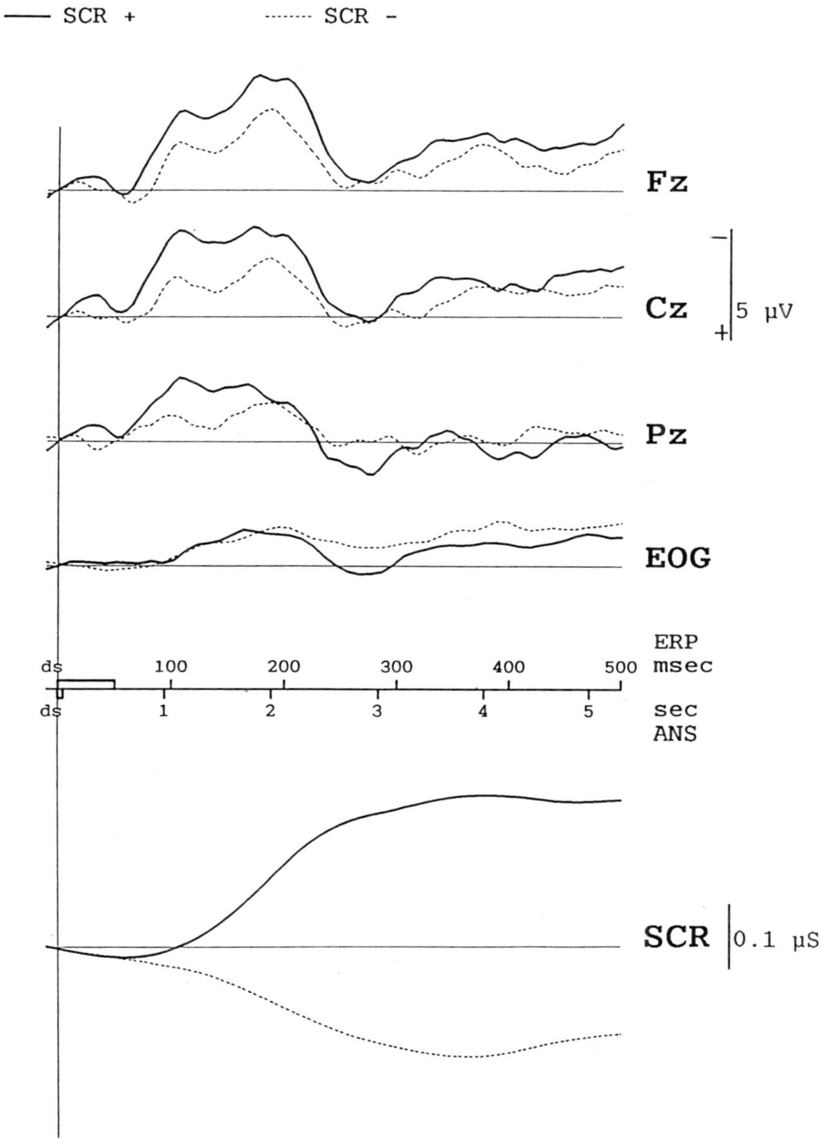

FIG. 4.40 Grand-average ERP, EOG, and skin-conductance response (SCR) curves for pitch-deviant tones for trials classified according to whether a SCR occurred (SCR +, thick line) at a trial or not (SCR −, dashed line). (From Lyytinen, Bloomberg, & Näätänen (in press). Copyright © in press by The Society for Psychophysiological Research. Reprinted with permission.)

course be questioned on the grounds of easiness of the reading task: The subject might have had some freely allocatable spare capacity to attend also to irrelevant auditory stimulation, at least occasionally (chapter 2). Duncan and Kaye's (1987) subjects, however, searched for and circled words related to a specified theme in a matrix of letters, certainly an involving task. Nevertheless, deviant stimuli elicited a well-defined MMN, quite similar to that obtained by Sams, Paavilainen, et al. (1985) in their reading condition (Fig. 4.19) with an almost identical stimulus paradigm. Duncan and Kaye's MMN was not followed by a P3a, however, whereas a distinct P3a was observed by Sams and his colleagues. This P3a might reflect a transitory attention switch to irrelevant stimulus deviation, which is probably more likely to occur with less demanding primary tasks such as reading.

Corroborating evidence was obtained by Lyytinen et al. (in press) who used a difficult problem-solving task (Raven matrices) as the primary task. In these conditions, MMN was elicited by slight frequency deviations without an accompanying P3a. Moreover, very recently, Alho, Woods, Algazi, and Näätänen (in press) found that the amplitude of the frequency MMN was not affected by the difficulty of a concurrent visual primary task (Fig. 4.41).

Hence, task-irrelevant oddball stimulation elicits MMN even when the subject is performing a highly demanding primary task. The next question is whether this MMN is enhanced by instructing the subject to discriminate deviants among standards within this oddball stimulation. Such comparisons are, unfortunately, usually contaminated by an overlapping N2b component elicited by deviants in active discrimination (Section 6.1). This N2b is small when a slightly deviant stimulus is delivered at a very low probability, however. ERPs recorded under such conditions suggest that MMN is not affected by attention (Näätänen, Sams, et al., 1983; Näätänen et al., 1982).

In anterior electrode locations, the N2b-overlap problem is reduced, because the MMN component is usually largest at these locations, whereas N2b is largest centrally (Section 6.1). In addition, MMN polarity reversal at the mastoid recordings, with the nose as reference, enables an assessment of the MMN component with no, or only very little, N2b overlap.

The results obtained with the MEG, which is blind to N2b and therefore suffers from no N2b overlap problem, also suggest that attention does not affect the MMN amplitude in oddball conditions (chapter 7).

2. *Drug effects.* Several previously reviewed studies have demonstrated differential drug effects on frequency MMN and on ERP measures (dealt with in chapter 6) that are indicative of attentive or controlled processing.

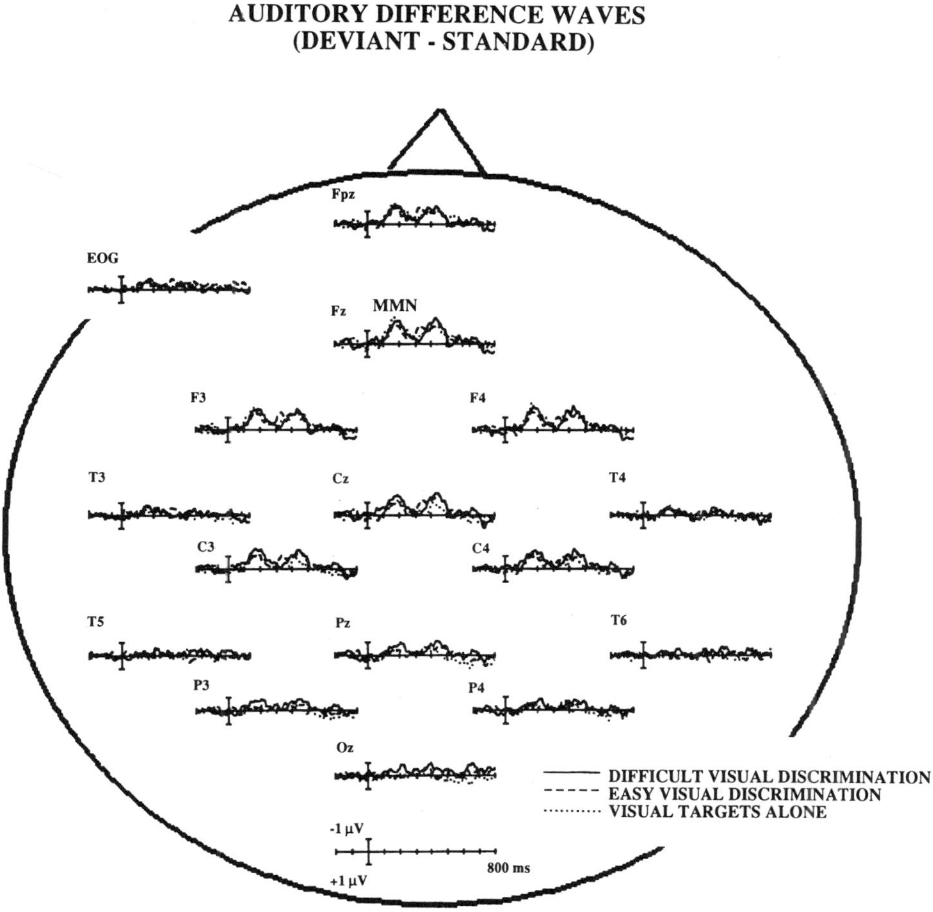

FIG. 4.41 Grand-average difference waves (deviant-stimulus *minus* standard-stimulus ERP) at different scalp sites for 1,050-Hz deviant tones occurring among 1,000-Hz standard tones during difficult (solid lines) and easy (dashed lines) visual discrimination tasks and during a visual simple-RT task where an infrequent target stimulus was presented alone with no intervening visual standard stimuli. (Adapted from Alho, Woods, Algazi, & Näätänen, in press. Copyright © in press by Elsevier Science Publishers BV [Biomedical Division]. Reprinted with permission.)

This provides further converging, though indirect, evidence for the attentional insensitivity of the frequency MMN.

3. *Memory-trace duration as a function of attention.* Complementary evidence for the MMN attentional insensitivity is provided by a very similar ISI–MMN relationship when stimuli were attended and when they were ignored (Mäntysalo & Näätänen, 1987). Thus the decay of the stimulus

representation in sensory memory, as inferred from these data, appeared not to depend on attention. This suggests that attention can, in these conditions, neither improve the quality of sensory information contained by these traces nor prolong their duration.

4. *Sleep and anesthesia.* Human and animal studies that suggest the existence of a sleep MMN were already reviewed. Moreover, MMN was elicited even in anesthesized cats.

5. *Dichotic listening.* MMNs elicited by frequency deviants within the attended and ignored inputs in dichotic stimulus presentation are very similar in amplitude and latency when a relatively slow stimulus rate is used (Näätänen et al. 1978, 1980). More recently, Alho, Sams, Paavilainen, Reinikainen, and Näätänen (1989), using a much shorter ISI (410 msec onset-to-onset), obtained corroborating evidence. A short ISI forces the subject to focus attention exclusively on relevant stimuli (Hillyard, Hink, Schwent, & Picton, 1973).

Very recently, however, Woldorff, Hackley, and Hillyard (1991) reported that when attention is very strongly focused on input to one ear, MMN is almost eliminated for intensity decrements in the input for the opposite ear (Fig. 4.42). The authors consequently interpreted their data as suggesting an early attentional suppression of sensory processing in full absence of attention. In these data, however, N2b overlap did not permit a separate measurement of the MMN component in the attended input (Näätänen, 1990).

Despite this problem, Woldorff et al. (1991) were, however, probably right in that the intensity MMN can be attenuated by withdrawal of attention. This result was corroborated by Näätänen, Paavilainen, Tiitinen, Jiang, and Alho (in press) who also used a very fast rate of stimulus presentation. The frequency MMN recorded in the very same blocks was not attenuated by withdrawal of attention, however.

In this study, both frequency and intensity deviants were presented within both dichotic input streams, with an instruction to count one type of deviant in a designated input. To avoid the N2b-overlap problem, the MMN component was also estimated by measuring the polarity-inverted "MMN" at the mastoids (with nose reference), where N2b does not reverse its polarity and is of negligible amplitude (Sams et al., 1990). In addition, ERPs to deviants of the unattended channel were compared with ERPs elicited with identical stimuli in a reading condition. The ISI used was random, with a range of 70–200 msec.

The frequency-MMN difference waves are shown in Fig. 4.43. The deviant-standard negativities were much larger for the attended than unattended channel, especially at the midline, corroborating Woldorff et al.'s (1991) results. This difference seems to be due to N2b, however, as the

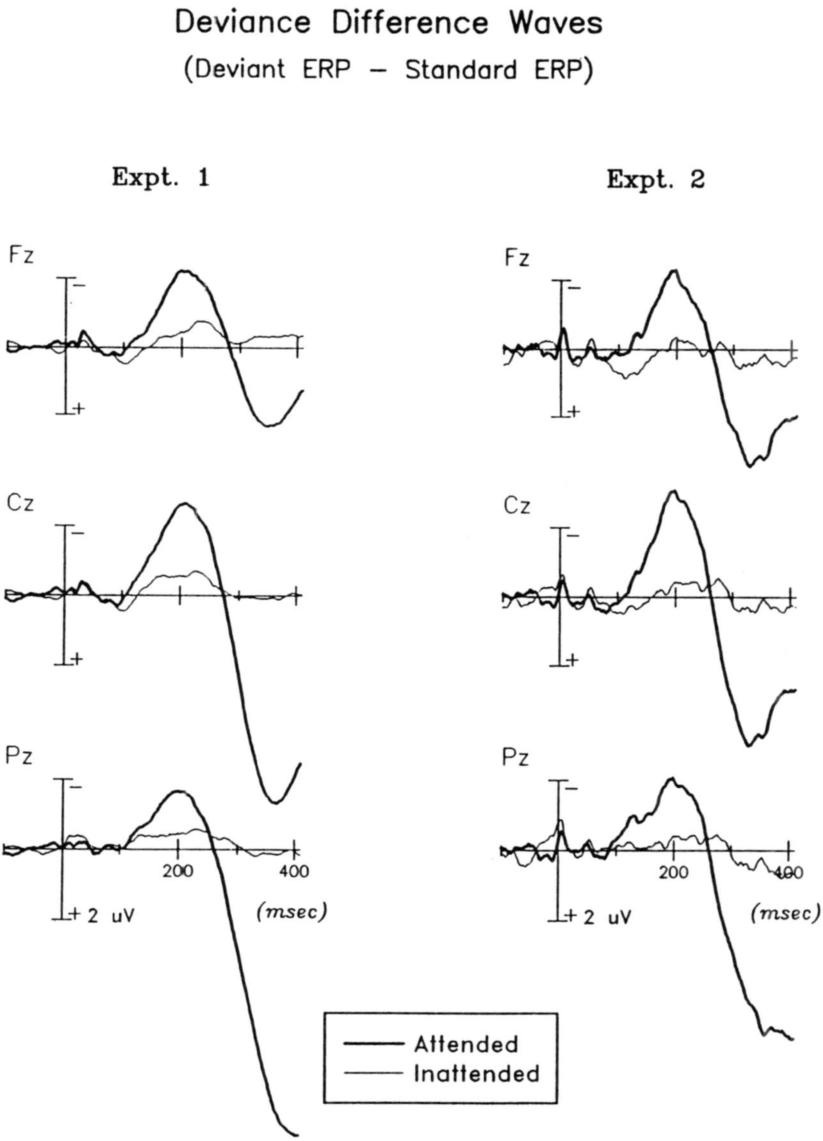

FIG. 4.42 Grand-average frontal (Fz), vertex (Cz), and parietal (Pz) ERP difference waves (deviant-stimulus ERP *minus* standard-stimulus ERP) from Experiment 1 (left column) and Experiment 2 (right column) separately for attended (thick line) and unattended (thin line) input in dichotic conditions. Deviant stimuli were slightly weaker in intensity than standard stimuli. Waveforms are collapsed across the ear of stimulation. (From Woldorff, Hackley, & Hillyard, 1991. Copyright © 1991 by The Society for Psychophysiological Research. Reprinted with permission of the publisher.)

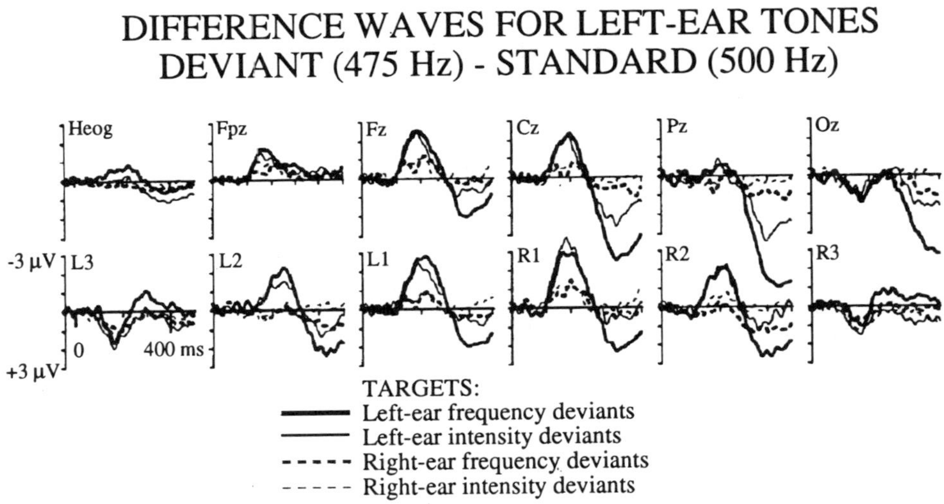

FIG. 4.43 Grand-average frequency-deviation ERP difference waves for left-ear tones at different scalp sites. The left-ear standards were 500 Hz, the right-ear standards 1,000 Hz; intensity was 80 dB SPL for both. There were two types of deviants both in the left ear (frequency deviants: 475 Hz, 80 dB; intensity deviants: 500 Hz, 70 dB) and the right ear (frequency deviants: 1,050 Hz, 80 dB; intensity deviants: 1,000 Hz, 70 dB). One of the four deviants at a time was the target to be counted. The difference waves (frequency-deviant ERP *minus* standard-stimulus ERP for the left ear) are from the different conditions as follows: (1) The left-ear frequency deviant itself as the target (thick solid line); (2) the left-ear intensity deviant as the target (thin solid line); (3) the right-ear frequency deviant as the target (thick dashed line); (4) the right-ear intensity deviant as the target (thin dashed line). (Heog refers to the horizontal EOG; L3 and R3 to left and right mastoids, respectively; L1 and L2 to equidistantly spaced electrode locations between Fz and L3 over the left hemisphere, R1 and R2 to homologous sites over the right hemisphere.) (From Näätänen, Paavilainen, Tiitinen, Jiang, & Alho, in press. Copyright © in press by The Society for Psychophysiological Research. Reprinted with permission.)

amplitude of the polarity-inverted "MMN" at the mastoids and the occiput showed no significant attention effect. The inverted MMN was quite large even in response to the "wrong" deviant in the input to the "wrong ear." It was also found that these deviants in attend conditions elicited MMN that was similar in size to that elicited while the subject was reading.

So, it indeed appears that the frequency MMN was not affected by withdrawal of attention. On the other hand, the intensity MMN was absent, or very small, in the unattended channel, corroborating Woldorff et al. (1991), and much smaller than MMN elicited by these intensity deviants in the reading condition (Fig. 4.44).

It appears, consequently, that the frequency MMN does not depend on attention, whereas the intensity MMN can indeed be modulated by attention. This difference might, however, be due to a relatively smaller, as

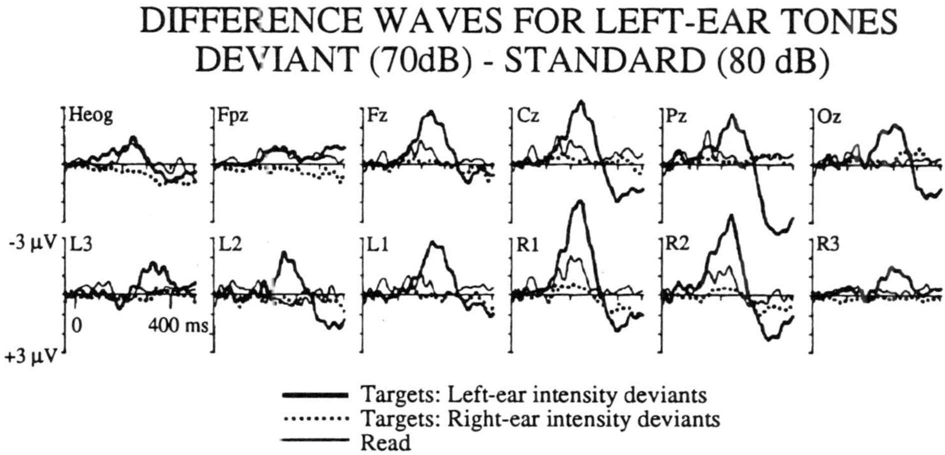

FIG. 4.44 Grand-average intensity-deviation (standards 80 dB, deviants 70 dB SPL) ERP difference waves for left-ear tones at different scalp sites from the study whose frequency-deviation data are illustrated in Fig. 4.43. Thin lines show these difference waves in a reading condition, thick lines from a condition in which the left-ear intensity deviant itself was the target, and dotted lines from a condition in which the right-ear intensity deviant was the target. (The data are from the replication blocks.) For explanation of electrode markings, see the legend of Fig. 4.43. (From Näätänen, Paavilainen, Tiitinen, Jiang, & Alho, in press. Copyright © in press by The Society for Psychophysiological Research. Reprinted with permission.)

estimated from discrimination performance, intensity than frequency deviation (see Alho, in press).

Woldorff et al. (1991) interpreted the attentional reduction of the intensity MMN as an evidence for "the attenuation or gating of processing in unattended channels at an early sensory level" (p. 41). Näätänen (1991), however, proposed that the attenuation of the intensity MMN in the absence of attention is probably due to a suppressing influence on the intensity-MMN generator process itself rather than on the antecedent sensory-analysis and -storing functions.

MMN: Possible Applications

Because MMN seems to provide a feature-specific measure of sensory analysis, storing, and discrimination, one might expect that MMN could be used for diagnostic and clinical purposes. MMN might, for example, provide a means for feature-specific testing of auditory functions in different kinds of hearing disorders. Also, MMN might enable one to estimate individual perceptual capabilities that provide the basis for auditory discriminations necessary for the understanding of spoken foreign language or for musical perception and performance. This is suggested by the strong relationship between behavioral pitch-discrimination accuracy in active conditions and the amplitude of MMN in passive conditions found by Lang et al. (1990).

Furthermore, learning effects in the form of improved discrimination accuracy might be reflected in an increased sensitivity of the MMN-generator mechanism to stimulus deviation as suggested by Näätänen, Schröger, and Paavilainen's (1991) very recent results to be reviewed later (see also Näätänen, 1990; Verleger, 1990). MMN could consequently be used for objective measurement of practice effects, that is, neural changes underlying improved accuracy of discrimination, in various kinds of performances.

Early Diagnosis of Hearing and CNS (Central Nervous System) Maturation. Alho, Sainio, et al. (1990) proposed that MMN might be used for early diagnosis of hearing dysfunction. As already mentioned, these authors found an MMN kind of response in newborns. They presented acoustic stimulus blocks, consisting of standard tones of 1000 Hz and deviant tones of 1200 Hz, to healthy full-term newborns who were in quiet slow-wave sleep.

Figure 4.45 shows that deviant stimuli elicited a large MMN type of frontocentral negativity starting at about 100 msec from stimulus onset. The figure also shows that when the intervening 1000-Hz tones were omitted without changing the ISIs between the 1200-Hz tones, the latter tones elicited a response with a clearly different midline distribution.

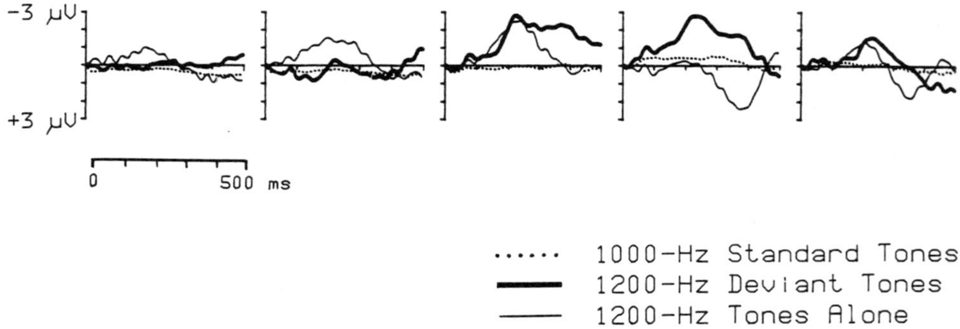

FIG. 4.45 Grand-average frontal (Fz), vertex (Cz), and parietal (Pz) ERPs of 8 healthy fullterm newborns to 1,000-Hz standard tones (dotted lines), 1,200-Hz deviant tones (thick lines), and to similarly timed 1,200-Hz tones presented with no intervening standard tones (thin lines). (Adapted from Alho, Sainio, Sajaniemi, Reinikainen, & Näätänen 1990. Copyright © 1990 by Elsevier Science Publishers, Ireland. Reprinted with permission.)

The authors concluded that if the deviant-stimulus negativity observed is indeed MMN, then this result suggests an early development of the brain mechanism involved in MMN generation. They further proposed that a possible MMN in newborns might provide a sensitive measure for an early diagnosis of cerebral dysfunction:

> As to practical applications of such a finding, the appearance of an MMN in a newborn might indicate proper cerebral processing of sensory input. Due to the complexity of the underlying generator process, the MMN might provide a sensitive measure for early diagnosis of brain dysfunction. Further, this measure might even be used to ensure adequate processing of the different auditory features critical to unhindered development of speech hearing and understanding. . . . (Alho et al., 1990, p. 154)

Kurtzberg and her colleagues (Kurtzberg, 1989; Kurtzberg, Stapells, & Wallace, 1988; Kurtzberg, Stone, & Vaughan, 1986; Kurtzberg, Vaughan, & Novak, 1986) described an ERP response, the "auditory discriminative potential," to phonetic deviation in newborns and infants of a few months in age. This was a frontally largest negativity that peaked at about 700–800 msec; it was elicited when the speech sound /da/ infrequently occurred in the sequence of frequent /ta/ sounds, or vice versa (Fig. 4.46). This negativity might be an infant analogue of the adult phonetic MMN. The authors themselves pointed to the resemblance of their negativity to

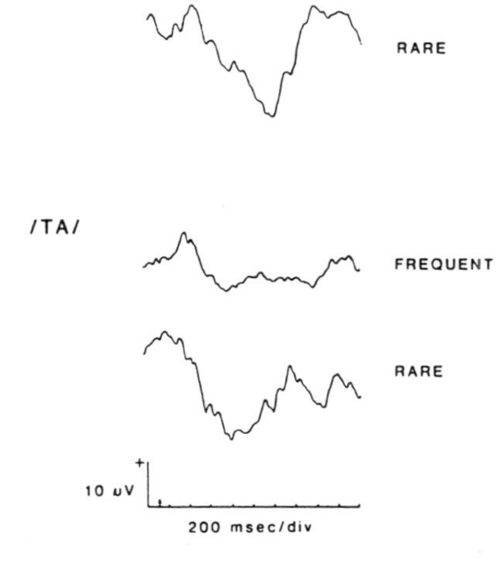

FIG. 4.46 Grand-average vertex (Cz) ERPs recorded from healthy full-term newborns to speech sounds /da/ (top) and /ta/ (bottom) when /da/ was the standard (frequent) and /ta/ the deviant stimulus (rare) or vice versa, in the oddball paradigm. Negativity downward. AEP refers to the auditory evoked potential. (From Kurtzberg 1989. Copyright © 1989 by Thieme Medical Publishers, Inc. Reprinted with permission.)

Courchesne, Ganz, and Nocia's (1981) "Nc," a frontally largest, late negativity that was elicited by infrequent visual stimuli in the oddball paradigm in 4–7-month-old infants.

Kurtzberg (1989) stated that the recording of the exogenous components and discriminative potentials "appears to be promising for predicting emerging language function in high-risk babies" (p. 258). Furthermore, Kurtzberg et al. (1988) found that their discriminative potential could provide early diagnostic information beyond that yielded by brainstem responses and the later exogenous components. The discriminative potential could only be elicited if those exogenous components were within the normal range.

According to Kurtzberg (1989), the discriminative potential is often the most robust marker of improvement in auditory processing after incoming auditory signals are amplified by means of a hearing aid. Figure 4.47 illustrates the absence of a discriminative potential in response to phonetic deviation presented without a hearing aid and the emergence of this potential when the hearing aid was installed.

Aging. Very recently, Lang and colleagues (in preparation) conducted an extensive study (138 subjects) of age effects on MMN to a frequency change recorded in a passive situation. The subjects' age varied from 20 to 82 years. No age effect was found, whereas the P3 latency, in keeping with previous studies (e.g., Goodin, Squires, Henderson, & Starr, 1978a; Emmerson, Dustman, Shearer, & Turner, 1989; Ford & Pfefferbaum, 1985; Pfefferbaum, Ford, Wenegrat, Roth, & Kopell, 1984; for a review, see Bashore, 1990), was systematically prolonged with age in a separate active oddball condition in these same subjects (Fig. 4.48). The authors were therefore able to conclude that the P3-latency increase with aging is not due to age effects on the automatic discrimination process that generates MMN but rather to age effects on some later process. This later process must be of perceptual-cognitive nature, judging from the fact that the P3 latency does not reflect response-related processes (Gopher & Donchin, 1986).

Aphasia. MMN might be useful in diagnosing aphasic patients. If deviant stimuli elicit no MMN, it might be taken as suggesting that corresponding feature-specific functions of auditory cortex are disturbed. On the other hand, if MMNs for different stimulus features are normal, it would indicate that the antecedent sensory-analysis, storing, and comparison (discriminative) functions are intact, and that the cause for aphasia must be more central. Aaltonen et al. (in press) studied aphasic patients with anterior or posterior left-hemispheric lesions (only two patients in each group). The anterior patients produced MMN to deviations in both pure tones and vowels, whereas the posterior patients showed, as already mentioned, no MMN to vowel deviation but showed a normal frequency

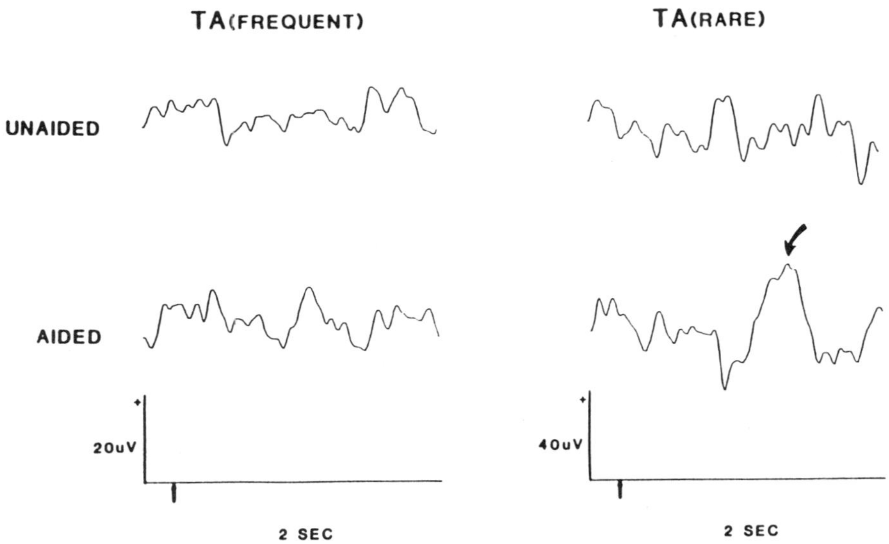

FIG. 4.47 Vertex (Cz) ERPs to speech sound /ta/ as the standard (frequent) stimulus (left) and as the deviant (rare) stimulus (right) in a 31-month old child whose click-ABR thresholds indicated a moderate to moderate-to-severe bilateral loss. (The other stimulus in both conditions was /da/.) Her unaided responses are very poorly formed, with no evidence of any kind of discriminative response. Tested with the use of her hearing aids, /ta/ presented as a deviant stimulus elicits a large positivity (at arrow) preceded by an MMN kind of negativity. (From Kurtzberg, 1989. Copyright © 1989 by Thieme Medical Publishers, Inc. Reprinted with permission.)

MMN (Fig. 4.49). Consequently, in these posterior patients, the problem appears to be at the level of sensory discrimination of phonetic stimuli or in processing even antecedent to this stage.

Diagnosis of Frontal-Lobe Patients. Alho et al.'s (1991) aforementioned tentative findings with frontal-lobe patients suggest that frontal lesions attenuate the amplitude of MMN recorded over the frontal cortex. These lesions might therefore affect the generator of the frontal MMN subcomponent, the one assumed to be involved in control of attentional direction. Consistently with this, as already mentioned, frontal lesions are usually associated with attentional disturbances (for a review, see Knight, 1990). MMN might consequently be used for diagnosing this functional damage. Moreover, MMN might help one to understand how and why the damage causes attentional impairment.

Schizophrenia. Very recent results of Shelley, Ward, Catts, Michie, Andrews, and McDonaghy (1991) showed that the MMN amplitude for duration deviation is considerably reduced in schizophrenics in comparison with controls.

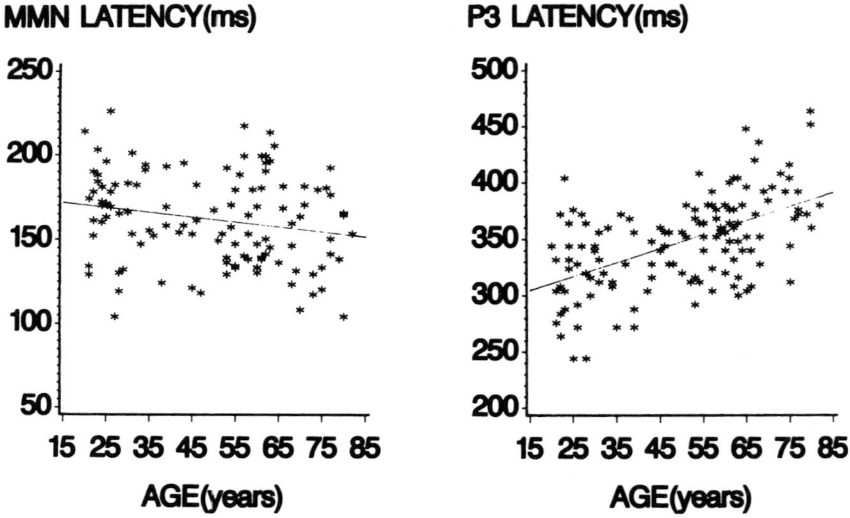

FIG. 4.48 The peak latencies of MMN at Fz (passive condition) and P3 at Pz (active condition) as a function of age, in cognitively healthy subjects. Each data point represents an individual subject. In the passive condition, the subject watching a TV program, the standard tone was 1,000 Hz and the deviant tone 1,100 Hz. In the active (discrimination) condition, the standard tone was 1,000 Hz and the deviant tone 2,000 Hz. A total of 138 persons (aged 20–82 years, 74 females and 64 males) were examined. MMN was not found in 16 cases (age range 29–65 years), P3 in 5 cases (age range 61–77 years). (From Lang, Mikola, Rinne, & Eerola, in preparation.)

MMN in Animals

Csépe and her colleagues (1987) demonstrated an animal analogue of the human MMN in the cat. These recordings were made with epidural electrodes placed over primary and secondary auditory cortices, auditory association cortex, and vertex area of freely moving cats. It was found that frequency deviants elicited a negativity that closely resembled the human MMN, but occurred at a considerably shorter latency (Fig. 4.50). As in humans (Näätänen et al., 1983), this negativity was larger with smaller probabilities.

As already mentioned, Csépe et al. (1987) found the cat MMN even in (slow-wave) sleep (see Fig. 4.51). These results were confirmed and extended by Csépe et al. (1988a) who found MMN in their epidural recordings over primary auditory cortex during slow-wave sleep and also during the low-theta (a hippocampal rhythm) phase of the paradoxical sleep. During the high-theta phase, on the other hand, no MMN, or only a very small one, was elicited.

MMN under pentobarbitol (Nembutal) anesthesia in the cat was demonstrated by Csépe et al. (1989). In wakefulness, responses to all different

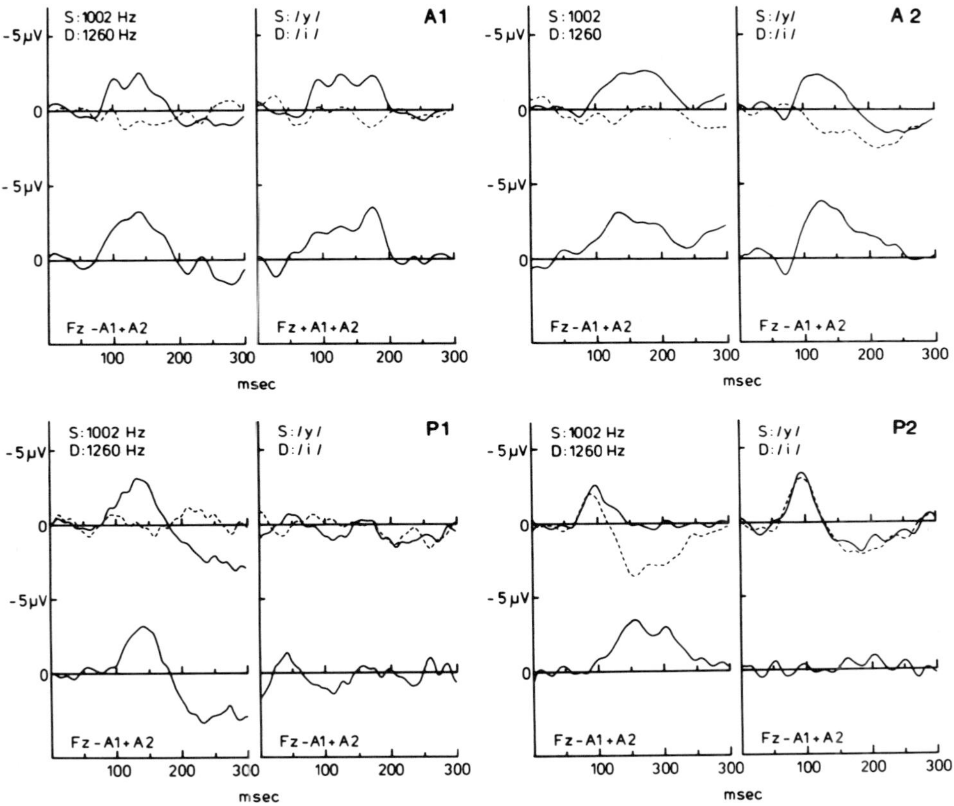

FIG. 4.49 Frontal (Fz) ERPs (rows 1 and 3) of four different patients (anterior lesions: A1, A2; posterior lesions: P1, and P2) to tone (left) and vowel (right) stimuli. ERPs to pure tones are from blocks in which the standard stimulus was 1,002 Hz and the deviant stimulus 1,260 Hz. ERPs to vowel stimuli are from blocks in which the standard stimulus was an /y/ and the deviant stimulus an /i/. ERPs to standards are presented with dotted lines, ERPs to deviants with solid lines. Rows 2 and 4 show the corresponding difference waves (the deviant-stimulus ERP *minus* the standard-stimulus ERP). (From Aaltonen, Tuomainen, Laine, & Niemi, in press. Copyright © in press by Academic Press Inc. Reprinted with permission.)

deviants started to deviate significantly from standards at a latency of about 30 msec over association cortex and at about 50 msec over the AI and AII areas. The MMN amplitude was enhanced with an increasing frequency difference but reached a plateau with a difference of 15%. Interestingly, the smaller the difference was, the larger was the cortical area (determined with recordings through 20 closely spaced electrodes arranged in the form of a matrix) showing a significant MMN.

In Nembutal anesthesia, there was no difference between responses to

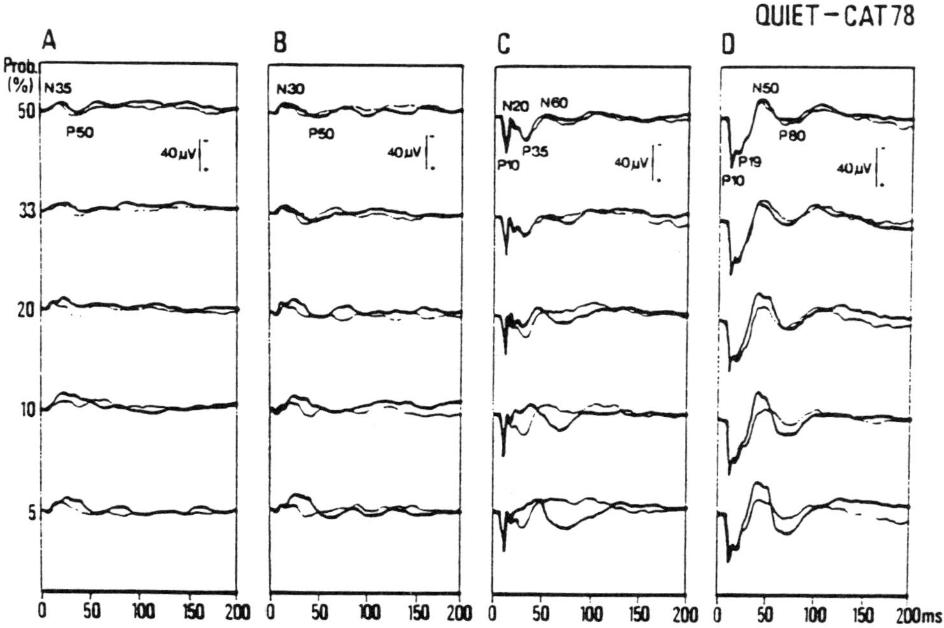

FIG. 4.50 Averaged ERPs of a cat recorded from the vertex (A), association cortex (B), and from the AI (C), and AII (D) areas of auditory cortex in wakefulness separately for blocks with different deviant-stimulus probabilities as indicated on the left. ERPs for standard stimuli (4,000 Hz) are shown with thin lines, ERPs for deviant stimuli (3,000 Hz) with thick lines. (From Csépe, Karmos, & Molnár, 1987. Copyright © 1987 by Elsevier Science Publishers, Ireland. Reprinted with permission.)

standard and deviant stimuli over association cortex. However, although the waveform of responses over primary auditory cortex became very simple, a small MMN-like negativity was elicited by deviants differing from standards by at least 10%. This statistically significant effect occurred at a short latency range at 60–70 msec.

On the basis of the differences in sensitivity to anesthesia and in onset latency observed, Csépe et al. (1989) suggested that the association-cortex and auditory-cortex MMNs might have different cerebral origins.

Csépe et al. (1988b, 1989) found early MMN kinds of effects from electrodes placed both in the medial geniculate body and hippocampus (Fig. 4.52). These MMNs corresponded in latency to the MMN recorded over nonspecific cortex, and were earlier than MMNs recorded over auditory-specific cortex. Both cortical and subcortical electrodes showed MMN also during slow-wave sleep, but only at lower deviant-stimulus probabilities and with a longer latency than in wakefulness.

Csépe et al. (1988b, 1989) concluded that the cat MMN has both cortical and subcortical (medial geniculate body) generators and, further, that

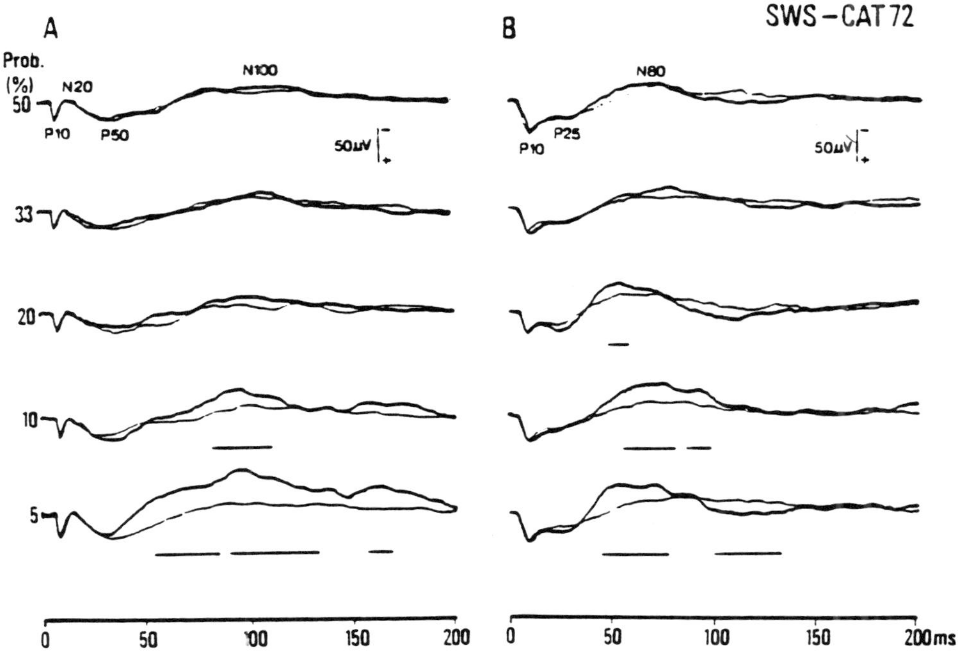

FIG. 4.51 Averaged ERPs of a cat recorded from the AI (A) and AII (B) areas of auditory cortex during slow-wave sleep (SWS) separately for blocks with different deviant-stimulus probabilities as indicated on the left. ERPs for standard stimuli (4,000 Hz) are shown with thin lines, ERPs for deviant stimuli (3,000 Hz) with thick lines. The horizontal lines drawn under the pairs of the traces show the significant ($p < .05$) differences between the two ERPs. (From Csépe, Karmos, & Molnár, 1987. Copyright © 1987 by Elsevier Science Publishers, Ireland. Reprinted with permission.)

MMN-like changes are not only generated in the sensory-specific system. In view of the different independent, or partially independent, generators of MMN kinds of waves suggested by their data, the authors proposed that "the incoming stimuli are processed in a multistage comparison way" (Csépe et al., 1989, p. 287).

It is, of course, uncertain to what extent these animal results can be generalized to humans, especially because the role of cortex in sensory processing is of considerably lesser importance in the cat than in humans. For example, frequency discrimination is still possible for the cat after bilateral ablation of the auditory cortex (Butler, Diamond, & Neff, 1957).

Very recently, as already mentioned, a monkey analogue of the human MMN was demonstrated by Javitt, Schroeder, Arezzo, and Vaughan (1991) and Javitt, Schroeder, Steinschneider, Arezzo, and Vaughan (in press). This MMN was elicited by an intensity decrement (Fig. 4.53).

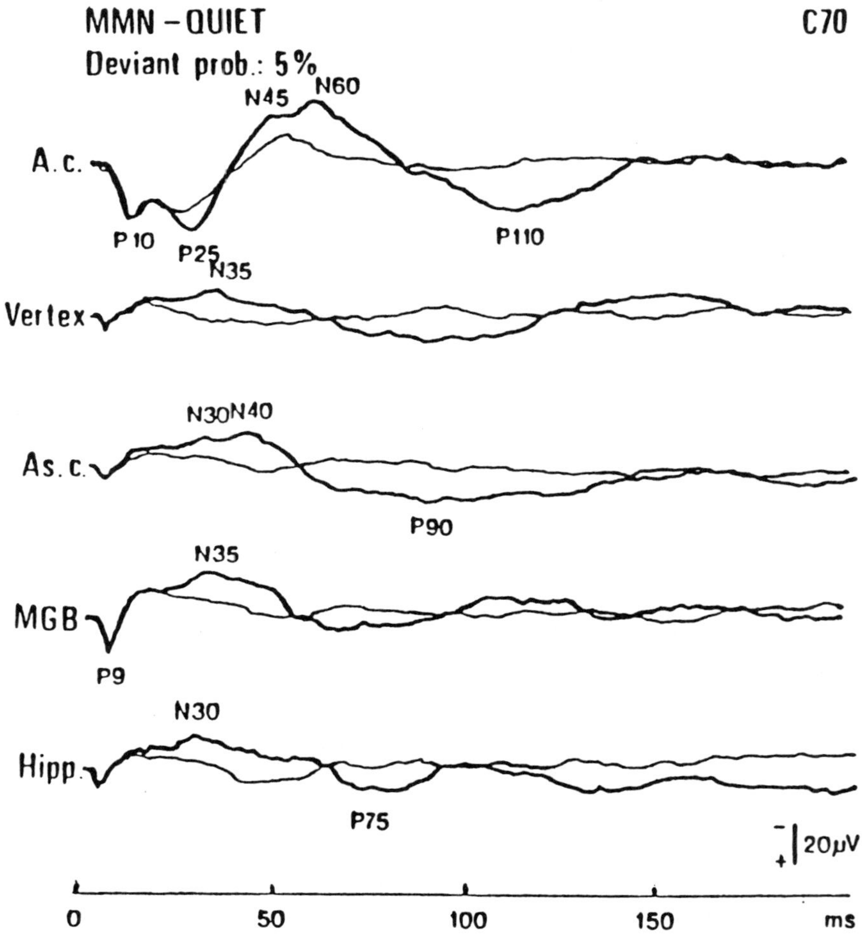

FIG. 4.52 Averaged ERPs of a cat recorded in the quiet waking state from the AII area of auditory cortex (A.c.), vertex, association cortex (As.c), medial geniculate body (MGB), and hippocampus (Hipp.) when the probability of the deviant stimulus was 5%. ERPs for standard tones (4,000 Hz) are shown with a thin line and ERPs for deviant tones (3,600 Hz) with a thick line. (From Csépe, Karmos, & Molnár, 1989. Copyright © 1989 by Springer-Verlag. Reprinted with permission.)

MMN in Other Sensory Modalities

A visual or somesthetic phenomenon analogous to the auditory MMN has not yet been satisfactorily demonstrated. Data suggesting that a visual MMN does not exist have been reported by Neville and Lawson (1987c) and Nyman et al. (1990). The latter authors' deviants differed from their standards in spatial frequency.

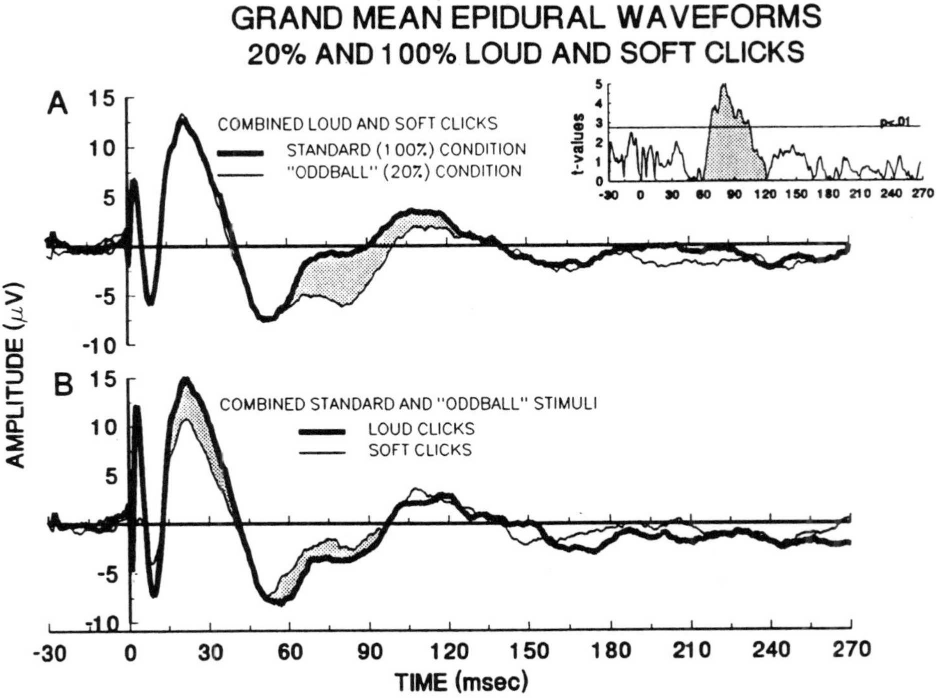

FIG. 4.53 (a) Grand-average ERP waveforms to deviant (20%; thick lines) and standard (100%; from separate blocks; thin lines) stimuli in monkeys. Standard stimuli were loud clicks and deviant stimuli were soft clicks, or vice-versa. The shaded area represents latency ranges during which paired waveforms were significantly different ($p < .01$). Inset: Paired t-tests of EP amplitude summed over 3-msec intervals for deviant versus standard stimuli. The horizontal line represents the $p < .01$ confidence level. (b) Grand-average waveforms for loud and soft clicks. The shaded areas represent latency regions during which paired waveforms were significantly different ($p < .01$). (From Javitt, Schroeder, Steinschneider, Arezzo, & Vaughan, in press. Copyright © in press by Elsevier Science Publishers, Ireland. Reprinted with permission.)

Czigler and Csibra's (1990) irrelevant stimulus was an occasional thickening of lines forming the frame inside which the standard and target configurations appeared. Subjects did not usually notice these line thickenings. These deviant stimuli elicited no MMN kind of negativity. However, when these stimuli with thicker frames were made targets, irrelevant, easily detectable deviant configurations inside the frame elicited an early negativity resembling the auditory MMN. Thus, the negativity was elicited by an irrelevant deviation in a visual stimulus whose other aspect was to be attended. This negativity seems therefore to be related to involuntary processing of stimulus deviation in vision. On the other hand, as also concluded by the authors, because of its apparent attention dependence, this negativity cannot be regarded, in the strict sense, as a visual analogue to the auditory MMN. For other related results, see Alho et al. (in press).

For a discussion on the possible existence of a visual MMN and on the proper conditions for its elicitation, see Sereno (1990) and Johnston and Hawley (1990) and, for some preliminary data suggesting a visual MMN, Cammann (1990).

As for a somatosensory MMN, some tentative evidence for its existence was provided by a very recent study of Hämäläinen et al. (in preparation). Their results are illustrated in Figs. 4.54, 4.55, and 4.56.

MMN and Memory Trace

To account for MMN to frequency deviation, Näätänen (1984) proposed that (a) some highly frequency-specific neuronal population is in a state of homogeneous inhibition at the arrival of the first stimulus (no MMN is elicited by this stimulus), unlike the afferent neurons that normally respond vigorously to the first stimulus; (b) this stimulus, at least a few repetitions of it, releases from inhibition the neurons specific to other frequencies

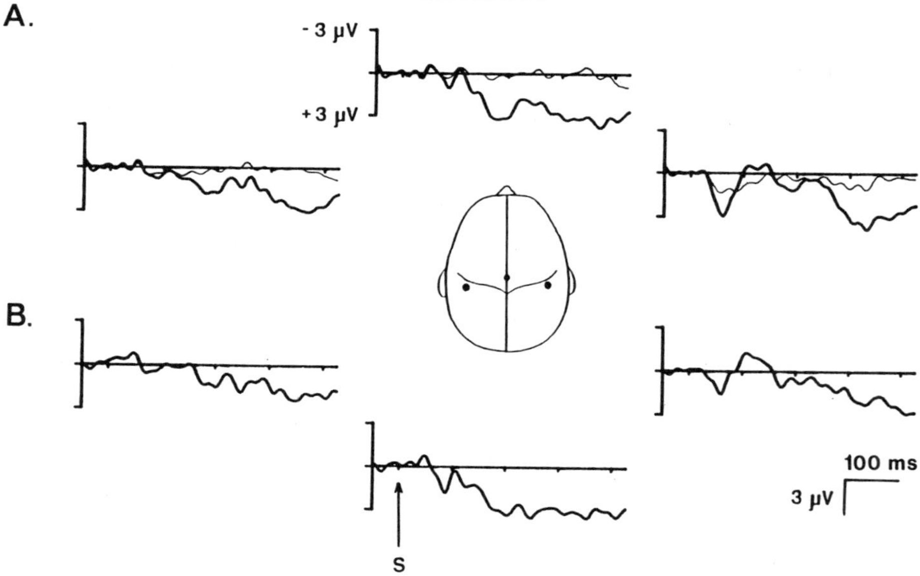

FIG. 4.54 (A) Grand-average somatosensory ERPs (four subjects) from scalp locations indicated in the inserted head to vibratory stimuli (30-Hz vibration of 300-msec duration). Standard stimuli ($p = 0.9$) were delivered to the tip of the left middle finger (thin lines) and deviant stimuli ($p = 0.1$) to the tip of the thumb of the same hand (thick lines), or vice-versa. Subjects were reading a book. (B) The corresponding difference waves. Observe the negativity in response to deviant stimuli in contralateral recordings (on the right) peaking at about 110 msec from stimulus onset, which might be a somatosensory MMN. (From Hämäläinen et al., in preparation.)

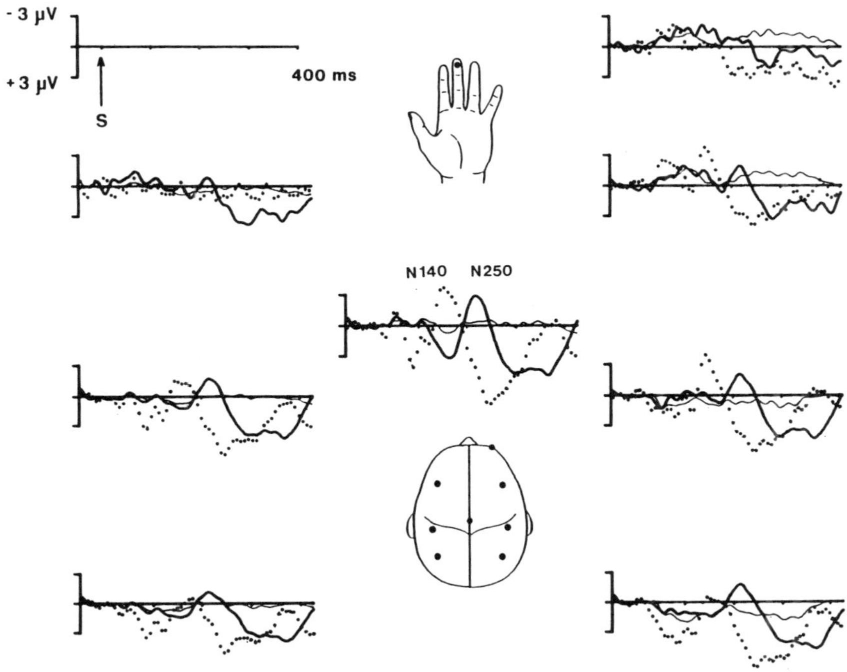

FIG. 4.55 Grand-average somatosensory ERPs (four subjects) from scalp locations indicated in the inserted head to vibratory 300-msec stimuli (30 Hz, $p = 0.9$; thin lines) and deviant stimuli (240 Hz, $p = 0.1$; thick lines). Both stimuli were delivered to the tip of the left middle finger. The dotted lines show responses to similarly timed deviant stimuli (240 Hz) when the standards were omitted. Subjects were reading a book. Notice the large N250 (N2b) deflection in response to deviants when presented among standards, and the large N140 (N1) deflection to the same stimuli when the standards were omitted. (From Hämäläinen et al., in preparation.)

(inhibition of inhibition) while neurons directly affected by this stimulus, those specific to its frequency, become refractory. This explains why the next stimulus elicits MMN if it differs from the first but does not if it does not differ; (c) repetitions of the same stimulus strengthen this stimulus-specific refractory pattern as well as increase excitability of the system for stimuli differing from this stimulus.

These suggestions are schematically illustrated in Fig. 4.57. The upper part of the figure shows the distribution of excitability of the tonotopically organized neuronal population generating the supratemporal N1 component before and after a few presentations of a tone of 1,000 Hz. The abscissa represents the locations of maximal sensitivity along the logarithmic (Romani et al., 1982) tonotopic system. The system gradually recovers in about 10–15 seconds after the cessation of stimulation. Observe the shallow form of the excitability-decrement profile.

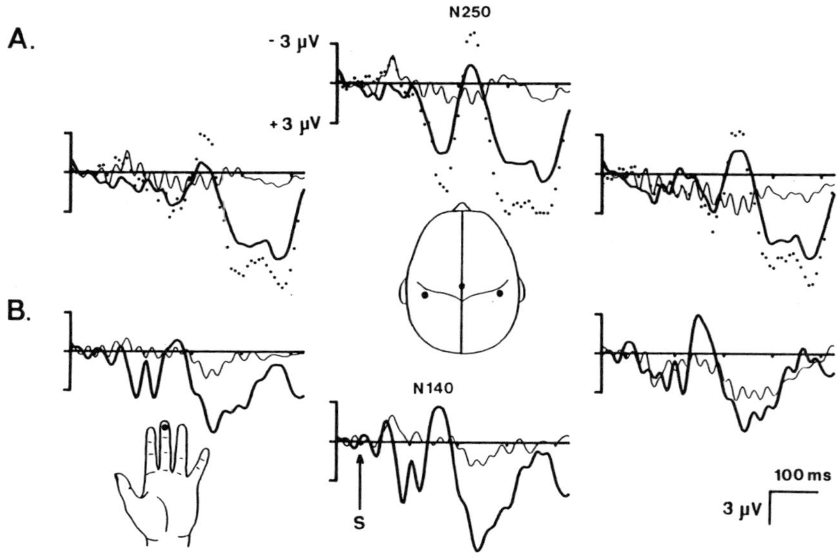

FIG. 4.56 (A) Grand-average somatosensory ERPs (two subjects) from scalp locations indicated in the inserted head to two vibratory stimuli, both lasting 300 msec, delivered to the tip of the left middle finger: deviant stimuli of 240 Hz ($p = 0.1$) and standard stimuli of 30 Hz ($p = .09$), when the subject was either counting the number of deviants (dotted lines), reading a book (thick lines), or playing a computer game with his right hand (thin lines). A control condition showed that the N250 attenuation observed with the computer game is not, at least totally, due to finger movements performed in playing the computer game. (B) The responses to similarly timed deviants, when the standards were omitted, and the subject was reading a book (thick lines) or playing a computer game (thin lines). These data suggest considerable attention "leak" to somatosensory stimuli during reading. (From Hämäläinen et al., in preparation.)

The lower part of the figure shows the distribution of excitability of MMN-generator neurons before and after a few presentations of a 1,000-Hz tone. The pre-stimulus excitability amounts to zero; therefore the first stimulus elicits no response whatever its characteristics. The first, and a couple of subsequent, stimuli, however, release the rest of the system from inhibition (lateral inhibition of inhibition), whereas the part of the system directly affected by the 1,000-Hz stimuli remains inhibited. Observe the sharp, deep profile of excitability distribution illustrating a total lack of MMN response to the 1,000-Hz stimulus. On the other hand, if a different stimulus is delivered (e.g., a tone of 1,200 Hz), a sizable MMN is generated because afferent excitation now reaches a neuronal population which is in an excitable state. As a consequence, the excitability of these neurons is reduced (but not down to the zero level by only one presentation of the deviant stimulus; see Sams et al., 1984) and that of the other neurons of the system increased (cf. Winkler et al., 1990). The previously entirely inhibited

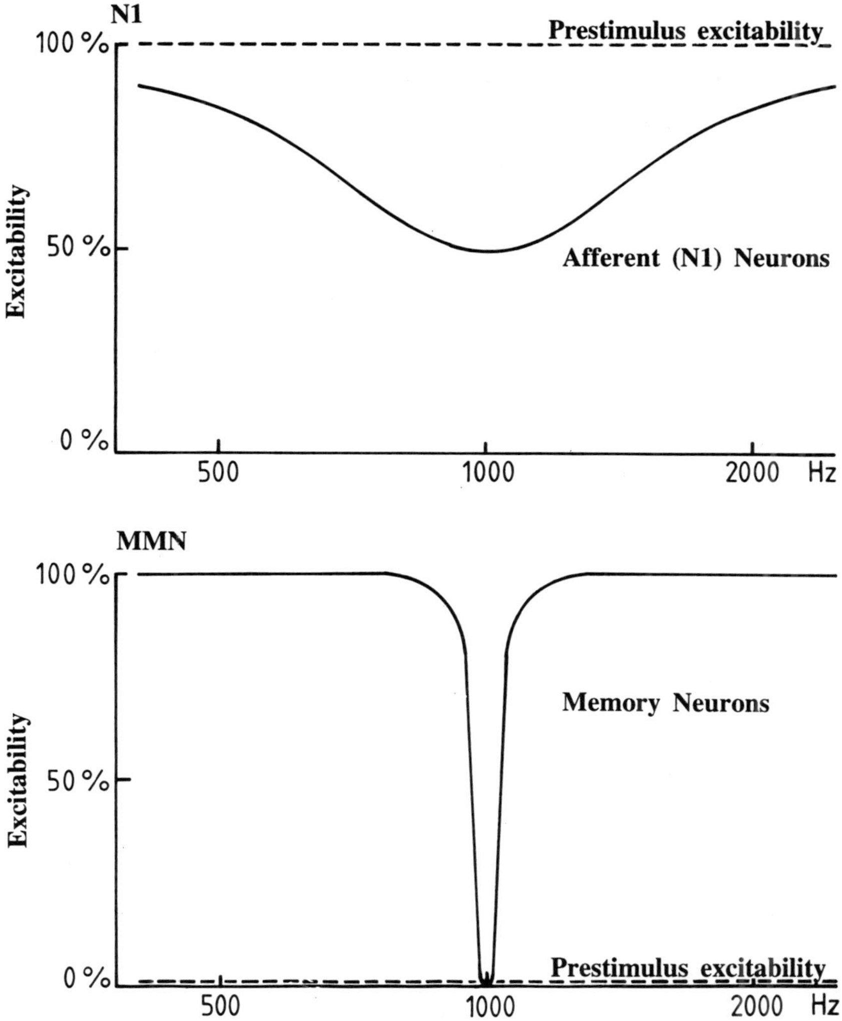

FIG. 4.57 A schematic illustration of opposite effects of auditory stimulation on the excitability of afferent and memory neurons in sensory analysis as suggested by Näätänen (1984). For details, see text. (Adapted from Näätänen, 1984. Reprinted with permission.)

neurons corresponding to the standard stimulus of 1,000 Hz now become partially excitable: a small MMN is elicited by the standard stimulus immediately after a deviant stimulus (Sams et al., 1984). Within 10–20 seconds from the cessation of stimulation, the system gradually returns to the initial pre-stimulation state of homogenous inhibition, and no MMN can be elicited by any stimulus.

Näätänen (1984) further proposed that the highly stimulus-specific pattern of the MMN mechanism suggested is the memory trace of auditory sensory memory. Interestingly, there is now some neurophysiological evidence for the model proposed. Javitt, Schroeder, Arezzo, and Vaughan (1991) found that the intensity-reduction MMN in monkeys (Javitt, Schroeder, Steinschneider, Arezzo, & Vaughan, in press) is associated with activation of pyramidal neurons in supragranular laminae of auditory cortex. These authors also found that injection of the selective NMDA receptor antagonist MK-801 abolished both the epidurally recorded MMN (following peripheral injection) and its intracortical correlate (following direct intracortical injection; Fig. 4.58). These findings suggest that NMDA receptor activation, which is controlled by the tonic level of neuronal

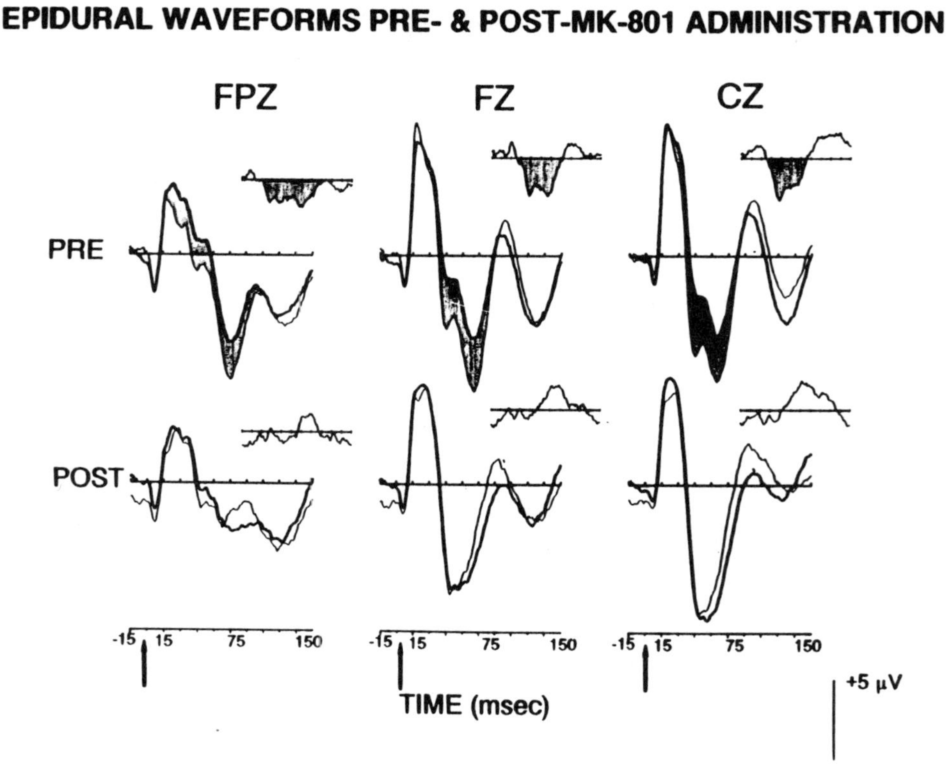

FIG. 4.58 Grand-average frontal-pole (FPZ), frontal (FZ), and vertex (CZ) ERP waveforms to soft clicks when presented as deviant stimuli (20%; thick lines) among loud clicks and when presented as standard stimuli (100%; thin lines). The upper (PRE) and lower (POST) halves of the figure show data obtained before and after MK-801 administration, respectively. Shaded regions represent MMN, which is eliminated by drug administration. Insets represent difference waveforms. (From Javitt, Schroeder, Arezzo, & Vaughan, Jr., unpublished data. Reproduced with permission.)

disinhibition, may be important for expression of the comparison process (D. Javitt, personal communication, April, 1991).

The memory system reflected by MMN data closely resembles echoic memory. Note these comparisons:

1. The system reflected by MMN contains, as does echoic memory, extensively processed sensory data, judging from the fact that even slight stimulus deviations elicit MMN, whereas repetitions of an identical stimulus do not.

2. Sensory information stored by the MMN system covers all stimulus features, even temporal, such as duration and order. Thus, strictly speaking, what is actually stored is sensory information on stimulus *events* rather than on mere static stimulus properties. This corresponds to the known properties of echoic memory and might, in fact, account for its ability to store verbal, melodic, and similar crucially time-based information.

3. Although the maximum duration of traces involved in MMN generation has not yet been established, the available results reviewed earlier (see also Section 5.1), taken together, suggest trace durations comparable to the duration of echoic memory as estimated from behavioral results (Cowan, 1984, 1988; Deutsch, 1975).

4. Echoic memory is a system with a large parallel-storing capacity (cf. Broadbent, 1958). MMN data in turn suggest that the underlying neural-trace system is able to develop at least two traces in parallel (Näätänen et al., 1978, 1980; Sams et al., 1984; Winkler et al., in press), possibly even several (Winkler et al., 1990).

5. Traces inferred from MMN data probably are attention-independent (Näätänen, 1990), just as echoic memory is described to be (Section 2.2).

6. As is the case with echoic memory (Section 2.2), the sensory-information contents of the traces of the MMN system can be outside of conscious experience. This can be inferred from MMN elicitation by a deviation in the unattended input or from the apparent simultaneous existence of traces of two or several stimuli. The contents of echoic memory can, however, enter conscious awareness, as everybody knows from everyday experience. It is probably the traces of the MMN system that provide these sensory data to conscious experience.

7. A sensory-memory representation of a stimulus can be prevented from developing by presenting an appropriate masking stimulus in close succession (Hawkins & Presson, 1986). Similar masking stimuli inserted in the MMN paradigm appear to prevent standards from developing their neural traces, as suggested by the failure of deviant stimuli to elicit MMN. This MMN attenuation or elimination was paralleled by severe deterioration of sensory memory of the standards (Winkler, Reinikainen, & Näätänen, 1991).

ERP and MEG (chapter 5) recordings suggest that this storage mechanism might be located in auditory cortex. As already mentioned, these recordings have localized, when appropriate analysis techniques have been applied, an MMN source in auditory cortex on the supratemporal plane. Neuronal traces underlying MMN generation might be located where MMN (its sensory-specific subcomponent) is generated (Näätänen, 1984, 1985, 1986b). This is supported by Paavilainen et al.'s (1991) results, which tentatively suggest that MMNs to deviations in different auditory attributes are generated in different loci of auditory cortex (Fig. 4.38).

There is one aspect of neural traces underlying MMN generation, however, that does not, as noted by Cowan, Winkler, Teder, and Näätänen (1991) seem to correspond very well to sensory memory: Even a single stimulus presentation results in sensory memory of the stimulus, whereas the trace inferred from MMN data seems to require reinforcement by corresponding sensory input before a deviant stimulus can elicit MMN (see the next section).

MMN and Long-Term Memory

In the preceding section, the comparison mechanism underlying MMN generation was described as a mechanism of a short time window only. This view holds that the current sensory input is compared with traces that depend only on very recent auditory events, those occurring up to a few seconds, maximally 15–20 sec, prior to that input (Näätänen, 1985, 1988a). The most recent results, however, might considerably widen that time window. They suggest that neural traces involved in MMN generation are, as proposed by several authors (Banquet, Smith, & Renault, 1990; Grossberg, 1990; Karmos & Csépe, 1990; Verleger, 1990), traces of a much longer duration that are only activated, rather than developed from the very beginning, by recent sensory events (cf. Cowan, 1988).

Such long-term stimulus effects on MMN generation were found by Näätänen, Schröger, and Paavilainen (1991). Following Port's (in press) suggestion, these authors used as their standard stimulus a complex spectrotemporal stimulus pattern resembling that used by Spiegel and Watson (1981). This stimulus was composed of 8 consecutive 50-msec segments of different frequencies as shown in Fig. 4.59. The deviant stimulus (10% of the stimuli) was an otherwise similar stimulus except that its sixth segment was of a higher (by 15%) frequency than the sixth segment of the standard stimulus (Fig. 4.59).

The session consisted of 3 phases, each including 6 blocks of 200 stimuli, during which subjects were reading. Each phase was followed by a discrimination test in which subjects' ability to discriminate deviants was measured.

It was found that MMN was elicited by the deviant stimulus in most subjects, at least in the later phases of the session (Fig. 4.60). This is remarkable, considering the fact that the frequency change occurred during

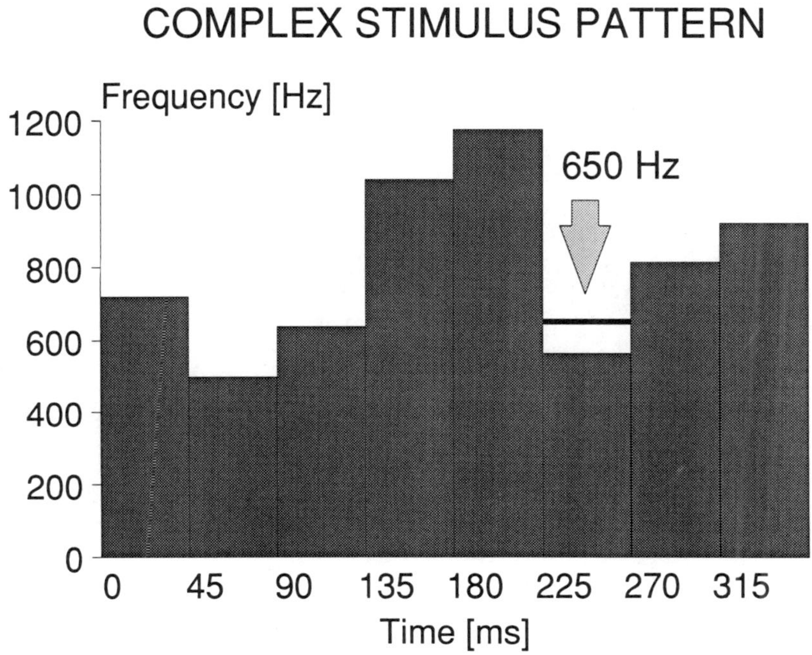

FIG. 4.59 The complex stimulus pattern used by Näätänen, Schröger, and Paavilainen (1991). The stimulus consisted of eight 50-msec segments of different frequencies. Each 50-msec segment included 5 msec rise and 5 msec fall times, so that the fall time of the previous segment overlapped with the rise time of the next segment. Thus the total stimulus duration was 365 msec. The deviant-stimulus pattern differed from the standard-stimulus pattern only by having a higher frequency sixth segment (650 Hz vs. 565 Hz). The frequency values of the segments were adapted from a 10-segment stimulus pattern used by Spiegel and Watson (1981; pattern A in their Table I, omitting, however, its 8th and 9th segments. (From Näätänen, Schröger, & Paavilainen, 1991.)

only about $\frac{1}{8}$ of the duration of the stimulus (Fig. 4.59). Further, this MMN, in general, was enhanced in amplitude and started earlier as the session progressed. There were, however, considerable individual differences in the MMN-amplitude enhancement, which seemed to be related to subjects' discrimination performance. Specifically, this enhancement occurred mainly with those subjects whose discrimination performance was initially rather poor but improved in the course of the session. In subjects with a good initial discrimination performance leaving no or only little "space" for improvement, the MMN amplitude was large already during the first phase of the session, but the latency became significantly shorter as the session progressed (Fig. 4.60).

The development of these long-term MMN effects during the course of the session appear to indicate that traces of a much longer duration than suggested by previous studies were involved. Because of the complexity of

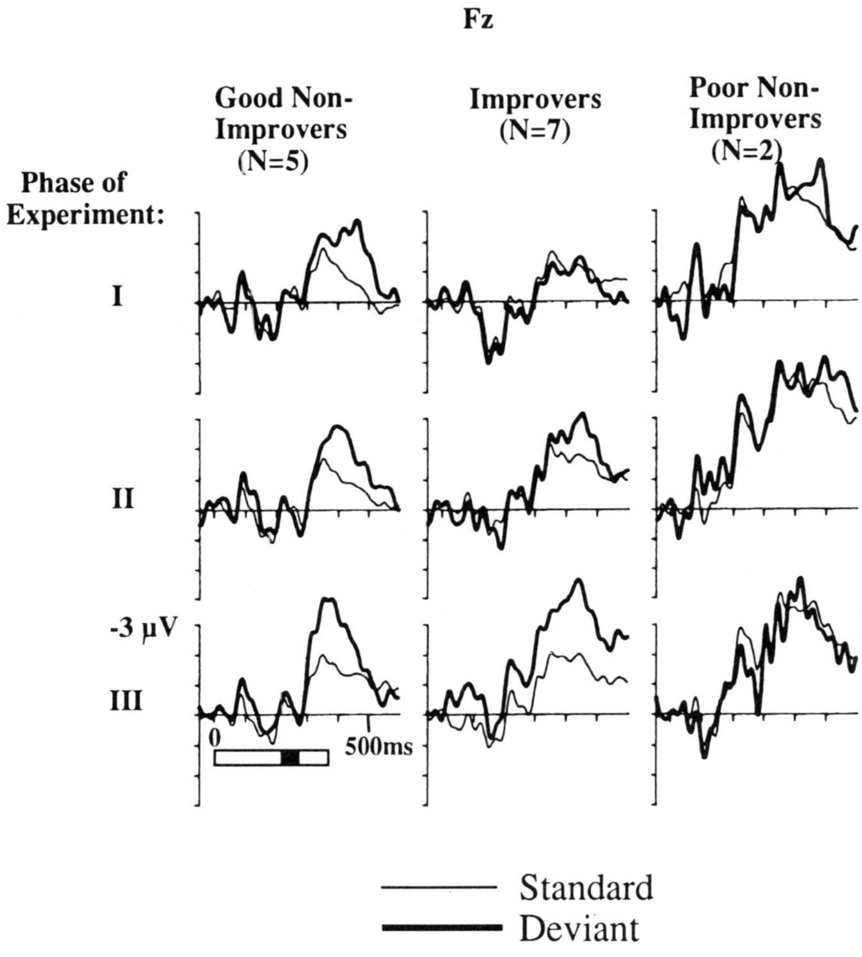

FIG. 4.60 Grand-average ERPs recorded at Fz from reading subjects to standard (thin lines) and deviant (thick lines) spectro-temporal stimulus patterns described in Fig. 4.59 in the 3 successive phases of a session (see text). In each phase, the subject was presented with 1,200 complex stimuli (90% standards, 10% deviants) in a random order. The constant onset-to-onset ISI was 975 ms. The 6th segment of the pattern (differing between standards and deviants) started at 225 msec (see bottom). After each phase, the subject's discrimination performance was tested, resulting in the formation of 3 groups of subjects. The left column shows grand-average ERPs of subjects with good initial discrimination leaving only a small space for improvement ("Good Non-Improvers"). The middle column shows grand-average ERPs of the subjects whose initial discrimination performance was less perfect but improved during the session ("Improvers"). The right column shows grand-average ERPs of the subjects whose performance remained poor throughout the session ("Poor Non-Improvers"). (From Näätänen, Schröger, & Paavilainen, 1991.)

the stimulus, the trace developing in the system initially represented probably only a rough or diffuse approximation of the spectrotemporal stimulus pattern used, but became more refined as the session progressed. This cumulative trace development continuing over a long period of time would indicate that the mechanism involved is able to store sensory information at least that long. Thus the trace that had developed, or started to develop, during the initial phase of the session in fact provided an above-zero starting point for the trace development in the later phases of the session. The qualitatively improved trace, that is, the increased accuracy of sensory information stored, apparently made it easier for the system to detect stimulus deviation against the background formed by the trace.

Consistently with this interpretation, the responses to standards and deviants remained very similar in the two subjects (Fig. 4.60, rightmost column) who initially performed very poorly in discriminating the two stimulus patterns and did not essentially improve in the course of the session. Furthermore, even their standard-stimulus response remained very large throughout the session, as if the system, because of its inability to develop a model for this complex spectrotemporal pattern, had always to treat it as a "new" stimulus.

In sum, the just-reviewed results seem to indicate that (a) a long-duration trace was gradually formed by the complex stimulus pattern (in most subjects), (b) long-term training or exposure effects occurred in the trace, and (c) this trace was involved in MMN generation.

One might, however, wonder how these long-term effects could be reconciled with results that suggest that MMN can only be elicited with relatively short ISIs in the block. This apparent conflict might be settled by assuming that (a) the system of neural representations underlying MMN generation in fact consists of long-duration traces, which (b) need to be activated strongly enough by a corresponding stimulus before MMN can be elicited by a deviant stimulus. Further, (c) if no long-term trace for a stimulus exists in the beginning of the block, several repetitions are needed before MMN can be elicited.

These predictions were very recently tested by Cowan, Winkler, Teder, and Näätänen (1991). They presented blocks of 9 standard stimuli, simple tones, of which one was randomly replaced by a deviant stimulus, a tone of a different pitch. The consecutive blocks were separated by a silent period of 11–15 sec in random and the standard stimulus of each block differed from that of the previous block. It was found that a deviant stimulus in position 4 in a block elicited MMN but failed to elicit it in position 2 (Fig. 4.61, right).

These results were complemented by data obtained from a condition in which the standard stimulus remained the same across the consecutive blocks of 9 stimuli. Now a deviant stimulus elicited a distinct MMN even

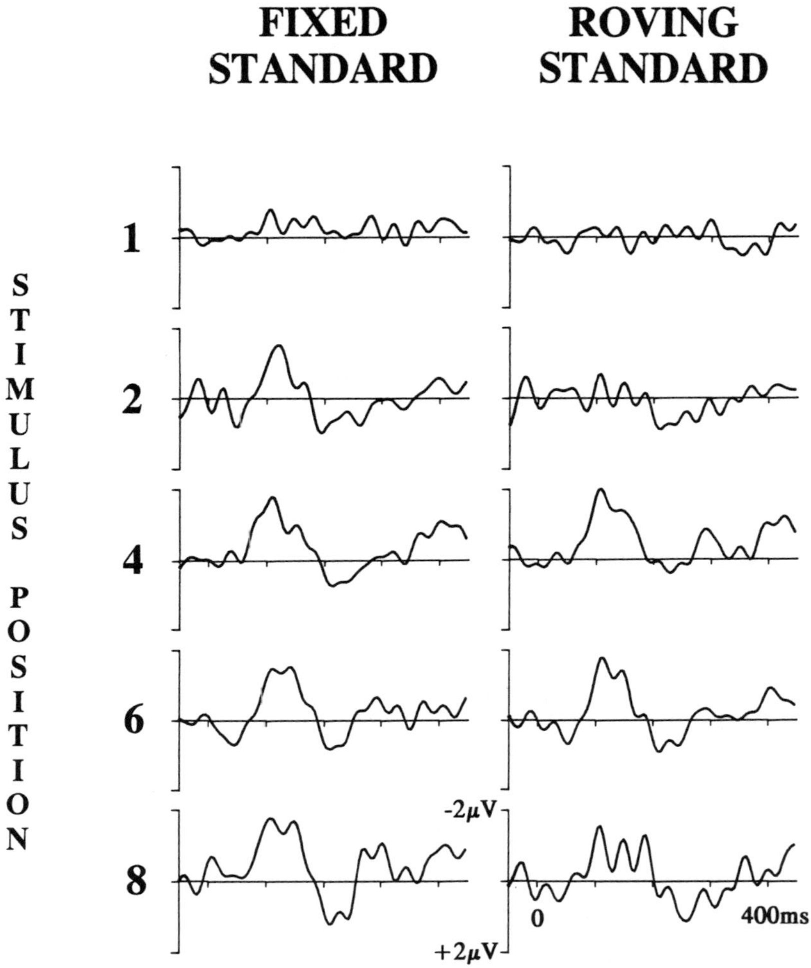

FIG. 4.61 Grand-average ERP difference waves (deviant-stimulus ERP *minus* standard-stimulus ERP) at electrode site F4 as a function of stimulus position in a block of 9 stimuli presented at onset-to-onset ISIs of 610 sec. (The silent interval between the blocks varied randomly from 11 to 15 sec.) Only one deviant stimulus occurred in each block, randomly in positions 1, 2, 4, 6, or 8. In the left are shown the difference waves of the sessions with standards that remained the same throughout the blocks. In the right are shown the difference waves of the sessions with standards which were changed between the blocks. The subject was reading during the experiment. (From Cowan, Winkler, Teder, and Näätänen, 1991.)

when presented in Position 2 (Fig. 4.61, left). This finding shows that the MMN-generation process gained from the presentation of the same standard stimulus in the preceding blocks.

A deviant stimulus presented in Position 1 elicited no MMN, however (Fig. 4.61, left), although the MMN elicitation in Position 2 suggests, as

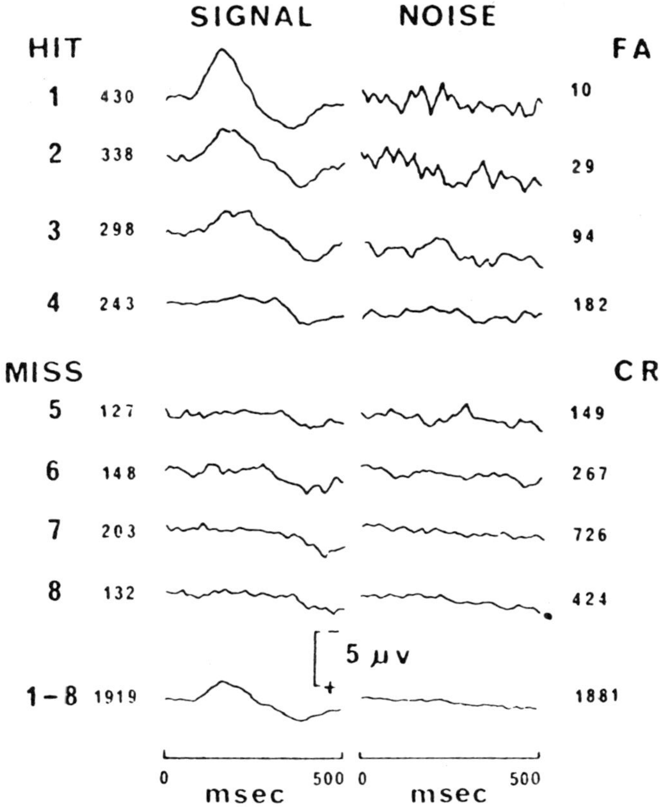

FIG. 4.62 Vertex (Cz) ERPs of one subject for each combination of confidence rating and presence/absence of a signal. The subject had to estimate whether a (threshold-level) signal was presented (probability .50) or not at a trial and to give a confidence rating for the estimate. Signal onset is at time zero in the left column. Numbers 1 to 8 at left indicate the confidence ratings in descending order. Subheadings FA and CR indicate false alarm and correct rejection, respectively. Bottom traces (1–8) show the overall average waveform across all eight ratings for trials when the signal was ("SIGNAL") or was not ("NOISE") presented. The number beside each trace indicates the number of trials included in each average. (From Squires, Hillyard, & Lindsay, 1973. Copyright © 1973 by the Psychonomic Society, Inc. Reprinted with permission.)

already mentioned, that some trace of the standard stimulus existed even at the moment of the delivery of the first stimulus in the block (Position 1). This indicates that the trace involved is a long-term trace and, further, that it needs to be activated by corresponding sensory input before the automatic deviance-detection response that generates MMN can be elicited. In addition, judging from ISI effects on MMN reviewed in the preceding, this activated phase of the trace decays in a few seconds. This would leave a passive long-term trace with an unknown decay function. These data consequently provide neurophysiological evidence for Cowan's (1988) recent suggestion that long-term and short-term memories are hierarchically organized, and that short-term memory is an activated part of the long-term storing system (see also Norman, 1968).

In sum, the results of the two studies reviewed indicate a development of new long-term stimulus representations as a function of predominant elements of auditory sensory events. Thus, MMN appears to provide a unique window to the adaptive dynamics of the system of sensory memory in humans. These changes are probably of greater adaptive significance with complex than simple stimuli. Simple stimuli such as pure tones are, presumably, accurately coded at the very first presentation; moreover, a long-term trace of a similar stimulus might well exist, due to the fact that such stimuli are relatively frequent. So, further repetitions could not improve the informational quality of the trace. (Yet they can strengthen and reactivate it, as suggested by Cowan, Winkler, Teder, and Näätänen's [1991] results.)

Consequently, with simple stimuli, there is not much space for long-term learning effects. In contrast, when complex stimuli such as Spiegel and Watson's (1981) spectrotemporal patterns are used, for most subjects, there is ample space for adaptive dynamic changes, as the initial stimulus encoding is deficient because of the complexity and unfamiliarity (lack of previous exposure) of the stimulus. It is important to realize that most auditory input that is biologically significant to an organism is of complex nature.

There might, in fact, be two basic types of adaptive modification in neural mechanisms activated by sensory input:

1. As discussed already, a long-term neural trace is formed for a stimulus occurring frequently enough. This would help in recognizing this stimulus among environmental variation as well as in detecting changes in it.
2. Receptive fields of neurons are shaped according to environmental variation; the system develops *differential* responsiveness for a new or enriched dimension of auditory variation when the exposure is continued for a certain length of time such as in a new language environment (see King & Moore, 1991). These changes of course improve the discrimination between the different stimuli exposing the system to this variation. In this adaptive modification of neural responsiveness to the new, or increasingly fine-grained, variation, neurons, which initially respond rather indiscriminatively to this variation, start to display a sharp "tuning" curve, one with a narrow maximum. In addition, these maxima for the different neurons will presumably develop to correspond to different levels of the dimension involved. In this way, the whole range of variation could become represented by the system in a fine-grained manner. Also, new neurons might be recruited to help deal with that variation.

In this manner, the system of auditory representations acquires and increases, presumably, its sensitivity to new variation. This kind of plasticity of neural mechanisms of sensory analysis might be greater with infants and young children than adults.

MMN: A Possible Expression of Extrapolatory Neural Activity

The MMN data reviewed in this chapter might in fact be interpreted as expressing a form of primitive intelligence of sensory systems. Namely, it appears possible that the sensory systems involved in storing of sensory information from the past events in fact use this information to form predictions of future events. The sensitivity of MMN to a change in temporal structure of stimulation, reviewed in the afore-going, in particular points to a possible extrapolatory nature of the neuronal population involved. According to this hypothesis, these neurons encode the repeating spatio-temporal response pattern of the system of afferent neurons and "project" it to the immediate future. Thus, for example, if a tone is repeated at constant ISIs of 1sec, then this rhythm is soon adopted by the population of extrapolatory neurons in the form of oscillatory changes replicating this rhythm in an anticipatory manner. This *time-variant* code thus forms a primitive "prediction" of the immediate sensory future. If sensory events correspond to this prediction (in this case, a stimulus occurs at its regular moment), then these extrapolatory processes are reinforced and become stronger and more accurate. In contrast, if the prediction is violated by sensory events (the stimulus is presented too early or a different stimulus is presented), then MMN is generated and the extrapolatory processes representing this prediction are weakened or terminated. At any moment of time, only a certain stimulus, or stimulus absence, would correspond to the state of the neuronal population, that is, its future-oriented code, with events deviating from this code at any instant triggering MMN.

The extrapolated events could, apparently, be also much more complex than just repetitions of the same stimulus with regular ISIs. For example, an alternation of two different stimuli at regular ISIs might also be encoded by the extrapolatory mechanism (cf. Nordby et al. 1988a). (If these two stimuli alternate in a block with irregular ISIs, however, then only the stimulus alternation is, presumably, encoded but not the ISI.) The extrapolatory function proposed might even involve such highly complicated spatio-temporal patterns as the 8-segment stimulus used in the study (Näätänen et al. 1991) described in the preceding section.

Consequently, according to the present interpretation, sensory neurons could be divided into two basic categories: (a) afferent neurons analyzing the present sensory input; (b) extrapolatory neurons forming predictions of future sensory events on the basis of repetitive spatio-temporal activation patterns of the system of afferent neurons, that are encoded in sensory memory. In this case, it would be this automatically generating prediction of sensory events rather than just a memory of past events that is continuously compared with the current sensory input.

4.5. MECHANISMS OF ATTENTION SWITCHING IN AUDITION

Besides extracting sensory information, automatic processing seems also to have, as already mentioned, a second function: causing attention switches to subjectively "silent," stimulus-specific products of automatic sensory processing. This passive-attention (James, 1890) function, already discussed in chapter 2, is, on the present hypothesis, based on automatic mechanisms which are partially separate from mechanisms of sensory-specific processing. Näätänen (1986a, 1986c, 1988a, 1990) proposed that passive attention, usually leading to conscious perception (see Libet, 1990), is based on: (a) automatic brain mechanisms with a special sensitivity to onset, offset, or change in acoustic input rather than to any specific sensory information; and (b) a high-priority access of signals ("interrupt signals") generated by these processing mechanisms to that controlling the direction of attention.

Conscious Perception of Discrete Stimuli. A discrete sound is, according to Näätänen (1986a, 1988a), consciously perceived because in addition to activating sensory-specific mechanisms encoding stimulus-specific features, the stimulus also activates separate onset-detector mechanisms. These mechanisms make, if some momentary threshold is exceeded, the preperceptual sensory data produced by the stimulus enter the limited-capacity system and therefore become, usually, consciously perceived (see also Loveless & Brunia, 1990). This threshold would depend, among other things, on the other ongoing processes and the direction and strength of the attentional focus.

On this hypothesis, specific stimulus features are analyzed by very early and fast, in part subcortical, neuronal events that are subjectively "silent." A direct access of the outcomes of all the processing of specific stimulus features occurring in parallel in the different sensory systems of the different modalities would "drown" the limited-capacity system with sensory overload. In addition, concentrated task performance, probably even sleep, would then be impossible, or at least very difficult—much more difficult than they are in reality (Näätänen, 1988a). Therefore a separate mechanism would be needed to control access of stimuli to the limited-capacity system.

Näätänen (1988a) proposed that this mechanism is expressed by the supratemporal N1 and, to a certain extent, the nonspecific N1 component. Evidence that some of the generators of the N1 wave may be involved in the control function proposed is summarized as follows (Näätänen, 1988a):

1. The N1 wave is considerably larger for longer than shorter ISIs (Section 4.3). Furthermore, this wave is especially large in response to the first stimulus in a block; its amplitude is often several times that for the second stimulus, and it attenuates thereafter, and reaches a constant amplitude rather soon. These facts roughly correspond to the subjective "obtrusiveness" of a sound when it is presented as the first stimulus of a block or at long ISIs. The strong response from N1 generators might also account for the fact that stimuli delivered at long ISIs to the "unattended" ear while listening to the opposite-ear input tend to catch our attention (Broadbent, 1982; Donald & Nugent, 1986; Newstead & Dennis, 1979).

2. The detection of threshold-level auditory stimuli strongly correlates with the N1 amplitude (Mast & Watson, 1968; Parasuraman & Beatty, 1980; Parasuraman et al., 1982; K. Squires, Hillyard, & Lindsay, 1973; K. Squires, Squires, & Hillyard, 1975). Such data, from the study of K. Squires et al. (1975), are illustrated in Fig. 4.62.

3. The N1 amplitude seems to be related to no other, more specific aspect of perception than to mere detection. As already reviewed, a dissociation between the N1 amplitude and (subjective) loudness as well as pitch has been demonstrated in several ways. In the same vein, Davis and Zerlin (1966) proposed that the mechanisms generating the N1 potential "do not lie on the direct path, so to speak, to psychological sensation but rather on a parallel path with other functions." (p. 116). See also Walter (1964).

4. N1 is especially sensitive to transient aspects (Gersuni, 1971; Graham, 1979; MacMillan, 1973) of stimulation, that is, to energy change per unit time, determined by intensity and rise/fall time (Loveless, 1983; Loveless & Brunia, 1990; Näätänen & Picton, 1987). Thus both stimulus onset and the offset of a long-duration stimulus elicit N1. These N1 amplitudes are also larger with shorter rise (onset N1) and fall (offset N1) times (Davis & Zerlin, 1966; Pfefferbaum et al., 1971). In addition, N1 reaches its maximum amplitude at a duration of 30–50 msec (Kodera et al., 1979; Onishi & Davis, 1968), whereas loudness summation lasts for a considerably longer time (Scharf & Houtsma, 1986). Moreover, the duration of the N1 component is not prolonged by prolonging the stimulus (in contrast to the sustained potential reviewed in Section 4.3).

5. Very similar N1 responses are elicited by a wide variety of acoustic stimuli such as clicks, tones, speech, and animal sounds (Gaillard & Lawson, 1984; Woods & Elmasian, 1986) when transient aspects of the stimuli are carefully controlled. Moreover, different kinds of auditory

stimuli elicit magnetic N1 responses with very similar sources in the supratemporal cortex (Hari et al., 1987). There is, however, MEG evidence also for stimulus-specific elements in the supratemporal N1 generator (Section 5.1.). Comparable ERP evidence, reviewed in section 6.2, also exists.

6. Stimulus-specific refractoriness of N1 established in several studies (Section 4.3) also suggests considerable stimulus-specificity, at least in a great deal of the neuronal population involved in the generation of the supratemporal N1 component. Hence that generator mechanism includes different stimulus-specific neuronal populations. This enables the system to generate an attention-trigger signal even when a continuous stimulus changes, for instance, in frequency, with no accompanying intensity change (Section 4.3).

7. N1 is reduced in sleep and disappears at Stage 4 (Section 4.3). This parallels the reduced obtrusiveness of discrete auditory stimuli during sleep, which is consistent with behavioral data and important for maintaining the sleep state.

Giard, Perrin, and Echallier's (1991) aforementioned recent results, however, show that the supratemporal N1 component is accompanied by a frontal component at a similar latency. This finding is illustrated in Fig. 4.63. These authors suggested that the generators of the frontal component, rather than those of the supratemporal component, might underlie the call-for-attention/conscious-perception function attributed by Näätänen (1986a) to the supratemporal component. However, it is also possible that the two components are jointly involved in the function proposed.

In addition, as already mentioned, the nonspecific component of the N1 wave might have a role in attention switching (Näätänen, 1988a; Näätänen & Gaillard, 1983; Näätänen & Picton, 1987; see also Loveless & Brunia, 1990; Verbaten, 1990). This component appears to be associated with a wide-spread transient arousal burst elicited by the stimulus. This arousal burst, or the activation of the generator mechanism of the component itself, together with the associated proprioceptive and other internal feedback, probably also subserves attention-switching to the eliciting stimulus. Because of the relatively slow recovery of this mechanism (Section 4.3), however, it cannot, presumably, operate with short ISIs.

It is also possible that the low-amplitude, transient, oscillatory 40-Hz response to stimulus onset mentioned in Section 4.2 (Bressler, 1990; Makeig, 1990; Makeig & Galambos, 1989a; Pantev, Makeig, Hoke, Galambos, Hampson, & Gallen, 1991) is generated by an attention-trigger mechanism with a function similar to that suggested for the previously discussed N1 components. Moreover, the event-related perturbation of the steady-state response (SSR) to 40-Hz stimulation (Makeig & Galambos,

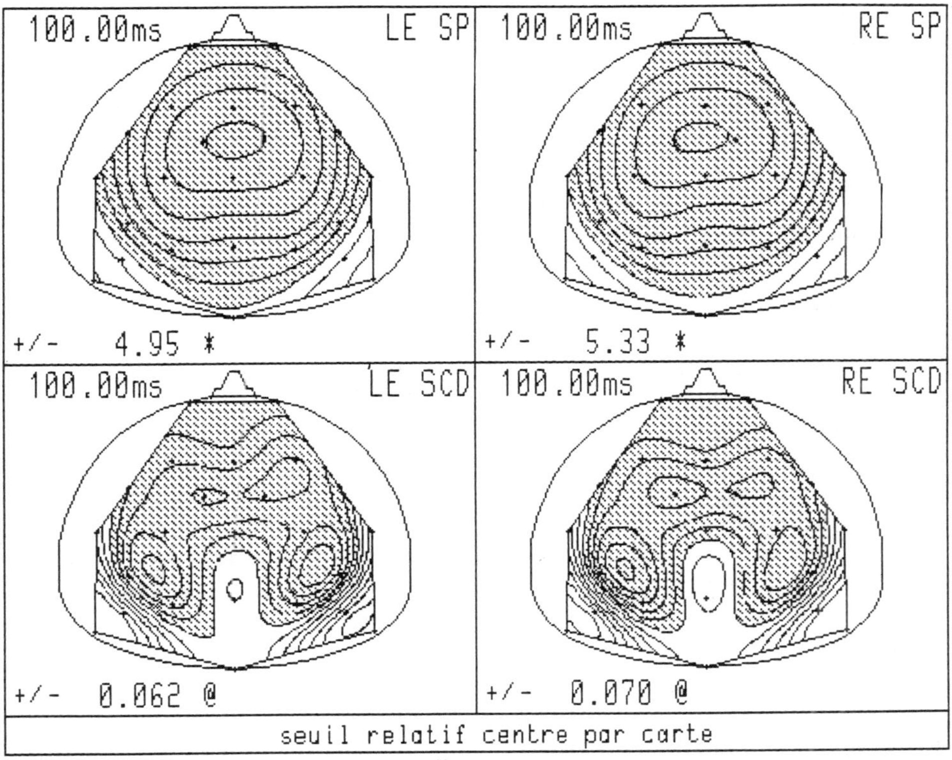

FIG. 4.63 *TOP:* Isopotential (SP) N1 maps for left-ear (LE) and right-ear (RE) standard tones of 1,000 Hz (intensity 70 dB HL, duration 50 msec including 10 msec rise-time) at the latency of 100 msec. The probability of the standard tones was 85% and that of deviant tones (1,100 Hz) was 15%. Stimuli were presented at constant ISIs of 1 sec in blocks of 20–25 stimuli. The break between the consecutive blocks was 1–2 min. The subject was reading a book during auditory stimulation. *BOTTOM:* Corresponding scalp current density (SCD) maps at the same latency. (Adapted from Giard, Perrin, & Echallier, 1991)

1989b; Rohrbaugh et al., 1989, 1990, 1991) examined in Section 4.2 might be related to the activation of the attention-trigger mechanism suggested.

The hypothesis of a stimulus-driven attention-trigger mechanism might also explain, according to Näätänen (1988a), why parallel monitoring for threshold-level stimuli from several different possible stimulus sources is as efficient as monitoring only one stimulus source at a time, provided that there is no overlap between stimuli or between one stimulus and a response to another stimulus (Moray, 1975; Shiffrin, 1975; Shiffrin & Grantham, 1974; Shiffrin, McKay, & Shaffer, 1976; Shiffrin, Pisoni, & Castaneda-Mendez, 1974; Sorkin & Pohlmann, 1973). For instance, Shiffrin and Grantham's (1974) subjects were as able to monitor three different sensory modalities (vision, audition, and touch) in parallel for the presence of a threshold-level stimulus as they were able to monitor for such a stimulus within one modality at a time. Such results have usually been interpreted in terms of active scanning by a limited-capacity device (see Broadbent, 1982). The present interpretation emphasizes a passive, stimulus-driven, attentional switch, instead of an active scanning. The attention-switch interpretation avoids the problem posed to active scanning by the lack of deterioration in detection accuracy. This deterioration could be expected to occur when a limited-capacity system has to monitor multiple parallel stimulus sources instead of only one.

Conscious Perception of Change in Continuous Stimulation. In reality, acoustic stimulation (e.g., speech) is often continuous rather than discrete, with changes occurring with no preceding "empty" intervals. A possible involvement of the supratemporal N1-generator activation in the chain of processes leading to conscious perception of these changes was suggested in the preceding text. As already reviewed (see Fig. 4.9), even minor frequency changes in a continuous tone elicit large N1 types of waves (Clynes, 1969; Kohn, Lifshitz, & Litchfield, 1978, 1980; Mäkelä, Hari, & Linnankivi, 1987; Näätänen et al., 1987a; Spoor et al., 1969). Thus, N1 is elicited by a merely qualitative change in a continuous stimulus. This can be accounted for by the change making the stimulus activate a new, or partially new, set of neurons in supratemporal auditory cortex (cf. the stimulus-specificity of this N1 generator already discussed). This phenomenon might be related to the event-related SSR perturbation examined in Section 4.2.

Conscious Perception of Change in Discrete Stimulation. Involuntary attention switches to physical stimulus changes, which did not occur to semantic stimulus changes, have been reported in numerous behavioral studies (Cherry, 1953; Lawson, 1966; Moray & O'Brien, 1967; Treisman, 1960; Treisman & Geffen, 1967; Treisman & Riley, 1969; Zelnicker, Rattock, & Medem, 1974). Such attention shifts can, presumably, be explained via the physical stimulus change automatically activating the MMN generator mechanism.

The evidence for the role of the MMN mechanism in these involuntary attention switches may be summarized as follows:

1. In agreement with the afore-mentioned results according to which physical but not semantic changes caused involuntary attention switches, MMN is elicited by physical but not semantic changes;
2. MMN tends to be followed by P3a (Section 4.4), a positive component that is surmised to signal attention switch (Näätänen et al., 1982; Snyder & Hillyard, 1976; N. Squires, Squires, & Hillyard, 1975). This P3a interpre-

tation is supported by results that show that when the primary task is very attention-demanding, MMN tends to occur with no concomitant P3a (Duncan & Kaye, 1987; Lyytinen et al., in press), whereas in easier primary tasks, such as reading, MMN of a similar size is usually followed by P3a (Sams, Paavilainen, et al., 1985a; see Section 4.4). Furthermore, P3a tends to be larger when MMN is larger and earlier (for instance, with wider deviations), that is, usually when stimulus deviation is more obtrusive.

3. Näätänen, Paavilainen, Alho, et al. (1989), however, found a much larger P3a to intensity increments than to equivalent intensity decrements, whereas these deviations elicited MMN of a very similar amplitude (Section 4.4). These data also suggest that P3a is associated with attention switch, as intensity increments were subjectively much more attention-catching than intensity decrements. The greater obtrusiveness of intensity increments probably resulted from intensity effects on N1 generators. As already mentioned, these generators were much more strongly activated by intensity increments than decrements. Therefore the attention-switch signal generated by the transient-detector system (stimulus onset) was, presumably, much stronger for intensity increments (while the attention-switch signal provided by the MMN-generator mechanism was equally strong for intensity increments and decrements).

4. Results from the active oddball condition suggest that the MMN-generator probably initiates the sequence of brain processes that leads to conscious discrimination of stimulus deviation and to the designated behavioral response. In one of these studies, Novak et al. (1990) showed that the late endogeneous sequence of ERP components and the RT are time-locked to the MMN occurrence. Furthermore, Lang et al. (1990) found a close relation between the subject's accuracy in behavioral discrimination of frequency change and the amplitude of MMN elicited by this change (Section 6.1).

Consequently, it appears that the preconscious discrimination of stimulus change generating MMN initiates the sequence of brain events leading to a conscious discrimination of this stimulus change. This seems to be the case both in active and passive conditions. Obviously, if MMN is indeed associated with preconscious discrimination, then the subcomponent involved would be the sensory-specific one. The frontal subcomponent of MMN (Giard et al., 1990) might in turn represent the next step, a "call" from the preattentive mechanisms to focal attention (Öhman, 1979; see also Öhman, in press) caused by the stimulus change (Giard et al., 1990; Näätänen & Michie, 1979a).

MMN and the Neuronal-Mismatch Process of the Orienting-Response Theory. Obviously, the process generating the sensory-specific subcomponent of MMN resembles the neuronal-mismatch process postulated by

Sokolov (1963, 1975) to account for the cerebral initiation of the orienting response (OR) (Section 2.6), although there are some important differences, too (Näätänen, 1984, 1986a). The MMN generator process indeed seems to provide the first cerebral event in OR initiation to physical stimulus change when stimuli are not delivered at ISIs too long for MMN elicitation. The cerebral mechanisms initiating the sequence of brain processes leading to an OR in the beginning of the stimulus sequence (the "initial OR"; O'Gorman, 1979), and to stimulus change when ISIs are very long, appear to differ from the OR initiation based on the activation of the MMN generator mechanism (Näätänen, 1986a; Näätänen & Gaillard, 1983; Näätänen & Lyytinen, 1989). In the case of the initial OR, the generator mechanism of the nonspecific N1 is probably involved (Kenemans, Verbaten, Roelofs, & Slangen, 1989; Näätänen, 1986a; Näätänen & Gaillard, 1983; Verbaten, 1990). For ORs to stimulus change in long-ISI blocks, see Näätänen (1986a).

4.6. AROUSAL PROVIDED BY AUTOMATIC PROCESSING IN AUDITION

In addition to its informational and attentional (attention-switching) aspects, automatic processing, depending on the physical features and timing of stimuli, may also cause a transitory increase in arousal (see Posner et al., 1976; Sanders, 1975). The mechanism of this effect is probably to a great extent based on the generator process of the nonspecific component of the N1 wave discussed in Section 4.3. The discharge of the neuronal population underlying the nonspecific component appears to trigger a widespread transitory arousal burst, facilitating sensory and, in particular, motor responses to the stimulus, probably also central integrative functions (Näätänen & Picton, 1987; Loveless & Brunia, 1990). This is supported, among other things, by the result that an auditory stimulus presented with long ISIs causes an increase in spinal excitability with a time course resembling that of the N1 wave (Fruhstorfer, Järvilehto, Lumio, & Soveri, 1970; Rossignol & Jones, 1976; Semjen, Bonnet, & Requin, 1973). This phenomenon is illustrated in Fig. 4.64.

As already mentioned, it has been proposed that the vigorous OR to the first stimulus in a sequence, the initial OR (O'Gorman, 1979), might be initiated by the cerebral mechanism generating the nonspecific N1 component (Näätänen & Gaillard, 1983). Consistently with this, the refractory period of this generator mechanism is very long but the response is strong when fully recovered (Section 4.3).

There are considerable cross-modal refractory influences on the nonspecific N1 component (Davis et al., 1972; Walter, 1964), suggesting that the

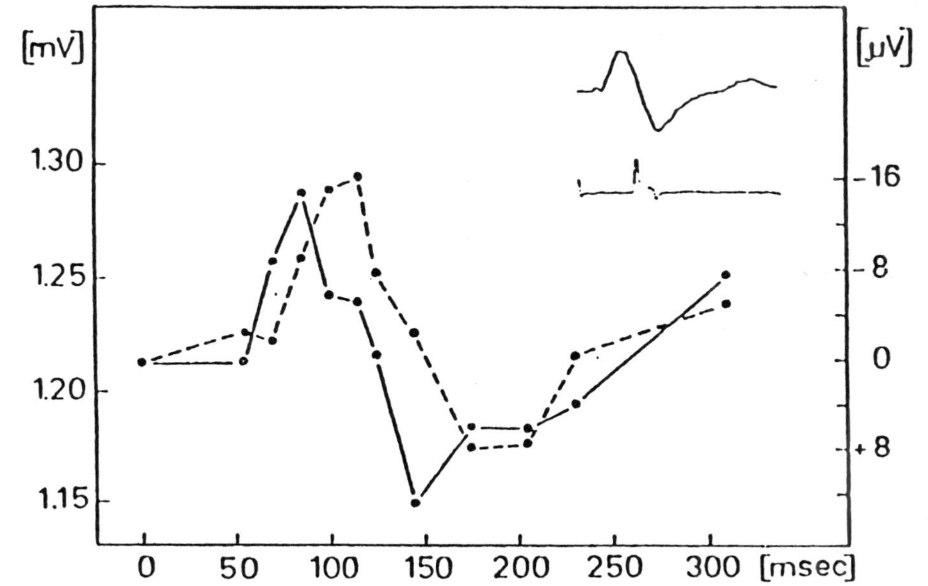

FIG. 4.64 Average amplitudes of the H reflex (solid line) and the vertex (Cz) ERP (dashed line) of one subject as a function of the interval between the click, presented at 0 msec, and the shock eliciting the H reflex. The millivolt scale belongs to the H-reflex, the microvolt scale to the ERP. In the right corner, a typical averaged ERP (above, time scale 480 msec) and a single H-reflex (time scale 120 msec) of this subject are shown. (From Fruhstorfer, Järvilehto, Soveri, Lumio, & Partanen, 1970. Unpublished data.)

generator mechanism consists of multimodal neurons. This is supported by results that show that rather similar negative components are generated at this latency range by stimuli of different sensory modalities (Allison, Matsumiya, Goff, & Goff, 1977, Gastaut, Regis, Lyagoubi, Mano, & Simon, 1967; Davis, Davis, Loomis, Harvey, & Hobart, 1939; Goff, Rosner, & Allison, 1962; Goff, Matsumiya, Allison, & Goff, 1969; Hari, 1980; Järvilehto et al., 1978).

The neuronal population underlying the nonspecific N1 component has not yet been localized, but, as already mentioned, Näätänen and Picton (1987; see also Velasco & Velasco, 1986; Velasco et al., 1985) proposed that this component is generated in the frontal motor and premotor cortex under the influence of the reticular formation and the VL (ventrolateral) nucleus of the thalamus.

In addition to arousing effects, stimuli may also have relaxing, even sleep-inducing, effects. These tend to occur when long sequences of homogeneous stimuli are repeated at constant ISIs (for a review, see Sokolov, 1963).

4.7. ERP INDICATIONS OF AUTOMATICITY DEVELOPED BY EXTENDED TRAINING

ERP data reviewed in this chapter suggest that a good deal of sensory processing is automatic in the sense of being independent of attention. An issue of central theoretical and practical importance is whether the range of automatic processing could be expanded by extended practice. This is the basic suggestion underlying Shiffrin and Schneider's (1977) and Schneider and Shiffrin's (1977) influential automatic versus controlled processing dichotomy discussed in Section 2.2. Extended consistent-mapping training was shown to lead to an amazing speed and lack of effort in detecting targets in visual multielement displays. This was interpreted as evidence for qualitative performance change, a shift from controlled to automatic detection.

This assumption has been tested with ERPs in several studies measuring the P3 amplitude which is commonly regarded as indicating the amount of limited-capacity perceptual-cognitive resources required by the processing of the eliciting stimulus (chapter 6). These studies have usually compared P3s elicited by targets or probes in consistent mapping with those elicited in varied mapping. Given that the P3 amplitude is indeed a valid measure of attentional resources needed in stimulus discrimination, the results seem to suggest that the two processing modes are not qualitatively different in the sense of automatic processing being capacity unlimited and controlled processing drawing on limited capacity. For example, Hoffman, Simons, and Houck (1983) found that P3 waves elicited by probes were of a very similar amplitude in consistent and varied mapping (see Fig. 4.65).

These results were replicated by Brookhuis et al. (1981), Dellen, Brookhuis, Mulder, Okita, and Mulder (1985), Gaillard and Arkel (1986), Kramer, Schneider, Fisk, and Donchin (1986), and Kramer and Strayer (1988).

Kramer et al. (1986), however, found that the P3 latency depended much less on memory-set size in consistent than varied mapping. In addition, the effect of the target probability on the P3 amplitude vanished in consistent mapping as the experiment progressed but it remained in varied mapping. These findings do suggest profound differences between the two processing modes proposed.

Hoffman, Houck, MacMillan, Simons, and Oatman (1985) found that consistent-mapping probes elicited a large P3 even when this task was combined with a perceptual-judgment task that was heavily favored by instructions. The authors suggested that subjects were not able to allocate resources from the consistent-mapping task to the concurrent task even when this reallocation would have been very favorable to their task performance.

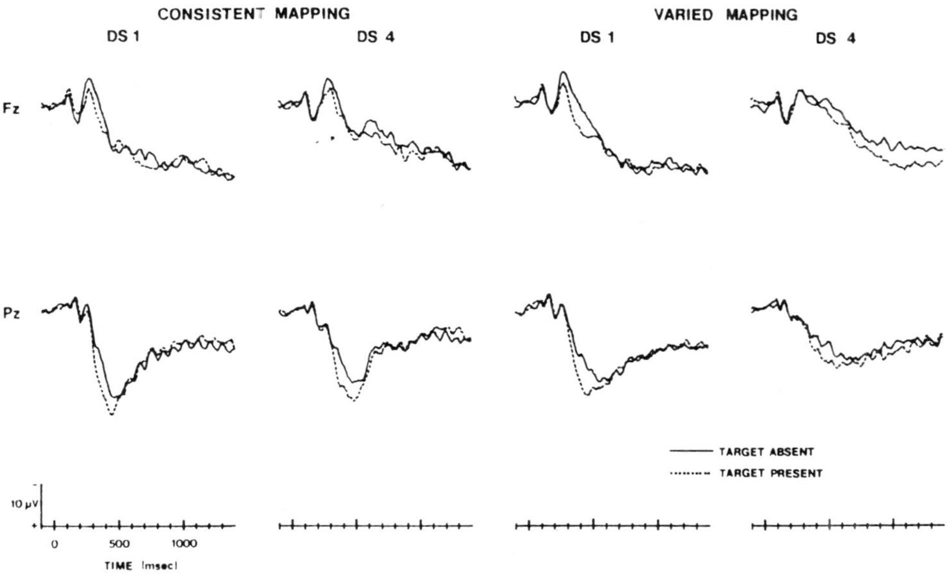

FIG. 4.65 Average frontal (Fz) and parietal (Pz) ERPs in consistent- and varied-mapping conditions for display sizes (DS) 1 and 4 when the display did not contain a target (solid line) and when it contained a target (dotted line). (From Hoffman, Simons, & Houck, 1983. Copyright © 1983 by The Society for Psychophysiological Research. Reprinted with permission.)

Strayer and Kramer (1990) also found large P3s in their consistent-mapping conditions even after extensive practice (23,000 trials; half with consistent and half with varied mapping) in order to achieve Schneider's (1985) "Phase 4" automaticity, "pure automatic" processing. On the other hand, these P3s were insensitive to manipulations of memory load (memory-set size) in the consistent-mapping task and of priority of this task relative to a concurrent recognition running-memory task. Consistent-mapping performance, too, was (relatively) unaffected by these manipulations. In contrast, these manipulations had large effects on P3 elicited in varied mapping when this task was paired with the running-memory task.

Strayer & Kramer (1990) propose that the large P3s in consistent-mapping conditions might reflect "the obligatory allocation of attention to task-relevant events during automatic processing" (p. 67). According to Shiffrin and Schneider (1977), in addition to automatic target detection, extended consistent-mapping practice also results in the development of automatic attention responses (section 2.2). In this case, the P3 would not reflect resources needed in target detection but those engaged as a consequence of target detection. This would implicate that the large consistent-mapping P3s could not be taken as evidence for resource demand of target detection per se in consistent mapping. The similarity of the P3 amplitude with low and high memory load is due, according to this interpretation, to the presumably high-priority nature of cerebral processes underlying passive attention: these processes forcefully take resources needed for their full-scale occurrence irrespective of the resource demand of the controlled activity going on at that moment.

5

Magnetoencephalography (MEG) and Automatic Processing

In the previous chapter, exogenous ERP components were described and discussed. The magnetoencephalographic (MEG) methods, introduced in Section 3.4, have provided important further information on different aspects of these components, in particular when both electric and magnetic responses were recorded in the same study. The same is true with regard to the mismatch negativity (MMN), also discussed in the previous chapter.

The advantage in using the MEG could perhaps be best understood in light of the following two basic properties of the methodology (see Section 3.4):

1. The magnetic responses are better than ERPs in localizing brain activity (but this advantage is of course limited to the activity visible to the MEG, and has recently diminished because of the fast progress of ERP-source analysis techniques (Scherg, 1990; Scherg & von Cramon, 1986);
2. The MEG sees only the tangential component of cerebral activity, and that mainly from the cortical level, depending, of course, on the strength of the signal (see Hari et al., 1988). This is considered by many as a drawback of the methodology but should be regarded as an advantage because it enables (a) a component-specific measurement with a strongly alleviated overlap problem and, related to this, (b) an application of deductive logic in the combined use of the MEG and ERP methodologies. As to the latter, for example, if an ERP deflection is an unknown mixture of two components and the MEG enables the determination of one of these, then by subtracting this known component from the sum (yielded by ERPs) of the two components, the other component could be determined. Consequently, the

interpretation of MEG data seems, in general, be more straightforward than that of ERPs (Hari, 1988).

5.1. MEG STUDIES IN AUDITION

Exogenous Components

Next, MEG results bearing on auditory exogenous ERP components are discussed. It is pointed out that they complement, due to the aforementioned advantages of the MEG method, the information yielded by ERP recordings.

1. Component separation. The MEG has significantly contributed to disentangling the different components of the auditory N1 wave (Section 4.3) by helping to determine the supratemporal N1 component (Elberling, Bak, Kofoed, Lebech, & Saermark, 1980; Hari et al., 1980). The magnetic response, when measured with an axial gradiometer, shows an anterior–posterior polarity reversal at the latency of N1 (as well as at some shorter and longer latencies), thus suggesting a vertically oriented current source at the level of the supratemporal cortex. Such data, from the study of Hari et al. (1987), in response to the onset (solid line) and offset ("Pause"; dashed line) of a noise burst are illustrated in Fig. 5.1.

Furthermore, as already mentioned, by enabling the determination of one component of an ERP wave composed of two components, the MEG also helps in estimating the other component. This is illustrated by the study of Hari et al. (1982) who investigated the ISI dependence of EEG and MEG responses to brief binaural tones. In different blocks, the ISI was either 1, 2, 4, 8, or 16 sec. At the shortest intervals, no significant differences in the N1 amplitude recorded at the different scalp locations were found. When the interval was prolonged, however, the vertex N1 became the largest, and the frontal amplitude was larger than the temporal amplitude. Only the vertex amplitude continued to increase as the interval was increased from 8 to 16 sec (Fig. 4.8).

It was also found that the amplitude of the magnetic response recorded at the same time as the N1—"N1m" or "M100"—increased with long intervals much less than did the electric response measured at the vertex. Hari et al. (1982) proposed that N1m was generated by current dipoles in the supratemporal cortex, and that these dipoles were best represented by the frontocentral electric recordings. Because of the increase in the amplitude of the vertex N1 at long ISIs, the authors also suggested that some additional sources are activated during infrequent stimulation, which are probably current dipoles perpendicular to the scalp near the vertex. The interpretation in terms of activation of additional sources was also sup-

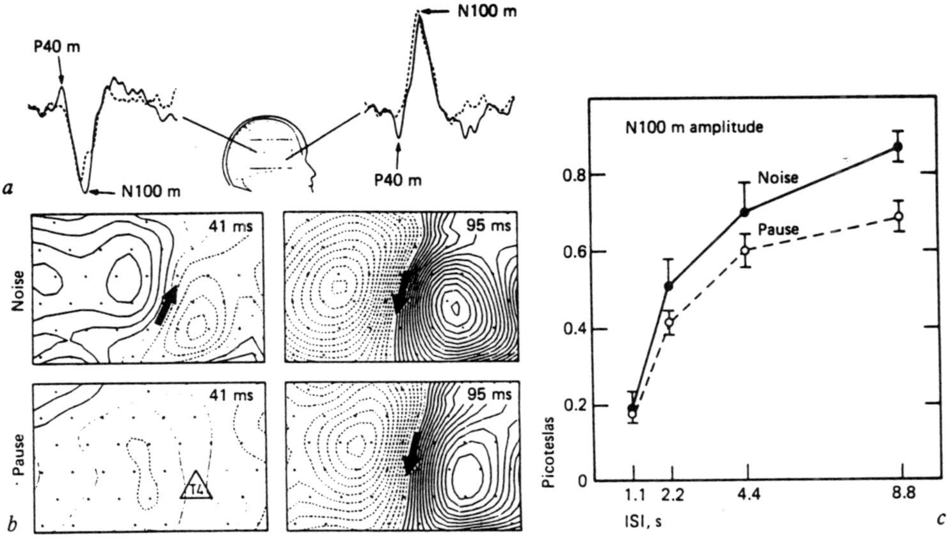

FIG. 5.1 (*a*) Examples of transient MEG responses to the onset of a noise burst (continuous line) and a pause in a continuous noise burst (dotted line) over the right hemisphere of one subject. (*b*) Field patterns during P40m and N100m elicited by noise and pause onsets. The isofield lines are separated by 50 fT. (*c*) ISI dependencies of the N100m responses to noise and pause onsets. (From Hari, 1990. Copyright © 1990 by Karger. Reprinted with permission.)

ported by the prolongation of the latency of the electric N1 when the ISI was increased from 1 to 16 sec, whereas the latency of the magnetic response remained stable.

Consequently, magnetic recordings have clearly shown that a current source located in the supratemporal cortex is activated at the time of the scalp-recorded N1 wave. A current dipole modeling the source would generate, in addition to the magnetic field, an electric field at the scalp with a negative polarity maximal in the frontocentral regions and a positive polarity below the level of the Sylvian fissure. This dipole corresponds to that proposed by Vaughan and Ritter (1970) and to the tangential dipole derived by Scherg and von Cramon (1986). Because the variation of the electric N1 as a function of different manipulations cannot be fully explained by the current dipole derived from magnetic recordings, radial dipoles, which the MEG cannot see, almost certainly exist (Näätänen & Picton, 1987). One such radial dipole—generated in the lateral surface of the temporal lobe—may underlie the T-complex of Wolpaw and Penry (1975). Another—perhaps generated in the region of the vertex by some relatively nonspecific system—may be necessary to explain the considerable amplitude enhancement of the electric N1 at very long ISIs (Näätänen & Picton, 1987).

As already mentioned, the P2 wave of the auditory ERP is also composed of at least two components (Vaughan et al., 1980). It appears that the MEG might be useful in an attempt to clarify this component structure, too (see Hari, 1990; Hari et al., 1987; Hoke, 1988; Hoke, Lehnertz, Lütkenhöner & Pantev, 1989).

2. Determination of component-specific effects. By providing a relatively pure measure of the supratemporal N1 component, the MEG enables one to study the effect of different factors specifically on this component. Thus, as already mentioned, Hari et al. (1982) could estimate the ISI effect separately on this N1 component by measuring the amplitude of its MEG equivalent N1m as a function of the ISI. In a subsequent study, Hari et al. (1987) found that the N1m amplitude may grow until the ISI is prolonged until at least 10 sec (Fig. 5.1).

Similarly, it was shown by Elberling, Bak, Kofoed, Lebech, and Saermark (1981) that with an increasing stimulus intensity, the N1m amplitude saturates much earlier than the amplitude of the electrically recorded N1. This saturation point in their study was at about 60 dB SPL (see also Pantev, Lütkenhöner, Hoke, & Lehnertz, 1986; Reite, Zimmerman, Edrich, & Zimmerman, 1982). This is probably the saturation point of the supratemporal N1 component. In a way analogous to the ISI prolongation, it is likely that after this component is saturated, further increases in stimulus intensity continue to recruit more and more neurons belonging to the generator mechanism of the nonspecific N1 component (Pantev et al., 1986). According to Bak, Lebech, and Saermark (1985), the strength of the N1m dipole moment is proportional to the square root of stimulus intensity.

3. Separation of contra- and ipsilateral responses. The MEG methodology has confirmed, and permitted a separate measurement of, the contra- and ipsilateral responses of the auditory cortex to a monaural sound (as well as a separate measurement of the responses of the two cortices to a binaural sound; Hari & Mäkelä, 1988; Pantev et al., 1986; Papanicolaou, Baumann, et al., 1990; Tiihonen, Hari, Kaukoranta, & Kajola, 1989). A separate evaluation of these two parallel responses with ERPs is complicated by the strong component overlap from sources in both hemispheres. Consequently, the ipsilaterally measured ERP tends to be only slightly smaller in amplitude than the contralateral one (Vaughan & Ritter, 1970), and the difference is much smaller than what could be expected on the basis of the known facts of neuroanatomy (Rosenzweig, 1951) and perceptual dominance (Näätänen & Picton, 1987). "Because of the broad extent of volume conduction and the high resistance of the skull, and because the auditory EP generators in the two hemispheres are probably similarly oriented, it would take an asymmetry of greater than 5 to 1 at the generator locations in the supratemporal plane before a 2 to 1 asymmetry would be recognizable at the scalp" (Näätänen & Picton, 1987, p. 394).

MEG studies have shown that:

1. Contralateral stimulation produces, in general, somewhat stronger fields than does ipsilateral or binaural stimulation (Elberling, Bak, Kofoed, Lebech, & Saermark, 1982; Hari & Mäkelä, 1988; Hoke, Lehnertz, Lütkenhöner, & Pantev, 1989; Mäkelä, 1988; Pantev et al., 1986; Reite, Zimmerman, & Zimmerman, 1981; Tiihonen, Hari, Kaukoranta, & Kajola, 1989). This contralateral advantage usually is relatively stronger than that shown by ERPs (for a review, see Näätänen & Picton, 1987)

2. The latency of N1m is about 5–10 msec (or even more; Papanicolaou, Baumann, et al., 1990) shorter for contra- than ipsilateral stimulation (Elberling et al., 1980, 1981; Hari & Mäkelä, 1988; Joutsiniemi, 1988; Mäkelä, 1988; Pantev et al., 1986; for comparable ERP results, see Butler, Keidel, & Spreng, 1969);

3. The equivalent current dipoles of N1m for contra- versus ipsilateral stimuli seem to differ from one another, suggesting that these responses are generated by somewhat different mechanisms in the auditory cortex (Elberling et al., 1982; Mäkelä, 1988; Pantev et al., 1986; Papanicolaou, Baumann, et al., 1990; Reite et al., 1981);

4. The equivalent current dipole is in right-handed subjects located in the left hemisphere somewhat posterior (usually about 10–15 mm, depending on the ear of stimulation) to the location of the corresponding dipole in the right hemisphere (which is related to the anatomical differences between the two hemispheres; Galaburda et al., 1978; Geschwind & Levitsky, 1968). In addition, the equivalent current dipole is, in right-handed subjects, generally stronger over the left than right hemisphere (Elberling et al., 1981, 1982; Kaukoranta, Hari, & Lounasmaa, 1987; Kuriki & Murase, 1989; for a review, see Hoke, Lehnertz, et al., 1989);

5. The relative positions of the left- and right-hemisphere dipoles in the anterior–posterior dimension, as well as their relative strength, may be reversed in left-handed subjects (Hoke, 1988).

4. Highly stimulus-specific responses. The MEG might also help to decompose responses known to date as ERP components into subcomponents, each representing an activation of highly stimulus-specific neurons in the auditory cortex. An example of these highly specific responses was provided by MEG data suggesting a tonotopic and amplitopic (intensity-related) organization of the auditory cortex.

The N1m' of Kaukoranta and colleagues (1987) also represents such a specific response. N1m' was elicited by vowel onset after all Finnish fricative consonants (/h/, /f/, /s/), and also by the transition of a noise stimulus to a square wave (Kaukoranta et al., 1987; Mäkelä, Hari, & Leinonen, 1988), at a latency of about 100 msec. N1m' was generated anteriorly to N1m in supratemporal auditory cortex (Kaukoranta et al., 1987). Because the response was even elicited by noise–square-wave transitions, it appears to reflect acoustic rather than phonetic stimulus features (Kaukoranta et al., 1987).

Another specific N1m response was demonstrated by Kuriki and Murase (1989). These authors found that the equivalent current dipoles for speech sounds /ka/ and /a/ differed in location in the left hemisphere but did not differ in the right hemisphere. The authors suggested that this interhemispheric asymmetry might indicate that "the magnetic responses include a component associated with linguistic processing in the auditory cortex" (Kuriki & Murase, 1989, p. 133).

A good deal of MEG data (e.g., Hari et al., 1987), however, suggest very similar loci of N1m generation for very different auditory stimuli. This is probably due, at least in part, to these different stimuli activating neurons with very wide receptive fields.

5. Source localization. The MEG has crucially helped in localizing the intracranial origin of different exogenous components of the auditory ERP by giving precise information about the "center of gravity" of the equivalent current dipoles calculated from the MEG data (however, the one-dipole model has mainly been used in these calculations, which may sometimes be quite misleading; see Section 3.4). As already discussed, the MEG has, in this sense, helped to determine that the supratemporal N1 component to stimulus onset is generated in the primary auditory cortex or in its immediate vicinity (and this separately for each hemisphere as well as for contra- and ipsilateral stimuli). In addition, N1m to stimulus offset is, MEG studies suggest, also generated in the Sylvian fissure, slightly anteriorly to the locus of generation of the onset response (Hari et al., 1987; Joutsiniemi, Hari, & Vilkman, 1989). Moreover, as discussed earlier, the MEG can locate some highly stimulus-specific neuronal populations contributing to the N1m response.

The MEG has also provided evidence about the site of generation of many other exogenous components of the auditory ERP. These data indicate that P2m, or M200, is generated anteriorly to the locus of the onset N1m (Hari et al., 1987; Hoke et al., 1989; Kuriki & Murase, 1989; Mäkelä et al., 1987; Pantev, Gallen, Hampson, Buchanan, & Sobel, in press; Papanicolaou, Baumann, et al., 1990; Papanicolaou, Rogers, et al., 1990; Pelizzone, Williamson, & Kaufman, 1985; Sams, Hämäläinen, et al., 1985). The MEG equivalent of the sustained potential (Section 4.3) is also generated on the supratemporal cortex, in a locus slightly anterior to that of the onset N1m and approximately corresponding to that of N1m to stimulus offset (Hari, Aittoniemi, et al., 1980; Hari, Pelizzone, et al., 1987; see also Joutsiniemi, Hari, & Vilkman, 1989). On the other hand, "P40m," an early response to stimulus onset, not elicited by stimulus offset (Joutsiniemi et al., 1989), seems to be generated in the vicinity of the locus for the onset N1m (Hari et al., 1987). P40m may be the magnetic equivalent of the electric P1. The "M50" of Reite, Teale, Neumann, and Davis (1987) and Reite, Teale, Zimmerman, Davis, and Whalen (1988) also seems to correspond to the electrical P1 (see Wood & Wolpaw, 1982).

Quite recently, the MEG has provided information about the loci of generation of even earlier, middle-latency, responses. Pelizzone et al. (1987) were apparently able to record the MEG equivalent of the electrical Pa at 30 msec, concluding that this response has a cortical origin. In addition, Mäkelä and Hari (1987; see also Tiihonen, Hari, et al., 1989) reported MEG evidence for a cortical (supratemporal) origin of the 40-Hz steady-state response (see Section 4.2). Furthermore, Hari, Hämälainen, and Joutsiniemi (1989) demonstrated that this steady-state response is satisfactorily explained by summation of responses evoked by single clicks. In addition, Scherg, Hari, and Hämäläinen (1989) found a magnetic cortical response at an even earlier latency of 19 msec in response to a filtered click.

A MEG equivalent of the 40-Hz oscillatory transient response mentioned in Section 4.2. (Galambos et al., 1981; Makeig, 1990; Makeig & Galambos, 1989a) was reported by Pantev, Makeig, et al. (1991). This response is illustrated in Fig. 5.2.

An auditory equivalent of the occipital alpha rhythm in vision was found by Tiihonen, Hari, Kajola, Karhu, Ahlfors, and Tissari (1991). This magnetic 8–10 Hz auditory rhythm had its equivalent source in the supratemporal auditory cortex in the vicinity of the equivalent current dipole of the supratemporal N1. In addition, this rhythmic activity differed in its reactivity from both the occipital alpha and the rolandic mu rhythm, the somatosensory equivalent of the occipital alpha. In contrast to the occipital alpha, the supratemporal rhythmic activity was not affected by the opening of the eyes. Also the clenching of the fist, which dampens the rolandic rhythm, did not affect the supratemporal rhythm.

The earliest MEG response was reported by Erné, Scheer, Hoke, Pantev, and Lütkenhöner (1987). This very small response occurred at the latency range of the auditory brainstem response, and its recording was only possible when all experimental parameters were simultaneously optimized. The authors reported that the magnetic equivalent of Wave V of the electric brainstem response reversed its polarity at homologous positions over both hemispheres.

6. Tonotopic organization of human auditory cortex. As already mentioned, the MEG methodology has revealed a tonotopic organization in the human auditory cortex. Using steady-state stimulation (sinusoidal amplitude modulation at 32 Hz), Romani, Williamson, and Kaufman (1982; see also Romani, Williamson, Kaufman, & Brenner, 1982) found that the depth of the equivalent current dipole logarithmically increased with the in-

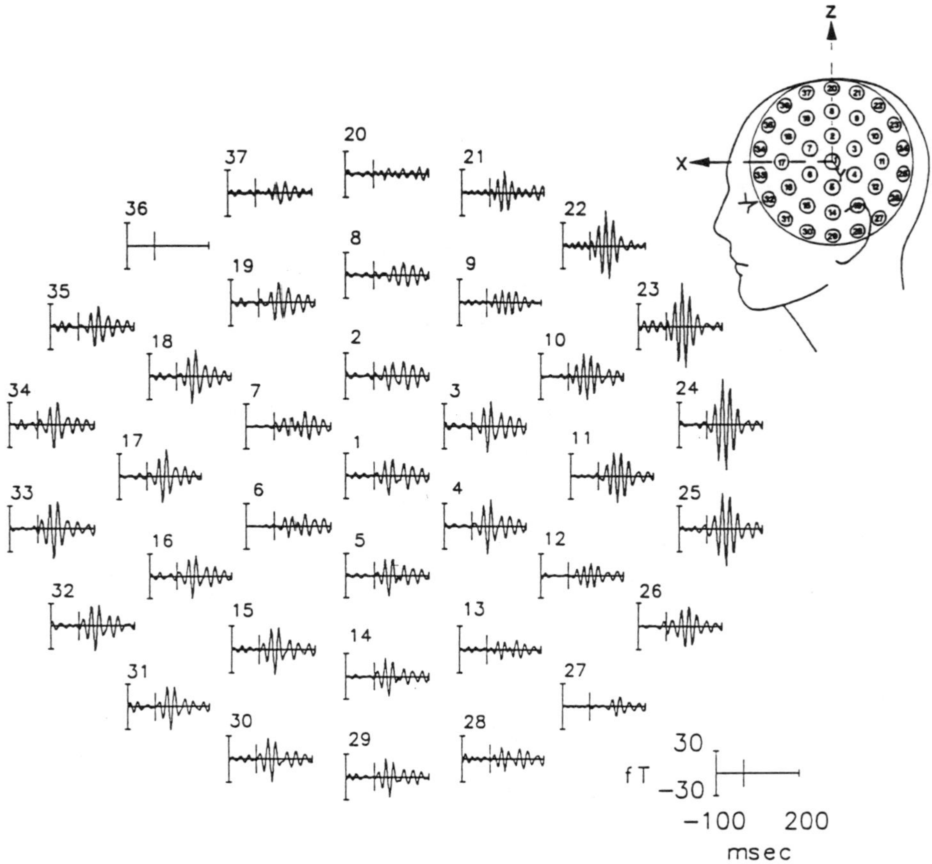

FIG. 5.2 Magnetoencephalographic (MEG) data illustrating the 40-Hz transient response from one subject recorded through 37 magnetic sensors from the left hemisphere. A 1,000-Hz tone burst of 80 dB nHL with 500-msec duration was presented at a constant (onset to onset) ISI of 4 sec. Digital bandpass filtering between 28 to 48 Hz. (From Pantev et al., 1991. Copyright © 1991 by the National Academy of Sciences, USA. Reprinted with permission.)

creasing frequency of the amplitude-modulated tone (Figs. 5.3 and 5.4). These data, consequently, suggest that the tonotopic organization of the cochlea is maintained at the level of the auditory cortex even in humans.

Furthermore, Elberling and colleagues (1982) found with transient (tone-burst) stimuli that the equivalent current dipole for N1m moved in the posterior direction with increasing tonal frequency. The recent results of Pantev et al. (1988; see also Pantev et al., 1990) also indicate that the locus of generation of N1m to transient stimuli depends on the frequency of the eliciting stimulus. With increasing frequency, the location of the equivalent current dipole became deeper and shifted in the posterior direction, thus

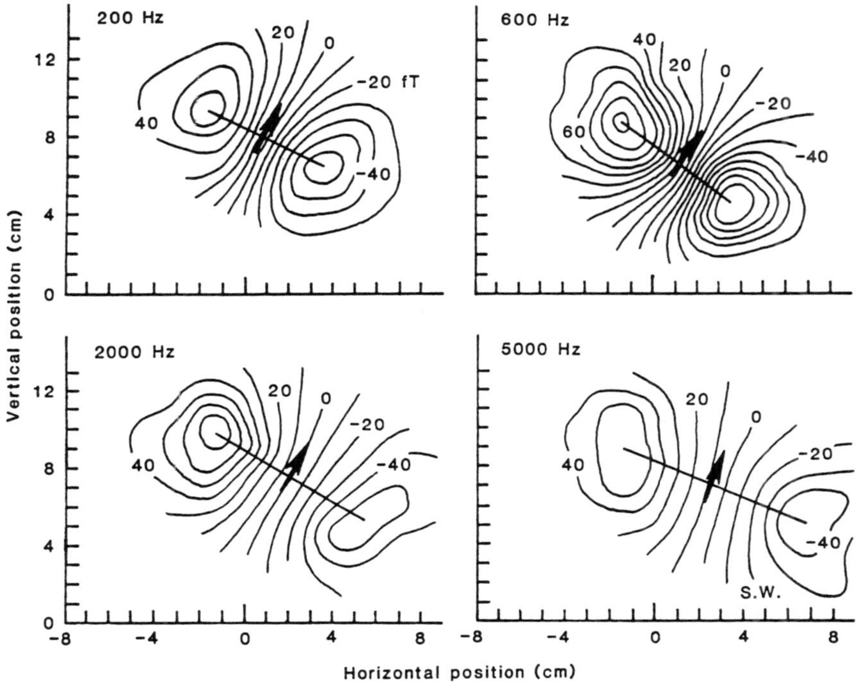

FIG. 5.3 Isofield contours for the component of the evoked magnetic field normal to the scalp detected over the right hemisphere of one subject. The origin is at the ear canal, the corner of the eye lies at position (0, 9), and the vertical axis points to the vertex. Arrows denote the position and orientation of the equivalent current dipoles for tones of 200, 600, 2,000, and 5,000 Hz. The sense of the arrow is arbitrarily chosen. (From Romani, Williamson, & Kaufman, 1982. Copyright © 1982 by the American Association for the Advancement of Science. Reprinted with permission.)

confirming Romani, Williamson, and Kaufman (1982); Romani, Williamson, Kaufman, and Brenner (1982); Elberling et al. (1982). The location of the equivalent current dipole for P2m did not depend on frequency.

Also Yamamoto et al. (1988) and Kuriki and Murase (1989) found that the equivalent current dipole of N1m shifts increasingly deeper with higher tonal frequencies. Further evidence for a tonotopic organization of the N1m generator was provided by Mäkelä, Hari, and Leinonen (1988). All studies have not found a tonotopic organization, however (Arlinger et al., 1982; Arthur et al., 1987; Tuomisto, Hari, Katila, Poutanen, & Varpula, 1983), or the source organization suggested (Hari & Mäkelä, 1986; Pelizzone et al., 1985) has been opposite to that concluded from the other studies (for a review, see Mäkelä & Hari, 1990).

Consequently, it is clear that the spatial resolution of MEG recordings is usually sufficient for revealing a tonotopic organization in the human auditory cortex. However, ERPs can also reflect this organization. Ber-

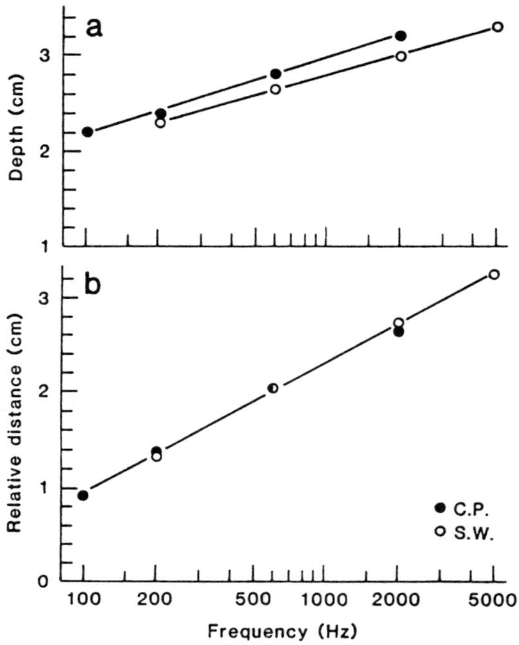

FIG. 5.4 (*a*) Depths beneath the scalp of the equivalent current dipoles representing cortical activity for two subjects plotted as a function of the logarithm of the tone frequency. (*b*) Cumulative straight-line distance between adjacent dipoles as a function of the logarithm of the frequency. (From Romani, Williamson, & Kaufman, 1982. Copyright © 1982 by the American Association for the Advancement of Science. Reprinted with permission.)

trand et al. (1988) obtained electrical-N1 data that suggested a tonotopic organization of the generator of the supratemporal N1 component (the tangential dipole). For corroborating evidence, see Woods et al. (1991) and Näätänen, Teder, Alho, and Lavikainen (1992). In contrast, the radial dipole, probably corresponding to the negative component of the T-complex, also implicated by Bertrand et al.'s (1988) data, did not depend on stimulus frequency.

7. Amplitopic organization of human auditory cortex. A neuron's response is not necessarily more vigorous with increasing stimulus intensity but may reach its maximum at a "submaximal" intensity and become weaker at still higher intensities (Brugge & Reale, 1985). In animals, topical mechanisms of intensity coding were suggested by Brugge and Merzenich (1973), Suga (1977), and Phillips, Orman, Musicant, and Wilson (1985). Some MEG evidence for an amplitopic (intensity-related) organization of the human auditory cortex was reported by Pantev, Hoke, Lehnertz, and Lütkenhöner (1989). In their study, the amplitude of the dipole moment (strength) increased for both N1m and P2m up to a stimulus intensity of 50–60 dB HL, remaining thereafter more or less constant or even decreasing. In addition, with increasing intensity, the location of the equivalent current dipole for N1m became more superficial and it changed in orientation. These systematic changes were not found for P2m but its dipole location in the tangential plane slightly shifted in the anterior direction with increasing intensity. This was also observed for N1m.

These data were interpreted as suggesting that the human auditory cortex is amplitopically organized. In this case, the location of the equivalent current dipole for N1m would be a function of two independent variables, the frequency and intensity of the stimulus (see also Yamamoto et al., 1988). Referring to the complex functional anatomy of the supratemporal auditory cortex, Mäkelä and Hari (1990), however, regarded the systematic shifts of source locations as a function of stimulus intensity as "unexpected."

8. Stimulus-induced reactivity increase. In Section 4.3, ISI effects on the electric N1 wave were reviewed. These studies clearly indicated that N1 becomes smaller as the ISI is shortened, almost vanishing with very rapid stimulus rates. Given this background, the effect of the stimulus onset asynchrony (SOA) on N1m to the second of paired stimuli observed by Loveless, Hari, Hämäläinen, and Tiihonen (1989) appears striking. The SOA of the paired stimuli, each a noise burst of 50 msec in duration, varied from 70 msec to 500 msec (randomly in the same block). The interpair interval varied from 1.2 sec to 1.4 sec.

It was found that the N1m amplitude was considerably larger for the second stimulus than for the first stimulus of the pair with SOAs of 70–230 msec. This effect was also observed with tone stimuli, regardless of whether they were identical or different in frequency. Moreover, it did not seem to matter whether the paired stimuli were presented to the same or different ears, which indicates involvement of a central mechanism.

These data consequently suggest that an auditory stimulus is followed by a brief period of facilitation during which the next stimulus elicits an enhanced response. (For related ERP findings, see Ciganek, 1964; Donald & Goff, 1973; Kitajima, Morotomi, & Kanoh, 1975; Rietveldt, Tordoir, & Hagenouw, 1967; for a review, see Rohrbaugh et al., 1990.) The facilitation observed might be related to the possible conscious-perception/attention-switching function of the supratemporal or other N1 components elicited by stimulus onsets and offsets (Section 4.5). Consistently with this, the facilitation also followed the offset of a continuous noise (Loveless et al., 1989).

In searching for an interpretation, the authors referred, as one possibility, to the disinhibition hypothesis of Mitzdorf (1987) based on visual-cortex responses recorded from unanesthesized cats. In these data, when two identical visual stimuli were presented in close succession, the response to the second was larger than that to the first. This facilitation was strongest with SOAs of 200–300 msec.

9. Physiological processes underlying subjective experience. Pantev, Hoke, Lütkenhöner, and Lehnertz (1989) studied the location of the equivalent current dipole of the N1m response elicited by three different tones: (a) a pure tone of 250 Hz; (b) a pure tone of 1000 Hz; (c) a complex tone composed of the fourth to the seventh harmonics of the 250-Hz tone (tones of 1000, 1250, 1500, and 1750 Hz). The perceptual pitch of this complex tone matched very well the pitch of the 250-Hz pure tone stimulus (the "missing fundamental").

It was found that the equivalent current dipole for the complex tone was located in depth closer to the dipole for the 250-Hz than to that for the 1000-Hz tone. All these locations were very close to one another, however. Pantev, Hoke, Lütkenhöner, and Lehnertz (1989) concluded:

> Thus it appears that neuromagnetic measurements have allowed the detection of an objective correlate of the purely subjective entity pitch. The results indicate that the spatial arrangement of the generators of the magnetic wave M100 reflects the pitch rather than the spectral contents of the stimulus. This finding suggests the following interpretation: If the perceived pitch of a complex auditory stimulus corresponds to that of a pure tone (missing fundamental) not contained in, and below the bounds of, the frequency spectrum of a complex tone (higher harmonics), then the virtual pitch will determine the place of maximal excitation. This implies that the tonotopic representation at cortex is different from that at the cochlear level, where frequency is the determining parameter, and that the pitch processor must be located peripheral to the generators of wave M100, which are supposed to be in the primary auditory cortex. . . . (p. 487)

As already reviewed (Section 4.3), Butler's (1972) refractoriness effects on the electrical N1, however, suggested that the supratemporal N1 generator is more closely related to the spectral contents than to the pitch of periodicity-pitch stimuli.

A neural correlate of perceptual experience has also been reported in MEG studies on tinnitus (ringing in the ear) (Hoke, Feldmann, Pantev, Lütkenhöner, & Lehnertz, 1989; Pantev, Hoke, Lütkenhöner, Lehnertz, & Kumpf, 1989). Judging from the selective suppression of P2m found in these studies, the persistent subjective sound heard by tinnitus patients might be traceable to a chronic activation of the neuronal population generating P2m: An elevated background activation would diminish a stimulus-elicited response from this neuronal population.

Auditory Responses Recorded with Large-Array Multichannel Biomagnetometers. The largest commercially available biomagnetometer to date (July, 1991) is the 37-channel device produced by Biomagnetic Technologies, Inc. (BTI). Its SQUID sensor array consists of 37 axially symmetric first-order gradiometer pick-up coils arranged in a hexagonal pattern. A 122-channel system covering the whole head, under construction by Neuromag Ltd. for the Low-Temperature Laboratory of the Helsinki University of Technology, is estimated to be in operation in 1992 (see Fig. 5.5).

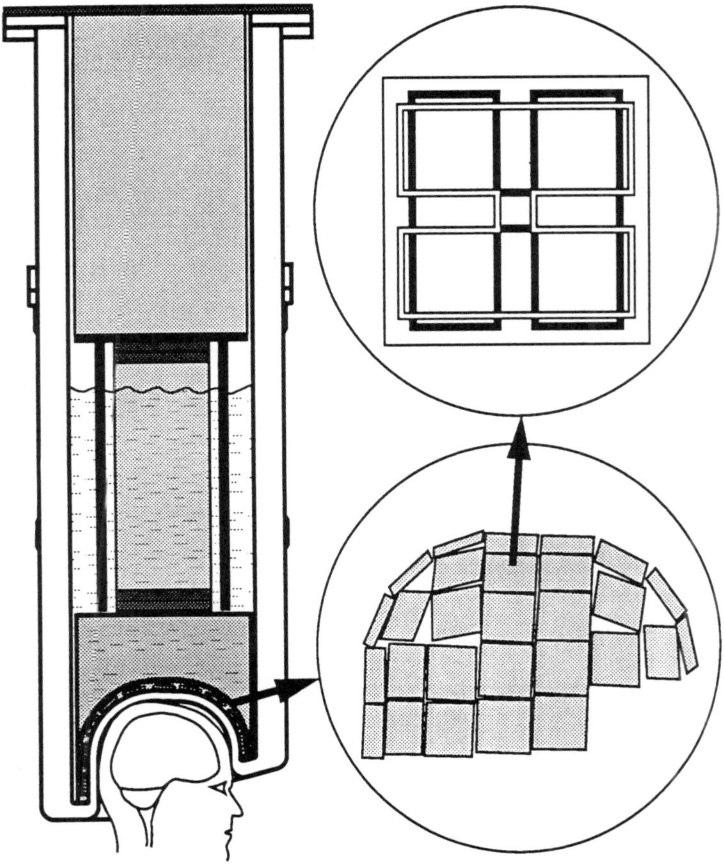

FIG. 5.5 A 122 channel MEG system of the Low-Temperature Laboratory of The Helsinki University of Technology constructed by Neuromag Ltd. The detection array of the new Neuromag-122 system comprises 61 two-channel thin-film gradiometer units evenly distributed over the whole head. Activity of several sources at any part of the cortex can now, for first time ever, be simultaneously followed. (Courtesy of Neuromag Ltd., Espoo, Finland.)

The great advantage of large-array systems is that the data needed for a map can be simultaneously recorded, because a wide enough area of the head can be covered simultaneously. With the 37-channel device, as well as with the 24-channel system of the Low Temperature Laboratory of the Helsinki University of Technology (Fig. 3.2), cortical activity of almost the whole cerebral hemisphere can be recorded simultaneously. This considerably enhances the speed and quality of MEG measurements. Such very recent data (Pantev, Gallen, Hampson, Buchanan & Sobel, in press), collected separately for each of the 30 consecutive sessions with a single subject over a period of 2 months, are presented in Fig. 5.6.

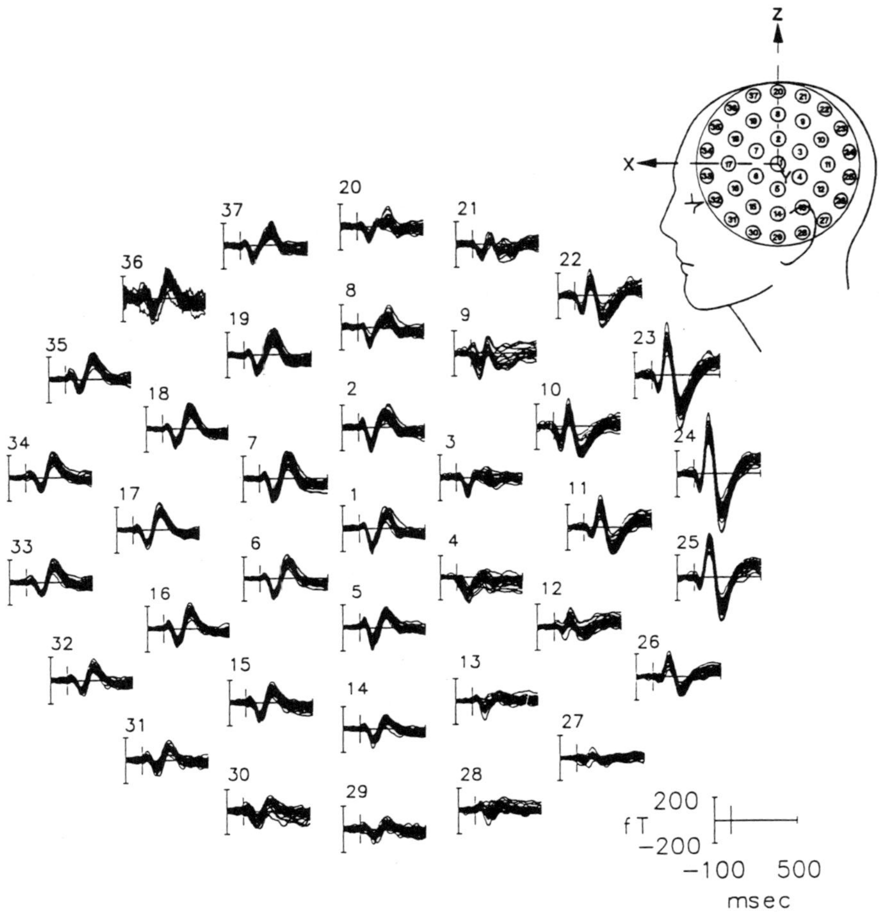

FIG. 5.6 Superimposition of the averaged MEG responses to a tone of 1,000 Hz presented at a constant ISI of 4 sec obtained in 30 consecutive sessions with one subject. The schematic placement of the large-array biomagnetometer is shown in the head inserted into the right upper corner. Stimulus onset is marked by the vertical line on the x-axis at the right lower corner. (From Pantev, Gallen, Hampson, Buchanan, & Sobel, in press. Copyright © in press by Elsevier Science Publishers, Ireland. Reprinted with permission.)

As shown by this figure, highly reproducible MEG waveforms were obtained. Equivalent current dipoles calculated for P1m, N1m, and P2m components were consistently located with standard deviations of only a few millimeters. These dipole locations for N1m and P2m are indicated in Fig. 5.7. A comparison with MRI (magnetic resonance imaging) showed that the equivalent current dipole source for N1m was located in the region of Heschl's gyrus and the transverse portion of the superior temporal gyrus (see Fig. 5.8).

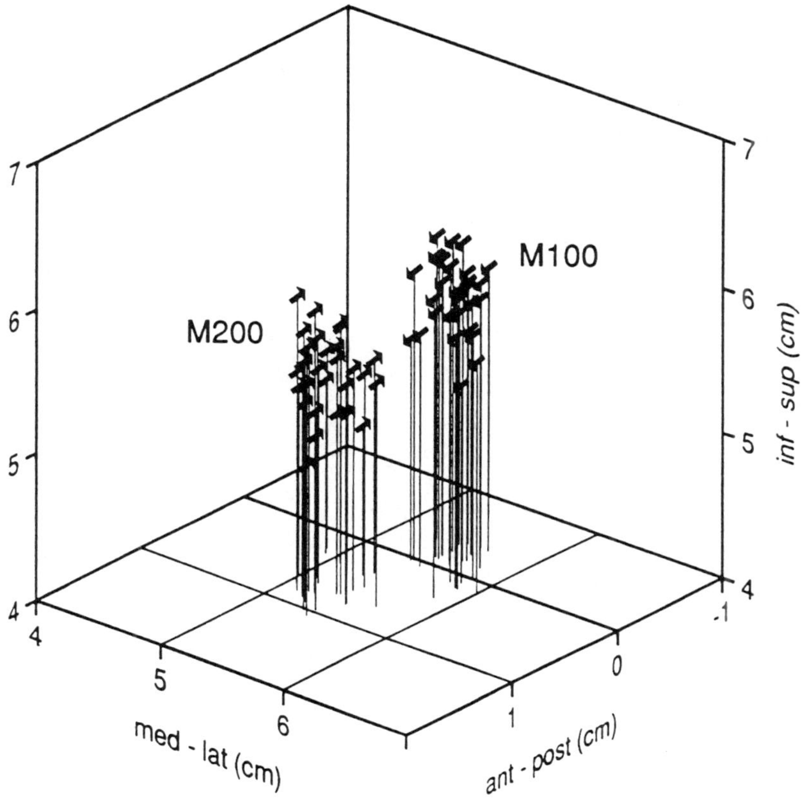

FIG. 5.7 Spatial separation of the M100 (N1m) and M200 (P2m) sources for the 30 different sessions (Fig. 5.6). The ECD locations of M100 and M200 are indicated by small arrows placed in a volume element of 3 × 3 × 3 cm. The axes values are related to the head frame center. (From Pantev, Gallen, Hampson, Buchanan, & Sobel, in press. Copyright © in press by Elsevier Science Publishers, Ireland. Reprinted with permission.)

Many other recent papers have also related MEG results to MRI or comparable structural information (Arthur et al., 1991; Kuriki et al., 1988; Leinonen & Joutsiniemi, 1988; Mäkelä, Hari, Valanne, & Ahonen, 1991; Paetau, Kajola, & Hari, 1990; Papanicolaou, Baumann, et al., 1990, Papanicolaou, Rogers, et al., 1990; Reite et al., 1988; Tiihonen et al., 1990; Yamamoto et al., 1988).

MEG Equivalent of the Mismatch Negativity (MMNm)

A MEG equivalent of MMN (MMNm), sometimes also called the mismatch field (MMF), to a slight frequency deviation was demonstrated by Hari,

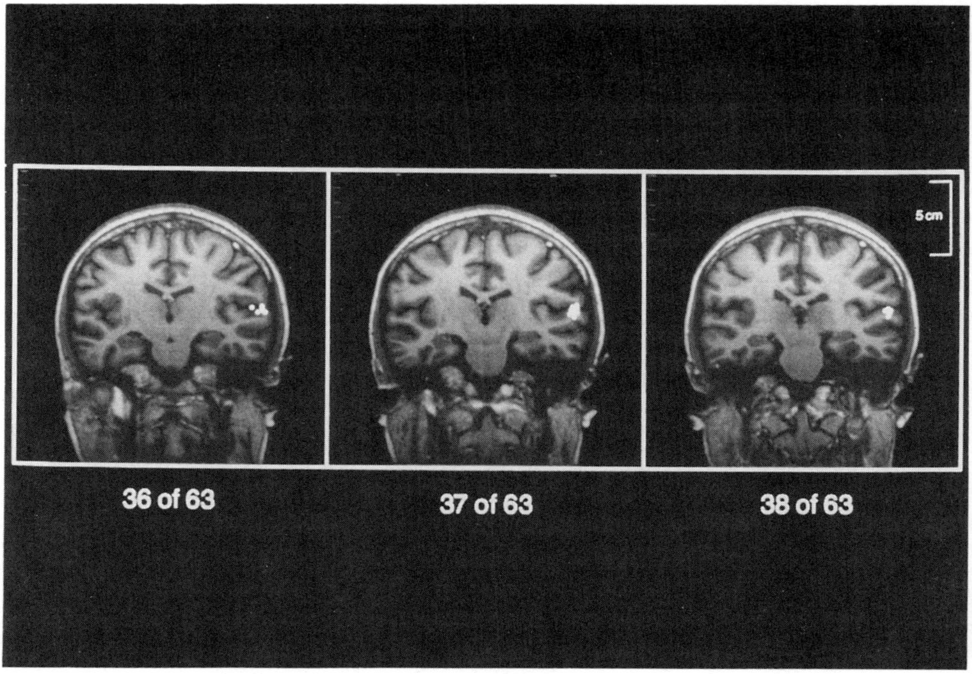

FIG. 5.8 Coronal overlays of the 30 different ECD locations (white dots) corresponding to the source of M100 (Fig. 5.7). The first of the two numbers indicates the slice number, the second one the total number of slices. (From Pantev, Gallen, Hampson, Buchanan, & Sobel, in press. Copyright © in press by Elsevier Science Publishers, Ireland. Reprinted with permission.)

Hämäläinen, et al. (1984; see also Sams, Hämäläinen, et al., 1985). The difference wave formed by subtracting the MEG response to standards from the MEG response to deviants reversed its polarity between recordings over the anterior and posterior parts of the Sylvian fissure, suggesting MMNm generation in or near the primary auditory cortex (Fig. 5.9).

Subsequent studies demonstrated MEG equivalents for intensity (Lounasmaa, Hari, Joutsiniemi, & Hämäläinen, 1989) and duration MMNs (Kaukoranta, Sams, Hari, Hämäläinen, & Näätänen, 1989) which also originated from the auditory cortex. Moreover, Sams, Kaukoranta, Hämäläinen, & Näätänen (1991) found that the equivalent current dipoles for frequency (see also Hari, Hämäläinen, et al., 1984; Hari, Rif, Tiihonen, & Sams, 1992), intensity, and duration MMNm differ from N1m in location. Evidence for dipole-location differences between the different MMNs was also obtained but only for some individual subjects (Fig. 5.10).

Sams and Näätänen (1991) found an MMNm to a reversal of the direction of a frequency glide, that is, the deviant stimulus was identical to the

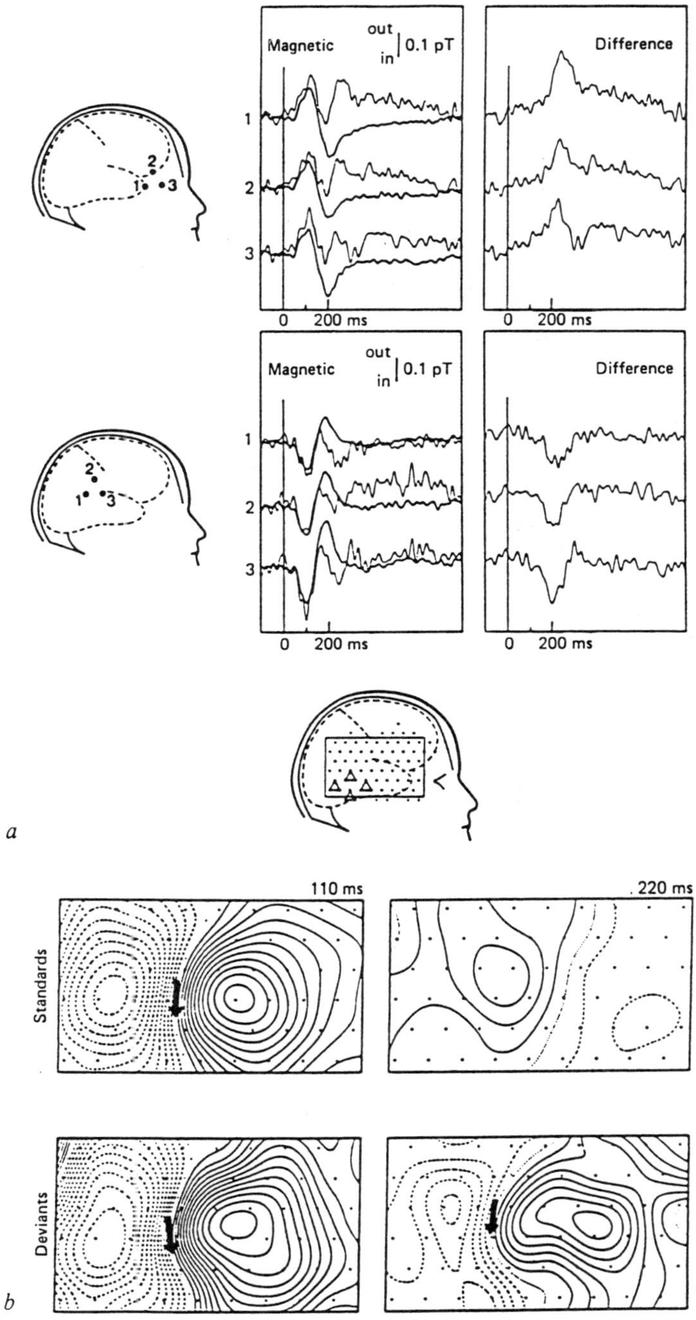

FIG. 5.9 *Top:* Magnetic responses of one subject to standard (thick lines) and deviant (thin lines) tones at the anterior (upper curves) and posterior (lower curves) ends of the right Sylvian fissure. The corresponding difference curves are shown on the right. *Bottom:* Isocontour maps of responses to standard (upper maps) and deviant (lower maps) tones at peak latencies of N100m and MMNm in one subject. The isofield lines are separated by 35 fT. The arrows illustrate the approximate locations of the equivalent current dipoles. (From Hari et al., 1984. Copyright © 1984 by Elsevier Science Publishers, Ireland. Reprinted with permission.)

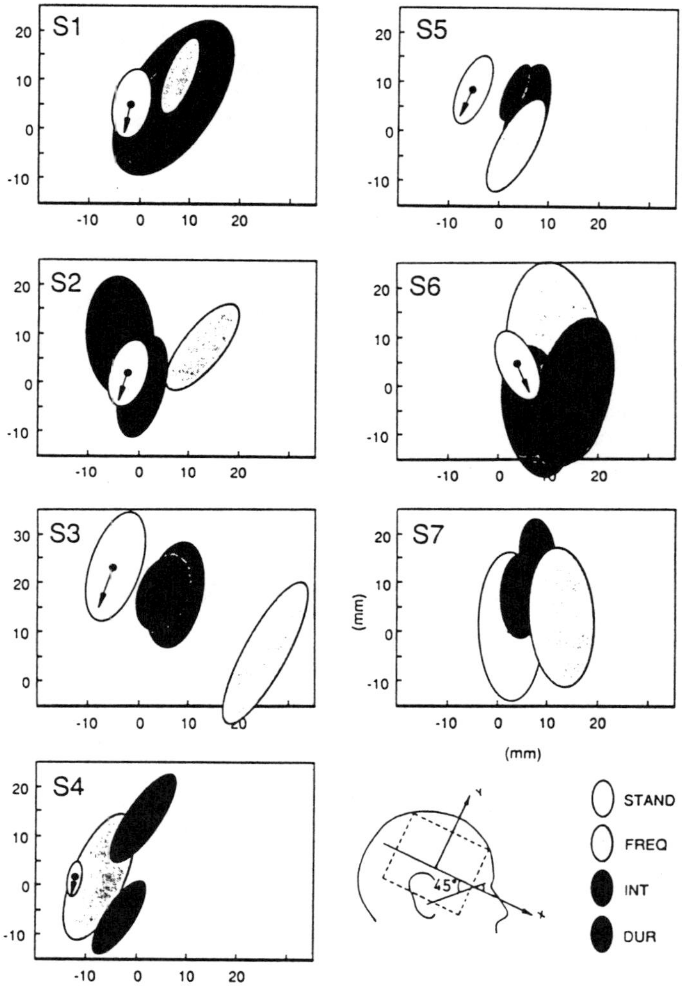

FIG. 5.10 The confidence areas for the 2-dimensional locations (on xy-plane) of the equivalent dipoles of seven individual subjects (S1-S7) for N1m to standards and for MMNm to frequency, intensity, and duration deviations. The orientation of the dipoles is indicated by the longer axis of an ellipsoid. The coordinate system is shown on the schematic head. The origin is 7 cm posterior to the outer canthus of the right eye. (From Sams, Kaukoranta, Hämäläinen, & Näätänen, 1991. Copyright © 1991 by The Society for Psychophysiological Research. Reprinted with permission.)

standard stimulus but was presented backwards. Because the frequencies covered by the standard and deviant stimuli were identical, the MMNm elicited by the deviant stimuli must be related to temporal stimulus information (see Section 4.4). This MMNm increased in amplitude with an increased slope of the frequency glide.

Another time-related MMNm was found by Hari, Joutsiniemi, Hämäläinen, and Vilkman (1989) who obtained MMNm to occasional too early stimuli in a sequence of regularly spaced stimuli. In addition, Joutsiniemi and Hari (1989) found a MEG response to an infrequent stimulus omission in this kind of stimulus sequence. Interestingly, the equivalent current dipole for this response was located in the frontal lobe. Due to its attentional sensitivity and the anterior locus of generation, the relation of this response to the electric MMN remains unclear, however.

MEG studies (Sams, Hämäläinen, et al., 1985; Lounasmaa, Hari, Joutsiniemi, & Hämäläinen, 1989) seem to also indicate that no MMN process is elicited by the first stimulus in the sequence, or by stimuli presented at very long ISIs. In a very recent study of Sams, Hari, Rif, and Knuutila (in press), MMNm was elicited with (constant) ISIs of 9 sec in a stimulus block, whereas the ISI of 12 sec was too long for most subjects. With very short ISIs, MMNm is probably considerably enhanced (cf. Hari, Lu, & Sams, submitted). These results suggest that MMN is not associated with stimulus infrequency per se but rather with stimulus change.

Evidence for Intermodal Integration in Responses of Auditory Cortex. Sams et al.'s (1991) standard stimulus was a simultaneous presentation of an auditory syllable /pa/ and a videotaped face articulating the same syllable. The deviant stimulus was the same auditory /pa/ paired with a videotaped /ka/, which was heard by subjects as either /ta/ or /ka/. This illusion is called the McGurk effect (McGurk & MacDonald, 1976).

Use of this incongruent stimulus combination as the deviant stimulus elicited an MMNm kind of effect in auditory cortex. (The effect was also elicited by the congruent stimulus combination when it in turn was the deviant event.) This is of considerable interest in view of the fact that the standards and deviants were acoustically identical (although they differed in the auditory percept produced). This result was interpreted as showing that visual information from articulatory movements has an entry to auditory cortex.

5.2. MEG STUDIES IN VISION

The first MEG responses recorded in the visual domain were the steady-state responses to very rapid visual stimulation (Brenner, Williamson, &

Kaufman, 1975; Reite, Zimmerman, Edrich, & Zimmerman, 1976; Teyler, Cuffin, & Cohen, 1975). The equivalent current-dipole source calculated from the data of Brenner et al. (1975) was located in the occipital cortex.

Transient patterned stimuli elicit a predominantly biphasic MEG response matching the latencies of the N1–P2 of the ERP (Beatty et al., 1986). The equivalent current dipole also for this transient MEG response was located in the occipital cortex. Unpatterned light flashes elicit somewhat earlier responses which have been recorded over the posterior scalp (Teyler et al., 1975; Zimmerman, Edrich, Zimmerman, & Reite, 1978).

The equivalent current dipole for left-hemifield stimulation is generally located to the right to the equivalent dipole for right-hemifield stimulation, and vice versa (Brenner, Okada, Maclin, Williamson, & Kaufman, 1981; Ilmoniemi et al., 1984; Janday, Swithenby, & Thomas, 1988; Lounasmaa, Williamson, Kaufman, & Tanenbaum, 1985; Richer, Barth, & Beatty, 1983). Both sources are very close to the midline, however, and seem to correspond to the visual primary cortex (Beatty et al., 1986).

Maclin and colleagues (1983) found that increases in the retinal eccentricity of visual steady-state stimulation shifted the location of the equivalent current dipole increasingly steeper in the visual cortex. This observation corresponds to the known retinotopic organization of area 17 in the primate brain (Beatty et al., 1986).

Kaufman and Williamson (1986) found that the equivalent current dipole source for an onset response shifted laterally as the lower quadrant instead of the upper quadrant of the visual field was stimulated. In addition, Aine et al. (1989), George, Aine, and Flynn (1988), and Ahlfors, Ilmoniemi, and Hämäläinen (in press) obtained evidence for multiple underlying sources for transient responses to stimuli presented to different quadrants of the visual field. Ahlfors et al. (1992) measured magnetic fields evoked by checkerboard-like sectorial patterns presented at 16 locations near the center of the visual field. The retinal area stimulated by each of these patterns was kept small in order to limit cortical responses to a small area. The results suggested that the occipital-lobe mechanism generating these responses at the latency of 80–100 msec from stimulus onset was retinotopically organized.

Tentative evidence that different neural populations in the visual cortex process chrominance and luminance information was obtained by Krauskopf et al. (1989). In addition, neural populations selective to spatial frequency within the visual cortex were suggested by the simultaneous magnetic and electric measurements performed by Okada, Williamson, and Kaufman (1982). Furthermore, Lounasmaa et al. (1985) demonstrated visually-elicited neural activity outside the visual cortical areas in response to a change in velocity of a moving visual pattern. This activity appeared to be located within or close to the Rolandic fissure (see also Kaufman & Williamson, 1989).

MEG evidence for an involvement of the visual cortex in visual imagery was obtained by Kaufman, Schwartz, Salustri, and Williamson (1990; see also Kaufman & Williamson, 1991). They found a suppression of alpha activity within certain specific regions of the occipital lobe during mental comparison of abstract figures. This result suggests that the magnetic alpha rhythm may well be due to many discrete sources in the occipital-parietal area.

Very recently, Lu and colleagues (1991) recorded MEG responses to pictures of human faces (Fig. 5.11). It was found that three different extrastriate areas seemed to be involved in this processing; an area near the occipital–temporal junction, a second in the inferior parietal lobe, and a

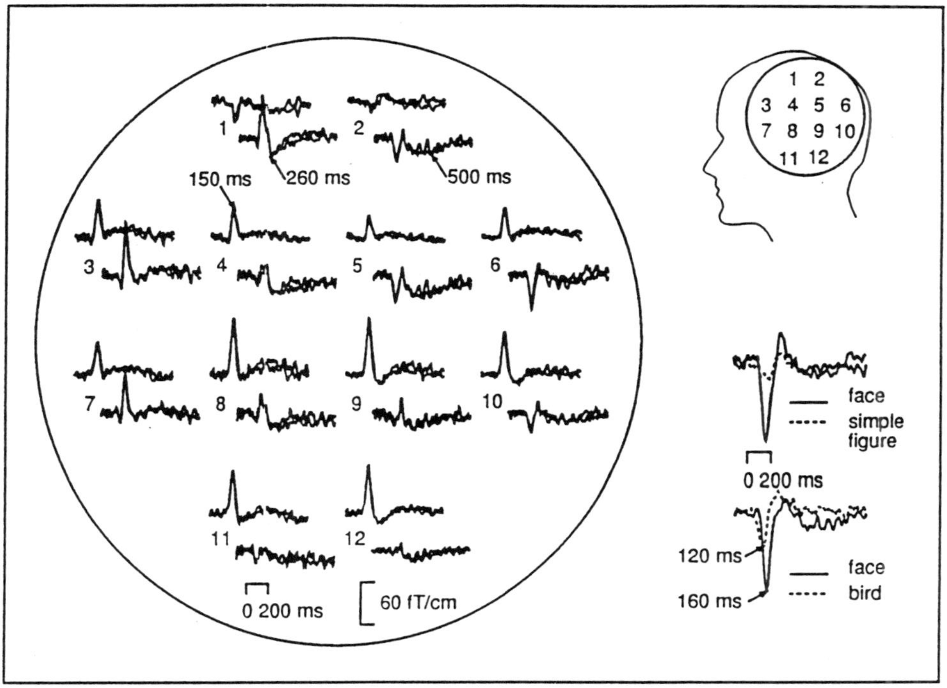

FIG. 5.11 Neuromagnetic responses to face stimuli over the left hemisphere of one subject, measured with a 24-channel SQUID gradiometer. The approximate location of the instrument is shown on the schematic head. Both traces in each pair were measured over the same location, the upper curves representing the magnetic field gradient in the vertical and the lower in the horizontal direction. The insert shows responses of the same subject from the right hemisphere to equiprobable face (solid lines) and simple (dashed lines) figures (upper illustration) and to face and bird stimuli (lower illustration). These signals were recorded over the same site in consecutive measurements. After averaging ($N = 100$ in each case), the responses were digitally low-pass filtered at 40 Hz. (From Lu et al., 1991. Copyright © 1991 by Pergamon Press PLC. Reprinted with permission.)

third in the middle of the temporal lobe (in this time order). The occipital–temporal and middle-temporal locations were not activated by the other types of stimuli used. The authors therefore suggested that these areas might have an important role in face perception.

5.3. MEG STUDIES IN THE SOMATOSENSORY SYSTEM

Brenner, Lipton, Kaufman, & Williamson (1978) demonstrated that fast-rate somatosensory stimulation of the median nerve elicits steady-state MEG responses over the contralateral primary somatosensory cortex (SI). The sources activated by the stimulation of the thumb and little finger were separated by 2 cm which corresponds to the known SI somatotopy (Penfield and Jasper, 1954). See also Okada, Tanenbaum, Kaufman, and Williamson (1984).

Transient responses to median-nerve stimulation have also been described (Hari, Reinikainen, et al., 1984; Kaufman, Okada, Brenner, & Williamson, 1981; Okada, Kaufman, Brenner, & Williamson, 1981). Responses recorded over the contralateral SI are large in amplitude, whereas those over the ipsilateral SI are negligible (Hari, Reinikainen, et al., 1984; Huttunen, Hari, & Leinonen, 1987; for a review, see Hari & Kaukoranta, 1985). Huttunen et al. (1987) found that for the early part of the contralateral response, the equivalent current dipole for median-nerve stimulation was lateral to that for ulnar-nerve stimulation, which again is in agreement with the known SI somatotopy. For early MEG responses, see also Hari and Kaukoranta (1985), Tiihonen, Hari, and Hämäläinen (1989), and Wood, Cohen, Cuffin, Yarita, and Allison (1985).

Wood et al. (1985) compared the early (20–30 msec) electric and magnetic responses to median-nerve stimulation. The responses were similar in waveform and their dipolar field patterns were centered over the contralateral primary somatosensory hand area but were rotated by 90° with respect to one another. The magnetic field pattern could be accounted for by a tangential current source in somatosensory area 3b in the posterior wall of the Rolandic fissure, whereas the electric responses appeared to be partly due to radial sources that could not be seen in the magnetic recordings.

Teszner, Hari, and Nicolas (1983) found that when the ISI of a stimulus block was prolonged from 1 to 8 sec, the MEG response to median-nerve stimulation increased in amplitude, whereas the field pattern of the response was not affected. Thus, the responses were, evidently, generated at SI with both short and long ISIs. In the simultaneous electric vertex recordings, a prominent "N130–P230 complex" with no magnetic counterpart was obtained with the long ISI. See also Huttunen, Hari, and Vanni (1987).

Kaukoranta and Reinikainen (1985) compared the ISI dependence of the electric and magnetic responses. The electric N1 recorded over the vertex peaked at 120 msec, whereas the main magnetic response reached its maximum amplitude at about 80 msec. In addition, the electric response increased more rapidly in amplitude with the increasing ISI than did the magnetic response (Fig. 5.12).

The authors concluded that the activity of the primary somatosensory cortex, which generated the MEG response, at least its main part, cannot be

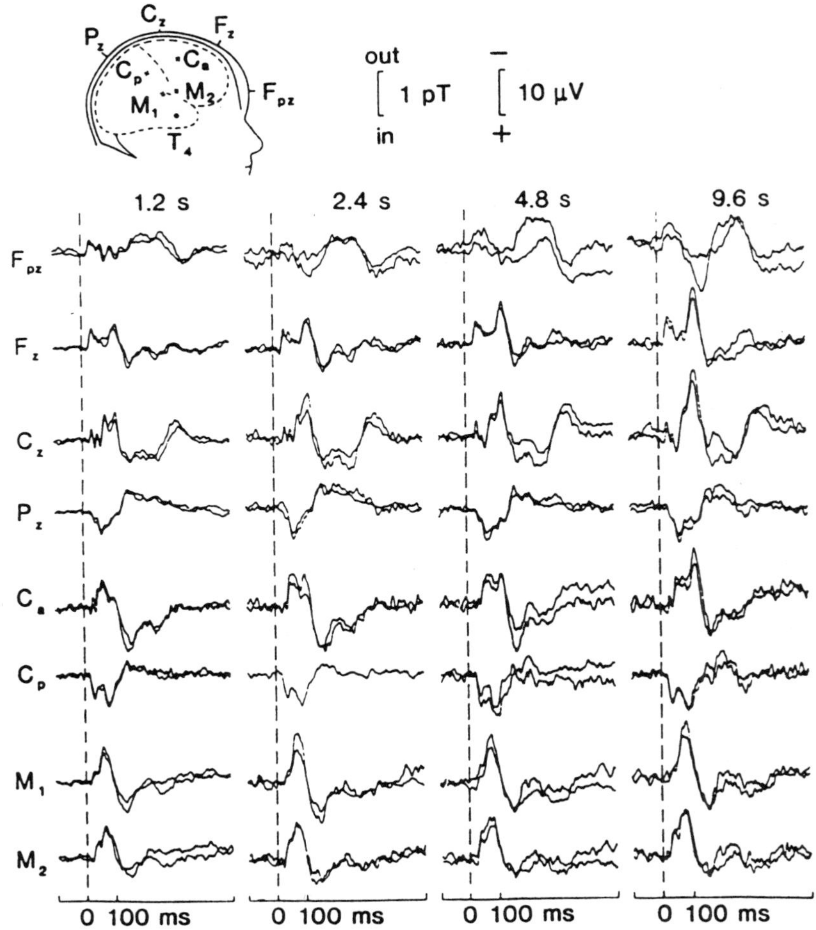

FIG. 5.12 Simultaneously measured electric, from different electrode locations (6 upper rows), and magnetic responses (2 lower rows) from one subject to somatosensory stimuli presented at different ISIs. (The ISI was constant within block.) The schematic head illustrates the recording locations. (From Kaukoranta & Reinikainen, 1985. Copyright © 1985 by the Low Temperature Laboratory of the Helsinki University of Technology. Reprinted with permission.)

the only source of the electric vertex response. Intracranial recordings of Goff, Allison, and Vaughan (1978) provide converging evidence.

Hari and Kaukoranta (1985) observed that when the stimulus rate is increased from 2 to 30 Hz, transient responses gradually change into steady-state responses.

As originally suggested by Okada et al. (1981), it is possible to record MEG responses also from the SII area (Hari, Hämäläinen, Kaukoranta, Reinikainen, & Teszner, 1983; Hari, Reinikainen, et al., 1984; Teszner et al., 1983; Kaukoranta, Hari, Hämäläinen, & Huttunen, 1986). Like SI responses, SII responses can be recorded both to median-nerve and peroneal-nerve (lower-limb) stimulation. Kaukoranta et al. (1986), using peroneal-nerve stimulation, found that SII responses to ipsilateral stimuli were weaker and had longer latencies than responses to contralateral stimuli.

MEG responses of the SI area elicited by stimulation of the lower limbs seem to emanate from sources that are consistent with the known SI somatotopy (Hari, Reinikainen, et al., 1984; Okada et al., 1984; Teszner et al., 1983).

Separate finger representations in the SII area were recently demonstrated by the MEG recordings of Hari, Hämäläinen, Hämäläinen, Kekoni, Sams, and Tiihonen (1990). See Fig. 5.13. Cutaneous electrical stimulation of the thumb or the middle finger elicited a response at around 100 msec. The field pattern of the response suggested a generator location in the secondary somatosensory cortex. When stimuli applied to the thumb served as standards and stimuli to the middle finger as deviants (or vice versa), responses to the deviants were almost 3 times as large in amplitude as those to the standards. This result does not demonstrate a somatosensory MMNm, however, because when the standards were omitted, deviants elicited responses very similar to those elicited by these deviants when interspersed with standards. Consistently with this, Huttunen, Hari, and Leinonen (1987) found no MMNm at SI when stimuli to the ulnar nerve served as standards and stimuli to the median nerve as deviants, or vice versa. (Both stimuli were applied to the wrist.)

Cerebral magnetic fields to the stimulation of the tongue were studied by Karhu, Hari, Lu, Paetau, and Rif (1991). The response consisted of two main deflections which peaked at about 55 msec and 140 msec from the onset of electric stimulation. The earlier deflection could be explained by a tangential dipole in the primary somatosensory cortex, whereas the dipole for the later response was about 1 cm lateral to the earlier response, probably in the SII area. The authors concluded from the results of this first MEG study with trigeminal-nerve stimulation that MEG allows noninvasive determination of the cortical tongue-representation area.

In addition, MEG studies with noxious stimulation, such as dental stimulation (Hari, Kaukoranta, Reinikainen, Huopaniemi, & Mauno, 1983;

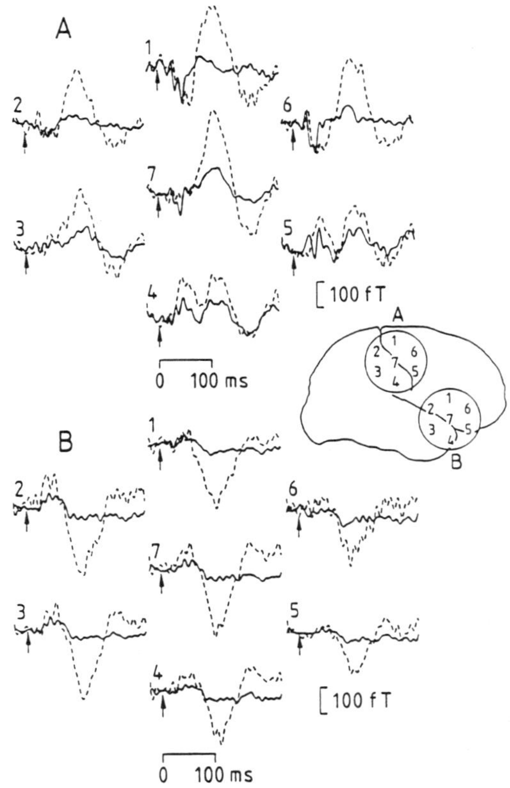

FIG. 5.13 Seven-channel MEG recordings in one subject at two locations (shown schematically on the inset brain) to electric pulses presented to the left thumb (standards, continuous lines) and middle finger (deviants, dashed lines). The arrows show the time of stimulus presentation. (From Hari et al., 1990. Copyright © 1990 by Pergamon Press PLC. Reprinted with permission.)

for a review, see Hari & Kaukoranta, 1985), seem to have contributed to understanding cerebral response patterns underlying the experience of pain.

Finally, a magnetic mu rhythm in man was described by Tiihonen, Kajola, and Hari (1989). This rhythm appeared to be mainly generated in the primary somatosensory hand-projection area. The frequency spectrum of the rhythm showed two distinct peaks, one around 10 Hz and the other around 21 Hz. The high-frequency activity was blocked by the clenching of the fist but was not affected by the opening of the eyes, in agreement with the electric mu rhythm.

6

Attention and Event-Related Potentials

In this chapter, effects of attention on the Event-Related Potentials (ERP) are examined. The stage for this examination was set in chapter 4 where the nature and extent of automatic, attention-independent processing was delineated on the basis of the available ERP evidence. These data seemed to establish that physical stimulus features, at least in the auditory modality, are extensively processed irrespective of the direction of attention.

The present chapter starts the analysis of the attention effects on ERPs by examining these effects first in the oddball paradigm. Attention in the oddball situation is usually introduced by instructing the subject to discriminate deviant stimuli among standard stimuli. This "one-channel attention" can, of course, involve other types of situations, for instance, listening to a speaker in the absence of a competing stimulus source. Thereafter, selective attention is dealt with, that in operation when attending to one out of two or several concurrent streams of input. Because of certain fundamental intermodal differences, ERP correlates of selective attention in different modalities are examined in separate sections. Theories of selective attention based on these data are also examined and evaluated.

6.1. AUDITORY ERPS AND ATTENTION: ONE-CHANNEL TASKS

This section examines ERPs recorded when the subject is concentrating on discriminating occasional deviant stimuli randomly interspersed among standard (frequent) stimuli. The left side of Fig. 6.1 schematically illustrates

ERP components elicited in the oddball paradigm, and the right side shows ERP waveforms arising as a result of summation of the components shown on the left side. The components and ERP waveforms of the "ignore" condition are illustrated on the upper half; those from the "attend" condition are shown on the lower half of the figure. (For the sake of simplicity, the N1 subcomponents are not separately illustrated.)

In the ignore condition, the main difference between ERPs to deviants and standards is MMN elicited by the deviants. MMN is under certain conditions (not illustrated in Fig. 6.1) followed by P3a (chapter 4) and, if the magnitude of stimulus deviation is wide, by N2b and some slower positivity.

The picture gets more complex when attention is introduced (Fig. 6.1, bottom). Yet the basic elements of the response, most notably the MMN component to deviants (Section 4.4), remain the same, or at least very similar, as in the absence of attention. The earliest difference (not shown in Fig. 6.1) from ignore conditions is probably a somewhat larger N1 amplitude for attend conditions (for both standards and deviants). This might be due to either a nonspecific increase in cerebral excitability during attention (Näätänen, 1967, 1975), a decreased threshold of the N1 attention-switching (conscious-perception) mechanism (chapter 4), or overlap by an attention-related endogenous negativity (see later).

The P2 wave to standards may also be somewhat larger in attend than ignore conditions, because of either an enhanced generator process of the P2 component or an overlap with an endogenous positivity in attend conditions (Näätänen et al., 1983; Sams, Paavilainen, et al., 1985).

N2b (for a review, see Näätänen & Gaillard, 1983) is usually elicited only in attend conditions. When a stimulus deviation is wide, N2b of a modest amplitude may, however, occur in ignore conditions (Näätänen et al., 1982). N2b might be related to brain events associated with transient arousal response and the OR (Loveless, 1983, 1986; Näätänen & Gaillard, 1983). N2b has a broad, central scalp distribution resembling, at least to some extent, that of the nonspecific N1 component (Näätänen & Gaillard, 1983; Sams et al., 1990). Pointing to this similarity, Loveless (1983) proposed that the two components might emanate from the same generator. However, topographical analyses of ERPs to auditory and visual stimulus deviations (Simson et al., 1977a, 1977b) and omissions (Simson et al., 1976) suggest that N2b is, in fact, modality-specifically distributed.

N2b is usually followed by P3a, also elicited by deviants in the attend oddball condition. The N2b–P3a association is very strong (Courchesne, Hillyard, & Galambos, 1975; Loveless, 1983, 1986; Näätänen et al., 1982; Renault & Lesévre, 1978, 1979; Snyder & Hillyard, 1976; K. Squires, Donchin, Herning, & McCarthy, 1977; N. Squires et al., 1975); therefore, the two have often been referred to as the N2–P3a or N2b–P3a wave complex. N2b can, however, occur without P3a (Knight, 1990; Ritter et al.,

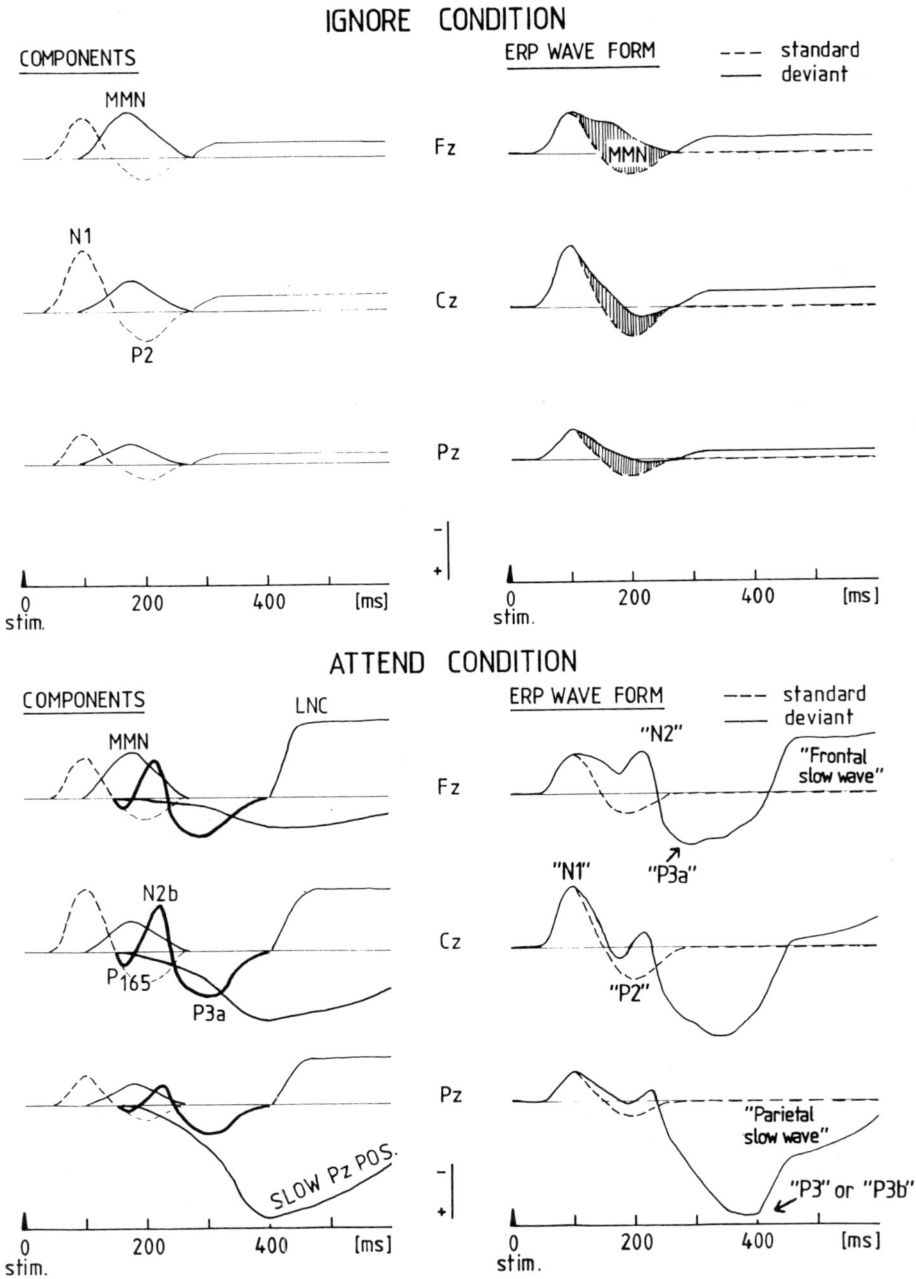

FIG. 6.1 A simplified schematic illustration of the frontal (Fz), vertex (Cz), and parietal (Pz) ERPs (right side) to standard (dashed line) and deviant (solid line) stimuli and the corresponding ERP components (left side) in the oddball paradigm. They are derived separately for the ignore (top) and attend (bottom) conditions. For a detailed explanation of the components and waves shown, see text. (Adapted from Näätänen, Sams, & Alho, 1986. Copyright © 1986 Elsevier Science Publishers BV [Biomedical Division].)

1991). P3a occurs without a preceding N2b, for instance in response to deviants in ignore conditions (Sams, Paavilainen, et al., 1985).

Fig. 6.2 shows ERPs to slightly deviant stimuli in Sams, Paavilainen, et al.'s (1985) discrimination condition. (The corresponding reading-condition data were illustrated in Fig. 4.19). The large negative peak after N1 in response to deviants in this figure is mainly composed of the N2b component. This is better seen in Fig. 6.3, showing difference waves

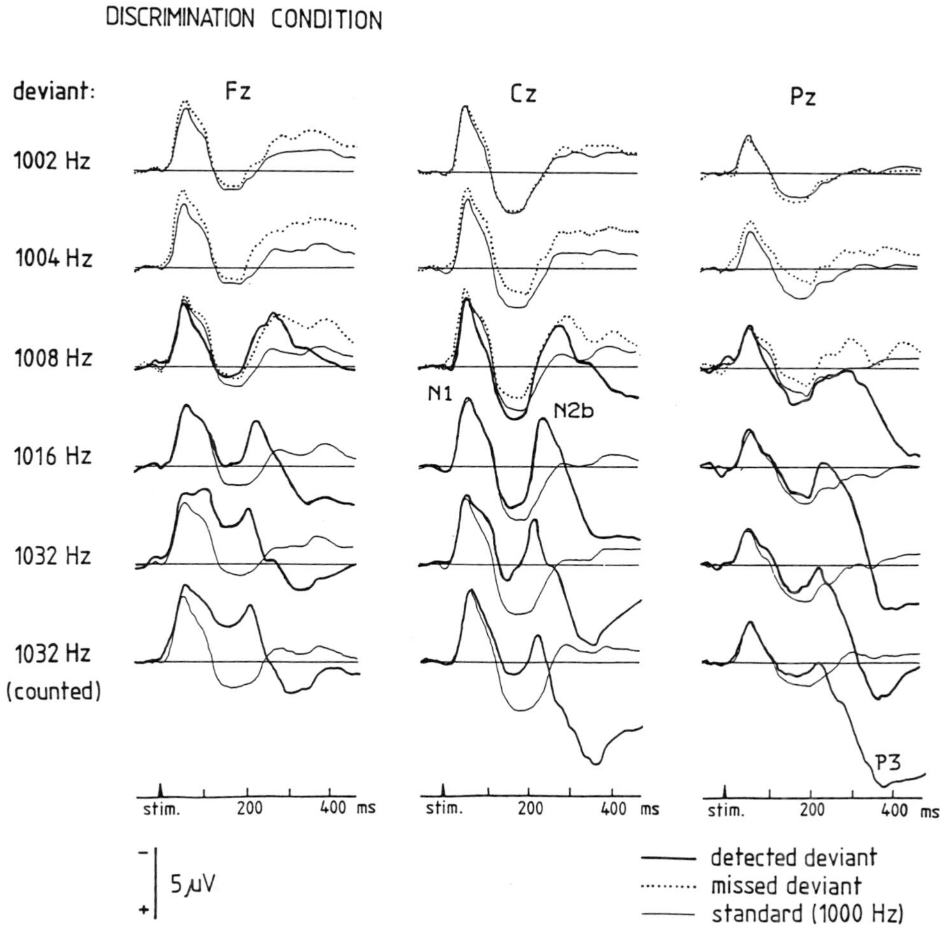

FIG. 6.2 Frontal (Fz), vertex (Cz), and parietal (Pz) grand-average ERPs to detected deviants (thick line), missed deviants (dotted line), and correctly rejected standards (thin line) in a discrimination condition when the standard stimulus was 1,000 Hz and the deviant stimulus, in separate blocks, 1,002–1,032 Hz. The subject was instructed to press a button upon discrimination of a deviant stimulus except when the deviant stimuli were to be counted (bottom row). (From Sams, Paavilainen, Alho, and Näätänen, 1985. Copyright © 1985 by Elsevier Science Publishers, Ireland. Reprinted with permission.)

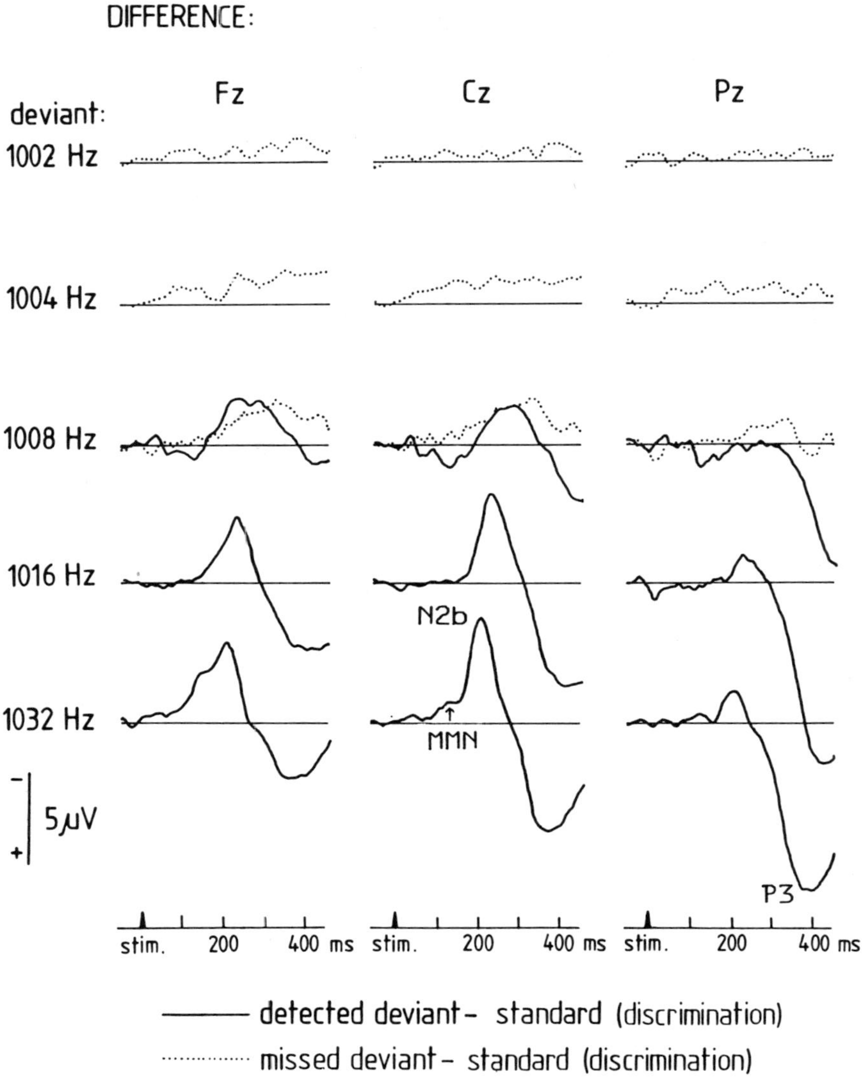

FIG. 6.3 Frontal (Fz), vertex (Cz), and parietal (Pz) grand-average difference waves obtained by subtracting ERPs to the correctly rejected standards from those to detected deviants (continuous line) and missed deviants (dotted line) in the discrimination condition when the standard stimulus was 1,000 Hz and the deviant stimulus, in separate blocks, 1,002–1,032 Hz. The subject was instructed to press a button upon discrimination of a deviant stimulus. (The same data as those presented in Fig. 6.2.) (From Sams, Paavilainen, Alho, and Näätänen, 1985. Copyright © 1985 by Elsevier Science Publishers, Ireland. Reprinted with permission.)

obtained by subtracting standard-stimulus ERPs from ERPs to detected deviants. The remaining sharp negativity provides quite a good estimate of the sum of the N2b and MMN components, for P2 is canceled in such a subtraction. The early portion of this negativity is mainly due to the MMN component, the late portion principally to the N2b component.

In Fig. 6.4, ERPs to deviants during reading were subtracted from those to detected deviants of the discrimination condition. Because the MMN component is canceled in this subtraction, the remaining sharp negative peak provides quite a reliable estimate of the N2b component. It is seen that the N2b latency becomes systematically shorter as the stimulus difference increases. The same is true with regard to the subsequent, posteriorly largest, late positivity.

N2b is preceded by a sharp positivity peaking at 150–160 msec from stimulus onset in Fig. 6.4. This positivity resembles Goodin, Squires, Henderson, and Starr's (1978b) and Goodin, Squires, and Starr's (1983) "P165" wave, which they obtained by subtracting the deviant-stimulus ERPs of their ignore condition from those of the attend condition. In the Sams, Paavilainen, and colleagues (1985) data, this positivity is not produced by a separate P165 component; rather, it emerges as a result of a complex summation of many overlapping components. If it were a separate component elicited by deviants in the discrimination condition, then it should be present in Fig. 6.3. In these data (Fig. 6.4), P165 probably emerges mainly because the exogenous P2 component (probably for both standards and deviants) was larger in the discrimination than reading condition (cf. standard-stimulus ERPs at Cz in Figs. 4.16 and 6.2). Novak and colleagues (1990) also found no evidence for a separate P165 component. Goodin et al. (1978b, 1983), however, reported that they found no significant P2 differences between standard stimuli in their attend and ignore conditions.

The most conspicuous aspect of the deviant-stimulus ERP under attend conditions is the late parietal positivity, as shown in Figs. 6.2, 6.3, and 6.4. This slow parietal process constitutes a major component of the "P3" wave, the aspect of the ERP that has received the greatest amount of research interest (Sutton, Braren, Zubin & John, 1965; for reviews, see Donchin & Coles, 1988; Johnson, 1988; Pritchard, 1981; Roth, 1983; Ruchkin & Sutton, 1983; Verleger, 1988). In the present context, the slow parietal positive component probably is the first ERP component that reflects not only stimulus deviation but also recognition that the stimulus is a target. This is suggested by oddball studies with two different deviant stimuli, one designated as a target and the other as a nontarget. In one of these studies conducted in the visual modality, Courchesne, Courchesne, and Hillyard (1978) reported a larger late positivity to the target than to an equally rare and deviant nontarget deviant. Corroborating results were

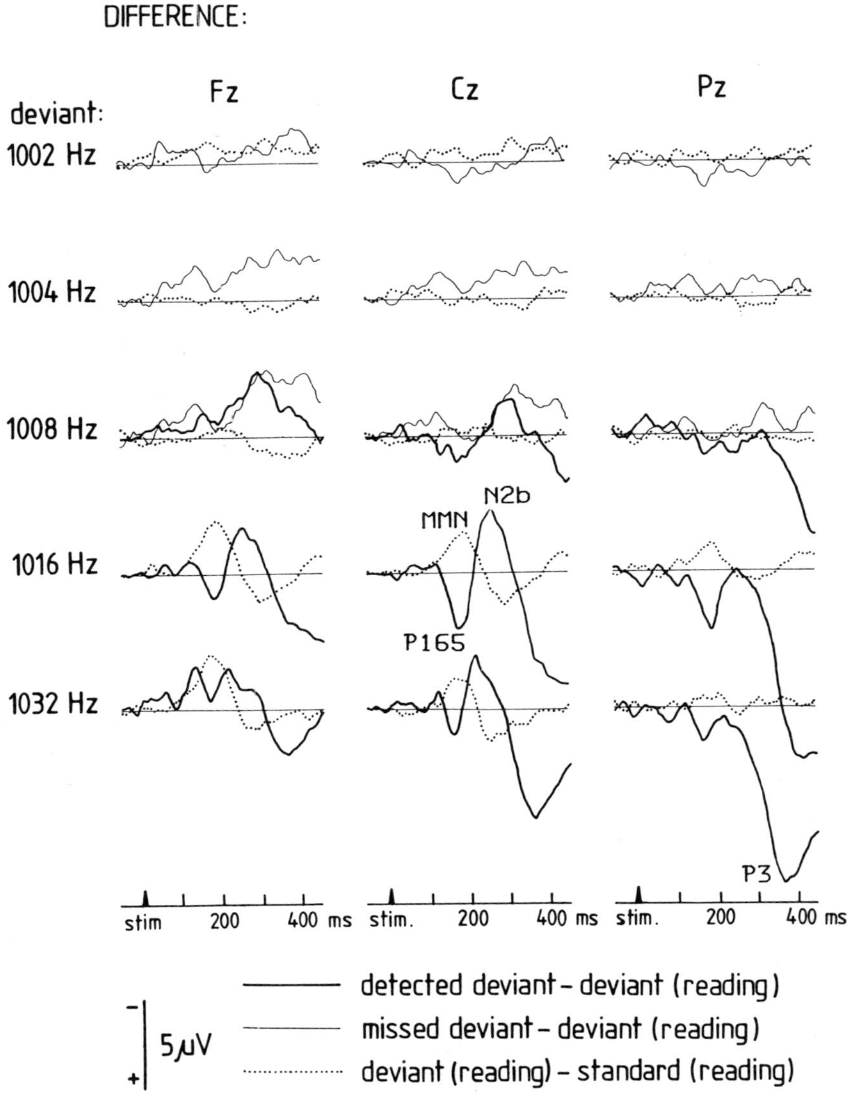

FIG. 6.4 Frontal (Fz), vertex (Cz), and parietal (Pz) grand-average difference waves obtained by subtracting (1) ERPs to reading-condition deviants from those to detected deviants in the discrimination condition (thick line), (2) ERPs to reading-condition deviants from those to missed deviants in the discrimination condition (thin line), and (3) ERPs to standards from those to deviants (dotted line) in the reading condition. The standard stimulus was 1,000 Hz and the deviant stimulus, in separate blocks, 1,002–1,032 Hz. The subject was instructed to press a button upon discrimination of a deviant stimulus. The same data as in Figs. 6.2 and 6.3. (Unpublished figure from Sams, Paavilainen, Alho, & Näätänen, 1985.)

provided by Courchesne, Hillyard, and Courchesne (1977) and Roth, Ford, and Kopell (1978).

On the other hand, Näätänen et al. (1982), presenting their equivalent target and nontarget deviants at a considerably smaller probability (2% each), found no significant difference in slow positivity elicited by the two deviants. The authors suggested that the very low probabilities used "may have resulted in all deviants eliciting 'significance responses' usually elicited only by targets, leaving no room for any specific target effect beyond the effect of stimulus deviance. This is tantamount to saying that highly infrequent environmental changes are 'biologically significant' (Sutton, 1979)" (Näätänen et al., 1982, p. 84).

Sams, Paavilainen, et al. (1985) averaged ERPs elicited by deviant stimuli at the discrimination threshold (deviants 1008 Hz, standards 1000 Hz) separately for the trials on which the deviant stimulus was and was not discriminated. Figures 6.2, 6.3, and 6.4 show that (a) the large, late positivity is elicited by discriminated 1008-Hz deviants only, the trace for the nondiscriminated targets remaining negative throughout the averaging epoch, and (b) the process generating this (statistically significant) negativity, possibly N2b, is initiated at the same time by the discriminated and nondiscriminated deviants, but it appears to last longer for the nondiscriminated deviants. In this case, the process apparently failed to reach the threshold for conscious discrimination (see also Loveless, 1986). A similar, though nonsignificant, long-duration shift is also seen for the clearly subliminal, 1004-Hz deviants.

Thus, if the process generating the possible N2b negativity succeeds in triggering slow positivity, then a conscious discrimination of stimulus deviation probably occurs on this trial, whereas if no positivity ensues, the preconscious discrimination process fails to result in conscious discrimination. Whether the N2b process is vigorous enough might in turn be determined by (a) the strength of the MMN-generating process preceding it, fluctuating as a function of the magnitude of stimulus deviation and the strength of the trace at the moment of the deviant stimulus (Section 4.4), and (b) the strength of temporary facilitatory coupling between the MMN and N2b generator processes; with increasing facilitation, the MMN generator process succeeds more easily in triggering the N2b process. This temporary facilitatory connection might constitute the central element in the neurophysiological basis of an attentive set to discriminate physical stimulus changes in the oddball task (discussed later).

The last component elicited by deviants in the oddball attend condition is a slow frontal negativity, with an onset latency of about 400–500 msec (Rohrbaugh, Syndulko, & Lindsley, 1978, 1979). This is the slow negative component that in S1-S2 paradigms explains the early, frontally distributed, slow negativity (Gaillard, 1976, 1978; Loveless & Sanford, 1974a, 1974b;

Näätänen & Gaillard, 1974) and precedes the S2-related, anticipatory negativity, the "true CNV" (Hillyard, 1973; Näätänen & Michie, 1979b; Ruchkin, Sutton, Mahaffey, & Glaser, 1986).[1] In most conditions, the slow frontal negative and parietal positive components tend to co-occur. Therefore, these two together are usually referred to as the "slow wave" (N. Squires et al., 1975). The two elements of the slow wave can, however, be dissociated (Loveless, Simpson, & Näätänen, 1987).

It is not yet quite clear which aspects of the attend condition the various ERP components elicited by deviants are related to. However, the following suggestions for the auditory ERP might be put forward:

- MMN and P3a are related to physical stimulus deviation but not to stimulus significance, for instance, whether the stimulus is a target or not. For MMN (but probably not for P3a; Ritter et al., 1991), this stimulus deviation can also be a repetition of the previous stimulus in a regularly alternating stimulus pattern, that is, a deviation against the temporal patterning of stimulation (Nordby et al., 1988a). Whereas MMN usually is elicited independently of attention, P3a elicitation often depends on attention.
- N2b is usually elicited by a physical stimulus deviation but may also be elicited by stimulus repetition, even when this repetition signifies no deviation in temporal patterning of stimulation (Näätänen, 1986d; Ritter et al., 1991; see also the data of Duncan-Johnson & Donchin, 1982). Thus, N2b might be related to expectancy violation (Näätänen, 1986d). In essence, N2b seems to be elicited by infrequent events in attended input. (Only wide deviations in unattended input may elicit an N2b; Näätänen et al., 1982.) N2b is not related to stimulus significance, however, in the sense of the stimulus being a target. This is shown by the aforementioned result that, given an attentive set, N2b is elicited by both target and nontarget deviants in one-channel situations (Alho, Lavikainen, Reinikainen, Sams, & Näätänen, 1990; Näätänen et al., 1982; Nordby et al., 1988a).
- The slow parietal positive component might be specifically related to stimulus significance, for it responds differentially to target and nontarget deviants, at least when they are not very infrequent (Näätänen et al., 1982). Furthermore, this positivity is elicited by the target irrespective of whether it is a stimulus deviation or repetition (Ritter et al., 1991; Sams et al., 1983, 1984). This component probably cannot be elicited in the absence of attention.
- The slow frontal negative component seems to be related to both

[1]However, most of the S2-related negativity is, as maintained by Rohrbaugh and Gaillard (1983), composed of the movement-related slow negative component called the "Bereitschafts-potential" (BP) (Kornhuber & Deecke, 1965).

stimulus change and significance (McCallum, Barrett, & Pocock, 1989; Näätänen et al., 1982; Sams et al., 1983, 1984).

It appears that the previously discussed complex sequence of late endogenous components, starting with N2b and the early phase of the slow parietal positivity (Näätänen, 1975; Sams, Paavilainen, et al., 1985), is triggered by the cerebral process generating MMN when the deviant stimulus is an auditory change. As already mentioned, Novak et al. (1990) suggested that this late sequence of brain processes generating the post-MMN endogenous components, as well as the processes underlying the release of motor response, are time-locked to the MMN generator process. Previously, it was observed by Renault and Lesévre (1979) that the duration of their ramp-like negativity ("N2a") determined the latencies of the subsequent components. This N2a was elicited by stimulus omissions in a sequence of regularly spaced visual stimuli. This N2a cannot, however, be regarded as a strict equivalent for the auditory MMN (see Czigler & Csibra, 1990; Näätänen & Gaillard, 1983).

Further converging evidence for the MMN generator process initiating the sequence of brain processes leading to conscious discrimination of stimulus deviation was provided by Lang et al. (1990). These authors showed that behavioral discrimination between sequential auditory stimuli is probably based on the mechanism generating MMN. In their study with high-school pupils of 17 years in age, three groups of pupils were formed on the basis of accuracy in pitch discrimination: those with "good," "mediocre," or "poor" "pitch ears." In the subsequent MMN recordings, performed while the subject was reading, the standard stimulus was of 698 Hz and the frequency of the deviant stimuli was different in different blocks.

In the good pitch-discrimination group, a clear MMN was found with a frequency difference of 19 Hz. For some subjects, even 12 Hz was enough. With the poor performers, the average threshold of MMN elicitation seemed to lie somewhere between 50 and 100 Hz. The moderate performers took an intermediate position between the two extreme groups (Fig. 6.5). The frequency difference of 25 Hz (about 3%) seemed to discriminate most effectively between the three groups.

In contrast, with large frequency differences, all groups produced very similar responses to deviant stimuli. This is probably due to the large frequency deviation eliciting a large response from the N1 generators, an effect also observed by Novak et al. (1990) and Scherg, Vajsar, and Picton (1989; see also Scherg & Picton, 1990).

The Lang et al. (1990) study consequently demonstrated that MMN recorded in a passive condition predicts the accuracy of discrimination performance. This suggests that the cerebral mechanisms involved in passive discrimination, as expressed by the MMN generator process, are also

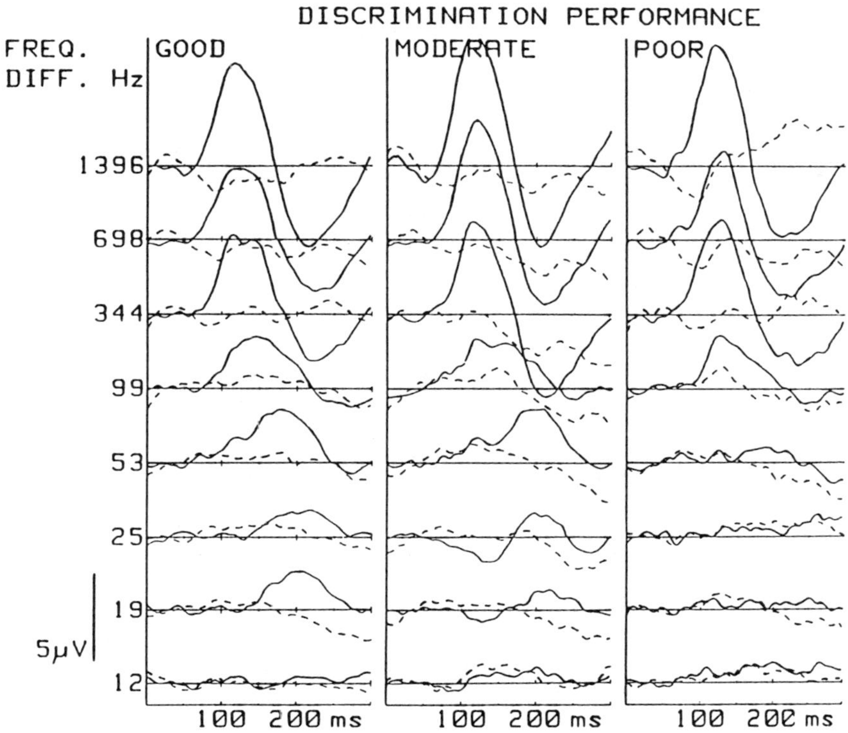

FIG. 6.5 Grand-average frontal (Fz) ERPs to standard (dashed line) and deviant (solid line) stimuli of subjects with good (left), moderate (middle), and poor (right) discrimination performance for different levels of separation between deviant and standard stimuli as indicated on the left. The standard stimulus was 698 Hz, the deviant stimulus, in different blocks, 710–2,094 Hz. (From Lang et al., 1990. Copyright © 1990 by Tilburg University Press. Reprinted with permission.)

involved in active discrimination. Thus, in the oddball task, the MMN generator process appears to represent the first, preconscious, step in discriminating stimulus deviation and to trigger the chain of further cerebral processes, which lead to conscious discrimination of stimulus deviation. These further processes generate, apparently, the post-MMN endogenous ERP components. (As discussed previously, the N2b process has, apparently, to exceed some threshold, however; otherwise the endogenous sequence is prematurely terminated and no conscious discrimination occurs.) If this MMN generator process of an individual is sensitive, it can trigger the chain of the further processes even when the frequency change is small; with a less sensitive MMN process, this chain of further processes is not triggered by a small frequency change, and no conscious discrimination occurs.

Consequently, as already suggested, attention in an oddball task might be characterized as "internal monitoring" of the possible occurrence of the MMN process, that is, as a temporary functional link between the MMN-generator mechanism and the limited-capacity system (Näätänen et al., 1982). The presence of this link is reflected by a facilitatory link between the MMN mechanism and further cerebral processes, so that even a very weak MMN process is sufficient to trigger those further processes. This link is also reflected by the aforementioned result that those later processes, as well as the motor response, seem to be time-locked to the MMN generator process (Näätänen et al., 1982; Novak et al., 1990). The earliest of the further processes triggered by the MMN generator mediate, presumably, between the preconscious discrimination of stimulus deviation by the MMN mechanism and the conscious discrimination of this deviation by the limited-capacity system. The critical borderline between the preconscious and conscious processes in discriminating a stimulus deviation under attentive set might lie in the connection between the N2b generator process and those of the subsequent positivities.

6.2. AUDITORY ERPS AND ATTENTION: MULTI-CHANNEL TASKS (SELECTIVE ATTENTION)

In this section, possible selective-attention effects on the obligatory components of the auditory ERP are first examined. Thereafter, endogenous effects of auditory selection attention are dealt with.

Obligatory Components: The "N1 effect" of Selective Attention

Early Studies. The early search for ERP correlates of selective attention in humans was centered around the N1 wave. Several studies conducted in the early 1960s presented their to-be-attended and -ignored stimuli in a predictable, usually alternating, order and reported that the N1 (N1–P2) amplitude was larger for attended than for ignored stimuli. The most frequently cited of these studies was that of Spong, Haider, and Lindsley (1965), conducted in D. B. Lindsley's laboratory at UCLA, Los Angeles, pioneering in the field at that time. This study compared ERPs elicited by auditory and visual stimuli when either stimulus category, as designated by instructions, was to be attended.

When performing the visual task, attending to flashes and ignoring clicks, the subject received bright flashes, requiring no response, and occasional dim flashes, which required the pressing of a key. The clicks that alternated with the flashes (ISI 1 sec) were all of the same intensity and were to be ignored. In the auditory task, the subject was required to press a key in response to occasional weak clicks interspersed among more numerous louder clicks. Flashes alternating with the clicks during the auditory task were all of the same intensity and were to be ignored.

It was found that when the subject was attending to visual stimuli, the nontarget flashes elicited much larger (occipital) ERPs than the same flashes did when clicks were to be attended. Similarly, when the subject was attending to auditory stimuli, (temporal) ERPs to nontarget clicks were larger than when flashes were to be attended.

As pointed out by Näätänen (1967), the enhanced amplitudes of ERPs to relevant stimuli may in fact have resulted from differentially enhanced nonspecific or general arousal or "activation," due to anticipatory and preparatory processes immediately prior to a relevant stimulus. These differential prestimulus processes or states were made possible by the alternating order of presentation of the stimuli, which allowed the subject to know the sensory modality of the stimulus that would come next. Näätänen proposed that "alertness" and "activation" will be high when the subject knows that a stimulus of the relevant modality is about to be presented, and will be low when a stimulus of the irrelevant modality is about to be presented.

Basically similar paradigms to that of Spong et al. (1965) were used, among others, by Davis (1964), Satterfield (1965), Satterfield and Cheatum (1964), and, within the visual modality, by Chapman (1965), Chapman and Bragdon (1964), and Sheatz and Chapman (1969). Most of these authors regarded their results as providing an ERP correlate for selective attention, stimulus relevance, or related psychological phenomena, and in the literature these works were frequently cited as evidence for such relationships. A similar remark to that made with respect to the Spong et al. study can, however, be also made with respect to these studies. For a review of these works and the details of this criticism, see Karlin (1970) and Näätänen (1967).

Näätänen (1967) conducted three experiments to separate the specific and non-specific effects of attention on ERPs from each other. The first experiment was aimed at studying ERPs to stimuli of an irrelevant modality during attention directed to another modality. "It might be that all kinds of stimuli, even of a completely irrelevant sense modality, elicit evoked potentials with enhanced amplitudes, if presented during attention directed to one sense modality" (p. 60). (Chapter 4 already reviewed evidence for a correlation between vigilance or arousal and the N1 amplitude.) Attention to vision was introduced periodically by presenting a sequence of a warning flash (SI) and an irregularly timed (1, 2, or 3 sec after S1) imperative flash (S2) requiring a rapid key press. In addition, a click was presented randomly, in a minority of the trials, either 1 or 2 sec after S1 (always before S2). It was found that these clicks elicited larger ERPs than did physically similar clicks presented during the intertrial interval when the subject was relaxed again. Hence, this result suggested that selective attention may also produce non-specific ERP effects.

Näätänen (1967, 1970) also demonstrated that when relevant and irrelevant stimuli are presented in an alternating order and at regular (1 sec) intervals, the CNV (Fig. 6.6) and the flattening of the background EEG selectively precede relevant stimuli. Such CNVs differentially preceding relevant stimuli in attention paradigms with a predictable stimulus order have been confirmed by Donchin and Smith (1970), Wilkinson and Ashby (1974), and, in the visual modality, by Corby and Kopell (1973).

These prestimulus changes in Näätänen's study took place mainly with those subjects whose ERP amplitudes were enhanced for relevant stimuli. The EEG flattening indeed was a nonspecific phenomenon: For example, the occipital EEG tended to be of a significantly lower amplitude before relevant than irrelevant auditory stimuli; that is, when the subject presumably paid attention to auditory stimuli than when he or she did not do so.

It was concluded that if the task offers some basis for anticipation of the

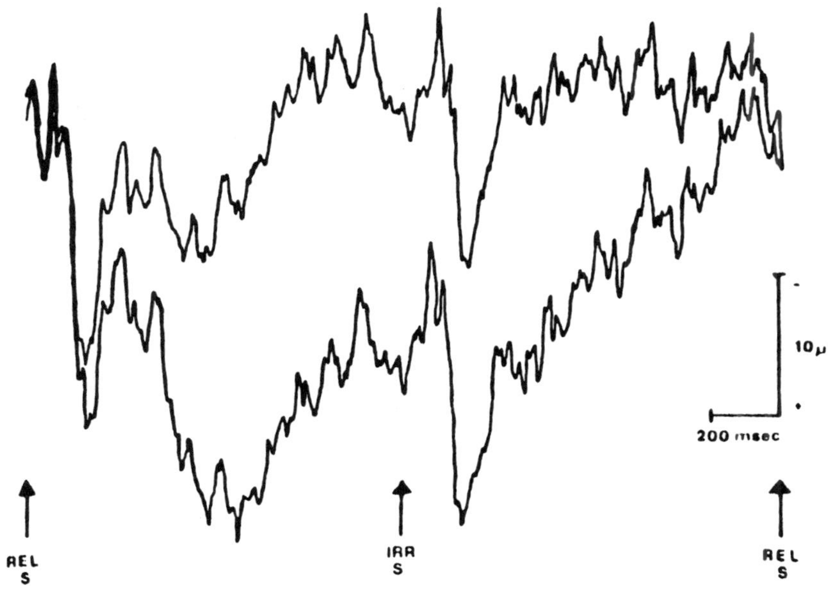

FIG. 6.6 The upper curve represents an averaged vertex (Cz) record of one subject during the 2-sec interval between two successive relevant stimuli (weak clicks) intervened by an irrelevant stimulus (strong click), with the bandwidth setting of 1–70 cps. The ISI was constant at 1 sec. The lower curve represents the same averaged vertex record when the bandwidth was .3–70 cps. (From Näätänen, 1967. Reproduced with the permission of the Finnish Academy of Science and Letters.)

relevant events, the subject "works periodically, maximizing his or her alertness and activation at the anticipated presentation of the relevant stimuli, to make the detection or discrimination required as efficient as possible. If the task is easy, cues for improved performance are not utilized as unnecessary." (Näätänen, 1967, p. 166).

A further experiment of Näätänen (1967) followed Spong et al.'s (1965) design, but the order of relevant and irrelevant stimuli was randomized and, instead of the 1-sec constant ISI, ISIs were randomly either 1, 2, or 3 sec. Because the subject now had no basis to predict above the chance level which kind of stimulus would come next, the possible differential preparation was eliminated. This also eliminated the auditory attention effect: There were no significant differences in the vertex and temporal ERPs between relevant and irrelevant clicks. On the other hand, in the visual task, a later attention effect was found, relevant flashes evoking vertex and occipital potentials with enhanced P2 or P3 waves.

This study was replicated by Hartley (1970), who obtained mainly corroborating results. He remarked that the slow stimulus rate makes it possible for subjects to handle the information on both channels should they wish to do so, and which they might do even if experimental instructions do not require it.

The "N1 Effect" of Hillyard and Colleagues. The first valid demonstration of the "N1 effect" of selective attention was provided by Hillyard, Hink, Schwent, and Picton (1973) in their now classic study. In this modification of the Wilkinson and Lee (1972; see also Debecker & Desmedt, 1971) short-ISI paradigm, Hillyard et al. also used very short ISIs to force their subjects to attend exclusively to relevant stimuli. The left-ear tones (1500 Hz) were of a considerably higher pitch than the right-ear tones (800 Hz). Both inputs included occasional, randomly placed, slightly higher-pitched tones which were to be counted in a designated ear.

It was found that the vertex N1 deflection was larger in response to attended than ignored stimuli (Fig. 6.7). Hillyard et al. regarded their N1 effect as an enhancement of the "N1 component" and proposed that it reflects Broadbent's (1970, 1971) stimulus-set mode of attention:

> A stimulus set preferentially admits all sensory input to an attended channel (stimuli having in common a simple sensory attribute, such as pitch, position in space, receptor surface, or the like) for further perceptual analysis while blocking or attenuating input arriving over irrelevant channels (for example, the unattended ear) at an early stage of processing. (Hillyard et al., 1973, p. 180)

The authors stressed the short onset latency of the effect as critical evidence:

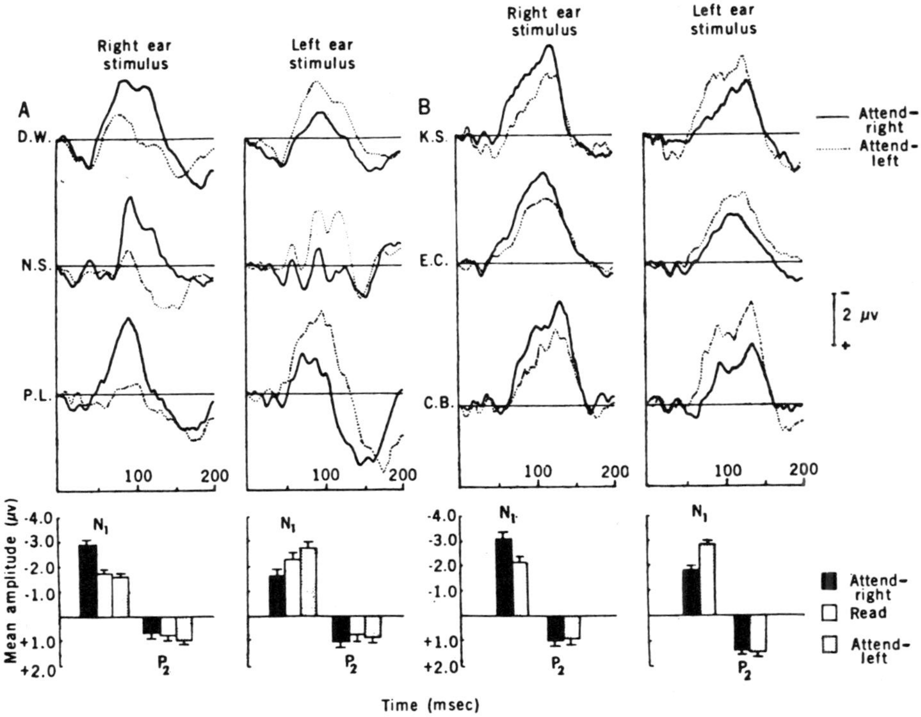

FIG. 6.7 (A)Vertex ERPs from three subjects in Experiment 1. Each tracing is the averaged response to 1,024 stimuli that were presented to each ear under attend-right (solid lines) and attend-left (dotted lines) conditions. Stimulus onset is at beginning of each tracing. Baselines were drawn through the mean voltage over 0 to 10 msec. Bar graphs give the mean and standard error (10 subjects) of the baseline to peak amplitudes of N1 and P2 evoked via each ear under three experimental conditions. (B) ERPs from three subjects in Experiment 2, with bar graphs giving mean amplitudes over all ten subjects. (From Hillyard, Hink, Schwent, & Picton, 1973. Copyright © 1973 by the American Association for the Advancement of Science. Reprinted with permission.)

> The early latency of the attention effects upon N1 (evident at 60 to 70 ms in most subjects) suggests that the underlying attentional process is a tonically maintained set favoring one ear over the other rather than an active discrimination and recognition of each individual stimulus. (Hillyard et al., 1973, p. 179)

This study was regarded by Näätänen (1975) as the only one demonstrating an attention effect at the N1 latency without providing a basis for the subject to predict the order of relevant and irrelevant stimuli. In achieving this result, the authors themselves emphasized the following features of their design: (a) relevant and irrelevant stimuli differed from one another both in spatial localization and pitch attributes, making them easily distinguishable; (b) the fast rate of stimulus presentation; and (c) the difficulty of the task, which ensured that subjects really had to be selectively attentive in order to cope with the task requirements.

P3 peaking at 250–400 msec was found for targets and occasionally also for deviants in the unattended input. The authors proposed that this P3 reflected Broadbent's (1970) response-set mode of attention, which they described as a subsequent processing stage in which "sensory information is compared against memorized 'templates' or 'models' . . . for selected stimuli which are not distinguishable simply by virtue of belonging to a particular sensory input channel" (Hillyard et al., 1973, p. 180). According to Näätänen and Michie (1979a), however, this view is not consistent with Broadbent's original description of the response set (chapter 2). The latter is not a later mechanism performing finer discriminations of physical stimulus differences after the stimulus-set mechanism has made an initial selection based on gross physical stimulus differences.

Further Research on the "N1 Effect." Since this pioneering study, considerable research effort was expended to clarify the conditions and limits of the N1 effect (for reviews, see Hillyard, 1981; Hillyard & Picton, 1979; Näätänen, 1982; Näätänen & Michie, 1979a; Picton, Campbell, Baribeau-Braun, & Proulx, 1978). This research showed, among other things, that even pitch (Schwent, Snyder, & Hillyard, 1976) or spatial differences alone (Hink, Fenton, Pfefferbaum, Tinklenberg, & Kopell, 1978; Schwent & Hillyard, 1975; Schwent et al., 1976) between relevant and irrelevant stimuli sufficed for the N1 effect to emerge. Furthermore, the effect could be obtained even when the subject was attending to one of five (Hink, Fenton, Pfefferbaum, et al., 1978) or four (Schwent & Hillyard, 1975) concurrent stimulus sequences arising from different apparent spatial locations. Also, Schwent, Hillyard, and Galambos (1976) and Parasuraman (1978) reported that the ISI has to be short for the N1 effect to emerge. Hink, Hillyard, and Benson (1978) went on to show that the N1 effect could even be obtained with syllabic stimuli. Donald and Young (1982) found that it takes some 30–45 sec from the beginning of a session for the N1 effect to emerge.

The interpretation of the N1 effect as an enhancement of an N1-generator process was, however, questioned by Näätänen (1975), Näätänen et al. (1978), and Näätänen and Michie (1979a). This controversy is discussed later.

Short-Latency Obligatory Components

The selective-filtering hypothesis of selective attention has a long tradition in research on the physiological basis of higher mental functions. Many prominent authors at different times have expressed a view that selective attention might be based on selective inhibition or blocking of afferent sensory impulses (e.g., Adrian, 1954; Hernández-Peón, 1955, 1961, 1966; Hernández-Peón, Scherrer, & Jouvet, 1956; Horn, 1952; Jouvet & Courjon, 1958; Lindsley, 1960, 1961; Palestini, Davidovitch, & Hernández-Peón, 1959; Scheibel, 1980; Skinner & Yingling, 1977; Tello, 1904, cited in Horn, 1965; Yingling & Skinner, 1977). These authors have mainly proposed some kind of efferent control mechanism by means of which the brain selectively monitors its own input traversing along different afferent sensory pathways. Such a control, or gating, could occur at any level of sensory pathways—at the peripheral receptor, at the first synapse in the central nervous system, or in the thalamus, the final relay structure of the sensory pathways before the cerebral cortex (Picton, Stuss, & Marshall, 1986). Such a gating function could also be located at the cortical level (see Section 6.3).

The subcortical-gating hypothesis of attention was tested in numerous animal experiments. Many of these studies (e.g., Glenn & Oatman, 1977; Hernández-Peón et al., 1956; Oatman, 1971, 1976; Oatman & Anderson, 1977, 1980) reported results that were interpreted as suggesting early mechanisms of selective attention in animals. The popularity of the peripheral-filtering hypothesis was further increased by demonstrations of mechanisms of efferent sensory control in different sensory modalities (Bonfils, Remond, & Pujol, 1986; Dallos, 1981; Desmedt, 1975; Evans, 1982; Guinan & Gifford, 1988a, 1988b; Liberman, 1988; Liberman & Brown, 1986; Møller, 1983; Towe, 1973; Weinberger, 1971). It is, however, not known whether any of these mechanisms are involved in selective attention (Hirschhorn & Michie, 1990; Näätänen & Michie, 1979a; Picton et al., 1986).

The possible existence of a selective-filtering mechanism was regarded by Näätänen (1975) as a basic question in attention research. He stressed the passive, tonic nature of selective filtering with respect to any individual stimulus; the differential treatment of the "relevant" and "irrelevant" impulses would be traceable to prestimulus events resulting in what he called a selective sensory state. Such a prestimulus selective modulation of the afferent sensory system could be either inter- or intramodal, within the limits of functionally separate afferent and efferent systems. Differences in the size of ERPs to relevant and irrelevant stimuli would then simply reflect the selectively premodified state of the afferent system. If such a selective efferent control mechanism does not exist, then the chain of physiological events triggered by relevant and irrelevant stimuli could not reflect selective attention until certain (memory-dependent) discriminatory phases of stimulus processing are reached.

Näätänen (1975) suggested that the following conditions are likely to increase the probability that the possible filtering mechanism will be set into operation:

1. The relevant and irrelevant stimuli traverse along at least partially different afferent systems.
2. The subject has a clear, "vivid" representation of the relevant stimulus. Otherwise, it might not be possible to "tune" the filtering system accordingly.
3. Expectancy (Näätänen & Merisalo, 1977; Niemi & Näätänen, 1981; Sanders, 1966), that is, the momentary subjective probability of the immediate delivery of the relevant stimulus, is high (which usually is the case with temporally predictable relevant stimuli and also with very short ISIs).
4. The subject works under time stress, so that there is a need for a very early stimulus analysis (Näätänen, 1975, pp. 294–295).

The discovery of the auditory brainstem response (ABR) (Section 4.2) opened an opportunity to test some of the most extreme versions of the selective-filtering hypothesis. These studies (Collet & Duclaux, 1986; Collet, Hellal, Chanal, & Morgon, 1988; Connolly, Aubry, McGillavary, & Scott, 1989; Davis & Beagley, 1985; Gregory, Heath, & Rosenberg, 1989; Hillyard, Woldorff, Mangun, & Hansen, 1987; Hirschhorn & Michie, 1990; Osterhammel, Shallop, & Terkildsen, 1985; Picton & Hillyard, 1974; Picton, Campbell, et al., 1978, 1981; Woods & Hillyard, 1978) show that ABR is not modified by selective attention. Such data, of Woldorff, Hansen, and Hillyard (1987), are presented in Fig. 6.8. Attended and ignored stimuli elicited identical ABR although a clear N1 effect was obtained to attended stimuli.

Lukas (1980, 1981; see also Brix, 1984) has, however, reported a selective-attention enhancement of ABR, but there are reasons to question this interpretation (Connolly et al., 1989; Donald, 1983; Näätänen, 1990; Wiederhold, 1986).

Hackley, Woldorff, and Hillyard (1987), in a study combining reflex and ERP measurements, obtained interesting results that they interpreted, together with findings from prior studies of reflexes (Balaban, Anthony, & Graham, 1985; DelPezzo & Hoffman, 1980; for a review, see Anthony, 1985; Hackley & Graham, 1983, 1987) and ERPs during selective attention, as indicating that "evoked auditory activity in the lower brainstem is obligatory and invariant with attention, whereas later activity mediated in the upper brainstem can be modulated by attention" (Hackley et al., 1987, p. 632).

It can be concluded that the weight of the available evidence clearly indicates that ABR as recorded from the scalp is not modulated by selective

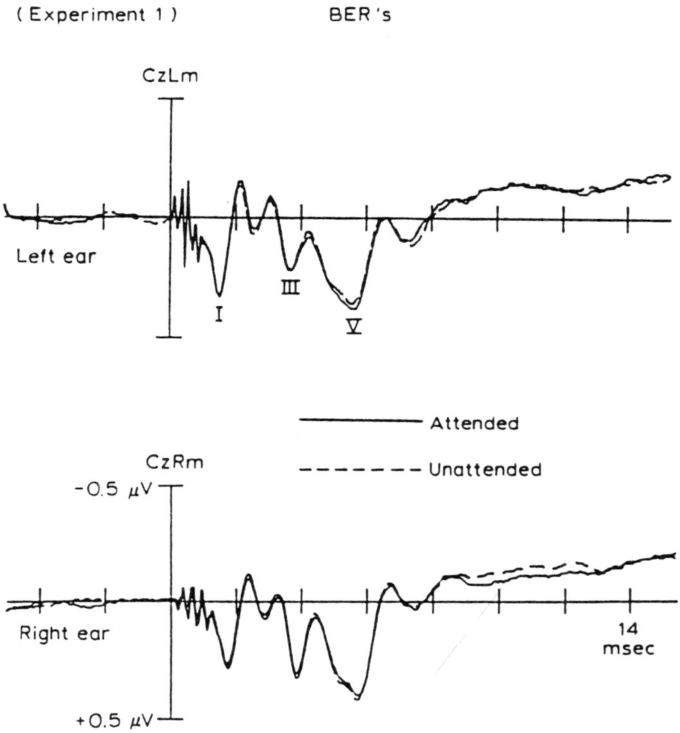

FIG. 6.8 Grand-average brainstem responses (BER) recorded between the vertex (Cz) and the ipsilateral mastoid with bandpass 30–3,000 Hz. Responses to left-ear standard tones are at top, those to right-ear standard tones at bottom. In each plot, the solid line is the response when the tones were attended and the dashed line is the response to the same tones when they were unattended. The high-frequency signal in the first millisecond of the records is stimulus artifact picked up by magnetic induction from the headphones. (From Woldorff, Hansen, & Hillyard, 1987. Copyright © 1987 by Elsevier Science Publishers BV [Biomedical Division]. Reprinted with permission.)

attention. On the other hand, there are some data pointing to a possible selective-attentional modulation of the middle-latency responses (MLR). Woldorff et al. (1987) presented 5000-Hz tone pips to the left ear and 3400-Hz tone pips to the right ear in random order and at very short ISIs, and the subject's task was to press a button upon detecting an occasional softer tone pip within the input to a designated ear. The authors found an early positive enhancement, the "P20–50 effect," which clearly preceded the N1 effect in response to attended stimuli. The P20–50 effect is illustrated in Fig. 6.9.

These results, more fully reported by Woldorff and Hillyard (1991), were replicated by Hackley et al. (1987). In addition, Woldorff and Hillyard

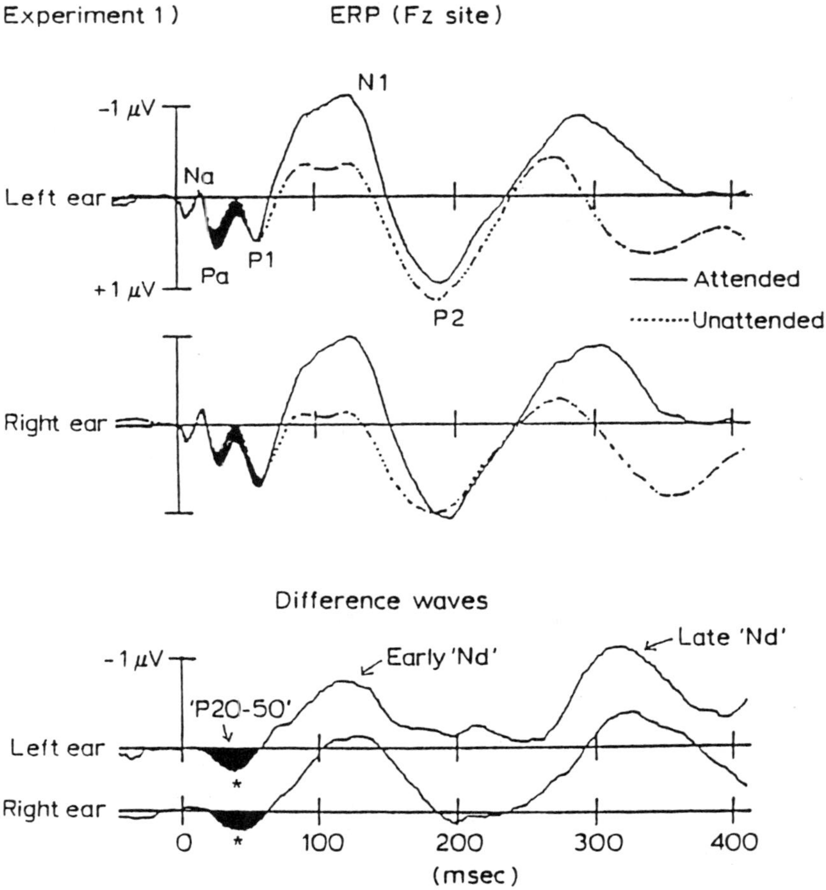

FIG. 6.9 Grand-average frontal (Fz) ERPs to left- (top row) and right-ear (2nd row) stimuli in dichotic attention condition. Both mid-latency (pre-P1) and long-latency (from P1) activity can be seen. Bandpass 0.01–100 Hz. Solid lines represent the ERPs when the tones were attended and dashed lines when they were unattended. The P20–50 attention effect (darkened area) appears as an enhanced positivity between 20 and 50 msec in the ERP to attended stimuli. This can also be seen in the difference waves (attended-stimulus ERP – unattended-stimulus ERP), shown at bottom. (From Woldorff, Hansen, & Hillyard, 1987. Copyright © 1987 by Elsevier Science Publishers BV [Biomedical Division]. Reprinted with permission.)

(1991) found that the magnitude of the P20–50 effect correlated with the magnitude of the subsequent N1 effect in across-subject comparisons.

According to Woldorff et al. (1987), the P20–50 effect peaked "around or just after" the Pa wave (see Section 4.2), which probably reflects early activity in or near primary auditory cortex. The authors, however, hesitated to attribute the P20–50 effect to enhanced activity of the generators of the Pa wave: "Whether the P20–50 derives from an enhancement of Pa generators, or whether it is a separate, broader wave that originates from a different set of sources, is not clear" (Woldorff et al., 1987, p. 152; see also Woldorff & Hillyard, 1991).

The very early onset of the effect led Woldorff et al. (1987) and Woldorff and Hillyard (1991) to interpret their results as strongly supporting the "early selection hypothesis" (reviewed by Johnston & Dark, 1982; see also chapter 2).

McCallum, Curry, Cooper, Pocock, and Papakostopoulos (1983) also reported a very early selective-attention effect, with an onset latency at about 26 msec, perhaps even earlier than that. This effect, which occurred in free-field listening, was negative in polarity, however. The relatively long duration of the effect suggests that it might be endogenous (see later) rather than an enhancement of the activity of a generator of any obligatory component.

On the other hand, Linden et al. (1987) found no evidence for selective-attentional modulation of the steady-state response (see Section 4.2). Corroborating preliminary data were reported by Spydell, Pattee, and Gouldie (1985). Linden et al. (1987) concluded that it is possible that selective attention affects MLRs when stimuli are "discrete" but not when they are presented at a rapid rate (around 40/sec) required for an optimal steady-state response. Hillyard et al. (1973) and Picton & Hillyard (1974) have also reported that selective attention did not affect MLRs.

In conclusion, as to selective-attention effects on early exogenous ERP components in audition, the available evidence strongly suggests that ABRs are not affected. On the other hand, there exists some promising evidence for an early selective-attention effect at the MLR-latency range, but it is not entirely clear whether the effect is due to a modulation of an exogenous component or to an overlap of an endogenous component. In view of the relatively long duration of the effect, the latter alternative appears more plausible.

Consequently, with regard to subcortical gating, the starting-point question of this section, ERPs in humans provide no supporting evidence, judging from the attention-insensitive ABRs. A selective-attention modulation of MLR, on the other hand, is not ruled out, but here we are, presumably, already dealing with cortical-level sensory mechanisms (Section 4.2).

However, in a very recent study, Giard, Collet, Bouchet, and Pernier (1991) reported supporting evidence for the peripheral-filtering model of attention. These authors found that selective auditory attention modifies the otoacoustic emissions in the human cochlea.[2] Otoacoustic emissions (Kemp, 1978) are probably generated by means of active contractions of the

[2]A similar claim was previously made by Puel, Bonfils, and Pujol (1988) and Froehlich, Collet, Chanal, and Morgon (1990), but their effect might, as observed by Froehlich et al., well be due to non-specific rather than stimulus-specific effects of selective attention.

outer hair cells in the organ of Corti (Brownell, Bader, Bertrand, & de Ribeaupierre, 1985). The outer hair cells are known to receive a strong efferent innervation from the medial efferent system (War & Guinan, 1979). Giard and her colleagues, in their study in which attended and ignored stimuli differed both in frequency and ear of entry, found that the spectrum of otoacoustic emissions evoked by attended tones was increased in the frequency bands corresponding to the attended frequencies. The authors concluded that selective auditory attention "filters the sensory input at the periphery by tuning the cochlear receptor". This effect was predicted by Scharf (1990).

Endogenous Effects: The Processing Negativity

Näätänen, Gaillard, and Mäntysalo (1978) described a slow endogenous negative component related to selective attention, which they termed the *processing negativity* (PN). The effect, recorded over the vertex and both left and right auditory cortices, was not produced by a modulation of an exogenous ERP component; rather it was a new component emerging during selective attention. Their selective dichotic-listening task resembled that of Hillyard et al. (1973) but differed from it, among other things, in having a considerably longer and constant (800 msec) ISI and no pitch difference between the inputs to the opposite ears. In Experiment 1, the subject counted occasional louder tones, in Experiment 2, higher-pitch tones, of the designated input.

In these data, selective attention did not affect the peak amplitude of the N1 deflection, but the N1 peak was followed by a small negative displacement of the ERP to attended standards relative to that to unattended standards. This displacement began at 150 msec, during the descending limb of the N1 deflection, and persisted for at least 500 msec.

In their subsequent, similar study—but now adding a large pitch difference between the dichotic inputs, Näätänen et al. (1980) obtained very similar results. This time, however, PNs recorded over the temporal areas were just as large as those over the vertex, leading Näätänen and Michie (1979a) to suggest that PN is, at least in part, generated in sensory-specific auditory regions. The addition of the pitch difference between the two input channels eliminated any sign of a P3 wave in response to deviants in the irrelevant input. Without the pitch difference, these deviants elicited P3s that were almost half of the amplitude of P3s elicited by target deviants (Näätänen et al., 1978.)

Näätänen et al. (1978) proposed that PN is an endogenous component generated by a cerebral mechanism different from that of the N1 component and, further, that even Hillyard et al.'s (1973) N1 effect might have been caused by PN rather than by an intensification of the generator process of the N1 component. Hillyard et al.'s considerably shorter ISIs might have shortened the PN latency, because subjects had to process stimuli faster in order to perform the task, so that PN overlapped the N1 component, causing an artificial increase in its measured amplitudes.

Such an early PN onset was demonstrated by Näätänen, Gaillard, and Varey in an experiment in 1977 (Näätänen & Michie, 1979a) in which attended and ignored inputs of quite a different frequency were delivered to the opposite ears. In this experiment, PNs obtained with three different constant ISIs, namely 250, 800, and 2000 msec, were compared with one another. Figure 6.10 shows data for the 800-msec ISI. It is seen that the attentional displacement commences as early as at about 70 msec from stimulus onset in vertex data, therefore overlapping the exogenous N1 component and producing an apparent "N1 effect."

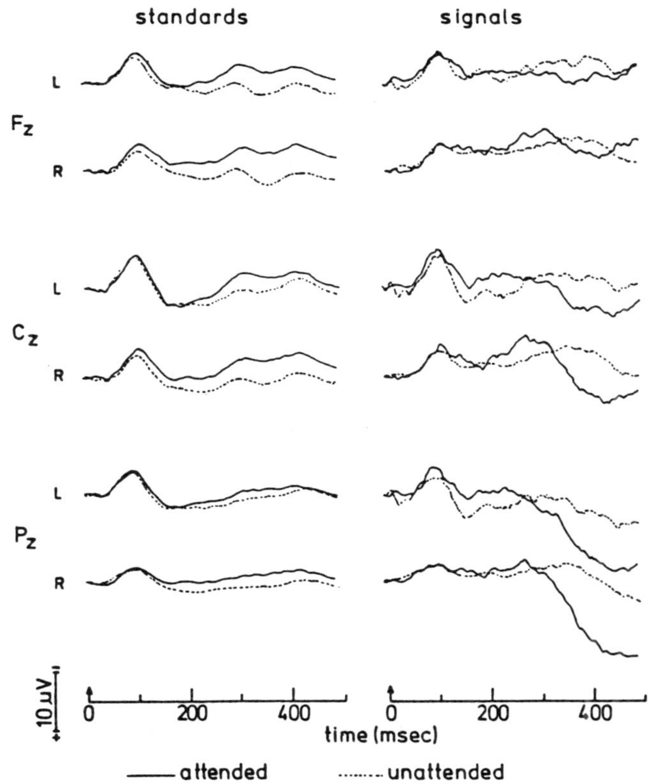

FIG. 6.10 Grand-average frontal (Fz), vertex (Cz), and parietal (Pz) ERPs to standards and deviants ("signals") separately for left- (L) and right-ear (R) stimuli when attended (solid line) and when unattended (dotted line). ISI 800 msec. (From Näätänen and Michie, 1979a. Copyright © 1979 by Elsevier Science Publishers BV [Biomedical Division]. Reprinted with permission.)

Corroborating results were provided by a rather similar study of Näätänen, Gaillard, and Varey (1981). An early onset of the negative displacement was found for each ISI, but a significant one at the N1 peak latency only with the 250-msec ISI.

Processing Negativity in Different Paradigms. PN was soon verified in many laboratories (e.g., Okita, 1979; Parasuraman, 1980), and was also observed by Hillyard and his colleagues (Hansen & Hillyard, 1980; Hillyard, 1981). Hansen and Hillyard suggested, however, that a "genuine" N1 enhancement was also present in their data. They presented a randomized sequence of binaural "high-pitch" and "low-pitch" (300 Hz) tones. The frequency of the high-pitch tone was, in different blocks, either 350, 400, or 700 Hz. Their targets, to be searched among the designated tones and responded to by a button press, were otherwise similar to these tones but of a longer duration.

Figure 6.11 shows Hansen and Hillyard's (1980) data separately for the low and high tones. A long-duration negative displacement can be observed commencing well before the N1 peak for the two largest frequency differences.

The right side of Fig. 6.11 presents this attention effect as revealed by subtracting the ERP to unattended stimuli from that to attended stimuli. This difference wave was called "Nd" (negative difference). With a greater pitch difference, both the onset and peak latencies of Nd were shorter and the Nd duration longer. The late portion of Nd had a topography anterior to that of the early Nd.

These data therefore confirmed that there are, in fact, two partially overlapping components in the attention effect, as originally proposed by Näätänen and Michie (1979a). The earlier, frontocentral component was dominant with small pitch differences, whereas the later, frontal one was disproportionally enhanced with larger pitch differences. However, in contrast to Näätänen and Michie (1979a), the authors suggested that the earlier component might be a possible "genuine" N1 enhancement. The later, slower one was identified as PN of the type observed by Näätänen et al. (1978). For the sake of clarity, the different long-latency negative components of the auditory ERP involved in attention research are listed in Table 6.1.

These two components of the ERP attention effect were corroborated by Näätänen et al. (1981), Arnsten et al. (1983), Okita, Konishi, and Inamori (1983), and Hansen and Hillyard (1984). In these data, too, the topography of the later component was anterior to that of the earlier one.

In sum, two selective-attention effects have been described with an onset at the N1 latency range: the "N1 enhancement"—in the sense of a strengthened generator process of some obligatory N1 component (Hillyard

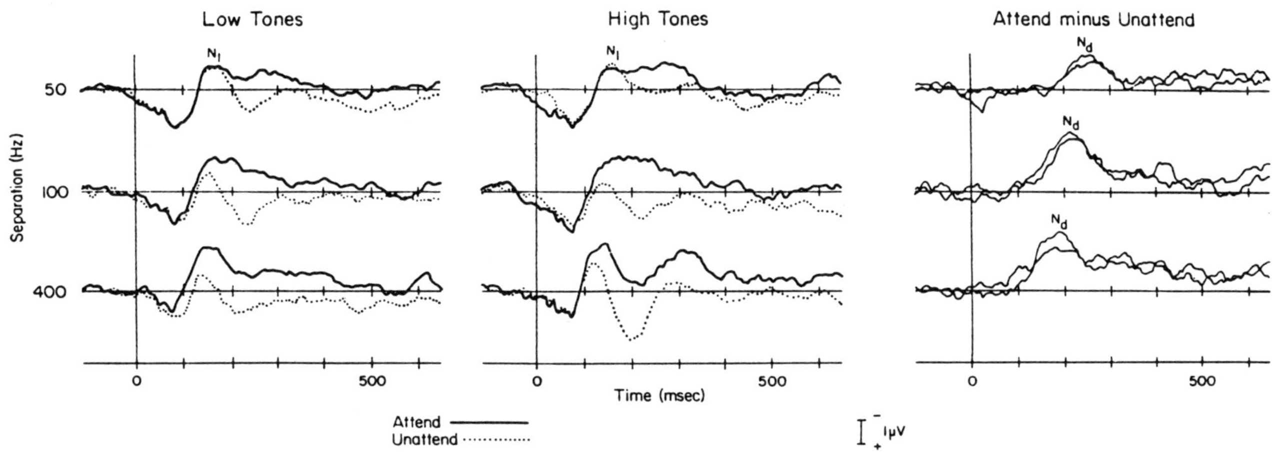

FIG. 6.11 Grand-average vertex (Cz) ERPs to standard tones at three different interchannel frequency separations between two binaural tones (low and high) of which one is to be attended and the other ignored. ERPs at left are to 300 Hz (low) tones and at center are, in different blocks, to 350, 400, or 700 Hz (high) tones. ERPs to attended tones (solid line) and unattended tones (dotted lines) are overlapped. Tracings at right are superimposed difference waves between ERPs to attended and unattended tones. (From Hansen, & Hillyard, 1980. Copyright © 1980 by Elsevier Science Publishers, Ireland. Reprinted with permission.)

TABLE 6.1
Different long-latency negative components of the ERP in studies of automatic and attentive processing of auditory stimuli.

Component	*First reported (or separated from other components)*	*Dependence on attention*
Supratemporal N1	Vaughan & Ritter (1970)	Some dependence on attention but possibly no selective-attention effect
Nonspecific N1	Hari et al. (1982) Velasco et al. (1985) Velasco & Velasco (1986)	Some dependence on attention but no selective-attention effect
T-complex N1	Wolpaw & Penry (1975)	Probably affected by selective attention
Frontal N1	Glard, Perrin, & Echallier (submitted)	Elicitation probably attention-independent; selective-attention effect unlikely
Sustained potential	Picton et al. (1978 a, b)	No or slight attention-dependence
Mismatch negativity (MMN)	Näätänen et al. (1978)	No or slight attention-dependence
sensory-specific and frontal components	Giard et al. (1990) Näätänen & Michie (1979a)	
N2b	Näätänen et al. (1982)	Strong attention-dependence
Processing negativity (PN)	Näätänen et al. (1978)	Full attention-dependence
early and late PN (Nd)	Hansen & Hillyard (1980) Näätänen & Michie (1979a)	
Frontal slow wave ("O wave")	Loveless & Sanford (1974a, b)	Some attention-dependence
CNV	Walter, Cooper, Aldridge, McCallum, & Winter (1964)	Full attention-dependence
Bereitschaftspotential	Kornhuber & Deecke (1965)	Full attention-dependence

et al., 1973)—and the processing negativity (Näätänen et al., 1978). Even to date, it is not yet settled whether we have here one and the same effect or two different effects, the issue at stake being whether all ERP effects of auditory selective attention are due to PN or whether some obligatory N1 component is selectively enhanced to attended stimuli in some conditions. This long-term controversy is further discussed later.

As shown by the Hansen and Hillyard (1980) binaural study just reviewed, PN can be obtained when relevant and irrelevant stimuli originate from the same spatial position and differ only in pitch. Further, Hansen, Dickstein, Berka, & Hillyard (1983) demonstrated that the attentional displacement for speech sounds originating from the same location is similar in morphology and scalp distribution to that to tone pips, though delayed. The speech sounds were binaural computer-synthesized CV (consonant-vowel) syllables that were clearly identified as /ba/, /pa/, /da/, or /ga/. Two stimuli always appeared in the same block, either the two first syllables, the two last syllables, or tones of 300 and 350 Hz. The subject's task was to detect occasional longer duration stimuli within the designated input.

Figure 6.12 shows that the attention effect for speech sounds was similar to that for tones, but delayed. Obviously, if the pitch difference between the two tones had been smaller, then the timing of the attention effect would probably have been more similar for the tones and speech sounds (cf. Hansen & Hillyard, 1980). The authors suggested that the attentional mechanisms brought into play when selecting complex phonetic stimuli for further analysis are similar to those engaged when selecting between tones of different frequencies.

Woods et al. (1984) presented dichotic prose passages, one spoken by a male voice and the other by a female voice, each including four probe stimuli: digitized irrelevant speech sounds ("a" and "but") spoken by the same voice, and tone bursts at the mean fundamental and second-formant frequencies of the voice.

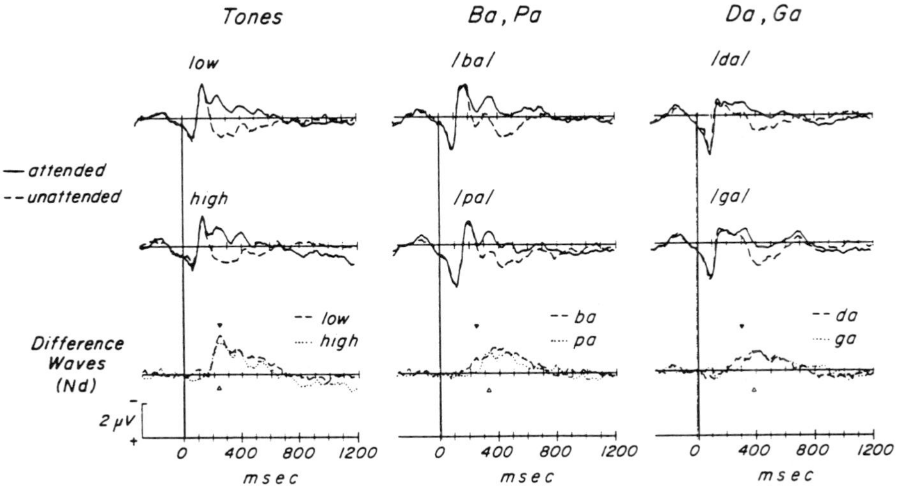

FIG. 6.12 Grand-average frontal (Fz) ERPs elicited by each of the six binaural standard (short-duration) stimuli as indicated in the figure when attended and when unattended. The subject was instructed to discriminate occasional longer duration stimuli among the to-be-attended input. The difference waves at the bottom of each column were derived by subtracting the ERP to unattended stimuli from the ERP to attended stimuli for the stimulus pairs shown above. (From Hansen, Dickstein, Berka, & Hillyard, 1983. Copyright © 1983 by Elsevier Science Publishers BV [Biomedical Division]. Reprinted with permission.)

It was found that a long-duration negative displacement followed speech probes but not tone probes presented in the attended input. The 2nd-formant probes in the attended message instead disclosed an enhanced P2 or P3a type of sharp positivity. A similar effect was not found for the tone burst at the fundamental frequency, owing presumably to a lesser physical deviance. These effects are illustrated in Fig. 6.13.

The stimulus to be attended does not have to be constant over the stimulus block for an Nd to emerge. Okita (1979; see also 1987) found a short-latency negative displacement when subjects attended to stimuli that kept slowly changing in spatial position and pitch, somewhat resembling real-life conditions in which we attend to a moving sound source. The stimulus to be ignored kept moving in the opposite direction both in spatial position and pitch.

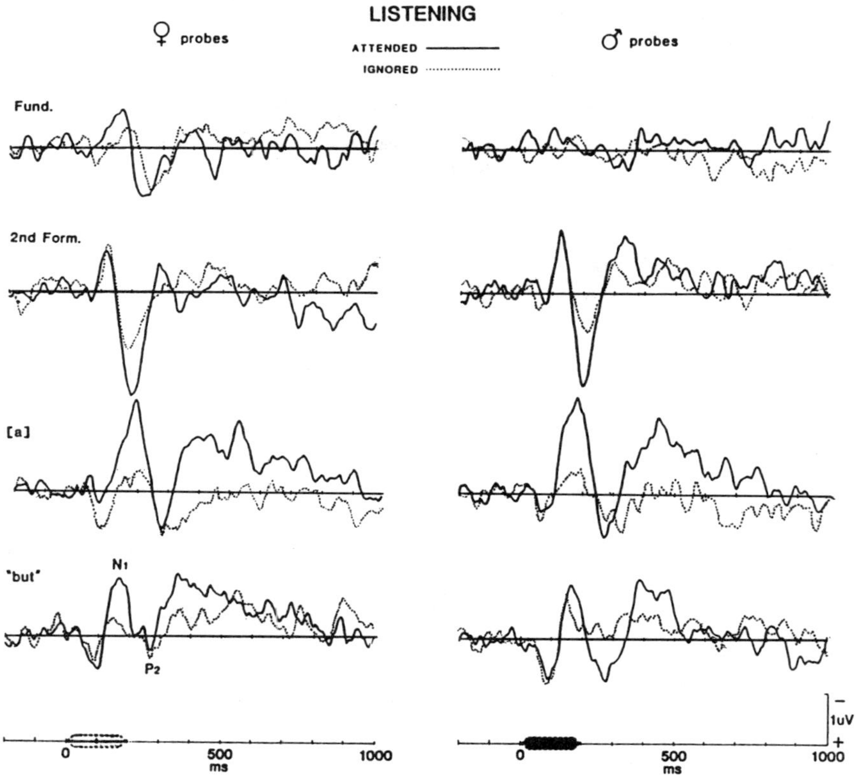

FIG. 6.13 Grand-average vertex (Cz) ERPs in response to different probe stimuli (fundamental (Fund.), second formant (2nd Form.), and speech probes /a/ and but) mixed with female (left column) and male (right column) prose passages when these dichotically presented passages were attended (solid line) and when they were unattended (dashed line). (From Woods, Hillyard, & Hansen, 1984. Copyright © 1984 by the American Psychological Association. Reprinted with permission.)

PN also occurs when a multidimensional discrimination is required in order to identify relevant input among irrelevant input. Hansen and Hillyard (1983) defined their relevant stimuli on two stimulus attributes, so that a stimulus had to originate from a designated location and had also to be of a designated pitch in order to be a relevant stimulus. Thus, stimulus blocks were composed of four (equiprobable) tones: "high left," "low left," "high right," and "low right."

The relevant tones, having a designated pitch and location, were called the "P + L +" tones. (The subject's task was to discriminate occasional longer-duration tones in this input.) The irrelevant "P + L −" tones had the same pitch as, but a different location from, the "P + L +" tones, whereas the irrelevant "P − L +" tones had the same location as the "P + L +" tones but differed from them in pitch. The "P − L −" tones differed from the "P + L +" tones in both pitch and location. The attentional ERP displacements (Nd) for the P + L +, P + L −, and P − L + tones were determined by subtracting the ERP to the P − L − tones separately from the ERPs to each of the former stimuli. In some sequences, both pitch and location differences were large. In others, the pitch difference was large and location difference was small, or vice versa.

Hansen and Hillyard (1983) found, in addition to a large and long-duration negative displacement for the P + L + tones, a shorter-duration displacement for the P − L + tones when the pitch difference was small ("Pitch Hard, Location Easy") and for the P + L − tones when the location difference was small ("Pitch Easy, Location Hard") (Fig. 6.14). However, when the difference in the nonmatching (−) feature was large, there was only a very small "Nd" for the P − L + or P + L − stimuli when the difference in the other attribute was also large ("Pitch Easy, Location Easy"), and none when the difference in the other attribute was small ("Pitch Easy, Location Hard," or "Pitch Hard, Location Easy") (Fig. 6.14).

The pattern of data obtained suggests that there were two separate components of the attentional displacement, one associated with each feature, when the stimulus satisfied the designated levels in both features. These separate components were demonstrated by first comparing ERPs for stimuli satisfying and not satisfying the designated level in the "Easy" feature (large difference), resulting in a large, early displacement (see Fig. 6.14), and then comparing ERPs to the two stimuli both satisfying the easy feature but only one of them satisfying the difficult feature also. The latter comparison reveals a late Nd of a low amplitude associated with satisfying the more difficult feature also (Fig. 6.14).

On the other hand, if the stimulus failed to satisfy an Easy dimension—this can be ascertained by the subject at an early latency,—then the attentive (task-dependent) processing of the difficult, slower, dimension was terminated early. This is suggested by the lack of a negative displacement between responses to stimuli of which one satisfied the difficult dimension

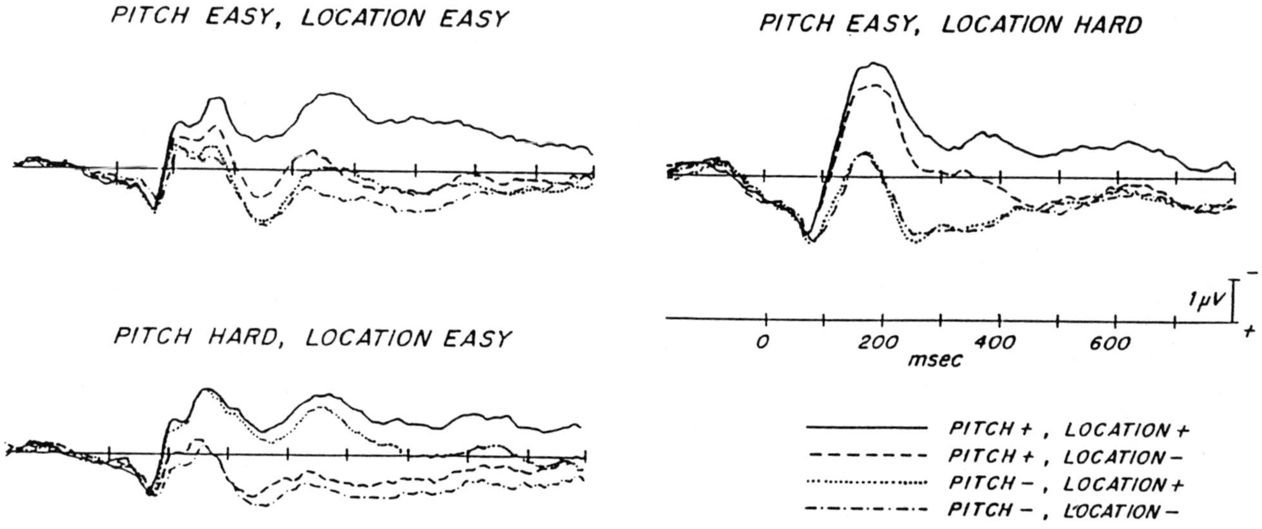

FIG. 6.14 Grand-average frontal (Fz) ERPs elicited by standard tones that possessed both the attended pitch and location attributes (pitch +, location +), only one attended attribute (pitch +, location −, or pitch −, location +), or neither attribute (pitch −, location −) in three different dichotic selective-attention conditions as indicated above the superimposed traces. (From Hansen and Hillyard, 1983. Copyright © 1983 by the American Psychological Association. Reprinted with permission.)

and the other not while both failed to satisfy the easy dimension. (See in particular the right side of Fig. 6.14.)

Hansen and Hillyard (1983) proposed that the overall pattern of their results was "consistent with parallel, self-terminating models and holistic models of processing and contradicts models specifying either serial or exhaustive parallel processing of these dimensions" (p. 1).

"Channel Separation" and the Processing Negativity. As already reviewed, Hansen and Hillyard's (1980) Nd was larger and earlier with an increased (frequency) difference between relevant and irrelevant stimuli ("channel separation") but was obtained even with quite a small channel separation (16.6%). Corroborating evidence was provided by Hansen and Hillyard (1983), Alho, Sams, et al. (1986; Alho, Töttölä, Reinikainen, Sams, & Näätänen, 1987), and Michie, Bearpark, Crawford, and Glue (1990), and with location difference by Hansen and Hillyard (1983) and Alho, Donauer, et al. (1987).

Alho, Donauer, et al.'s (1987) data are shown in Fig. 6.15. The difference between the apparent sound locations was manipulated by varying the intensity difference between the left and right inputs delivered through earphones. When the location difference was large, the negative displacement started earlier and was larger than when the location difference was small (Fig. 6.15, left). The right side of the figure shows analogous pitch-separation data.

McCallum et al.'s (1983) attention effect occurred, as already mentioned, at a very short onset latency (at 26 msec or even shorter) when the location difference was very large. They delivered their sound stimuli by using four loudspeakers positioned so that the sound either came from the left, right, front, or back of the subject. This short onset latency was only found for

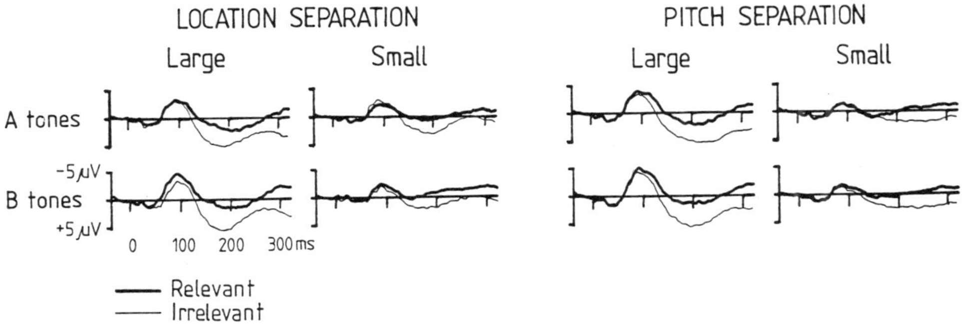

FIG. 6.15 Grand-average vertex (Cz) ERPs to A and B tones when they were relevant (thick lines) and when they were irrelevant (thin lines) for "large" and "small" location (on the left) and pitch (on the right) separations. (From Alho et al., 1987. Copyright © 1987 by Elsevier Science Publishers BV [Biomedical Division]. Reprinted with permission.)

the left–right dimension but not for the front–back dimension. This suggests that differences along some dimensions are inherently more difficult or slower to discriminate than those along others.

Alho, Töttölä, et al. (1987) found the attention effect even when the to-be-attended stimuli were of 500 Hz and those to be ignored of 527 Hz and vice versa, a difference of only 5.4%. Some subjects showed the effect even when the difference was only 9 Hz (1.8 %).

Channel separation can also be increased by introducing an additional difference, one involving a second stimulus dimension, between relevant and irrelevant stimuli. In Alho et al.'s (1989) study, this additional difference increased the Nd amplitude. In addition, Michie, Solowij, Crawford, and Glue (1990) found that their Nd commenced earlier when relevant and irrelevant stimuli differed on two dimensions (location and pitch), compared with when they differed in one dimension only.

Processing Negativity and the Inter-Stimulus Interval. Hillyard et al. (1973; see also Schwent, Hillyard, & Galambos, 1976; Parasuraman, 1978) regarded a short, irregular ISI as essential in producing their "N1 effect." According to them, this ISI schedule caused high stimulus load, which forced subjects to process stimuli selectively. Furthermore, Näätänen and Michie (1979a) proposed that the PN-onset latency depends on the ISI, so that with short ISIs, PN onset occurs early enough to overlap N1 peak and thus enhance its amplitude.

Subsequent research has indeed shown that, when variable ISIs are used, the ISI effect on the Nd latency is substantial. The mean ISI in Parasuraman's (1980) "short-ISI" blocks with dichotic stimuli was 500 msec, and in his "long-ISI" blocks it was 1 sec. He found that Nd started about 40 msec earlier in the short-ISI blocks, whereas its amplitude was unaffected. Corroborating results were obtained by Hansen and Hillyard (1984), who used mean ISIs of 400 msec and 2 sec (Fig. 6.16). This result was interpreted as indicating a faster and more efficient rejection of unattended-channel stimuli from further processing when stimuli are delivered more rapidly. This was supported by the fact that at the slow rate, ERPs to deviants of the unattended channel showed a slow frontal negativity and parietal positivity that did not occur at the fast rate.

On the other hand, when constant ISIs are used, the ISI effect on the Nd latency appears to be considerably more modest (Näätänen et al., 1981).

Teder, Alho, Reinikainen, and Näätänen (in press) compared attention effects with four different random-ISI schedules: 60–100, 120–200, 360–600 msec, 600–1000 msec (onset to onset). Standard and deviant stimuli were tones of 300 and 330 Hz, respectively, and the ear of entry was random. The subject's task was to press a button each time a deviant stimulus appeared in a designated ear.

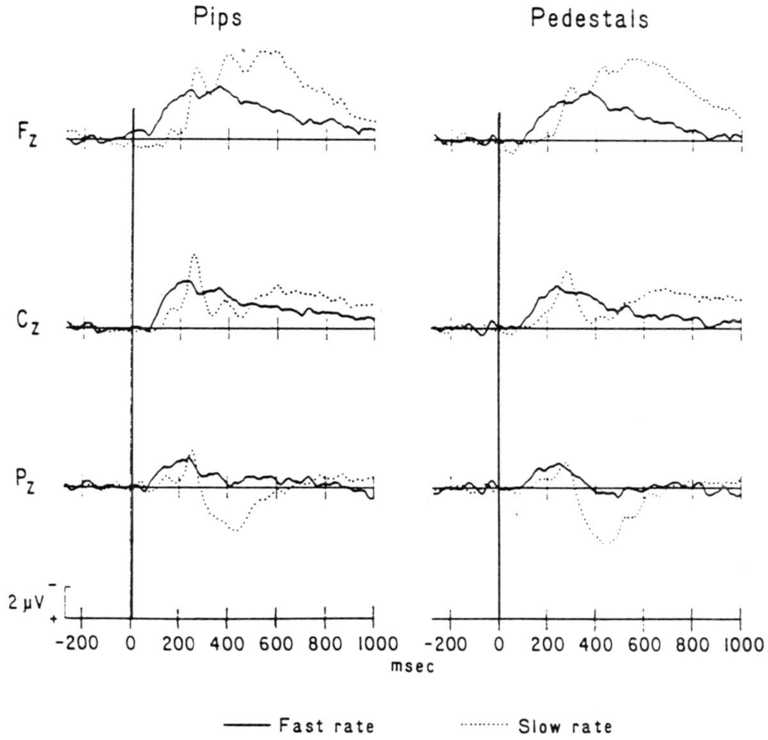

FIG. 6.16 Grand-average frontal (Fz), vertex (Cz), and parietal (Pz) ERP difference waves obtained by subtracting ERPs for unattended standards from those to attended standards, the two stimuli originating from separate loudspeakers, separately for pip and pedestal standards at fast (solid lines) and slow (dotted lines) rates of presentation. Stimulus onset is denoted by the vertical line. (From Hansen & Hillyard, 1984. Copyright © 1984 The Society for Psychophysiological Research. Reprinted with permission.)

Fig. 6.17 displays vertex ERPs (top) and Nds (bottom) separately for each ISI schedule. It can be seen that the early Nd phase peaks later with the two longer-ISI than with the two shorter-ISI schedules. In addition, Nd is considerably larger with the two longer-ISI than with the two shorter-ISI schedules. This might result from an elicitation of a second Nd phase with the two longer ISIs. This second phase is apparently due to activation of a new generator, which is supported by differences in distribution found between the early and late parts of Nd in these data. Consequently, it appears that the late PN component is, in contrast to the early PN component, enhanced with longer ISIs. This is also supported by the results of Näätänen et al. (1981) and Woods (1990).

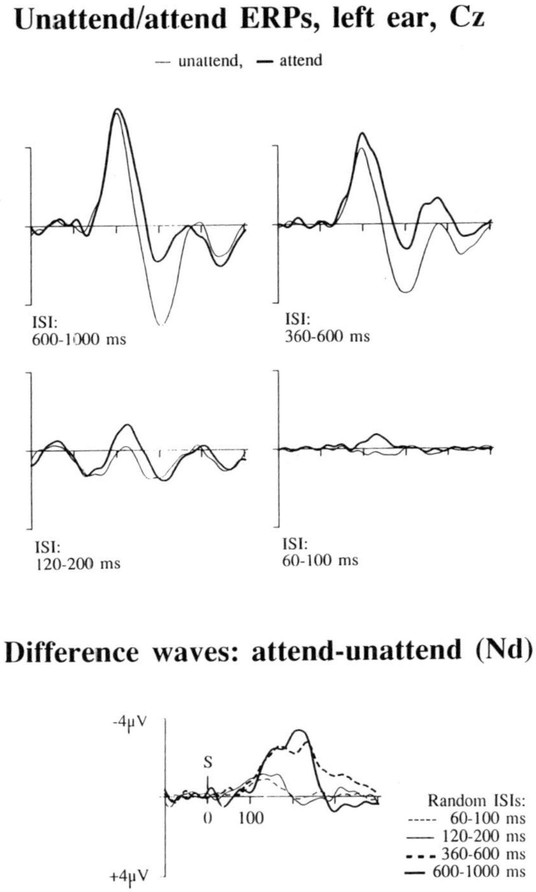

FIG. 6.17 TOP: Grand-average vertex (Cz) ERPs to unattended and attended tones for left-ear stimuli in a dichotic attention study with 4 different random-ISI conditions as indicated below the tracings. S = stimulus onset. BOTTOM: Superimposition of difference waves obtained by subtracting ERPs to unattended stimuli from those to attended stimuli, separately for each ISI condition shown above. (From Näätänen & Teder, 1991. Copyright © 1991 by Scandinavian University Press. Reprinted with permission.)

Processing Negativity and the Relevant-Stimulus Probability. In the majority of the previously reviewed PN studies, two equiprobable stimuli were presented, the subject's task being to attend to one of the stimuli. Thus, the relevant-stimulus probability was .50 in these studies. Alho, Lavikainen, et al. (1990) wished to determine the probability effect on Nd. Their stimulus blocks consisted of randomized "low," "medium," and "high" binaural tones. In the 1/3 conditions, the three tones were equiprobable. In the 1/6 conditions, the low and high tones each occurred at a probability of 1/6, and the medium tones at the complementary probability of 2/3. In the 1/30 conditions, the low and high tones each occurred at a probability of 1/30 (the medium tones at 28/30). In a half of the blocks, the "low" tones, and in the remaining blocks, the "high" tones were to be counted.

It was found that Nd was smaller with smaller relevant-stimulus probabilities (Fig. 6.18). With the smallest probability, only a negligible Nd was left. It is not clear, however, to which extent the Nd decrease was due to the diminished probability and to which extent to the accompanying increase in the ISI between relevant stimuli, that is, to the event and temporal probabilities.

Berman, Heilweil, Ritter, and Rosen's (1989) results are consistent with

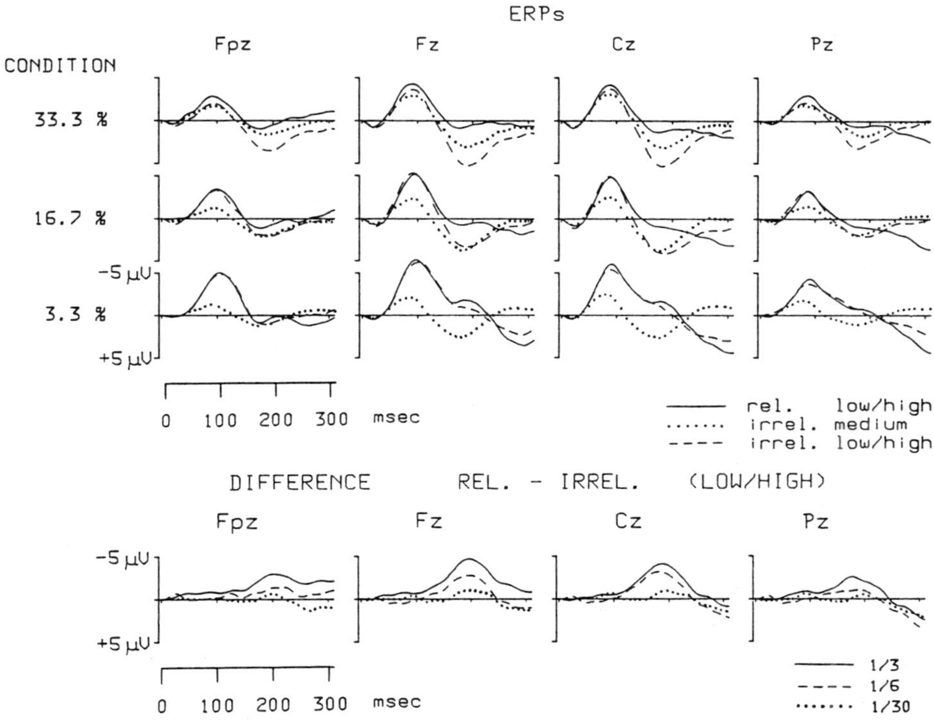

FIG. 6.18 TOP: Grand-average frontal-pole (Fpz), frontal (Fz), vertex (Cz), and parietal (Pz) ERPs to relevant low/high (continuous lines), irrelevant medium (dotted lines), and irrelevant low/high (dashed lines) binaural tones when the low and high tones each occurred at a probability of either 1/3, 1/6, or 1/30. The complementary medium-tone probabilities were 1/3, 2/3, and 28/30, respectively. Stimulus onset at 0 msec. BOTTOM: Corresponding difference waves obtained by subtracting the grand-average ERP to irrelevant low/high tones from the ERP to the same stimuli when relevant. (From Alho, Lavikainen, Reinikainen, Sams, and Näätänen, 1990. Copyright © 1990 The Society for Psychophysiological Research. Reprinted with permission.)

those of Alho, Lavikainen et al. (1990) in that the Nd amplitude, in contrast to the amplitude of N2 types of negativities (for a classification, see Näätänen, 1986d), is not attenuated by increase in stimulus probability. This suggests that Nd is indeed generated by a brain process measuring stimulus similarity, whereas the other memory-dependent negativities are generated by processes responding to difference.

Intracranial Generators of the Processing Negativity. Näätänen et al. (1978, 1980) suggested, on the basis of the relatively large Nds over temporal cortex (electrode sites T3 and T4), that PN might be generated in auditory cortex. Curry et al.'s (1983) Nd over sites C3 and C4 (near the auditory areas) tended to be even larger than that recorded over the vertex. Corroborating evidence was also provided by Renault, Baribeau-Braun, Dalbokova, and El Massioui (1986) and by Maiste and Picton (1987). Näätänen (1982) proposed that the early PN component is generated in sensory-specific cortex and the late component in frontal regions. This is consistent with Hansen and Hillyard's (1980) aforementioned two Nd phases, with the later being distributed more frontally than the earlier one. Corroborating data were obtained in several studies (e.g., Näätänen et al., 1981; Okita, Konishi, & Inamori, 1983; Woods & Clayworth, 1987).

Woods and Clayworth (1987) found that the early Nd differed in scalp topography from N1 recorded under passive conditions by being more frontal and less contralateralized than the passive N1 (see also Maiste & Picton, 1987). In addition, Nd was relatively smaller over temporal cortex than the passive N1. Moreover, Alho, Paavilainen, Reinikainen, Sams, and Näätänen (1986) and Teder et al. (in press) reported that the passive N1 (the supratemporal component) inverts in polarity at the mastoids when the nose is used as the reference, as initially observed by Vaughan and Ritter (1970), whereas the early Nd does not.

Knight et al.'s (1980; Knight, Hillyard, Woods, & Neville, 1981) lesion data also suggest that the exogenous N1 and the early Nd emanate from different generators. These authors showed that dorsolateral prefrontal lesions can reduce Nd without affecting the exogenous N1. Further converging evidence for separate generators was provided by Woods and Courchesne's (1987) between-subject comparisons, which dissociated the amplitude of N1 recorded under passive conditions from the early-Nd amplitude.

Giard, Perrin, Pernier, and Peronnet (1988) applied scalp-current density analysis to their ERP data obtained by using a dichotic design very similar to that of Näätänen et al. (1978). The first phase of Giard et al.'s (1988) Nd (which they called Nd1), a small negativity peaking at 80–85 msec, was interpreted as an enhancement of some exogenous N1 component. Interestingly, this early effect, apparently originating in the supratemporal auditory cortex, showed a frequency-specific locus of generation:

When the subject attended to high (2000-Hz) tones, the effect was maximal over the frontal region of the left hemiscalp, whereas when low (1000-Hz) tones were attended, the effect was maximal over the central region of the right hemiscalp.

This result has very recently been extended by Giard and her colleagues (M.H. Giard, personal communication, June 1991): The Nd1 effect of attention was again found, with a topography suggesting an origin in the supratemporal auditory cortex. Very interestingly, this topography varied with the frequency of the attended stimulus (500, 1,000, 2,000, 4,000 Hz), and this variation resembled the tonotopic variation of N1 elicited by the same tones when ignored. These results were interpreted as expressing attentional modulation of the N1-generator activity in the tonotopically organized areas of the supratemporal cortex.

The negativity corresponding to the notion of the early Nd in Giard et al.'s (1988) study, starting at about 110 msec from stimulus onset and lasting some 200 msec (their Nd2), was bilaterally generated and appeared to originate, at least its main part, from auditory, but not supratemporal cortex. This was followed by a third phase of negativity (Nd3), which apparently corresponds to the late, frontal Nd. The generator of this third negative phase appeared to be deeply located in the frontal lobes. On the other hand, Knight et al. (1981) and Woods and Knight (1986) interpreted their lesion data as suggesting that the frontal lobes do not generate attentional negativity but rather that the right frontal lobe facilitates the generator of this negativity, which is located elsewhere.

Some animal experiments are illustrative here, too. Benson and Hienz (1978) recorded single-unit responses from auditory cortex of rhesus monkeys performing a dichotic-listening task that they had learned in 3 months. This task was very similar to that used with human subjects, except that the monkey pressed a response key to each stimulus delivered to a given ear. Fourteen out of 77 units showed significantly greater rates of evoked discharges to a stimulus when it was attended than when it was unattended. These selective increases in the firing rate began in primary auditory cortex at 23.2 msec, on the average, whereas the latencies for units of auditory cortex outside the primary area were on the average 12 msec longer. These firing-rate increases, sometimes lasting until 200 msec after stimulus onset, might be associated with the sensory-specific portion of Nd.

In sum, the generation of the early Nd phase in auditory cortex appears to be well established. This is further supported by MEG studies of auditory selective attention, to be reviewed in chapter 7. On the other hand, the frontal-lobe origin of the late Nd phase must yet be considered unsettled. The rCBF data, to be reviewed in chapter 8, provide indirect support by revealing strong activation of different frontal structures during selective attention.

Selective Attention and Late Positivities in Audition

Target stimuli, occasional deviant stimuli in the designated input to be discriminated and responded to, elicited large P3 waves in the studies reviewed, whereas Nds for targets and standards of the designated input were very similar (Maiste & Picton, 1987; Alho et al., 1989; for a review, see Näätänen, 1982). (Equivalent deviant stimuli in the to-be-ignored input elicited no P3 waves or only small ones.) An increase in target-stimulus probability attenuated the P3 amplitude for these stimuli in selective dichotic listening (Donald & Little, 1981). These facts are consistent with the main thrust of the P3 literature, according to which (Näätänen, 1990):

1. Deviant stimuli elicit P3 waves when the stimulus sequence is to be attended but do not elicit them, or elicit much smaller ones, when the stimulus sequence is not attended (for reviews, see Donchin et al., 1978; Johnson, 1988; Pritchard, 1981; Roth, 1983).
2. These P3 waves are smaller for higher target-stimulus probabilities (Duncan-Johnson & Donchin, 1977).

One might well assume that the P3-amplitude difference between deviants in attended and unattended inputs (P3 differential) might indicate the degree of attentional selectivity (see Hansen & Hillyard, 1984). Moreover, the target-P3 latency and amplitude might reflect aspects of further processing of the to-be-attended stimuli, that occurring after their initial selection. Hillyard et al.'s (1973; see also Hillyard & Picton, 1979; Hink, Hillyard, & Benson, 1978) hierarchical model predicts a short target-P3 latency when a relevant stimulus can, as indicated by an early Nd onset, be very rapidly selected for further processing. Consequently, the model predicts that the Nd-onset and P3 latencies correlate with each other.

Unfortunately, the data available do not provide much support for these predictions. When there was a large N1 effect, the P3 differential was smaller than when the N1 effect was weaker, and vice versa (Schwent, Snyder, & Hillyard, 1976; see, however, Hansen & Hillyard, 1984). Moreover, the emergence and decay of Donald and Young's (1982) N1 effect in their experiment did not correspond to those of the P3 differential. Most conspicuously, the differential P3 response was almost immediate in the beginning of the session, whereas the N1 effect took some time to develop. This pattern of results was replicated by Hansen and Hillyard (1988) who, however, measured the attention effect as a slow negative displacement rather than a growth of the N1 amplitude. Similar time-course differences can also be observed developmentally: The "N1 effect" emerges at the age of 10–11 years, whereas the P3 differential is already there prior to age 6 (see Donald, 1983).

As already mentioned, by varying the frequency difference ("channel separation") between relevant and irrelevant stimuli, Hansen and Hillyard (1980) manipulated the Nd amplitude and latency. This did not, however, affect the P3 amplitude or latency to targets (hits). Nor did channel separation have a significant effect on the RT.

Similar results were obtained by Hansen and Hillyard (1983). As already reviewed, their subjects were instructed to press a button as quickly as possible upon detecting an occasional longer-duration stimulus among the to-be-attended stimuli defined on the basis of both their location and pitch ("channel cues"). According to Hansen and Hillyard (1983), these results:

> . . . would be expected if the channel cues and duration were processed in parallel from the outset, with the duration discrimination requiring the longest time to reach completion. If these cue analyses occurred serially, RTs should have been prolonged when the channel cues were made less discriminable. . . . The latency of the P300 wave to the targets was similarly insensitive to variation in interchannel discriminability, again implying that the analysis of duration was the bottleneck in target identification. . . . The present data . . . suggest that the P300 in this task is associated with the terminal decision that a stimulus is a target, which follows parallel analyses of its channel and target attributes. (pp. 15–16)

Novak et al.'s (1990; Novak, Ritter, & Vaughan, in press a; Novak, Ritter, & Vaughan, in press b) results, however, seem to indicate that P3 is in fact not associated with the terminal decision that a stimulus is a target. The target-P3 latency in their attend-oddball condition was very similar to that in their dichotic condition (composed of course of concurrent attend and ignore oddball sequences) with exactly the same stimulus parameters, although the RT was 123 msec longer in the dichotic condition. Evidently, the subject reached the decision as to the presence of a target much later in the dichotic than one-channel conditions, but this was not reflected by the P3 latency. This suggests that P3, in fact, is not time-locked to the terminal decision that a stimulus is a target. Instead, it is more likely, as already discussed in Section 6.1, that P3 as well as the other late endogenous components are time-locked to MMN (Novak et al., 1990; Novak et al., in press/a, in press/b).

This would also explain Hansen and Hillyard's (1980, 1983) finding that the target-P3 latency is not affected by the onset latency of the preceding Nds, and thus by channel separation. Due to the strongly, or fully, automatic nature of the frequency MMN, deviant stimuli probably elicited an MMN with similar time characteristics, irrespective of the magnitude of channel separation. Therefore, if P3 is indeed time-locked to MMN, then the P3 latency for target deviants is also unaffected by channel separation.

Is There a Real N1 Effect of Selective Attention?

It was established earlier that the predominant early selective-attention effect on auditory ERPs is caused by the emergence of PN, an endogenous negative component associated with selective attention. It is, however, not settled whether all early negative attention effects are due to PN or whether the exogenous N1 (some of its subcomponents) can be enhanced by selective attention under certain optimal conditions. As already mentioned, Hillyard et al. (1973) interpreted their selective-attention effect in terms of an exogenous N1 component on the grounds that the time course of the attention effect closely corresponded to that of the N1 elicited by unattended stimuli, but Näätänen (1975) suggested that despite the short onset latency of the "N1 effect," it might yet be endogenous. Furthermore, Näätänen et al. (1978) demonstrated such an endogenous attention effect, PN, which indeed can occur at a sufficiently short latency in order to overlap the exogenous N1 and to cause its "artificial" enlargement via summation (see Näätänen & Michie, 1979a).

Hansen and Hillyard (1980) accommodated both views. They proposed that their early Nd might be due to an enhanced exogenous N1 component and the late Nd to an endogenous effect, PN. Their early Nd, however, was clearly delayed in relation to N1 recorded in a reading condition, assumed to provide a reasonably good estimate for the exogenous N1 component (Näätänen, 1982).

As already mentioned, Woods and Clayworth (1987) and Alho, Paavilainen, et al. (1986) found that the scalp topography of the early Nd differed from that of N1 recorded in passive conditions. (For a penetrating analysis of the response-overlap problem in these short-ISI paradigms, see Woldorff, in press.) Moreover, as also mentioned, Knight et al.'s (1980, 1981) lesion data and Woods and Courchesne's (1987) between-subjects comparisons suggest that the two originate from at least partially separate generators.

Recently, however, work conducted in Hillyard's laboratory (Woldorff et al., 1987; reported more fully by Woldorff & Hillyard, 1991; Hackley et al., 1987, 1990) has demonstrated an early Nd that coincides very closely in time with the exogenous N1 component. Woldorff and Hillyard's (1991) data are illustrated in Figs. 6.19 and 6.20.

The Nd shown in Fig. 6.20 has two distinct phases with no temporal overlap; an early one, almost perfectly matching with N1 to ignored stimuli in timing (Fig. 6.19), and a later one, starting at about 250 msec from stimulus onset. In the early Nd, the authors distinguished two consecutive phases, "Nd80" and "Nd125," both larger in amplitude over the hemisphere contra- than ipsilateral to attended stimuli (Fig. 6.20). This supported their interpretation that attention enhanced exogenous ERP components, con-

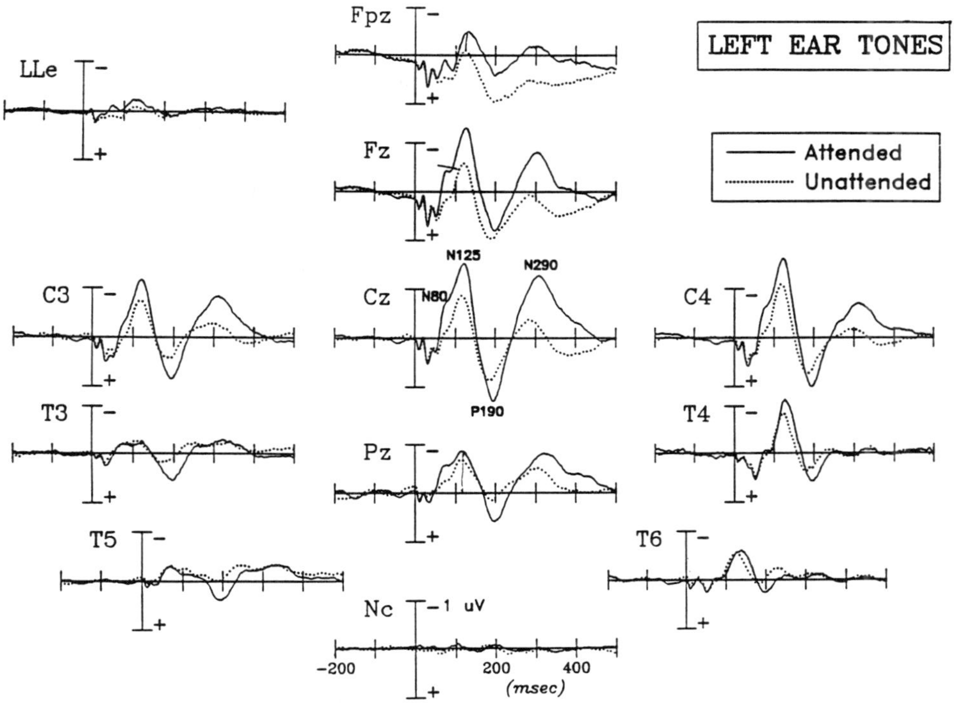

FIG. 6.19 Grand-average ERPs for attended (solid lines) and unattended (dotted lines) left-ear tones at different electrode sites as indicated in the figure in a dichotic attention study. Reference for all sites is the algebraic average of the mastoids. Nc = Noncephalic (balanced sterno-vertebral). LLe = Lower Left eye (below and to left of the left eye). (From Woldorff and Hillyard, 1991. Copyright © 1991 by Elsevier Science Publishers, Ireland. Reprinted with permission.)

sidering that unattended stimuli, too, elicited negativities at these same latencies and, further, that these negativities were larger contra- than ipsilaterally to eliciting stimuli. However, a careful examination of their published data indicates that both Nd80 and Nd125 were clearly anterior to the corresponding N1 phases for unattended stimuli (cf. Figs. 6.19 and 6.20; see also their Table 2). This suggests that at least a good deal of these Nd effects were, in fact, endogenous.

The early and late Nd phases were intervened by a sharp central positive attention effect "Pd190" (Fig. 6.20). It appears that a positive centroposterior component is here in fact superimposed on a relatively continuous attentional negativity (consisting of two or several overlapping negative components), cutting it into two parts. This is supported by the continuously negative anterior (Fpz) attention effect.

Although admitting that all their attention effects might, in fact, be of an endogenous origin, Woldorff and Hillyard (1991) regarded it as much more

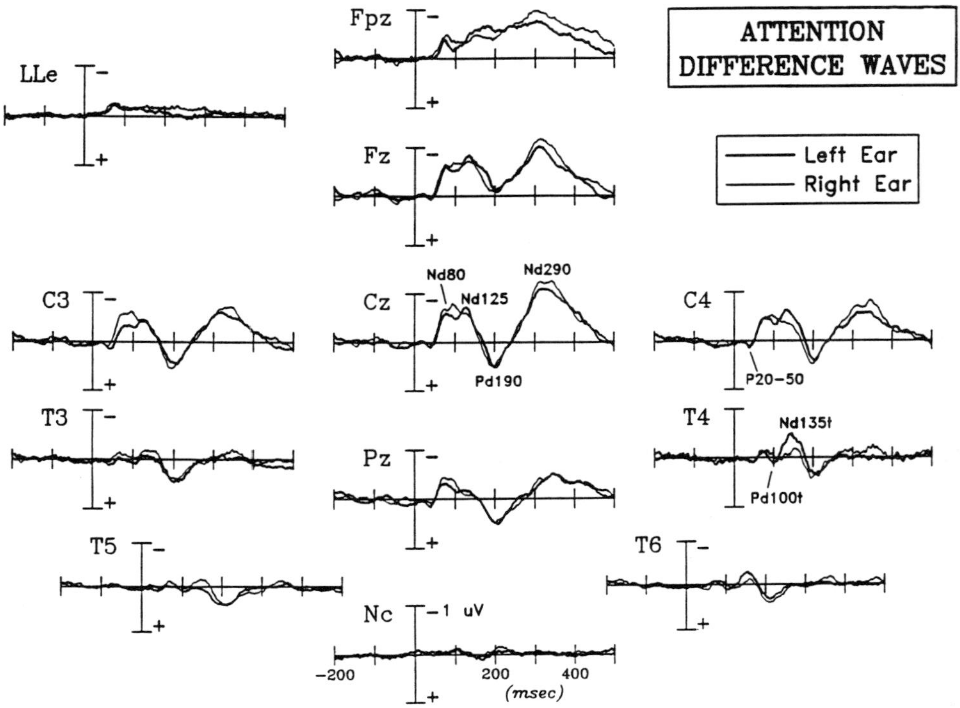

FIG. 6.20 Grand-average difference waves (attended-stimulus ERPs *minus* unattended-stimulus ERPs) separately for left-(thick line) and right-ear (thin line) tones at different electrode sites as indicated in the figure in a dichotic attention study. The same data as shown in Fig. 6.19. Reference for all sites is the algebraic average of the mastoids. Nc = Noncephalic (balanced sterno-vertebral). LLe = Lower Left eye (below and to left of the left eye). (From Woldorff & Hillyard, 1991. Copyright © 1991 by Elsevier Science Publishers, Ireland. Reprinted with permission.)

plausible that at least some of them were exogenous. The authors concluded that their results, as taken together, "provide strong support for the early selection hypothesis that attention can serve to selectively bias or gate stimulus processing before full perceptual analysis has occurred" (Woldorff & Hillyard, 1991, p. 170).

Näätänen, Teder, et al.'s 1992; (see also Näätänen & Teder, 1991) very recent results, in turn, suggest that even an Nd almost perfectly coinciding in time with the exogenous, apparently supratemporal, N1 component is generated by a separate mechanism. These authors presented tones of 300 and 6000 Hz to the subject's left and right ear, respectively, in random order with very short ISIs (varying from 60 to 200 msec). The subject was instructed to count occasional, slightly higher pitched tones within a designated input stream.

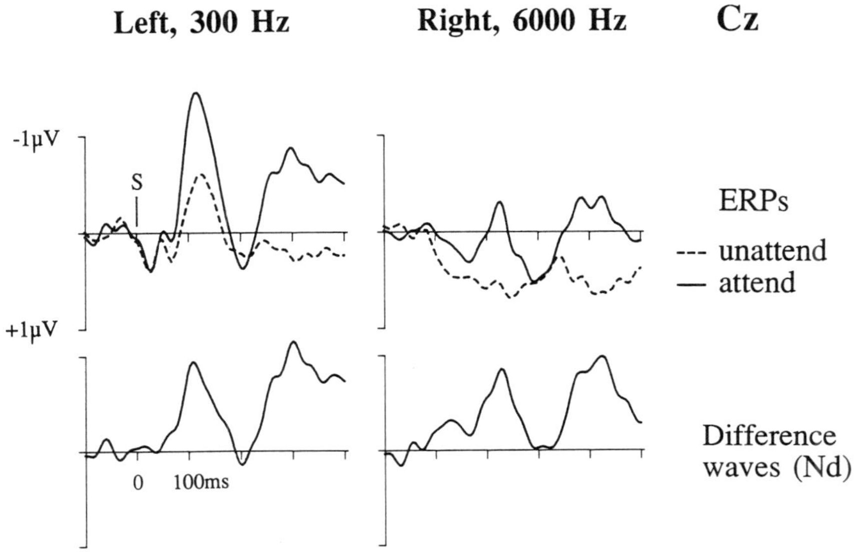

FIG. 6.21 TOP: Grand-average vertex (Cz) ERPs to attended (solid line) and unattended (dashed line) stimuli delivered to the left (300 Hz) and right ear (6,000 Hz) in a dichotic attention study. BOTTOM: Corresponding difference waves (ERPs to unattended tones subtracted from ERPs to attended tones). (From Näätänen, Teder, Alho, & Lavikainen, 1992.)

Figure 6.21 shows that vertex ERPs are much larger for low- than high-pitched tones. In fact, it is questionable whether any N1 was elicited by the 6000-Hz tones. On the other hand, the Nds for the two tones are very similar in amplitude. This pattern of data strongly suggests that the mechanisms of the exogenous N1 generation and those of the attention effect are different even with a nearly perfect temporal coincidence, for one would expect the attention effect to be at least roughly proportional to the strength of the generator response elicited in the absence of attention.

Endogenous attention effects may also precede the exogenous N1 components, providing further evidence for different mechanisms of these components and the attention effect. For example, as already mentioned, McCallum et al. (1983) showed that with a large spatial separation, Nd might begin well before the exogenous N1 commences.

Further converging evidence for the separability of the early-Nd and exogeneous-N1 mechanisms was recently provided by Woods, Alho, and Algazi (1991). In this study, the N1 scalp distribution for unattended tones varied with tone frequency (see also Bertrand et al., 1988), whereas that of the early-Nd distribution did not (Fig. 6.22). Corroborating results were obtained by Näätänen, Teder, et al. who, in their aforementioned study,

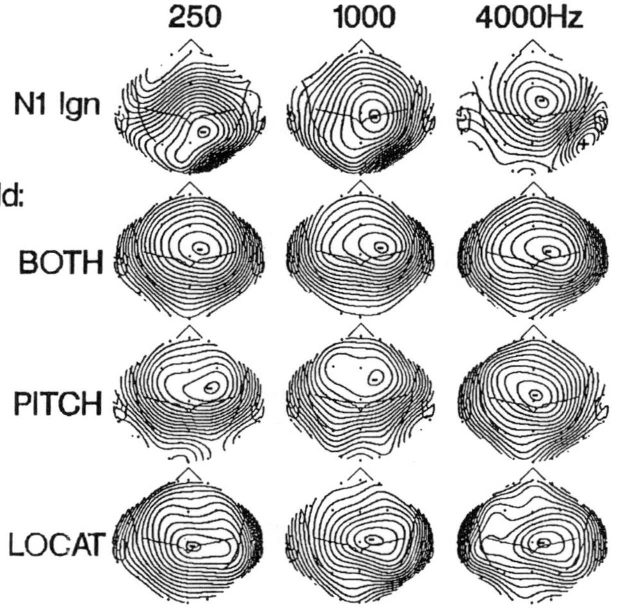

FIG. 6.22 ERP scalp distributions derived with spherical spline interpolation in an attention study in which attended and ignored stimuli differed either in pitch, location, or both. (a) *N1 Ign:* Mean voltages of ERPs evoked by unattended tones of different frequencies. Latency range 70–90 msec. (b) *Nd. Both:* Distributions of Nd mean voltage from 130–150 msec to standard tones with both attended pitch and attended location features separately for different tone frequencies. (c) *Pitch:* Distributions of mean Nd voltage from 130–150 msec to tones of attended pitch but unattended location separately for different tone frequencies. (d) *Locat:* Distributions of Nd mean voltage from 130–150 msec following tones of attended location but unattended pitch separately for different tone frequencies. Electrodes (dots) on the right were contralateral to the ear of stimulation. Contour lines are shown at 99% maximal voltage, and then at 6.25% steps through the total voltage range. (From Woods, Alho, & Algazi, 1991. Copyright © 1991 by Rapid Communications of Oxford Ltd. Reprinted with permission.)

found that the Nd scalp distribution was practically taken identical when high tones were attended and when low tones were attended (Fig. 6.23).

Moreover, Teder, Alho, Reinikainen, and Näätänen (in press) observed that even when there is an excellent temporal correspondence between the exogenous N1 and the early Nd in the averaged data, single-subject data may reveal considerable temporal dissociation (Fig. 6.24).

However, none of the previously reviewed studies rules out the possibility that some exogenous neuronal population contributing to the N1 wave also contributes to the Nd effect (see also Woldorff & Hillyard, 1991). This is

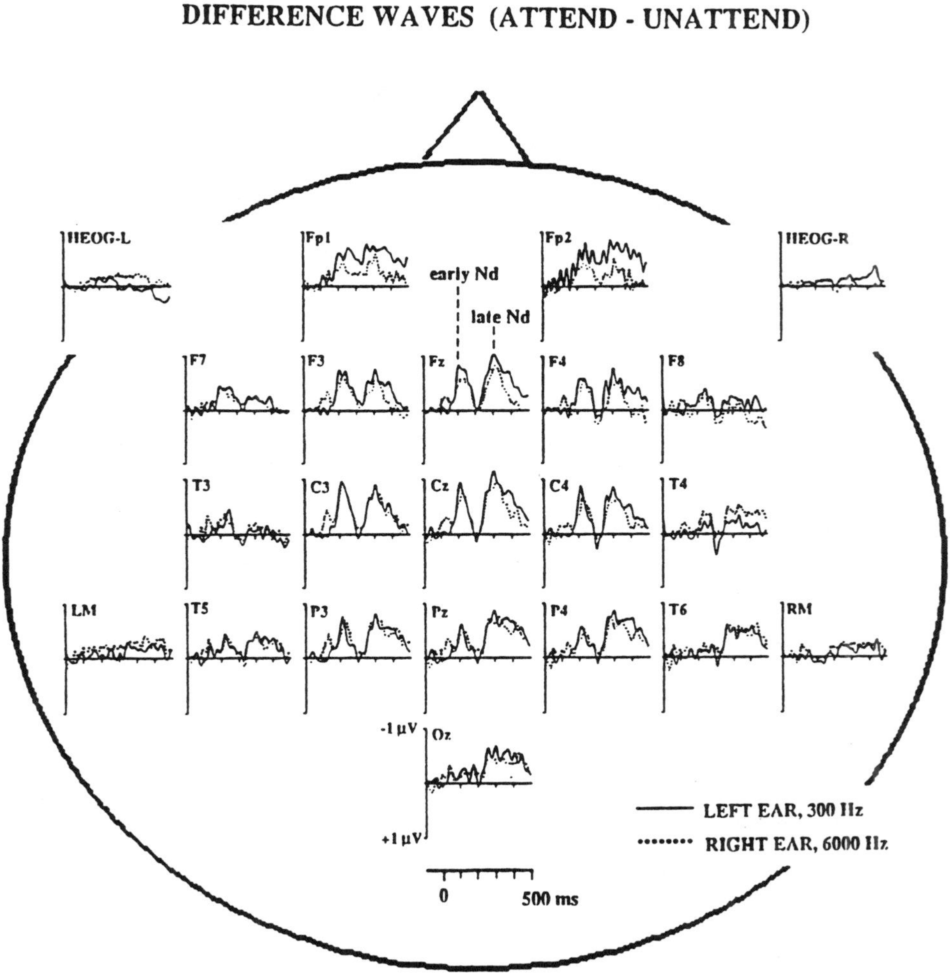

FIG. 6.23 The topographical distribution of the grand-average difference waves (attended-stimulus ERPs − unattended-stimulus ERPs) shown in Fig. 6.21 separately for the 300-Hz standard tones presented to the left ear (solid lines) and for the 6000-Hz standard tones presented to the right ear (dotted lines). (From Näätänen, Teder, Alho, and Lavikainen, 1992.)

because the supratemporal N1 component might actually be composed of different subcomponents, each generated by different, discrete neuronal populations (Giard et al., 1988; Hansen & Hillyard, 1980; McCallum & Curry, 1980; Näätänen & Picton, 1987; Näätänen et al., 1988; Woldorff & Hillyard, 1991; Woods & Clayworth, 1987).

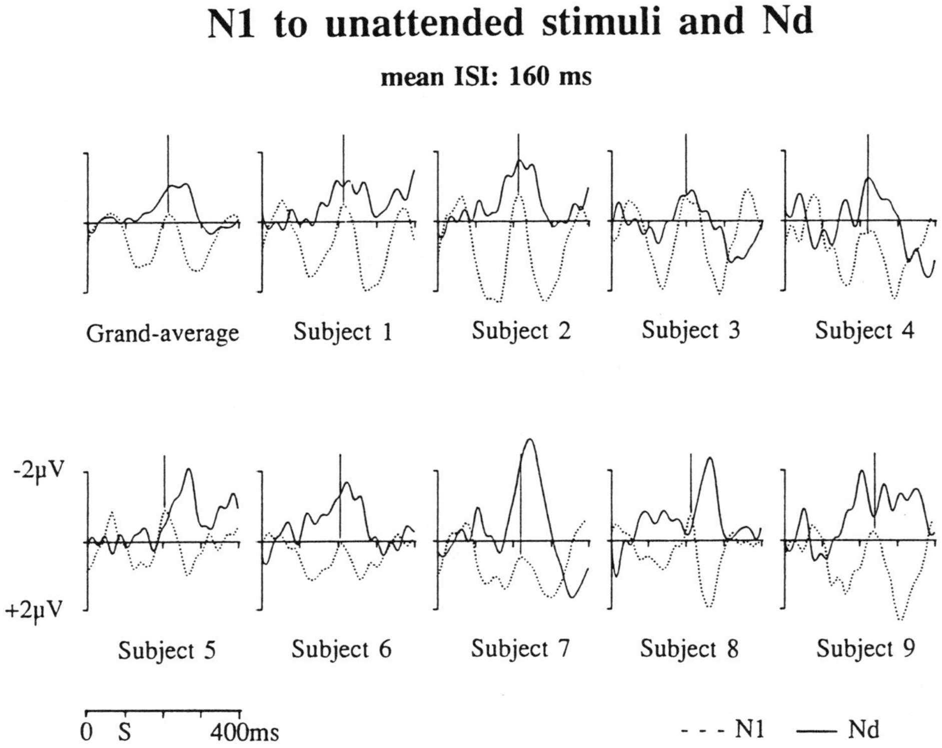

FIG. 6.24 Grand-average and single-subject vertex (Cz) N1 to unattended stimuli (dashed lines) and Nd (continuous lines) collapsed across left and right ears. Data from Condition 160 (ISI 120–220 msec). Stimulus onset at S. The N1 peak latencies are marked with vertical lines. (From Teder, Alho, Reinikainen, & Näätänen, in press. Copyright © in press by The Society for Psychophysiological Research. Reprinted with permission.)

The T-Complex and Selective Attention. As already reviewed (Section 4.3.), one component of the exogeneous N1 in audition emanates from the lateral aspect of the temporal lobe, that is, the negativity belonging to the Wolpaw and Penry (1975) T-complex. Woods, Alho, and Algazi (in press) found that this negativity was larger when subjects attended to the eliciting auditory stimuli than when they attended to concurrent visual stimuli (a difficult video game).

The T140 enhancement was more prominent over the right than the left temporal lobe, irrespective of whether the auditory stimulus block was delivered to the left or right ear. "One possible explanation is that the Nd140 reflects increased activity of generators in auditory association cortex, the same areas that show enhanced cerebral blood flow, particularly in the right hemisphere, when attention is switched from the visual to auditory modalities in intermodal attention tasks. . . ." (Woods, 1990, p. 189). Cerebral blood-flow studies of selective attention are reviewed in Chapter 8.

Woldorff and Hillyard (1991), in their previously reviewed study, also reported an attentional enhancement of the negativity belonging to the T-complex, that was larger over the right than left hemisphere (see Figs. 6.19 and 6.20).

If Nd140 really is due to an attentional modulation of the negative component belonging to the T-complex, then this complex should show right-hemispheric preponderance even when attention effects are not present. Unfortunately, the available data are not very clear in this respect (for a review, see Näätänen & Picton, 1987), but Wolpaw and Penry (1977) provided some data supporting right-hemispheric preponderance of the T-complex.

An attentional T140 enhancement during intermodal selective attention was also reported by Hackley et al. (1990). In addition, these authors found a large early Nd over the central scalp, which they interpreted as a composite of an exogenous-N1 enhancement and a PN. It is very difficult to decide whether an exogenous N1 component was enhanced, however. The authors also reported an enhanced "P2 component" when auditory stimuli were attended, but this effect, too, might be endogenous, judging from the considerably prolonged P2 peak latency for auditory stimuli when attended.

In conclusion, it appears that at least the main portion of the supratemporal N1 component is insensitive to attention. On the other hand, a possible attentional modulation of some of its subcomponents cannot be ruled out (Giard et al., 1988; Woldorff & Hillyard, 1991). As to the N1 component belonging to the T-complex, generated on the lateral surface of the temporal lobe, the three previously reviewed, very recent studies suggest that it may be modulated by selective attention.

The Interpretation of the Processing Negativity: The Attentional-Trace Theory of Selective Attention

Two main interpretations have been offered for the slow negative displacement examined in the foregoing. This attentional effect reflects either further processing performed for stimuli selected in the initial stimulus-set selection (Hansen & Hillyard, 1980; Näätänen et al., 1978, 1980; Näätänen & Michie, 1979a; Okita, 1979, 1981, 1989; Okita et al., 1983), this selection process itself (Harter & Guido, 1980; Harter & Previc, 1978), or both, so that the first component reflects this initial selection and the second component either the further processing of stimuli accepted in the initial selection or the maintenance of the selective-attention state (Näätänen,

1982). As already mentioned, Hillyard et al. (1973) interpreted their N1 effect in terms of the initial selection. Näätänen et al. (1978) and Näätänen and Michie (1979a) suggested that PN might also reflect an outcome of the initial selection, such as a subsequent orienting or transient-arousal response (see also Näätänen, 1987). According to Näätänen and Michie (1979a), it is possible that the negative attentional displacement is "associated with (voluntary or preparatory) *orienting* to an input when it has been found to meet the criterion of stimulus relevance" (Näätänen & Michie, 1979a, p. 130), regarding the frontal dominance of the effect as strongly supporting this interpretation. The authors proposed that the attentional displacement is caused by the activity of two generator systems: (a) those associated with orienting, this activity being "frontally dominated and modality nonspecific" (p. 131), and (b) the mechanisms of further stimulus processing, which are, at least to some extent, sensory specific.

The Attentional-Trace Theory. Näätänen (1982) proposed that the initial selection is performed with an "attentional trace." This was defined as a voluntarily maintained representation of the physical features of the relevant stimulus which separate it from the irrelevant stimulus. Thus, for instance, if relevant and irrelevant stimuli differ in pitch, then the attentional trace would represent the pitch of the relevant, but not that of the irrelevant, stimulus.

The initial selection performed with the attentional trace was described as a self-terminating *matching* (comparison) process on-line generating the early PN component. This matching process, triggered by each auditory stimulus while an attentional trace exists, is, on the theory, an automatic consequence of maintenance of this trace by some higher system. Hence, whereas the matching process itself is automatic, the maintenance of the attentional trace is a voluntary, controlled process.

It was further proposed that when an irrelevant stimulus is presented, the matching process terminates early, and sooner for more conspicuous differences between relevant and irrelevant stimuli. This was explained on the assumption that the attentional trace represents a gradually smaller and smaller range along some sensory dimension as processing proceeds for a given stimulus in the selective system (Näätänen, 1982). Consistently with this, Shelley (1991) has suggested that selection begins in polymodal areas that have neurons with wide receptive fields, and is continued by neurons with narrower receptive fields in the sensory areas (cf. Alho, 1987). See also the principle of reafference or recurrent excitation (Pandya & Yeterian, 1985; see also Woods, 1990).

Thus, on this hypothesis, the attentional trace is a recognition mechanism for relevant stimuli that is more sharply "tuned" to relevant stimuli for more advanced phase of processing of input. In addition, the early PN might reflect increased neuronal firing (see Benson & Hienz, 1978, reviewed earlier), which continues as long as the sensory input remains within the range of the attentional trace, that is, proceeds within the facilitated part of the receiving system. This principle is illustrated in Fig. 6.25. It should be pointed out that the range of the attentional trace depicted in Fig. 6.25 is set before stimulus delivery, and is not altered as the stimulus is processed.

Näätänen (1982) further proposed that the attentional trace might be located in auditory cortex, possibly in secondary sensory areas. "The very short onset latency points to a selective sensory state . . . already prevailing before and at the stimulus moment and causing the differential treatment of attended and unattended auditory stimuli. There must be a temporary bias somewhere in the sensory system toward the attended stimulus; otherwise

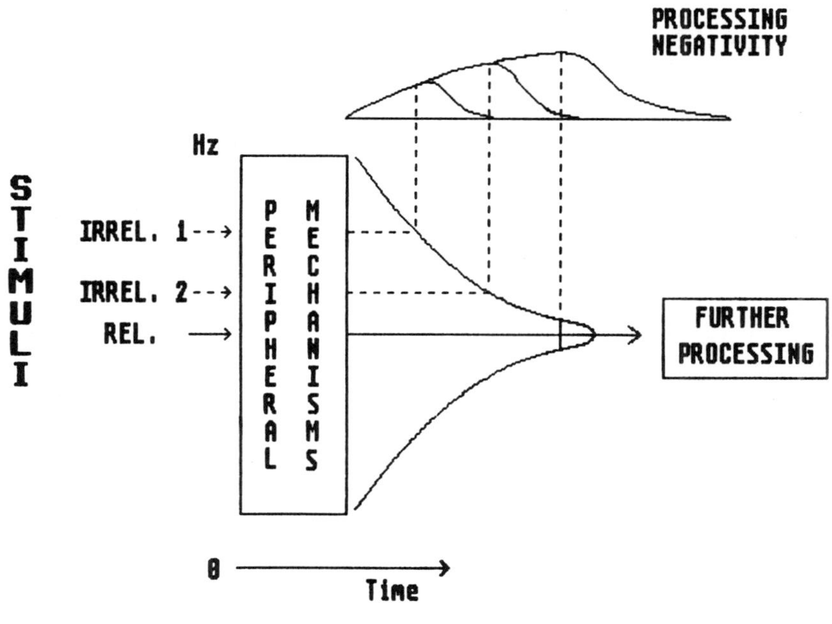

FIG. 6.25 A schematic illustration for the generation of the sensory-specific component of the processing negativity (PN) as dictated by the attentional-trace theory. The attentional trace is a controlled recognition mechanism for the to-be-attended stimuli in some sensory receiving system—in this case in a receiving system for auditory frequency—which is tuned more and more narrowly to the frequency of the attended ("relevant") stimulus for later processing in the sensory system involved. The relevant stimulus matches with the attentional trace throughout its processing in this system. A large, long-duration PN is therefore generated, and the input passes to the next prepared processing stage ("Further Processing"). The irrelevant stimuli also elicit some PN, for they match the wide-range, early part of the attentional trace. This matching phase of irrelevant stimuli lasts longer for smaller (Irrel. 2) than larger (Irrel. 1) differences between relevant and irrelevant stimuli.

an effect at a latency of 50 msec would be impossible" (p. 629). As already mentioned, Hillyard et al. (1973) interpreted their N1 effect in a similar way.

This selective state in the sensory system was described as resulting from selective rehearsal of the sensory-memory representation of the relevant stimulus. As suggested by MMN data (Section 4.4), each stimulus, after a few repetitions, automatically produces (activates) its trace in the sensory-storage system (Cowan et al., 1991). According to the attentional-trace theory, we can choose which trace, and which of its features, to rehearse. In the very beginning of the session, however, the attentional trace does not exist, because sensory memory does not contain a corresponding activated trace. In addition, the attentional trace, existing only during the maintenance or rehearsal activity, cannot be maintained very long in the absence of the corresponding stimulus, with the duration of sensory memory setting the upper limit.

The attentional trace depends, consequently, both on afferent (producing the activated sensory-memory trace) and efferent (rehearsal) input. Of these inputs, the efferent must be current and the afferent either current or recent. The efferent input signifies the voluntary aspect, the afferent the necessary environmental support. It would accordingly be impossible to develop an attentional trace by voluntary means only, without an activated sensory-memory representation of the relevant stimulus.

Thus, on the theory, only stimulus features that are frequently presented can be incorporated into the attentional trace. Of course, the subject rehearses only the stimulus feature that is needed for task performance. Therefore, stimulus features shared by relevant and irrelevant stimuli would not be rehearsed and hence represented in the attentional trace. If the subject chooses for rehearsal an infrequent stimulus, such as the target in most of these studies, this will not result in the development of the attentional trace, at least not of a strong one. This is due to infrequent sensory reinforcement of the level of the feature separating targets from "relevant standards."

Further, when fatigued or bored, or in the presence of distracting stimuli, the subject may be unable to continuously maintain the attentional trace, that is, every now and then an attentional lapse occurs. During these attentional lapses, the attentional trace is lost but can be called back as long as the corresponding stimulus has an adequate representation in sensory memory. In the maintenance of the attentional trace, temporal expectancies with regard to the relevant stimulus might also play a role (Näätänen, 1982).

The model was meant to explain attentional selection occurring in the typical ERP selective-attention paradigm in which discrete stimuli are intervened by "empty" intervals. The model can, however, be applied even when stimuli are continuous, such as when listening to one of two or several concurrent speakers. This is supported by the fact that Nd is obtained with individual syllables of the attended continuous speech message (Woods, Hillyard, & Hansen, 1984) and with tonal stimuli presented at very short (onset-to-onset) ISIs, such as those varying randomly between 60–100 msec (Teder et al., in press).

Therefore, the attentional trace appears to be maintained by the continuous, or almost continuous, matching process when the attended message is continuous. This would explain the relative ease of keeping one's mind selectively focused on a given speech message among competing ones: the cocktail-party phenomenon. The development of the attentional trace even in this situation is, evidently, based on sensory-memory data provided by the first few words uttered by the speaker to be listened to. For supportive behavioral results, see Treisman et al. (1974), who found that subjects need a few words before being able to tune their attention selectively to one of the concurrent dichotic messages.

Nd and Processing Negativity. An obvious implication of the model suggested is that PN is not obtained by subtracting the ERP to the unattended stimulus from that to the attended stimulus (Näätänen, 1982). This operation yields the PN differential (Nd; Hansen & Hillyard, 1980), not PN itself, because the common initial part is subtracted out. (During the generation of this common part until Nd onset, the system does not yet "know," presumably, whether or not the current sensory input being processed is relevant.) The total PN is perhaps best obtained by comparing attended-stimulus ERPs with those elicited when the whole stimulus block is ignored, the subject reading a book, for example (see Fig. 6.26). Thus, PN is an on-line rather than outcome expression of the matching process. For a distinction between these two categories of ERP components, see Ritter, Simson, and Vaughan (1983).

These suggestions are schematically illustrated in Fig. 6.26. On the top, ERPs to attended and unattended stimuli are superimposed. The ERP to attended stimuli is more negative than that to unattended stimuli, resulting in Nd (the second row). Nd starts earlier for a larger difference between relevant and irrelevant stimuli, because the irrelevant-stimulus PN is terminated earlier with larger than with smaller differences.

Nd is not always entirely due to PN differences between ERPs to relevant and irrelevant stimuli, however. This is because irrelevant stimuli may elicit some (relatively late) positivity (Alho, Töttölä, et al., 1987; Hansen & Hillyard, 1988; Michie, Solowij, et al., 1990; Näätänen et al., 1981; Solowij, Michie, Crawford, & Glue, 1990). This positivity was called the "rejection positivity" by Alho, Töttölä, et al. (1987).

The Frontal (or Fronto-Central) PN Component. This component, reviewed earlier (see Fig. 6.16), begins later, lasts longer, and is often larger in amplitude than the more central component (Hansen & Hillyard, 1980,

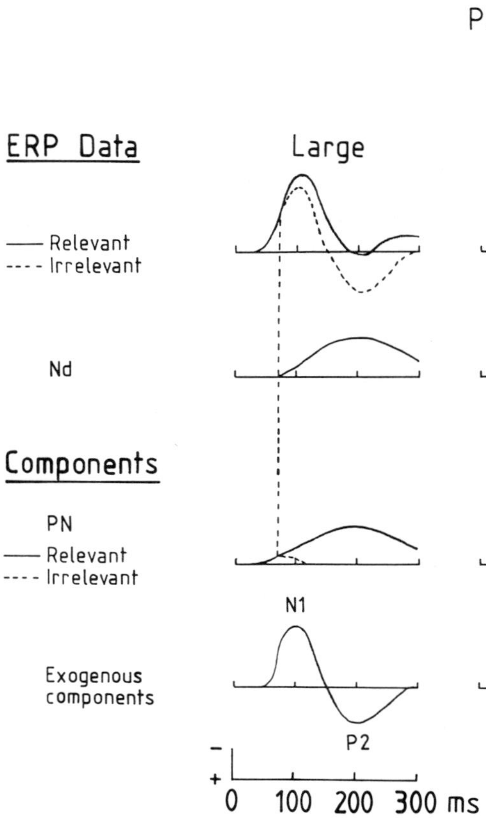

FIG. 6.26 A schematic illustration of the ERP and its different components at the vertex (Cz) when the subject attends to one of two equiprobable tones differing in pitch. "Large" refers to a condition in which this pitch separation is large; in "Medium," this separation is smaller, and in "Small," the two pitches are very close to one another. (Stimuli are presented with short, random ISIs.) *First row:* ERPs to the relevant (continuous lines) and irrelevant (dashed lines) tones. *Second row:* The corresponding Nds obtained by subtracting the irrelevant-stimulus ERP from the relevant-stimulus ERP. The Nd-onset latency increases and amplitude decreases with diminishing pitch separation. *Third row:* These pitch-difference effects on Nd are due to the increase and prolongation of PN to irrelevant stimuli (dashed lines) with diminishing difference, the PN to relevant stimuli (solid lines) being similar for all differences. *Fourth row:* The attenuation of the exogenous N1 and P2 components (identical for relevant and irrelevant stimuli) with diminishing pitch difference. The ERPs shown in the first row are composed of the summation of these exogenous components with the corresponding PNs (third row). (From Alho, Töttölä, Reinikainen, Sams, & Näätänen, 1987. Copyright © 1987 by Elsevier Science Publishers, Ireland. Reprinted with permission.)

1984). In addition, in contrast to the early component, the late component is enhanced with increasing ISIs (Näätänen et al., 1981; Teder et al., in press; Woods, 1990).

Näätänen (1982; see also Hansen & Hillyard, 1983) proposed that the frontal component might reflect further processing of stimuli accepted in initial selection. This further processing can be characterized as a prepared mental reflex (Woodworth, 1938; Logan, 1979) maintained by the limited-capacity system in a state of readiness, to be released if a stimulus is accepted by the attentional-trace system (Fig. 6.25). Logan (1979) suggested that the role of the limited-capacity system in repetitive tasks is to set up a program for stimulus analysis rather than to carry out the information-processing stages that convert a stimulus to a response.

Alternatively, the frontal component might reflect selective rehearsal of the stimulus to be attended (Näätänen, 1982). This is supported by the very long duration of the frontal component, its larger amplitude for longer ISIs (Hansen & Hillyard, 1984; Näätänen et al., 1981), and also by the frontal topography itself, insofar as the frontal areas are essential to voluntarily directed attention (Knight, 1984, 1990; Luria & Homskaya, 1970; Picton et al., 1986; Stuss & Benson, 1986; Tucker & Williamson, 1984; Woods, 1990; see also the rCBF results reviewed in chapter 8). Further, Näätänen and Picton (1987) have associated the frontal PN component with "executive" cerebral activity. It is, however, also possible that the frontal component is activational in nature, generated by transient cerebral arousal (Näätänen, 1987, 1990) belonging to an orienting response to a relevant stimulus (Näätänen & Michie, 1979a).

Shelley, Ward, Michie, Andrews, Mitchell, Catts, and McConaghy (1991) found that the late, frontocentral Nd phase was substantially attenuated, whereas the early (also frontocentral) phase was not, by extended practice in a complex multidimensional task similar to that employed by Hansen and Hillyard (1983). For corroborating results, see Hansen and Hillyard (1988) and Woods (1990). Furthermore, Ciesielski, Courchesne, and Elmasian (1990) reported that the late Nd phase was almost entirely absent in autistic subjects whose auditory focused-attention performance was as good as, or better than, that in normals. Consequently, it may be concluded that the later, fronto-central PN component is much more labile than the sensory-specific component.

Maiste and Picton (1987) varied the difficulty of discriminating targets among standards presented to a designated ear. They found that the late component was enhanced by increased task difficulty, whereas the early component was not affected.

The late Nd phase shows several interesting similarities with the event-related perturbation of the steady-state response (SSR) examined in Section 4.2. These similarities include the time course of the two effects (compare Figs. 4.5. and 4.6. with Figs. 6.10 and 6.16; see also Rohrbaugh et al., 1990,

1991). Also, as already reviewed (Section 4.2), the SSR latency-reduction response observed by Rohrbaugh and his colleagues (Rohrbaugh et al., 1991) was attenuated with continued stimulus presentation (Session 2 vs. Session 1) and enhanced with attention, increased task difficulty, auditory (rather than visual) stimuli, and long ISIs. These factors seem, as already reviewed, to affect the frontal component in a similar way. Consequently, the two phenomena might share, at least in part, a common cause. Possibly, both are related to a transient arousal response (see previously).

It is noteworthy that Grossberg, in an innovative series of theoretical publications (see, e.g., Grossberg, 1982; 1984), has proposed a theory of information processing which in a number of essential features resembles the attentional-trace theory reviewed here, although the two theories were developed totally independently.

Studies Testing the Attentional-Trace Theory: The Early PN as Generated by an On-Line Matching Process. The theory proposes that: (a) the early PN is generated by initial selection in which relevant stimuli are accepted for further processing and irrelevant stimuli are rejected; and (b) this selection occurs as a comparison process in which sensory input is compared with a voluntarily maintained representation of the relevant stimulus (the attentional trace). This comparison process is initiated by each stimulus and continues longer, the more similar the stimulus is to the one represented by the attentional trace (Näätänen, 1990).

These assumptions receive support from several studies. Figure 6.27 superimposes Hansen and Hillyard's (1980) irrelevant-stimulus ERPs shown in Fig. 6.11. It can be seen that the smaller the frequency difference between relevant and irrelevant stimuli, the longer the peak latency and duration of the irrelevant-stimulus negativity. This is not due to corresponding changes in N1-generator activity, for this activity is known to be weaker for smaller differences and to not vary in latency and duration with the difference (Näätänen & Picton, 1987). Rather, as proposed by Näätänen (1990), an endogenous negative component partially overlaps, and sums with, the N1 component in these data. The overlapping component appears to be PN to the irrelevant stimulus, which is larger and lasts longer for smaller differences.

This effect consequently accounts for Hansen and Hillyard's (1980) later Nd onset with smaller differences (Fig. 6.11), that is, the later separation of the traces for relevant and irrelevant stimuli. This later Nd onset is hence not due to a later PN onset to relevant stimuli with smaller stimulus differences. This suggests that the early PN is generated by a comparison or matching process in which relevant stimuli are selected, rather than by further processing of the relevant stimuli. In the latter case, irrelevant stimuli could elicit no PN.

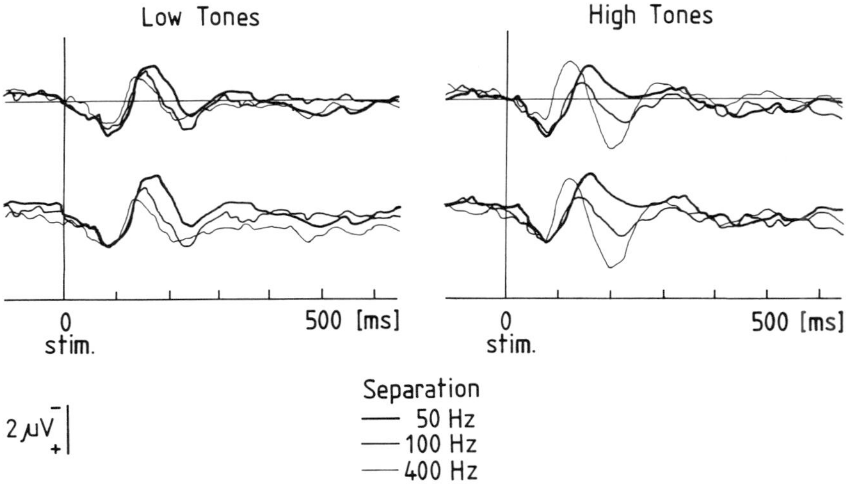

FIG. 6.27 Grand-average vertex (Cz) ERPs to unattended low (left) and high (right) binaural tones for different frequency separations (50, 100, or 400 Hz) between these unattended tones and attended tones superimposed either at the stimulus moment (top traces) or at the P1 peak (bottom traces). See the legend of Fig. 6.11. (Adapted from Hansen & Hillyard, 1980. Copyright © 1980 by Elsevier Science Publishers BV [Biomedical Division]. Reprinted with permission.)

Results supporting this conclusion were also obtained by Alho, Donauer, et al. (1987), Alho, Paavilainen, et al. (1986), Alho, Töttölä, et al. (1987), Berman, Friedman, and Cramer (1990), Born, Brüninger, et al. (1987), Gaillard & Verduin (1985), Hansen & Hillyard (1983, 1988), and, with the MEG, Hari, Hämäläinen, Kaukoranta, Mäkelä, Joutsiniemi, & Tiihonen (1989; see chapter 7).

In one of these studies, Alho, Paavilainen, et al. (1986) administered stimulus blocks that consisted of three equiprobable tones of different pitch: "low," "medium," and "high," and the subject counted one of them. The difference between the tones was, in different blocks, either "large," "medium," or "small." All stimuli were presented to the subject's right ear. Figure 6.28 shows that the counted (low) stimulus elicited a more negative ERP, starting at 100–150 msec from stimulus onset, than did the same stimulus when one of the other stimuli was counted. In addition, the ERP to the irrelevant low stimulus was more negative when the medium stimulus was being counted than when the high stimulus was counted (Fig. 6.28). Thus, the low stimulus elicited the largest attentional negativity when counted but elicited some of this negativity even when the adjacent stimulus was counted. An analogous pattern of data was obtained for the high stimulus.

Moreover, ERPs to the irrelevant (low or high) tones were more negative

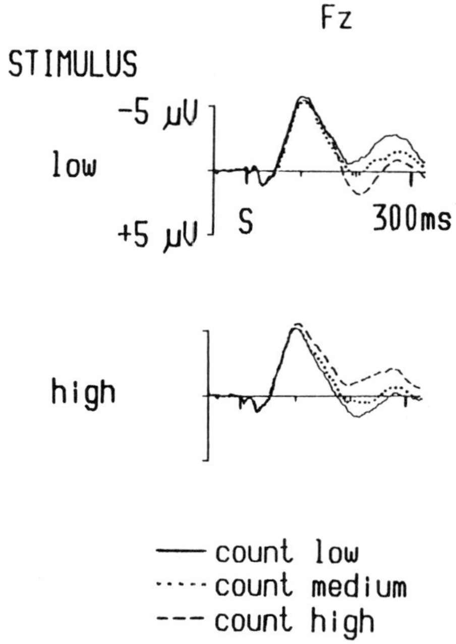

FIG. 6.28 Grand-average frontal (Fz) ERPs to low (top) and high (bottom) right-ear tones when low (460 Hz, solid line), medium (500 Hz, dotted line), or high (543 Hz, dashed line) tones were to be counted. (From Alho, Sams, Paavilainen, & Näätänen, 1986. Copyright © 1986 The Society for Psychophysiological Research. Reprinted with permission of the publisher.)

with smaller than with larger stimulus differences in a block (see "high stimulus" in Fig. 6.29). This further suggests that irrelevant stimuli elicited PN and, further, that this PN was larger for smaller differences. (A control experiment showed that this effect was not due to more frequent discrimination errors in blocks with smaller stimulus differences.) In further support of the theory, the relevant-stimulus PN probably was rather similar, regardless of the magnitude of the stimulus difference (see low, counted stimulus in Fig. 6.29). The ERP difference at the N1 peak latency is due to the greater refractoriness of the N1 generator when the three stimuli are more similar to one another (Section 4.3).

Consequently, these data indicate that an irrelevant stimulus elicits some PN and, further, this PN is larger with smaller differences between this irrelevant stimulus and the relevant stimulus. Alho, Donauer, et al.'s (1987) study with apparent spatial differences between relevant and irrelevant tones provides further support. With a small spatial difference, Nd started later and was smaller than with a large spatial difference. This appeared to result from a larger PN to irrelevant stimuli for smaller spatial differences. Similar results were obtained with frequency differences.

PN elicitation by irrelevant stimuli was also suggested by Alho, Töttölä, et al. (1987). Of their two equiprobable tones, one always was 500 Hz. The high tone was, in separate blocks, a tone varying from 503 Hz to 1229 Hz. Either the high or low tone was task-relevant. The Nd amplitude was larger,

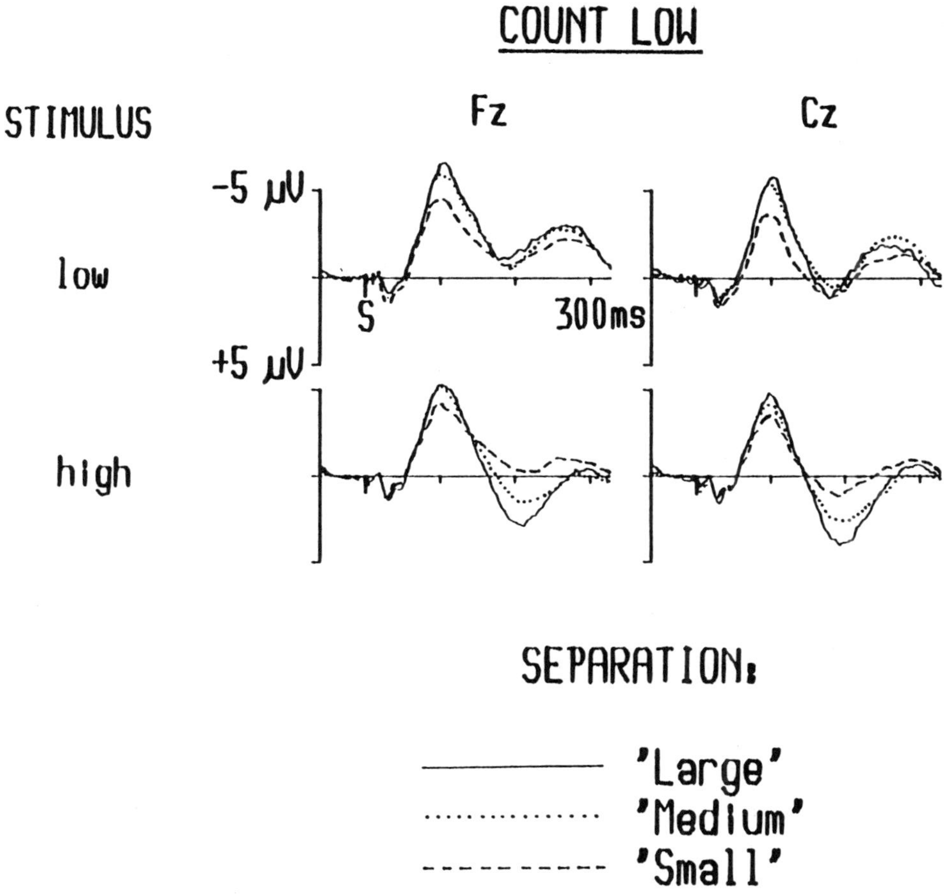

FIG. 6.29 Grand-average frontal (Fz) and vertex (Cz) ERPs to low (top) and high (bottom) tones when low tones were counted as a function of the frequency difference between the relevant (counted) and irrelevant (uncounted) tones in a block. The solid lines indicate the ERPs when the frequency difference was "large," the dotted lines when it was "medium," and the dashed lines when it was "small." (From Alho, Sams, Paavilainen, & Näätänen, 1986. Copyright © 1986 The Society for Psychophysiological Research. Reprinted with permission.)

and the onset latency shorter, for larger frequency differences. Some Nd was even found for a difference as small as 9 or 27 Hz (Fig. 6.30). The pitch-difference effects on Nd again resulted from PN to the irrelevant stimulus being larger in amplitude, and in this study also longer in duration, with smaller pitch differences, whereas the relevant-stimulus PN was unaffected.

Also in line with the theory, the relevant-stimulus ERP was more negative

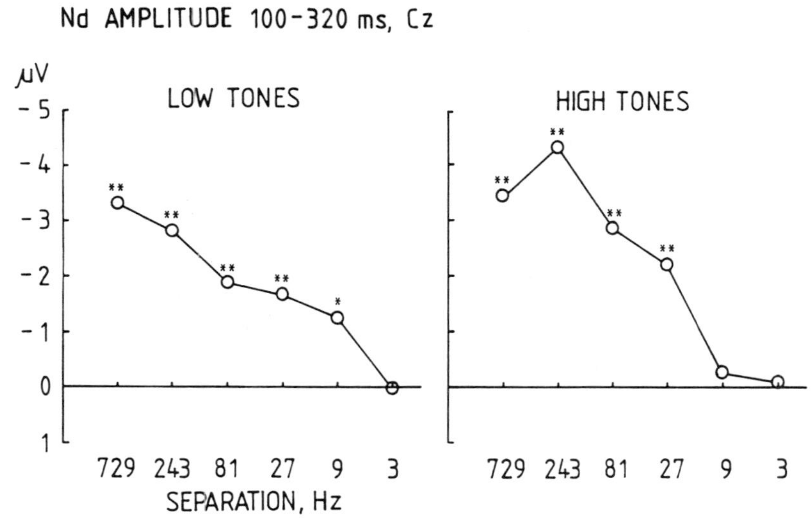

FIG. 6.30 Vertex (Cz) mean Nd amplitudes across subjects for the "low" (on left) and "high" (right) tones as a function of the difference between the two tones in a block. Blocks of equiprobable low (500 Hz) and high tones were presented, one of the tones being designated relevant at a time. The task was to count how many times at least 4 consecutive relevant stimuli occurred in a block. In separate blocks, the high tone was either 503, 509, 527, 581, 742, or 1229 Hz. The Nd was obtained by subtracting the irrelevant-stimulus ERP from that elicited by the same stimulus when relevant. (From Alho, Töttölä, Reinikainen, Sams, & Näätänen, 1987. Copyright © 1987 by Elsevier Science Publishers, Ireland. Reprinted with permission.)

than the ERP to an identical stimulus when the subject was reading. Moreover, the irrelevant-stimulus ERP of the attend conditions was initially more negative than the reading ERP to an identical stimulus, and this negative difference lasted longer for smaller frequency differences. This pattern of data hence provides strong support for the suggestion that even irrelevant stimuli during focused attention elicit some early PN, and that therefore Nd obtained by subtracting the irrelevant-stimulus ERP from that to relevant stimuli does not reveal the whole PN.

Corroborating evidence was provided by Born, Brüninger, et al. (1987), Gaillard and Verduin (1985), McCallum et al. (1989), Michie, Bearpark, et al. (1990), and Michie, Solowij, et al., 1990). Converging MEG evidence is reviewed in chapter 7. Further support is provided by some ERP studies of visual attention, to be reviewed in Section 6.3.

In addition, Hansen and Hillyard (1988), in their previously reviewed study, showed that in the very beginning of the stimulus block, both relevant and irrelevant stimuli elicit a large PN; therefore, Nd is then absent or only very small (see Fig. 6.31). With subsequent stimulus presentations, Nd emerged, however, which was due to a progressive PN attenuation for

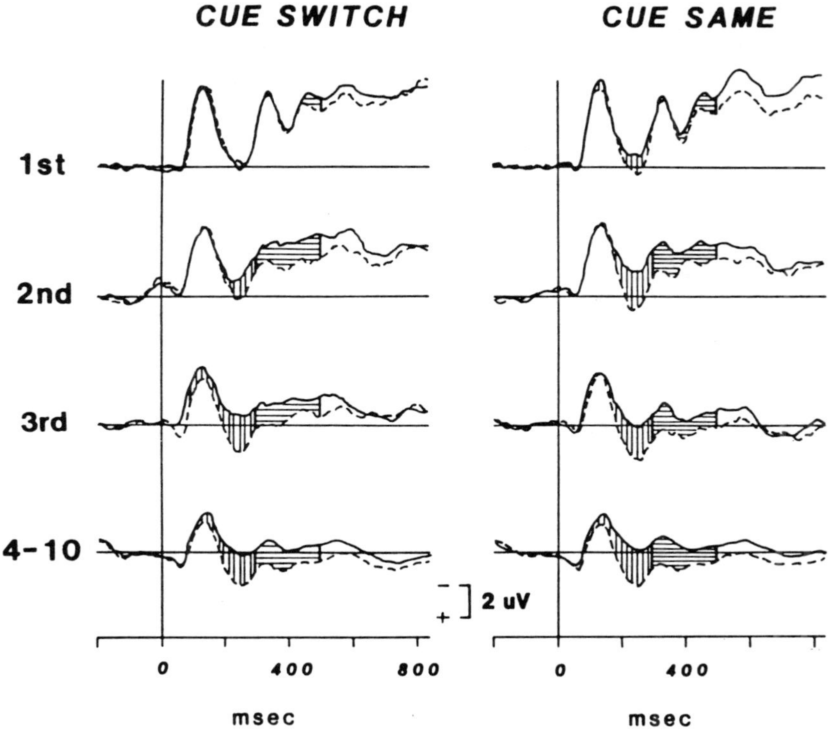

FIG. 6.31 Grand-average frontal (Fz) ERPs elicited by short-duration (standard) binaural tone stimuli at successive ordinal positions in the cued trains. The solid-line ERPs are to attended tones and the dashed lines to unattended tones. The vertical and horizontal shadings demarcate the latency windows of the early (100–300 msec) and late Nd (300–500 msec) measures, respectively. ERPs in the left column are from trains in which the cue directed attention to the tones opposite in frequency to that of the previous train (cue-switch); those in the right column are from trains for which the attended frequency was the same as the previous train (cue-same). (From Hansen & Hillyard, 1988. Copyright © 1988 The Society for Psychophysiological Research. Reprinted with permission.)

irrelevant stimuli rather than to a PN enhancement for relevant stimuli. Concurrently, the attentional focus got sharper, as suggested by a parallel decrease of RT and P3 latency to targets as well as increase in detection accuracy.

One can also try to interpret PN by varying the further processing required. If PN reflects this further processing, as suggested by Hansen and Hillyard (1980), Okita (1979, 1981), and Näätänen and Michie (1979a), then one could expect a larger PN for a more difficult further processing. Parasuraman (1980) varied the difficulty of discriminating targets from standards presented to a designated ear. Hardly any effect on the Nd amplitude was found, although the discrimination performance (d') was affected (see Näätänen, 1982).

In another study using a dichotic paradigm, Maiste and Picton (1987), as already mentioned, found that the early PN component was not affected but that the later, frontal component was enhanced by increased difficulty of "within-channel" target discrimination. This result consequently suggests that it is the late, rather than the early, component that reflects further processing. As already proposed, the enhancement of the late component with increased task difficulty might also be due to a stronger arousal response caused by task-relevant stimuli.

In addition, Alho, Lavikainen, et al. (1990), presenting sequences of three equiprobable binaural stimuli differing in frequency, compared Nd when further processing was and was not required. Further processing involved discriminating deviant stimuli of a slightly longer duration among stimuli of a designated frequency. When no further processing was required, the subject only counted all relevant stimuli. As shown in Fig. 6.32, the early Nd was quite similar when further processing was and was not required.

In conclusion, the previously reviewed studies indicate that the early PN component reflects initial selection. Further processing seems to affect PN,

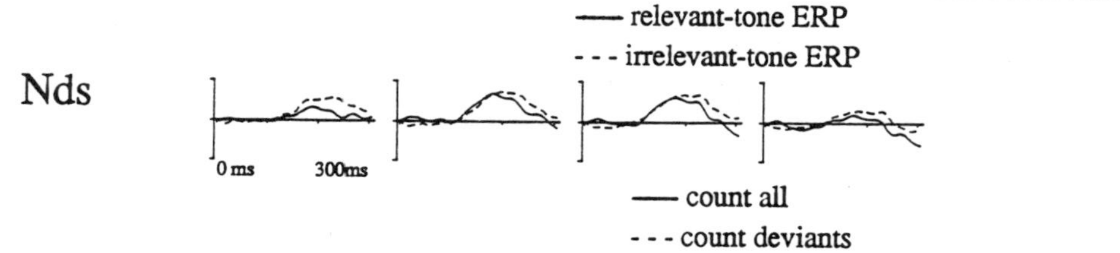

FIG. 6.32 Frontal-pole (Fpz), frontal (Fz), vertex (Cz), and parietal (Pz) grand-average ERPs to relevant (solid lines) and irrelevant (dashed lines) tones and the corresponding Nds (relevant-tone ERP *minus* irrelevant-tone ERP; bottom) when subjects counted all relevant tones (top row) and when they counted deviant tones among all relevant tones (second row). Blocks of 3 equiprobable binaural tones of different frequencies (423, 500, and 590 Hz) were delivered of which one of the extreme tones at a time was designated relevant. (From Alho, Lavikainen, Reinikainen, Sams, & Näätänen, 1990. Copyright © 1990 The Society for Psychophysiological Research. Reprinted with permission.)

at least under some conditions, but the PN component affected is probably the later, frontal one. The early component appears to be fully accounted for by initial selection, being an on-line reflection of this selection process itself.

Studies Testing the Attentional-Trace Theory: Features Represented. On this theory, only the stimulus features that separate relevant and irrelevant stimuli are rehearsed, that is, enter the attentional trace (Näätänen, 1982). There would be no sense in rehearsing a stimulus feature in which the two stimulus classes do not differ. To study this prediction, Alho et al. (1989) presented relevant and irrelevant stimuli differing in pitch either monaurally to a given ear ("constant location") or randomly to either ear ("random location"). It was hypothesized that if stimulus location is represented in the attentional trace even though selection occurs on the basis of the pitch, then Nd should be larger with constant location because of a better correspondence, on average, between a stimulus of the designated pitch and the attentional trace for with random locations a good deal of these stimuli would, obviously, result in a partial match only. On the other hand, if the subject in those conditions tries to maintain both locations in the attentional trace, that is, to divide attention between them, this should also result in an attenuated Nd, judging from the divided-attention results of the same study.

It was found that Nd was not affected by constant versus random location, which suggests, as already explained, that the spatial origin of the stimulus was not represented in the attentional trace. An analogous pattern of results was obtained when relevant and irrelevant stimuli presented to different ears were either constant or varied randomly in frequency (being either 1000 or 3000 Hz).

Studies Testing the Attentional Trace: Sensory-Specific Locus of Generation. The attentional trace was suggested to reside in auditory cortex, possibly in secondary auditory areas (Näätänen, 1982). A sensory-specific locus is consistent with the function attributed to the attentional trace: a rapid, accurate discrimination of different sounds even when they differ only very little from one another. ERP data suggesting early-PN generation in auditory cortex were already reviewed. Corroborating MEG data are reviewed in chapter 7.

The principal location of the attentional trace in auditory association rather than primary areas is supported by the only modestly, if at all, larger Nds over the hemisphere contralateral to the ear of entry of attended stimuli than those over the ipsilateral hemisphere (e.g., Maiste & Picton, 1987; Woods & Clayworth, 1987; see, however, Woldorff & Hillyard, 1991). Furthermore, association cortex shows considerably more attentional lability than primary cortex in animal single-unit recordings (for a review, see Woods, 1990). Although only a small number of neurons in primary auditory cortex show attentional lability (e.g., Hocherman, Benson, Goldstein, Heffner, & Hienz, 1976; Beaton & Miller, 1975), in association areas, both increases and decreases in neuronal firing rates frequently occur during conditioning (Diamond & Weinberger, 1984) and attention (Hocherman et al., 1976).

The attentional trace presumably involves an area in auditory cortex specific to the feature represented by this trace. Thus, its location may differ as a function of whether stimuli are selected, for example, on the basis of pitch or spatial position. This is supported by Woods, Alho, and Algazi's (1991) aforementioned results (Fig. 6.22). These authors presented tone pips varying randomly in pitch (250, 1,000, or 4,000 Hz) and ear of delivery. Subjects attended to a designated pitch/ear combination (P + L +) in order to discriminate occasional shorter-duration targets among these stimuli. It was found that, in addition to a large, long-duration Nd to P + L + stimuli, stimuli sharing only pitch (P + L −) or location (P − L +) with attended stimuli also elicited some early Nd. Interestingly, the "pitch-specific" early Nd, that elicited by P + L − stimuli, was more frontally and symmetrically distributed than the "location-specific" early Nd (P − L + stimuli). This finding suggests that attention to pitch modulates different cortical areas than attention to location.

Consequently, in the case of a two-dimensional attentional trace, (that is, relevant stimuli are defined by two features), the trace is probably distributed to two loci in auditory cortex, one for each feature. This is also consistent with Nd additivity when relevant stimuli are defined by both their pitch and spatial locus of origin compared with when they are defined only by their pitch or locus (Alho et al., 1989).

Very recently, Alho, Niittyvuopio, Paavilainen, Summala, and Näätänen (1992) found that in early-blinded subjects, the Nd topography in selecting stimuli on the basis of the ear of entry is posterior to that in normals. This suggests that auditory functions may "occupy" posterior neuronal populations that normally are in the service of visual functions. These data are illustrated in Fig. 6.33. For analogous ERP evidence for neural plasticity in deaf individuals, see Neville and Lawson (1987a, 1987b).

The present inferences about the attentional trace have so far been only indirect, that is, based on responses elicited during selective attention which seem to reflect an interaction between current sensory information and rehearsed sensory information. On the other hand, the rCBF might more directly indicate the selective sensory state resulting in the generation of differential responses to attended and unattended stimuli (chapter 3). These studies are reviewed in chapter 8.

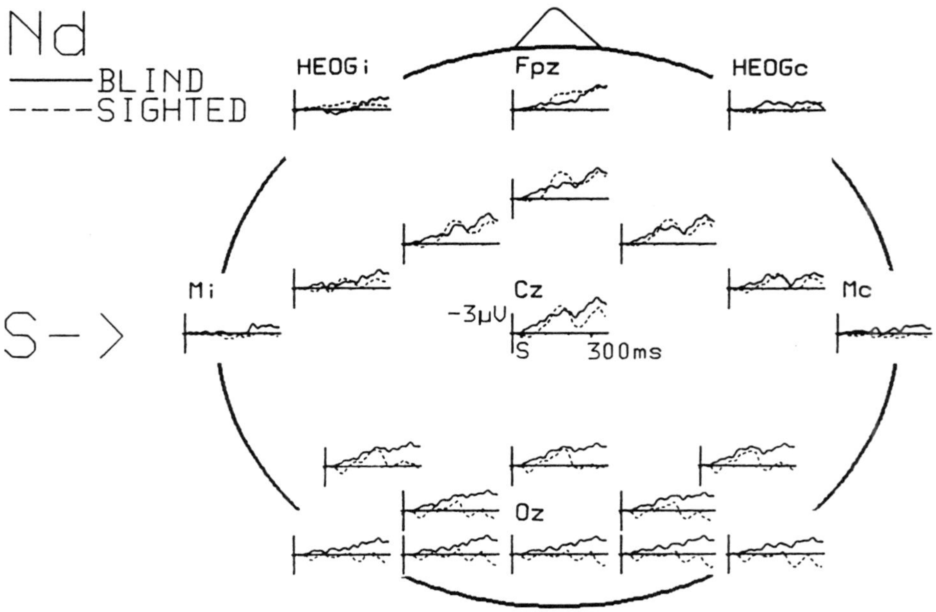

FIG. 6.33 Grand-average Nds obtained by subtracting the ERP to unattended standard stimuli from the ERP to attended standard stimuli at different electrode positions separately for early blind (solid lines) and sighted (dotted lines) young adults. In different blocks, the subject was instructed to attend either to the left- or right-ear stimuli in order to detect occasional 630-Hz deviant tones among 600-Hz standard tones. Data averaged across the left- and right-ear stimuli. Nd waves for electrodes contralateral to the stimulated ear are shown on the right side of the head. (From Alho, Niittyvuopio, Paavilainen, Summala, & Näätänen, 1992).

Studies Testing the Attentional-Trace Theory: Sensory Memory as Its Informational Basis. The development of the attentional trace depends, according to the theory, on the availability of sensory data from the relevant stimulus to the selection mechanism (Näätänen, 1982). A rapid, precise selection process requires a precise representation of the stimulus to be selected (of the feature defining the relevant stimulus) at the moment of sensory input. The sensory information contained in the attentional trace is therefore most likely to originate from sensory memory (its activated part). This proposal generates the following predictions (Näätänen, 1990):

1. Nd cannot be elicited by the first relevant stimulus of the sequence, that is, before the (activated) sensory data corresponding to this stimulus exist in sensory memory.
2. Nd cannot occur with very long ISIs, those that exceed the span of the

activated sensory memory; furthermore, Nd (the early phase) should also be earlier and larger for shorter ISIs between the relevant stimuli.

3. When targets are infrequent changes embedded within frequent stimuli (relevant standards), there should be no Nd between ERPs to targets and relevant standards. The level of the attribute of targets separating them from relevant standards (e.g., a slightly higher pitch) is delivered at ISIs that are too long for this level to be represented in the attentional trace, if this trace is based on stimulus-activated sensory memory. On the other hand, if the target probability is considerably increased, then the target level of that attribute may be incorporated into the attentional trace, causing an Nd between ERPs to the target and the relevant standard. In this case, the attentional trace has become two-dimensional, that is, it has incorporated two stimulus attributes.

The first prediction is supported by Donald and Young's (1982) N1 effect (measured only at the N1 latency) that did not emerge in the very beginning of a session but instead needed some 30–45 sec to develop. Further support was provided by Hansen and Hillyard (1988). Their short stimulus sequences (on average about 6 sec), separated by silent 5-sec breaks, consisted of two equiprobable binaural tones differing in pitch. Before each sequence, the lower or higher tones were designated as task-relevant by introducing a discrimination task involving these stimuli. A long-duration Nd was obtained for all relevant stimuli except the one occurring in the first position of the sequence when this first stimulus differed in pitch from the relevant stimuli of the preceding sequence. However, when the attended pitch was the same as in the previous sequence, even the first relevant stimulus elicited Nd, though a small and delayed one (Fig. 6.31).

These results suggest that the attentional trace depends on recent sensory reinforcement, and that although the trace may persist several seconds with no reinforcement, it considerably decays within 5 seconds after the last relevant stimulus. (In addition, changing the attentional focus appears to require a post-instruction presentation of a new to-be-attended stimulus even in the presence of adequate sensory-memory data; Näätänen, 1990).

Further corroborating evidence was obtained by Woods (1990) (Fig. 6.34) and by Wagner et al. (in press), who found a considerably larger Nd when the preceding stimulus was relevant than when it was irrelevant (see also Hansen & Hillyard, 1988).

Unfortunately, as pointed out by Woldorff and Hillyard (1991), when stimuli are presented with very short ISIs, sequential ERP analyses conducted in order to test the sensory-memory hypothesis are problematized by strong refractoriness effects. These authors found that their Nd80 to a relevant stimulus was smaller when the preceding stimulus was also relevant than when it was irrelevant. In contrast, their Nd125 was larger when the

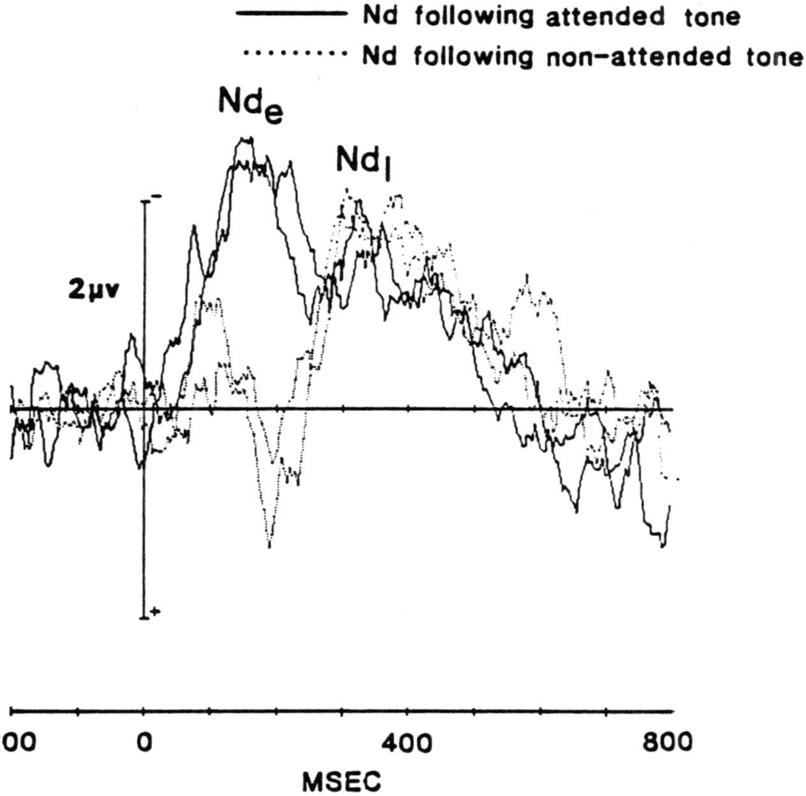

FIG. 6.34 Stimulus-sequence effects on the early (Nd$_e$) and late Nd (Nd$_l$) obtained by subtracting the unattended-tone ERP from the attended-tone ERP in a dichotic attention study. The tracings show grand-average vertex (Cz) Nds when the preceding tone was an attended tone (solid lines) and when the preceding tone was an unattended tone (dashed lines). The Nds were averaged over tone frequencies and ears. Traces are superimposed from the first and second halves of the experiment. (From Woods, 1990. Copyright © 1990 by Oxford University Press. Reprinted with permission.)

preceding stimulus was relevant, and, further, this effect was stronger for shorter (120–220 msec) than for longer (220–320 msec) ISIs between the two stimuli.

In general, these sequential analyses support the dependence of the attentional trace on sensory memory, its activated phase. On the other hand, Okita (1987) regarded his results as contradicting this assumption, but they need not be so interpreted (see Näätänen, 1990).

The second prediction involved the ISI–Nd relationship: The early Nd phase should be earlier and larger for shorter ISIs between relevant stimuli. Consistently with this, as already mentioned, Parasuraman (1980) and

Hansen and Hillyard (1984) found that the Nd onset and peak latencies were considerably shorter for shorter than for longer mean ISIs (Fig. 6.16). On the other hand, the early-Nd amplitude was not affected.

With long ISIs, no Nd, or only a small and delayed one, is predicted by the theory. Consistently with this, Hansen and Hillyard (1988) obtained only a very small and delayed Nd to a relevant stimulus after a period of 5–6 sec with no relevant stimuli (Fig. 6.31). Moreover, McCallum et al. (1983) found only a very small Nd in their free-field study in which a relevant stimulus was presented every 23.4 seconds on average. This interval appears to exceed the time span of sensory memory—at least, its activated phase (see Cowan, 1984), but the Nd observed was possibly elicited only when a relevant stimulus followed the previous relevant stimulus at a much shorter than average interval (Näätänen, 1990).

Alho, Lavikainen, et al.'s (1990) study on the effect of the relevant-stimulus probability on Nd was reviewed earlier. Their mean ISI between consecutive relevant stimuli was in different conditions either 1.5, 3.1, or 15.3 sec. As shown in Fig. 6.18, Nd was greatly attenuated when the mean ISI between the relevant stimuli was prolonged.

Hansen and Hillyard (1984) wished to clarify why the Nd onset is delayed when the ISI is increased (Fig. 6.16). They considered two possibilities, already proposed by Schwent, Hillyard, and Galambos (1976). According to the "memory hypothesis," memory for the physical features of relevant stimuli fades with long ISIs, whereas on the "load hypothesis," Nd is then delayed because of the diminished processing load.

To decide between these two hypotheses, Hansen and Hillyard (1984) delivered "pedestal" stimuli: brief intensity increments of continuous tones originating from the "relevant" and "irrelevant" loudspeakers. In this way, they provided continuous reinforcement of the pitch and location attributes of the relevant (and irrelevant) stimuli.

Nevertheless, the prolongation of the mean ISI caused an Nd delay similar to that found when no pedestals were used. The authors therefore proposed that the Nd was delayed with longer mean ISIs because of decreased processing load, regarding this result as inconsistent with the attentional-trace theory. They remarked, however, that subjects perhaps "failed to utilize the continuous cues provided by the pedestal stimuli because they faded into a steady and monotonous 'background' " (Hansen & Hillyard, 1984, p. 403).

Another possibility is that because of the strong time uncertainty with long, irregular ISIs (Karlin, 1959; Klemmer, 1956; Niemi & Näätänen, 1981), subjects were not willing or able, despite the availability of the requisite sensory information, to maintain the attentional trace the way they could when they have the same amount of sensory information but are under much less time uncertainty (Näätänen, 1990). The ISI of the long-ISI condition varied irregularly from 1.25 to 2.75 sec, and that between consecutive relevant stimuli, of course, varied considerably more.

Hansen and Hillyard's (1988) later results in turn supported the attentional-trace theory in showing that Nd is not elicited in the beginning of a stimulus sequence, thus depending, apparently, on sensory reinforcement of relevant stimuli.

The third of the aforementioned predictions was that the target level of a stimulus attribute can be represented by the attentional trace only if this level is presented frequently enough. Typically, the subject is listening, say, to left-ear stimuli in order to discriminate occasional pitch deviants among them. In accordance with the prediction, when ERPs to occasional deviant (target) and standard stimuli are compared, no Nd is obtained (Hink, Fenton, et al., 1978; Hink, Hillyard, & Benson, 1978; Maiste & Picton, 1987; Alho et al., 1989). Consistently with this, very little or no Nd is observed under active oddball conditions when ERPs to low-probability targets are compared with those to standards (see Näätänen et al., 1983; Sams, Paavilainen, et al., 1985).

Complementarily, the theory also predicts that if the probability of the target-level attribute is increased up to a certain limit, then this level can also be incorporated into the attentional trace which then becomes two-dimensional. This prediction is supported by Hansen and Hillyard's (1983) previously reviewed study with four equiprobable stimuli: left high-pitch, left low-pitch, right high-pitch, right low-pitch tones, the subject's task being to discriminate occasional increases in the duration of the designated tones. In accordance with the prediction, the designated tones elicited ERPs with separate Nds for both spatial and pitch attributes.

Corroborating data were provided by Alho et al. (1989; see also Michie, Bearpark, et al., 1990), who found Nd additivity when relevant stimuli were defined by both their pitch and ear of origin.

Finally, if MMN provides a measure, though an indirect one, of (the activated phase of) sensory memory, then it is possible to test whether this memory is involved in attentional selection by comparing MMN and PN, which are assumed to be measures of sensory memory and of the use of this memory in selective attention, respectively (Näätänen, 1990):

1. Both MMN (a substantial part of it) and the early PN are negativities generated in auditory cortex.
2. Both MMN and PN indicate that fine-grained, precise sensory information is represented by the generator mechanisms involved.
3. The decay of this sensory information in the absence of the corresponding stimulus might occur in both systems at roughly the same rate.
4. Both sensory-memory (as judged from MMN data) and selective-attention (as judged from the Nd emergence in the beginning of the session) systems need a few stimulus repetitions before they can function optimally.

These similarities suggest that stimulus selection based on sensory stimulus features uses sensory memory (its activated phase). Sensory data contained by the neural traces underlying MMN generation make, on the present hypothesis, the attentional trace possible. There are, however, several fundamental differences between the two stimulus representations postulated:

1. The attentional trace depends strictly on voluntary choice and allocation of effort, that is, voluntary attention, whereas the sensory-memory trace involved in MMN generation is automatically formed by auditory stimuli.

2. The attentional trace involves consciousness; it is produced and maintained by "focusing the mind" on certain critical stimulus feature(s), whereas information stored by the trace of MMN generation is preconscious (but reaches consciousness if attention is directed to it).

3. The neural traces underlying MMN encode all auditory stimulus features, irrespective of their relevance to the task to be performed, whereas the attentional trace only encodes task-relevant features, that is, those defining relevant stimuli (Alho et al., 1989).

4. Apparently, only one attentional trace (though it may be distributed to different feature-specific analysing mechanisms) can exist at any given moment, whereas there can be two concurrent passive neuronal models, probably even more (which may also be distributed to different feature-specific mechanisms). Hence, the attentional trace is a "single-channel" concept, belonging to the realm of controlled processing (chapter 2), whereas the trace involved in MMN generation is a result of parallel automatic processing.

5. The trace of MMN generation is associated with sensory memory (Cowan et al., 1991), whereas the attentional trace, according to Näätänen (1982, 1987), is instead a working-memory construct (Baddeley, 1986; see also Broadbent, 1984).

6. The attentional trace is controlled by frontal activity (see later; see also the rCBF literature reviewed in chapter 8), whereas the MMN mechanism of auditory cortex is not, and might, on the contrary, control some frontal activity (chapter 4).

7. The trace of MMN elicitation is involved in a response that measures the difference between the eliciting stimulus and the one represented by the trace, whereas the mechanism using the attentional trace responds best to a stimulus similar to the one represented. These opposing processing modes can be characterized as the difference and similarity modes of processing, respectively.

8. This is, in turn, related to the opposite probability dependencies of MMN and PN: A probability decrease enhances the MMN amplitude (Section 4.4) while attenuating the PN amplitude (Alho, Lavikainen, et al., 1990; Berman et al., 1989).

9. Consistently with this, a stimulus can elicit a concurrent MMN and PN, there even being no amplitude reduction of these components due to

temporal overlap (e.g., Alho et al., 1989). This indicates that the generator mechanisms of the two components are, at least in part, functionally separate.

10. This separability is further supported by the differential sensitivity of MMN and PN to various drugs (Born, Bothor, et al., 1987; Born, Brüninger, et al., 1987; Born, Fehm-Wolfsdorf, et al., 1986; Born, Kern, et al., 1987; Born, Kern, et al., 1989; Pietrowsky et al., 1990).

In sum, the evidence just reviewed supports the assumption that sensory memory (its active phase, apparently a prerequisite for MMN elicitation; see Cowan et al., 1991) is essential for the attentional trace. The sensory-specific stimulus-selection mechanism postulated, the attentional trace, is apparently set up by using sensory information stored by the neural traces of the sensory-memory system.

Studies Testing the Attentional-Trace Theory: Frontal-Lobe Control of the Attentional Trace. The theory proposes that the sensory-specific attentional trace is maintained and controlled by a frontal-lobe mechanism. In the foregoing, data indicating a later, frontal or frontocentral PN component were reviewed. This component might reflect the aforementioned, well-established involvement of frontal lobes in selective attention. Reduced Nd amplitudes in frontal-lobe patients suggest an involvement in particular of the right prefrontal cortex in selective attention (for a review, see Knight, 1990). Okita et al.'s (1983) larger frontal Nd over the right than the left frontal cortex also suggest right-hemisphere frontal dominance in control of attention.

The data from frontal-lobe patients do not indicate (though do not rule out; Knight, 1990) that a PN component is generated in frontal cortex, however (Knight, 1990; Knight et al., 1981; see also Woods & Knight, 1986). According to Knight et al. (1981), the frontal lobes might instead exercise a modulating influence on the mechanism of the attentional negativity located elsewhere. Giard et al.'s (1988) scalp-current density analysis, however, suggests a deep source in the frontal lobes for the late PN component.

The rCBF data, to be reviewed in chapter 8, further support the proposal that frontal lobes maintain and control the attentional trace.

It is, however, also possible, as already mentioned, that the frontal PN component is mainly associated with an orienting or arousal response (Näätänen & Michie, 1979a; Näätänen, 1987).

6.3. SELECTIVE ATTENTION AND VISUAL ERPS

In chapter 2, behavioral research and theory of visual selective attention was reviewed. In the present section, ERP studies of selective attention in vision are examined. These studies have provided new, important information about the nature, timing, and locus of selective processes in vision. Also, the special status of the spatial position of the stimulus as a selection cue (for a review, see Johnston & Dark, 1986), discussed in chapter 2, has shown up in a particularly striking manner in these studies. This primary status of spatial location is testified by the fact that the associated ERP signature of selection by location is an enhancement of exogenous components, an effect not produced by any other type of stimulus selection (e.g., selection on the basis of color). This section begins with ERP findings associated with visual-spatial attention; thereafter, ERP signs of selective processing in vision based on other stimulus attributes are also examined.

ERPs and Visual-Spatial Attention

The predominant finding in these studies, which is examined hereafter, is that all stimuli presented to the attended location in the visual field elicit enhanced exogenous P1 and N1 components. If attention indeed enhances these exogenous components, rather than produces endogenous components (the processing negativity), then gain-theory types of attention theories (see Näätänen, 1986e; Mangun & Hillyard, 1988, 1990a) would be supported. These theories suggest that selective-attention effects occur as early as in processes preceding the development of initial stimulus representations; therefore, these representations could, on this type of theory, be modulated by attention.

If the exogenous P1 and N1 components in the ERP to an attended visual stimulus are indeed enhanced, then the question arises as to whether attention effects, in the chain of processes elicited by a visual stimulus, first occur in the generator processes of these components or in some, still earlier processes. In the latter case, the P1 and N1 effects would result, at least in part, from attentionally modulated afferent input to the P1 and N1 generators (see Eason, Harter, & White, 1969; Skinner & Yingling, 1977; Mangun & Hillyard, 1990a). Consequently, this section starts by examining studies on very early attention effects.

Eason, Oakley, and Flowers (1983) reported enhancing effects of spatial selective attention on electroretinogram (ERG) measures N20–P60, P60–N90, and P60–N120. On these grounds, the authors proposed that spatial attention in vision is mediated by efferent control of afferent pathways, which differentially modifies synaptic transmission at a precortical level extending as far down to the periphery as to the retina. Mangun, Hansen, and Hillyard, (1986), however, failed to replicate this effect, even though they used a more sensitive ERG measure than that of Eason and his colleagues. (Mangun et al., however, did not obtain the usual P1 effect of attention in their study.)

It appears that there is no firm electrophysiological evidence for an attentional modulation of subcortical visual processing in humans. On the other hand, the evidence for the attentional enhancement of the early exogenous P1 is very strong; therefore, the earliest ERP effect that has been reliably established in vision starts at about 70–90 msec from stimulus onset or somewhat later (Eason, 1981; Harter, Aine, & Schroeder, 1982; Harter, Anllo-Vento, & Wood, 1989; Harter, Millter, Price, LaLonde, & Keyes, 1989; Hillyard & Münte, 1984; Hillyard, Münte, & Neville, 1985; Hillyard, Simpson, Woods, Voorhis, & Münte, 1984; Mangun & Hillyard, 1987; Mangun, Hillyard, & Luck, in press; Neville & Lawson, 1987c; Rugg, Milner, Lines, & Phalp, 1987; Wijers, Lamain, Slopsema, Mulder, & Mulder, 1989; for a review, see Wijers, 1989).

Evidence for an attentional enhancement of the exogenous N1, at some 150–200 msec from stimulus onset, is strong, too (e.g., Eason et al., 1969; Hillyard & Münte, 1984; Hillyard, Münte, & Neville, 1985; Hillyard et al., 1984; Mangun & Hillyard, 1987, 1988, 1990a, 1990b; Mangun et al., 1986; Mangun, Hansen, & Hillyard, 1987; Mangun et al., in press; Neville & Lawson, 1987c; Rugg et al., 1987; Voorhis & Hillyard, 1977; for a review, see Wijers, 1989).

These P1 and N1 effects are illustrated by Mangun and Hillyard's (1990a) recent data, shown in Fig. 6.35. Their stimuli were bars flashed at a fast rate and in random order to locations either 5° to the left or right of a fixation cross that had to be visually fixated throughout the whole stimulus block lasting 1–2 min. The subject's task was to discriminate the height of the bars at one location, ignoring the flashes at the other, and to press a button upon detection of an occasional slightly shorter bar.

Figure 6.35 presents the response to a left flash. This response begins as a P1 wave over the contralateral occipital scalp with an onset latency of 80–100 msec. This P1 wave is considerably larger in amplitude when the stimulus is presented to the corresponding location in the opposite field. This effect occurs similarly for standards and deviants. (Some studies have, however, reported larger ipsi- than contralateral P1 responses; e.g., Rugg et al., 1987; Wijers, Lamain, et al., 1989.[3]) The N1 and N2 peaks are also enhanced in response to attended stimuli. In the words of Mangun and Hillyard (1990a):

> The effect of attention is manifest as an amplitude modulation of these peaks without any changes in their latencies, polarities or waveshapes. Such a result

[3]In a very recent study with split-brain patients (Mangun, Luck, Gazzaniga, & Hillyard, 1991), normal P1 and N1 waves were elicited by lateralized flash stimuli over contralateral occipital cortex but, in contrast to normal controls, were absent over the occipital cortex ipsilateral to the stimulated visual field. This result indicates that these early ERP components over the ipsilateral hemisphere in normal subjects are generated by callosally mediated activation of the ipsilateral hemisphere following the initial registration of the visual information in contralateral occipital cortex.

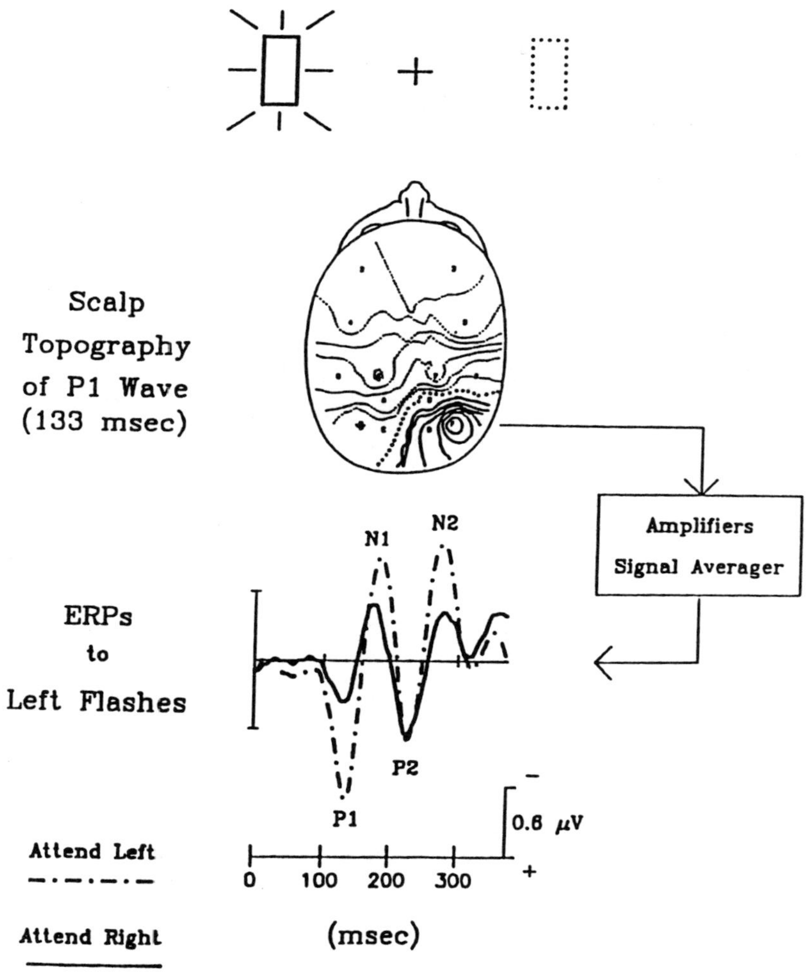

FIG. 6.35 Attention effects on the visual ERP in a typical spatial attention task. Stimuli (illustrated on top) were bars flashed on a video screen in random order to locations 5 degrees to the left or right of fixation (+) with short, irregular ISIs. The subject was instructed to attend to the bars at one location and to press a button upon detection of an occasional, slightly shorter bar (target) at this location. In the bottom, ERPs to left flashes when attended (dot-dash lines) and ignored (attend right; solid lines) are shown. (From Mangun & Hillyard, 1990a. Copyright © 1990 by Guilford Press. Reprinted with permission.)

is consistent with a mechanism of sensory gating, since it implies that the principal effect of attention on the neural generators of these sensory-evoked components is simply to increase or decrease their level of activation. These attention-related changes in activity are presumed to be the result of descending neural influences on either the inputs to the early ERP generators or the activity of the generators themselves. (p. 274)

The gain-increase type of explanation of the P1 effect was further supported by the scalp topography observed. This attention effect indeed seemed to manifest itself as an amplitude enhancement of the P1 generator process, its cerebral locus remaining the same.

Corresponding to the anatomical projection of the geniculostriate pathway to visual cortex, the P1 attention effect reached its maximum amplitude approximately over extrastriate visual cortex (Areas 18 and 19). The authors concluded that these data are in line with a radially oriented dipole generator located in extrastriate cortex. According to Mangun and Hillyard (1987, 1988, 1990a, 1990b), P1 has an amplitude maximum over ventrolateral prestriate cortex. Consistently with this, recent single-unit recordings in monkey visual cortex have demonstrated attention-sensitive neurons in the extrastriate area V4 (e.g., Moran & Desimone, 1985). Mangun and Hillyard (1990a) suggested that spatial attention involves a mechanism of sensory gain control operating at or before the level of extrastriate visual cortex.

On the other hand, Wijers, Lamain, et al.'s (1989) results are inconsistent with the interpretation of the early positive selective-attention effect on the visual ERP in terms of the exogenous P1 component. Their P1 amplitude was considerably larger as stimuli were delivered to higher positions in the visual field, whereas the amplitude of their P1 attention effect did not depend on the stimulus position.

In the foregoing, the P1 enhancement was interpreted as reflecting enhanced sensory input from a stimulus presented to an attended location. An alternative interpretation might be proposed, however. This is based on the fact that the attention effect on the P1 amplitude is observed in averaged data. This leaves open the possibility that the P1 component in single-trial responses actually is not enhanced but attention increases the degree of temporal synchronization of the individual responses to stimulus onset. Also, attention might sometimes synchronize a spontaneous rhythm such as the alpha rhythm which might then overlap the ERP. This might have happened for example in the data illustrated in Fig. 6.39 where one can see many consecutive waves with approximately the same frequency.

Mangun et al. (in press) propose that the P1 attention effect may represent "attentional control of processing along the 'ventral stream' of visual projections to the temporal lobe that carries out functions of feature analysis and object recognition." This is consistent with monkey data suggesting separate dorsal and ventral processing systems or "streams" that originate in primary visual (striate) cortex and appear to play different roles in visual perception (for a review, see Desimone & Ungerleider, 1989). The dorsal processing stream, which projects through prestriate areas V2 and MT to the posterior parietal lobe, is likely to have an important role in encoding the spatial aspects of visual inputs and in guiding visuomotor performance. The ventral stream, relaying through the prestriate areas V2,

V3, and V4, seems to convey information about stimulus form, color, and pattern to the inferior temporal lobe. Single-unit recordings from these areas of occipital cortex have shown that spatial attention strongly affects visual-evoked activity in both dorsal (posterior parietal lobe) and ventral streams (prestriate area V4 and inferior temporal lobe) but not in prestriate area V2 or in the striate cortex itself (Desimone & Ungerleider, 1989; Mangun et al., in press; Wurtz, Goldberg, & Robinson, 1980).

The generators of the attention-sensitive P1 and N1 components were localized with an improved accuracy over previous studies by Mangun et al. (in press). In this study, rectangular bars were presented at a rapid rate in random order to all four quadrants of the visual field in order to activate discrete zones of the primary visual cortex while the gaze was fixed on a central cross. The subject was instructed to attend exclusively to one of the four locations at the time and to press a button when an occasional, shorter bar occurred at that location.

It was found, in keeping with previous studies, that attending to a given location enhanced the P1, N1, and N2 amplitudes of ERPs elicited by stimuli (both standards and targets) presented to this location. The P1 amplitude was again largest over the occipital area contralateral to the visual field of stimulus presentation. Current-source density (CSD) maps for the P1 component revealed a focus over the contralateral occipital scalp, with a maximum located about 5 cm lateral to the mid-sagittal plane (Fig. 6.36). Importantly, this focus for a given stimulus remained in the same location irrespective of whether this stimulus was or was not attended. This supports the "sensory-gain" hypothesis (Harter & Aine, 1984; Mangun & Hillyard, 1988, 1990a) of spatial attention, suggesting that this form of attention modulates the magnitude of sensory-evoked activity in the visual pathways without engaging additional neural generators, at least in the latency range of the P1 wave (Mangun et al., in press).

The current-density focus for the P1 attention effect was "highly similar" in location irrespective of whether the stimulus occurred in the upper versus lower quadrant of the visual field. This contradicts the hypothesis that the P1 attention effect might originate in striate cortex, because the CSD distribution and/or polarity would change in this case, due to the opposed orientation of the cortical gyri representing the upper and lower visual fields (Regan, 1988). Mangun et al. (in press) concluded that these invariant and sharply localized CSD distributions instead suggest a generator in lateral prestriate cortex, directly underlying the maximum scalp focus.

The authors also related their scalp-CSD distributions to the underlying cortical anatomy revealed by the subjects' magnetic-resonance imaging (MRI) scans. Figure 6.37 shows the relative locations of the CSD foci for the P1 and N1 attention effects for the left hemisphere. It can be seen that the P1 focus was located ventrolaterally to the N1 focus, which appeared to lie approximately over the border of the occipital and posterior parietal

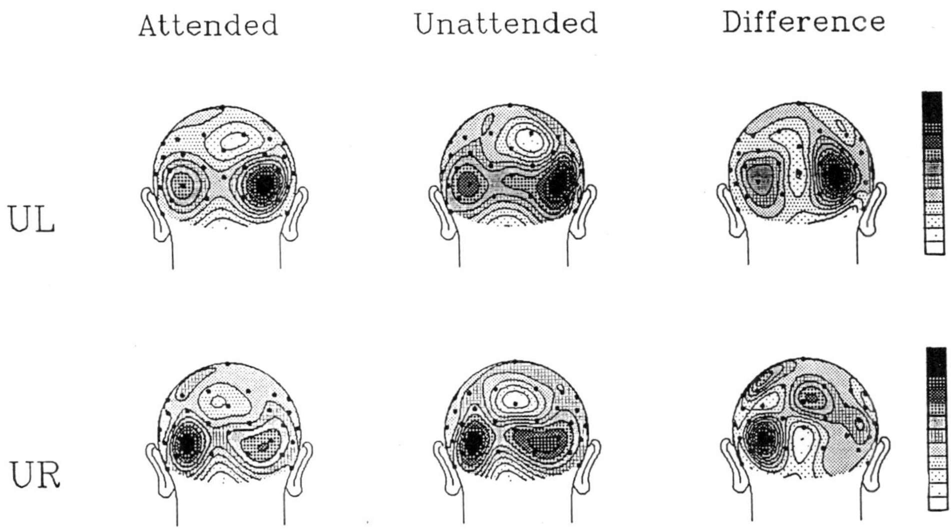

FIG. 6.36 Grand-averaged current-source densities (CSD) for the P1 wave (at 108 msec) in response to upper left-(UL) and upper right-hemifield (UR) stimuli when attended and when unattended. Stimuli occurred equiprobably in the four quadrants, the subject attending to one of these positions. The right column shows the CSD distribution of the attention-related P1 difference map (attended-stimulus ERP – unattended-stimulus ERP). Darker zones represent increasing magnitude of current source. Lightest zones represent current sinks (negativity). (From Mangun, Hillyard, & Luck, in press. Copyright © in press by Lawrence Erlbaum Associates.)

lobes. These locations support Mangun and Hillyard's (1990a) assumption that the P1 attention effect is caused by modulation of sensory flow in the ventral, prestriate visual processing stream, whereas the N1 attention effect reflects attentional control over the dorsal projection to the parietal lobe (Harter & Aine, 1984). In line with this proposal, as Mangun and Hillyard (1990a) pointed out, the P1 attention effect commences at a latency that corresponds to the average latency (about 70–80 msec) of evoked unit discharge in the monkey prestriate area V4 (e.g., Robinson & Rugg, 1988).

Mangun et al. (in press) derived further support for the suggestion that the P1 and N1 attentional enhancements are related to separate attentional systems from the fact that these enhancements may be dissociated under certain conditions. These dissociations seem also to indicate that the P1 and N1 attention effects do not simply arise from the modulation of a common input source at an earlier level.

Neville and Lawson (1987c) compared ERP effects of attending to central versus peripheral locations of the visual field. The target was an occasional apparent movement in the attended stimulus produced by an immediate second flash in an adjacent location to that of the first flash. When attention was directed to central stimuli, the attentional N1 enhancement

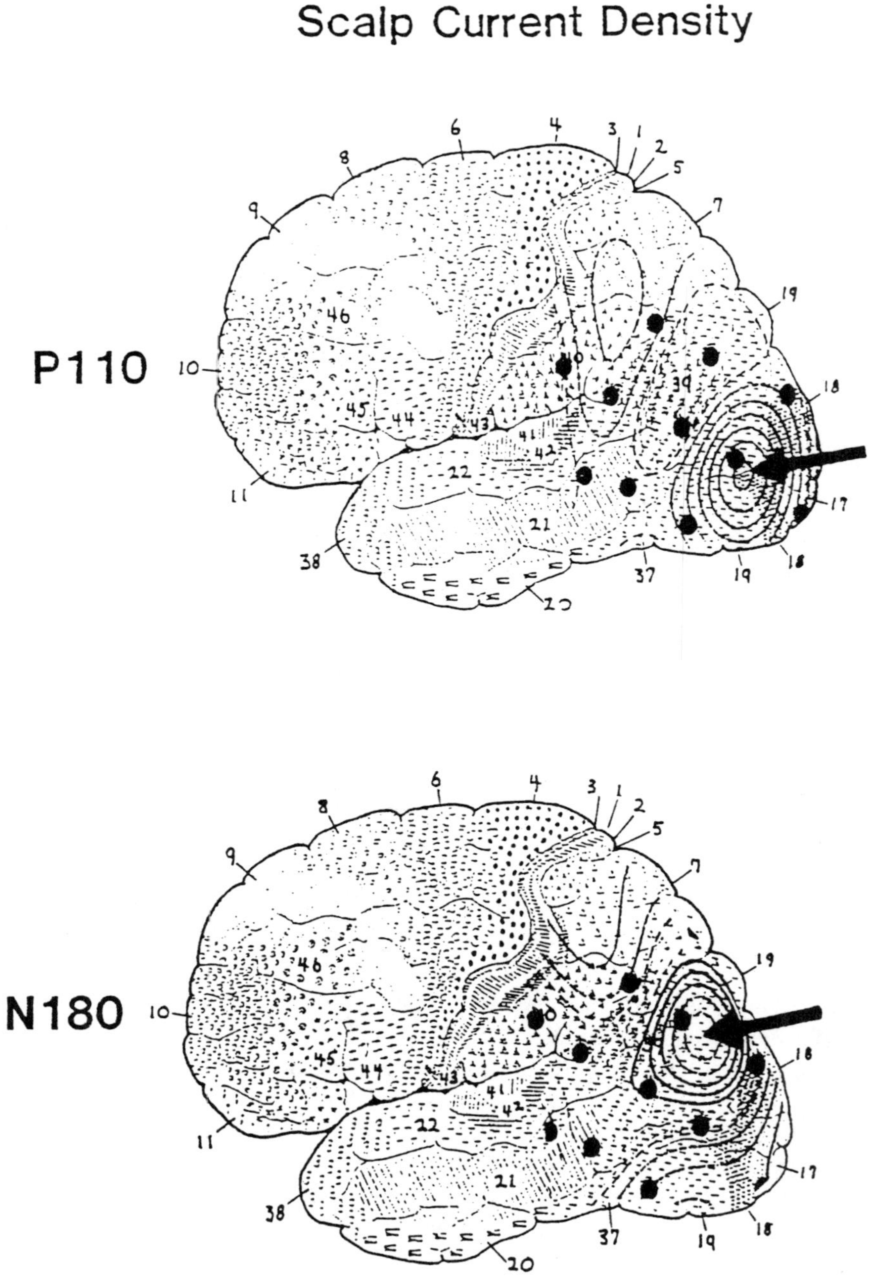

FIG. 6.37 Grand-average current-source density (CSD) contours for P1 (P110) and N1 (N180) attention effects to upper right-hemifield stimuli superimposed upon a left-hemisphere cytoarchitectonic map in the study whose results are shown in Fig. 6.36. The CSD-sink maximum for the N1 attention effect is located dorsally to the CSD source for the P1 effect. (From Mangun, Hillyard, & Luck, in press. Copyright © in press by Lawrence Erlbaum Associates.)

was most pronounced over the occipital regions and was of equal magnitude over the two hemispheres. In contrast, when peripheral stimuli were attended, the major N1-amplitude increase occurred over the temporoparietal area contralateral to the stimulus.

The authors therefore suggested that attention to central and peripheral stimuli is associated with modulation of activity in different neural pathways. Furthermore, they regarded their results as "compatible with the hypothesis that attention to the center of the visual field modulates activity in the retinogeniculate pathway that projects to striate cortex while attention to the visual periphery is associated with activity in the visual pathway that includes projections to parietal cortex of the contralateral hemisphere" (Neville & Lawson, 1987c, p. 263).

The attention effects for the peripheral stimuli observed by the authors were larger in the temporo-parietal regions of the right hemisphere than the left. These asymmetries, together with the behavioral data indicating that detection of the direction of motion tended to be more accurate for targets in the left than the right visual field, suggested to the authors that the right hemisphere played a greater role than the left in their task. In addition, these data are, according to them, consistent with reports of differential effects of left- and right-hemispheric lesions, suggesting that the right parietal areas contribute more to attentional processes than do the homologous areas of the left hemisphere (Heilman & van den Abell, 1980; Mesulam, 1981, 1983; see also Mountcastle, 1978; Yin & Mountcastle, 1977).

Neville and Lawson (1987c) also found that the N1 attention effect to the moving (target) stimuli was 2–3 times in amplitude that for the stationary (standard) stimuli in the visual periphery, whereas for central stimuli, this was only observed at a reduced level and as limited to the parietal region. This suggests a special sensitivity of the visual system to peripheral movement discussed in Section 2.2.

Slow Negativity Associated with Spatial Attention in Vision. The enhancement of the exogenous components P1 and N1 is not, however, the only ERP signature of attention to a certain locus or region of the visual field: In some studies a slow, PN type of negativity is also elicited by stimuli at the attended location. For instance, Harter et al. (1982) found such a slow negativity (though they seemed to have obtained a P1 enhancement also) when the stimulus was presented to the attended hemifield. The early part of this negativity, prominent between about 125 msec to 300 msec from stimulus onset, was greater over the hemisphere contralateral to the attended visual field in the occipital (but not central) area.

Slow negative shifts in association with visual-spatial attention have also been observed by Czigler (1983), Eason (1981), Eason et al. (1983), Hillyard and Münte (1984), Rugg et al. (1987), Wijers, Lamain, et al. (1989), and Scheffers, Wijers, and Mulder (submitted). In some studies, the exogenous enhancements were observed posteriorly, whereas the anterior effects appeared as slow negativities (Mangun & Hillyard, 1987; Rugg et al., 1987). Okita, Wijers, Mulder, and Mulder (1985) found a late, slow frontocentral negativity when two relevant stimuli were diagonally presented in the same display of four, quite closely spaced letters arranged in a form of a square. Even slow positivities have been observed: anterior ones by Hillyard and Münte (1984) and occipital ones by Neville and Lawson (1987c).

Whether the spatial attention effect occurs as an enhancement of exogenous components or as a slow negativity seems to depend, among other things, on the magnitude of spatial separation between the relevant and irrelevant stimulus locations in the visual field. Hillyard and Münte (1984) found an exogenous type of an effect when this separation was large but a slow anterior negativity with quite a late onset (at about 200–225 msec) when that separation was small.

ERP Effects in Trial-By-Trial Cued (Selective-Set) Attention Tasks. The vast majority of behavioral studies of spatial attention have employed a trial-by-trial cueing or priming procedure (the selective-set paradigm; see chapter 2), in which a prior cue indicates the most likely location where relevant stimulus is about to occur (e.g., Posner, 1980; Eriksen & Yeh, 1985). As already reviewed, stimuli presented to the precued (attended) locations are detected and discriminated with higher speed and/or accuracy than are stimuli occurring at unattended locations (chapter 2). These behavioral effects have been attributed to improved sensory/perceptual processing of attended-location stimuli by some authors (e.g., Posner, 1980) and to such post-perceptual factors as decision bias by others (e.g., Shaw, 1984).

According to Mangun and Hillyard (1990a), if the early, modality-specific ERP components were modulated by spatial cueing, this would support an attention effect at the sensory/perceptual level. In their initial study of spatial cueing, Hillyard et al. (1985) observed no significant changes in the P1 component, but this probably resulted from the long (1.8 sec) interval between the cue and the stimulus presented at the cued location. In more recent studies with shorter intervals (Harter & Anllo-Vento, 1991; Harter, Millter, et al., 1989; Mangun, Hillyard, & Luck, in press; Mangun et al., 1987; Mangun & Hillyard, 1990a), stimuli presented at precued locations have indeed elicited ERPs with considerably enhanced P1 amplitudes (Mangun & Hillyard, 1990a).

The effect of spatial cueing on the P1 amplitude in a simple RT-paradigm is illustrated in Fig. 6.38 (Mangun & Hillyard, 1990a). An initial arrow cue presented at the fixation point indicated the most likely ($p = 0.75$) visual field (right or left) of a subsequent stimulus to which the subject was to

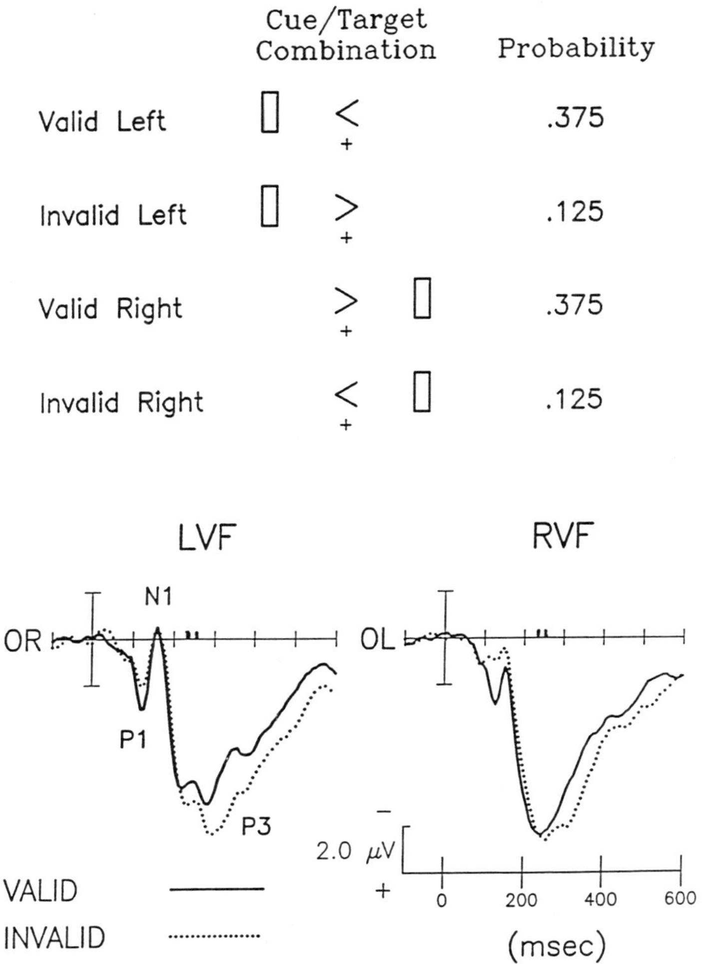

FIG. 6.38 Grand-average ERPs from the occipital scalp contralateral to the side of stimulation in an RT task in which a prior cue indicated the most likely location (left or right of the fixation point) of the stimulus (target) to be presented next. Subjects were instructed to make a simple RT response to both validly ($p = 0.75$) and invalidly ($p = 0.25$) cued stimuli. ERPs were averaged separately for valid and invalid stimuli in left (LVF) and right (RVF) visual fields. Lateral eye movements were monitored by a high-gain EOG to ensure that subjects did not deviate their eyes toward the cued location. (From Mangun, Hillyard, & Luck, in press. Copyright © in press by Lawrence Erlbaum Associates.)

respond by a rapid button press irrespective of whether the stimulus occurred on the cued (valid) or uncued (invalid) field. It was found that validly cued stimuli were responded to faster and elicited larger P1 waves than invalidly cued stimuli. In contrast, the validity of precuing did not affect the N1 amplitude.

The P1 amplitude to valid flashes, those presented to the cued visual field, was similarly enhanced and the RT to these stimuli speeded in Mangun and Hillyard's (1987, 1990a) choice-RT task in which subjects responded according to the height of the target bar, pressing with the right hand to tall bars and with the left hand to short bars. The P1 attention effect was maximal over the same lateral occipital scalp sites as in the sustained-attention tasks reviewed previously. Unlike in the simple-RT task, the N1 amplitudes were also enhanced to validly cued flashes.

Mangun et al. (in press) concluded that the enhanced P1 component to validly cued targets over the occipital cortex consistently observed in these studies indicates that advance cueing of target location facilitates sensory processing rather than merely biases subsequent decision processes. This parallels recent results according to which symbolic pre-cues, such as arrows, can improve the detectability of near-threshold-luminance targets at cued peripheral locations (Mangun et al., in press), an effect that is difficult to account for in terms of changes in decision bias (see Downing, 1988).

ERP Indicators of Pre-Stimulus Directing of Spatial Attention in Vision. Harter and colleagues, using a similar design to the one just described, have also observed enhanced P1/N1 amplitudes to targets occurring at cued locations (Harter & Anllo-Vento, 1990; Harter & Anllo-Vento, 1991; Harter, Anllo-Vento, & Wood, 1989; Harter, Millter, et al., 1989). Harter, Millter, et al. (1989) presented a central arrow cue that was followed by a target appearing equiprobably in the left or right visual field. The subjects, children of 6–9 years, were required to give a rapid finger-lift response to targets in the cued field and not to respond to targets in the uncued field. The enlarged P1-N1 amplitudes (measured peak-to-peak) obtained were again largest over the occipital scalp contralateral to the attended field.

Interestingly, the authors also found slow parietal-occipital negativities contralateral to the attended field (predominant over the right hemisphere) within the cue-target interval (600 msec), interpreted as signs of executive processes associated with the directing of attention (Näätänen & Picton, 1987). This contralateral potential commenced at about 200 msec from arrow onset and was larger over the right than left hemisphere. This right-hemisphere preponderance was initially strongest over the occipital area and then shifted to the central and parietal regions.

The ERP effect associated with directing visual-spatial attention was reversed in polarity at about 400 msec, that is, 200 msec prior to stimulus presentation. Now the contralateral posterior hemisphere became positive and the ipsilateral negative. The occipital-parietal positivity reached its amplitude maximum, accompanied by an ipsilateral negativity of a similar size, just before the onset of the stimulus-evoked P1. These late, slow effects were superimposed on a slow negative potential that appeared to be a CNV.

The slow positivity was interpreted as reflecting the modulation of cortical excitability in the regions receiving input from the relevant and irrelevant visual fields. Consistently with this proposal, the targets falling on the relevant visual field elicited enhanced P1 and N1 waves and, further, the magnitude of this enhancement, as well as the level of performance, was correlated with the amplitude of the slow positivity. As already mentioned, the modulation of cortical excitability was, according to the authors, initiated and controlled by executive processes directing attention, which were reflected by the preceding contralateral negativities preponderant over the right hemisphere.

Consequently, in this study, the earliest neurophysiological signs of the directing of attention were present as early as 200 msec from the onset of a cue indicating where attention should be directed, that is, well before the stimulus to be attended was presented. This accords with a number of behavioral studies of spatial orienting of attention (reviewed by Posner, Cohen, & Rafal, 1982) that indicate that spatial attention can be rapidly switched. Harter, Millter, et al.'s (1989) results also stress the role of the right hemisphere in directing visual-spatial attention, which is consistent with lesion and neuropsychological data implicating the importance of the parietal and prefrontal cortex, particularly of the right hemisphere, in spatial processing and in directing spatial attention (Heilman, 1979; Knight, 1985; Kolb & Whishaw, 1985; Mesulam, 1981; Posner et al., 1982).

Attention to Multi-Element Stimulus Arrays. In ERP studies of visual-spatial attention, stimuli have usually been presented separately to attended versus unattended locations. Although early ERP differences do emerge in such conditions, maximal attentional selectivity is perhaps not produced, insofar as a single stimulus presented to an "empty" visual field tends to draw attention automatically to it irrespective of whether this location was to be attended or not (see chapter 2). Indeed, stronger behavioral effects of spatial cueing have been found in situations where a multielement stimulus display was presented and a subset of those elements was precued (e.g., Jonides, 1981). Moreover, multielement arrays are more like natural visual scenes than are sequences of isolated stimuli (Mangun & Hillyard, 1990a).

Several recent studies in Hillyard's laboratory (Heinze, Luck, Mangun, & Hillyard, 1990; Heinze, Mangun, & Hillyard, 1990; Luck, Heinze, Mangun, & Hillyard, 1990) have investigated the differential processing of attended and unattended subregions within bilateral multielement displays. A bilateral stimulus having equal physical energy in the left and right visual fields would activate the two hemispheres more or less symmetrically. However, if attention is directed to the left or right half of a bilateral display, then the early ERPs should be enhanced over the hemisphere contralateral to the attended hemifield, if attention indeed acts by increasing the "gain" of the sensory pathways carrying information from the attended hemifield.

The results obtained support this prediction. In one of these experiments, Heinze, Luck, et al. (1990; see also Heinze, Mangun, & Hillyard, 1990) presented two pairs of letters simultaneously on each trial, one pair on each side of the fixation point. These bilateral arrays of letters, delivered at a rate of 2/sec, were composed of random letter combinations. Subjects were instructed to attend either to the left-side or right-side letter pairs and to press a button if the two letters on that side were identical. Letter pairs occurring on the unattended side could also be identical but were not to be responded to.

It was found that the left-hemisphere P1 was largest when the right hemifield was attended, and vice versa. In contrast, the N1 wave was not enlarged over the contralateral hemisphere.

Spatial Visual Attention: Spotlight or Gradients? In chapter 2, the metaphor of the "attentional spotlight" was introduced. The distribution of attention in the visual field was described by some authors in terms of a narrow spotlight (see Johnston & Dark, 1986) facilitating the processing of stimuli that fall within the boundaries of the spotlight and leaving other stimuli unfacilitated or suppressed to the same extent regardless of their proximity to the attentional spotlight. On the other hand, it has also been proposed that spatial attention is more broadly distributed in the form of an attentional "gradient" across the visual field. Such a gradient of attention would yield a maximal enhancement of perceptual processing with stimuli presented at the attended location, which would gradually diminish with distance away from that location (Mangun & Hillyard, 1987, 1988).

Mangun and Hillyard (1990a) presented task-irrelevant probe flashes at varying distances from an attended location. If the metaphor of the narrowly focused attentional spotlight is valid, then ERPs to the probe stimuli should not differ as a function of whether they are presented near (3–4 degrees) or far (8–9 degrees) from an attended location. On the other hand, if gradients of visual facilitation emerge around the locus of focal attention, then there should be ERP differences between probes presented near versus far from this locus.

It was found that the probes occurring near the attended location elicited larger P1, N1, and P2 waves than those elicited by the same probes when presented far from the attended location (in the opposite visual hemifield). Thus, spatial attention enhanced ERPs to irrelevant stimuli located some 3–5° away from the attended location. Mangun and Hillyard (1990a) concluded that this result does not support the analogy of visual spatial attention as a narrowly focused spotlight but instead as more broadly distributed attentional gradients.

Mangun and Hillyard (1987, 1988) obtained corroborating results in their study with three stimulus locations. Bar stimuli were flashed at a rapid rate and in random order to one of three upper-field locations: one in each of the lateral visual fields about 5° to the left and right of fixation and one on the vertical midline. Subjects attended to the stimuli at one of these three locations in turn, with their gaze always remaining fixed on a same central spot, trying to detect infrequent, slightly shorter bars at the designated location. If attention was distributed in a gradient-like fashion across the visual field, then the ERP to a stimulus occurring in the lateral visual field should decrease progressively as attention was focused first 5° and then 10° from that stimulus location.

Figure 6.39 shows the progressive decline in P1 and N1 amplitudes as attention was directed to locations at increasing distances from that of the evoking stimuli. The N2 wave was only found for stimuli occurring in the attended location (and thus did not show a graded response pattern). These findings suggested that spatial selective attention reflected in the P1/N1 waves is distributed as a rather broad gradient across the visual field, whereas the later processing indexed by N2 generation is more narrowly focused on the attended region.

Neville and Lawson (1987c), using quite a similar paradigm, found no ERP evidence for attentional gradients, however, but this is probably due to their three stimulus locations being much more widely separated from one another than those of Mangun and Hillyard (1987, 1988). On the other hand, when two stimulus positions are very close to each other, as in Hillyard and Münte's (1984) difficult condition (separation only 0.5°), early ERP signs of differential processing seem to be absent. However, stimuli in that study were presented 2° above the fixation point in order to diminish discriminability. (See also Wijers, Lamain, et al., 1989; Wijers et al., 1987.)

Mangun and Hillyard (1988) investigated the perceptual significance of these early graded amplitude changes by relating them to behavioral measures of the attentional gradient. The same stimuli were used as in their previous study (Mangun & Hillyard, 1987; reviewed earlier). Subjects were instructed to devote all of their efforts to the primary task of detecting infrequent, shorter target bars at the designated location and to press a button to them with their right hand. This time, however, a secondary task was also introduced, in which subjects were asked to press a second button with their left hand if they "happened to notice" (without actively trying to detect) a shorter target bar in either of the two irrelevant locations. Secondary target detections would thus yield a behavioral measure of perceptual processing of stimuli presented to to-be-ignored locations.

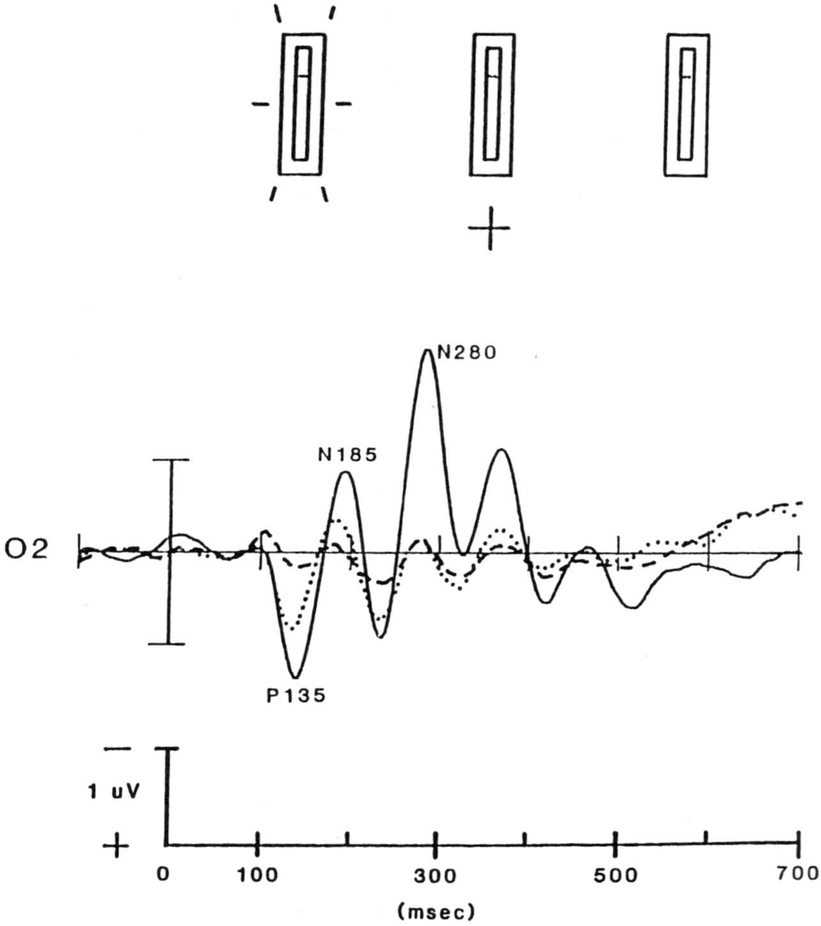

FIG. 6.39 Grand-average ERPs from right occipital scalp to left flashes when the subject was attending to the left (solid line), midline (dotted line), or right (dashed line) flashes. The subject was instructed to fixate a central fixation cross (+) while directing attention to the designated one of the three positions in order to discriminate occasional shorter target bars among standard bars presented in this location. These data suggest attentional gradients during visual-spatial attention. (From Mangun & Hillyard, 1990a. Copyright © 1990 by Guilford Press. Reprinted with permission.)

Mangun and Hillyard (1988) found, as they did in their previous study (Mangun & Hillyard, 1987), that the P1 and N1 waves were progressively attenuated as attended locations became increasingly distant from an evoking lateral stimulus (Fig. 6.40). This ERP-amplitude gradient was paralleled by a gradient of target detectability, as indicated by the d' measures. Consistently with this, Downing (1988) showed that d' scores for

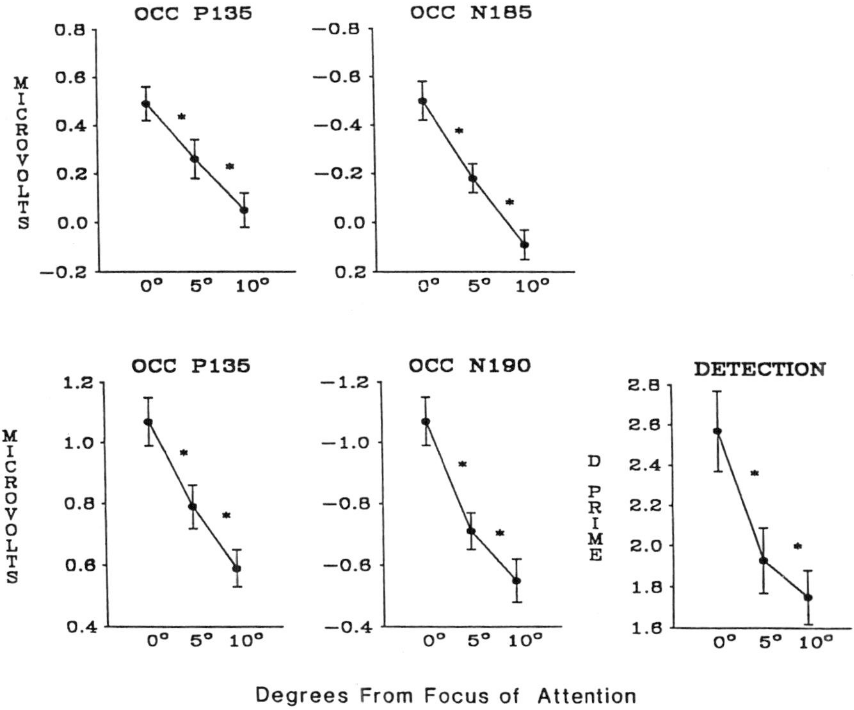

FIG. 6.40 Mean ERP (P1 and N1) and perceptual gradients during spatial attention (results from two experiments). *Top:* The mean amplitude of the P1 (P135) and N1 (N185) waves to lateral flashes as a function of the distance between the attended locus and the stimulated locus in the visual field. *Bottom:* The replication of this pattern of data for P1 and N1 in a second experiment. These ERP gradients were paralleled by a gradient of signal detectability (the rightmost panel at bottom). (From Mangun & Hillyard, 1990a. Copyright © 1990 by Guilford Press. Reprinted with permission.)

luminance detection tend to decrease in a graded fashion, as the distance between the expected and actual stimulus locations is increased (see also Downing & Pinker, 1985).

Rugg (1991) warned, however, that ERP data suggestive of attentional gradients need to be interpreted with caution. He maintained that a similar pattern of results is also obtained if subjects adopt a strategy of allocating attention to the to-be-attended location on the majority of trials and to a nearby location on a minority of trials:

> This would yield averaged ERPs to stimuli from each location that were composed of differing proportions of "attend" and "unattend" trials. Just as if an attentional gradient had existed, the averages would display a decline in the size of attention-related effects as the distance from the focus of attention

increased. As acknowledged by Mangun and Hillyard (1988), these alternative explanations, *attentional gradient vs. attentional switching,* have quite different theoretical consequences, but cannot be distinguished on the basis of averaged ERPs. (p. 223)

Wijers, Lamain, et al. (1989) presented randomized sequences of stimulus bars arising from eight positions arranged in a form of a hemi-circle around the fixation point. Subjects were required to attend to one stimulus location, the most peripheral left or right location, and to respond as fast as possible when the stimulus bar presented to this location was of a designated color.

It was found that P1 attention effects (largest ipsilaterally) extended to stimuli located at least 2° of visual angle from the locus of the relevant stimulus. However, no ERP evidence for a sloping attentional gradient was obtained; the relevant-location (Location 1) and adjacent-locations (Locations 2 and 3) attention effects were of similar magnitude, whereas no other location showed an intermediate effect, not even Location 4, which still was in the attended hemifield. This P1 enhancement was followed by a slow negative shift at about 175–350 msec from stimulus onset, which seemed to be limited to the stimulus positions where also the P1 effect was found.

An early color-selection effect (relevant stimuli were defined by both location and color) was also obtained that manifested in an early anterior positivity, occipital negativity. This effect occurred not only for the relevant location but also for all other locations within the same visual half-field, even for Location 4, where the spatial attention effect was not found. This early color-selection effect was followed by a later color-selection effect, which was a central N2b type of negativity confined to the relevant location and the adjacent location, and by a still later, parietal P3b positivity exclusively evoked by stimuli of the relevant color at the relevant location (targets).

In their (Wijers, Lamain, et al., 1989) divided-attention condition, all four stimuli of a designated hemifield were to be attended. The P1 attention effect was elicited by each stimulus of the designated hemifield and was of the same magnitude as in the focused-attention condition, but was not followed by the later, negative attention effect. The color-attention effect was also obtained for each stimulus of the attended hemifield.

The authors regarded the abrupt disappearance of the P1 and early color-selection effects across the boundary of the relevant and irrelevant hemifields (from Location 4 to Location 5) in divided attention as "rather surprising" in view of the small (0.15°) separation between these positions, on the one hand, and the extensive spread (at least 2°) of the attention effect to adjacent locations in the focused-attention condition, on the other hand. Moreover, it was about as hard to discriminate between Locations 4 and 5 in divided attention as between Locations 1 and 2 (also separated by 0.15°) in focused attention. Thus, the sharp drop-off of the ERP attention effects when the interhemispheric boundary was crossed, indicating high discriminability at the physiological level, was not reflected in behavioral measures. As stated by Wijers, Lamain, et al. (1989):

> This suggests that discriminability is not necessarily the decisive factor for the occurrence of P1 amplitude effects. Apparently, the attentional system may use the existing physiological segregation between the visual half-fields to enhance the resolution of spatial selectivity. This seems important evidence to support the idea that visual selective attention is dependent on characteristics of the perceptual system (e.g. the neural specificity theory of Harter & Aine, 1984). (pp. 241–242 see also Rizzolatti, Riggio, Dascola, & Umilta, 1987; Tassinari, Aglioti, Chelazzi, Marzi, & Berlucchi, 1987)

When divided attention involved one location in each hemisphere, no early (P1 or N1) effect of spatial visual attention was obtained, the first attention effect being a slow negativity commencing at about 200 msec (Okita, Wijers, Mulder, & Mulder, 1985).

Attention in Space: Intra-Hemifield Mappings. Mangun and Hillyard (1990a) attempted a more extensive mapping of the distribution of visual attention in space, especially in view of several recent behavioral studies (e.g., Hughes & Zimba, 1987) suggesting that natural boundaries, such as the horizontal and vertical meridians, may constrain the distribution of attention in the visual field. (See also the divided-attention results of Wijers, Lamain, et al., 1989, reviewed earlier). Vertically oriented white bars were flashed one at a time in random order to four locations: two "far lateral" and two "near lateral" positions located 6° and 2°, respectively, to the left and right of the midline. All these positions were in the upper visual field, such that subjects fixated a point in the center of the display located slightly below the lower edge of the stimuli. The subject was instructed to attend to one of the four locations at a time in order to detect occasional shorter target stimuli occurring at that location.

As for the far lateral stimuli, substantial attention effects were found: the P1, N1, and N2 amplitudes for these stimuli were largest when that location was attended and smallest when attention was directed to the far lateral stimuli of the opposite visual field (Fig. 6.41).

The P1 and N1 amplitudes for the far lateral stimuli showed a very different drop-off as attention was shifted away from these stimuli in 4° increments: Although the P1 amplitude progressively decreased as a function of this distance, the N1 amplitude did not show a progressive decrement but rather was similarly enlarged when these far lateral stimuli

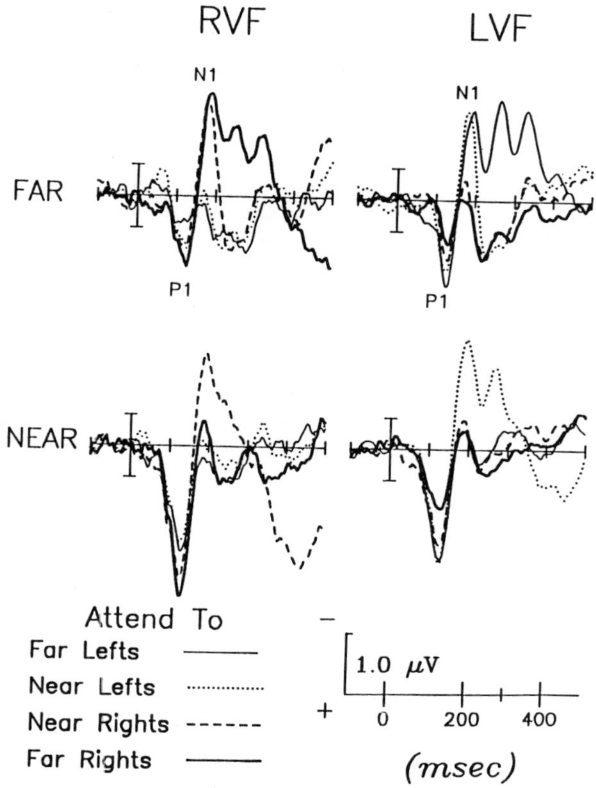

FIG. 6.41 Grand-average ERPs to far lateral stimuli (6 degrees eccentricity; top) and near lateral stimuli (2 degrees eccentricity; bottom) when the far lateral stimuli or when the near lateral stimuli were to be attended. ERPs are superimposed for the 4 attention conditions: Attend far left (thin solid lines), Attend near left (dotted lines), Attend near right (dashed lines), and Attend far right (thick solid lines). ERPs were recorded from lateral occipital sites contralateral to the field of stimulation (RVF = right visual field; LVF = left visual field). (From Mangun & Hillyard, 1990a. Copyright © 1990 by Guilford Press. Reprinted with permission.)

were attended and when the near lateral stimuli in the same half-field were attended. On the other hand, the N1 amplitude to the far lateral stimuli showed a sharp drop when attention was directed to either of the stimulus locations in the opposite visual half-field.

Consequently, the N1 amplitude for the far lateral stimuli suggested an all-or-none effect of the vertical meridian on the attentional enhancement. The N1 amplitude for the near lateral stimuli, however, showed a different pattern (Fig. 6.41, bottom): This amplitude was largest for attended near lateral stimuli and was sharply attenuated when attention was directed to any of the other three locations. For stimuli at all positions, the N2 wave was elicited only by attended stimuli, a general pattern of results found in all spatial attention studies of this type (Mangun & Hillyard, 1990a).

These results were interpreted as suggesting that the P1 wave indexes a tonic, pre-set spatial gating process, while the N1 wave is a sign of active orienting to relevant or potentially relevant events (see also Hillyard et al., 1985; Mangun et al., in press). In addition, the difference in the N1 response pattern to near versus far lateral stimuli would suggest that attentional orienting is more automatic or robust for stimuli at locations peripheral to the focus of attention (cf. section 2.2), whereas stimuli occurring medially to the focus of attention could be more effectively ignored. In the words of Mangun and Hillyard (1990a):

> Accordingly, the far lateral flashes would elicit an N1 of enhanced amplitude either when they were attended or when the near laterals (in the same hemifield) were attended, but the latter stimuli would not produce an enlarged N1 when the far laterals were attended. The division of a visual hemifield into medial and lateral regions may be relative to the focus of attention just as the left and right visual fields are defined relative to the point of eye fixation. Thus, the point at which attention is focused may define a boundary in visual space that serves as a reference for subsequent attentional orienting. (pp. 284–285)

ERPs and Allocation of Visual Spatial Attention. The early ERP amplitudes can be reliable indicators of the graded allocation of attention among multiple spatial locations. In Mangun and Hillyard's (1990b) letter-search task, semicircles of 4 letters each were flashed in random order to the left or right visual field at a rapid rate. The subject was instructed to respond by a button press to infrequent sets that contained a target letter "T" located in any of the four letter positions. Left-field targets were to be responded with the left hand and right-field targets with the right hand.

The subject's attentional "allocation policy" was manipulated by varying the relative percentages of attentional effort to be dedicated to the left versus right letter displays (Kinchla, 1980; Sperling, 1984). Five separate conditions were employed, with the left/right allocation of attention being: 100%/0%, 75%/25%, 50%/50%, 25%/75%, and 0%/100%. After some practice, subjects appeared to be able to allocate attention according to these numerical instructions, as suggested by their behavioral target-detection and RT trade-off curves (Fig. 6.43).

It was found that the P1 and N1 amplitudes progressively increased with greater attentional allocation to the eliciting stimuli (Figs. 6.42 and 6.43), the trade-off being clearly reciprocal. Importantly, the P1-amplitude enhancement with increasing percentages of attention allocation bore a monotonic (though not linear) relation with improved target detectability and decreased RTs (Fig. 6.43). The authors concluded that this orderly

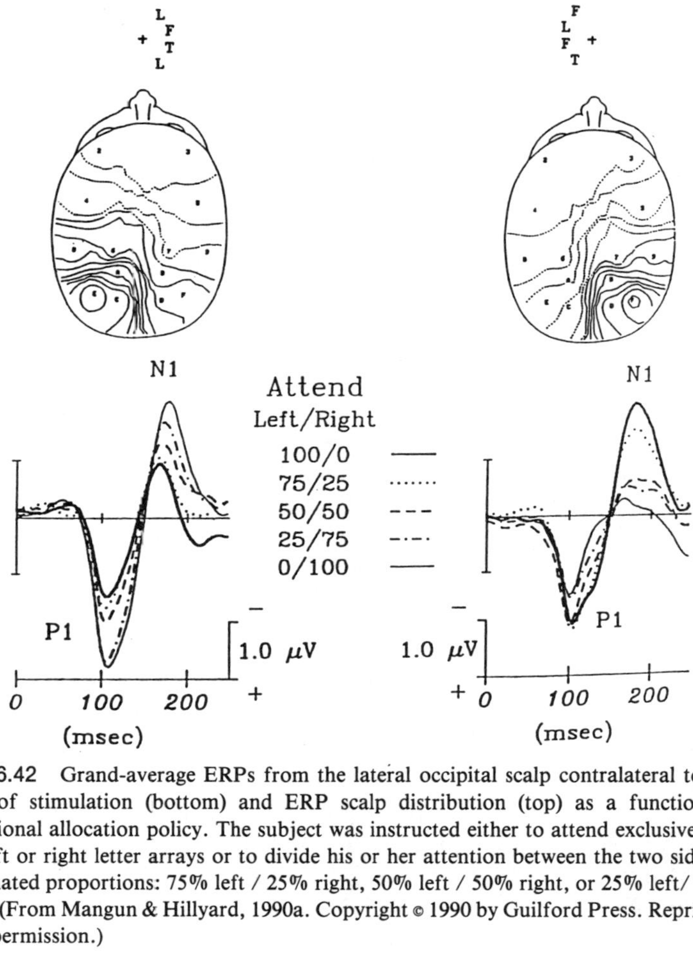

FIG. 6.42 Grand-average ERPs from the lateral occipital scalp contralateral to the field of stimulation (bottom) and ERP scalp distribution (top) as a function of attentional allocation policy. The subject was instructed either to attend exclusively to the left or right letter arrays or to divide his or her attention between the two sides in designated proportions: 75% left / 25% right, 50% left / 50% right, or 25% left/ 75% right. (From Mangun & Hillyard, 1990a. Copyright © 1990 by Guilford Press. Reprinted with permission.)

relationship provides a validation of these early ERP waves as indices of attentional allocation policy.

Visual-Spatial Attention: Effects on Auditory ERPs. The studies reviewed thus far have shown that a visual stimulus presented to (or near) the attended location elicits enhanced exogenous ERP components and, further, that this effect occurs regardless of whether or not this stimulus perfectly matches the to-be-attended stimulus in other attributes. This suggests the primacy of the spatial cue over the other visual stimulus attributes in visual selection. Now, one might further ask whether this spatial attention effect extends even beyond modality boundaries, so that auditory stimuli originating from the attended visual location also elicit an ERP attention effect. Such a result was predicted by Näätänen (1975).

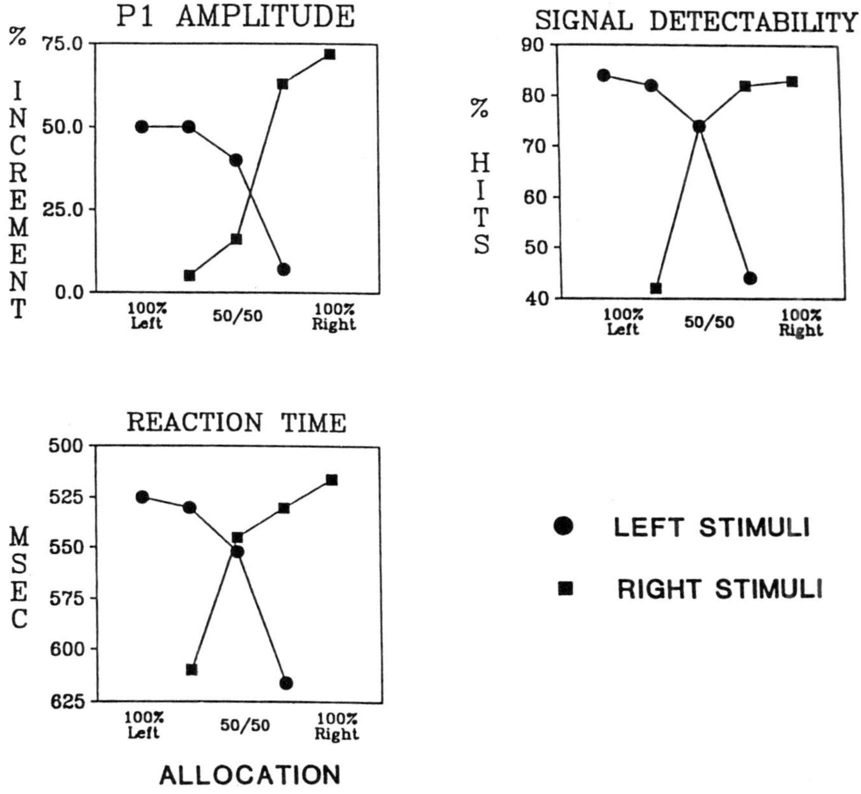

FIG. 6.43 The mean P1 amplitude (percent increment over the P1 amplitude for unattended stimuli), hit rate (the percentage of targets detected), and RTs (msec) for the left and right hemifield stimuli as a function of allocation of attention to these stimuli (100% left, through 50/50 to 100% right conditions). (From Mangun & Hillyard, 1990a. Copyright © 1990 by Guilford Press. Reprinted with permission.)

Hillyard et al. (1984) have, in fact, conducted an experiment of this genre. These authors presented tones and flashes in a rapid random sequence from the same spatial locations 30° to the left and right of fixation. The subjects of the "Auditory group" only attended to tones, whereas the "Visual group" attended only to flashes. Selective spatial attention was introduced by instructing the subject to perform a duration-discrimination task within the designated (either left or right) input of the correct modality. For each group, stimuli of the other modality were wholly irrelevant throughout the experiment to minimize any tendencies to switch attention to them.

It was found that flashes presented to the attended auditory location indeed elicited a larger N1 type of response than did flashes presented to the

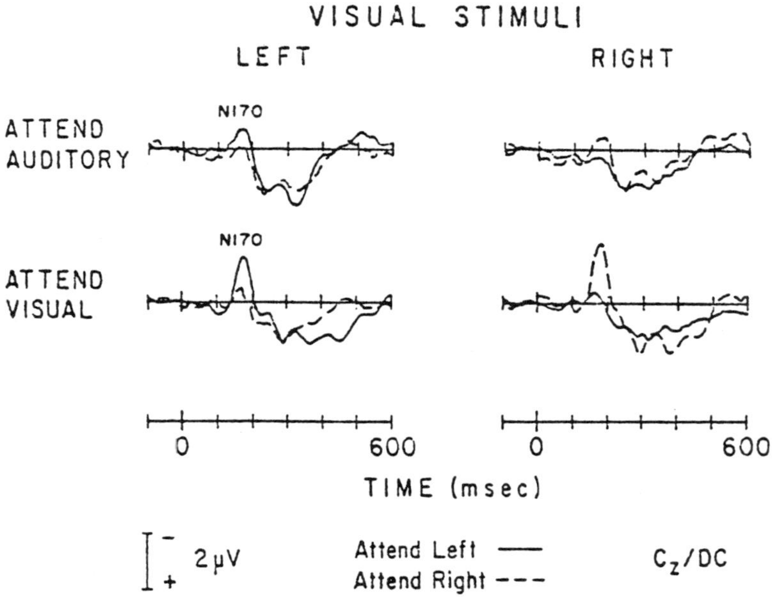

FIG. 6.44 Grand-average vertex (Cz) ERPs to flashes presented to the left and right visual fields in the "visual" (Attend visual) and "auditory" (Attend auditory) groups of subjects. The lower tracings show the effect of lateralized visual attention (attended vs. unattended visual field) on the visual ERP (visual group) and the upper tracings show the effect of lateralized auditory attention on the visual ERP (auditory group). (From Hillyard, Simpson, Woods, van Voorhis, & Münte, 1984. Copyright © 1984 by Raven Press. Reprinted with permission.)

unattended auditory location (Fig. 6.44). (The P1 amplitude was not affected by attention, however.) An analogous result was also obtained for auditory stimuli, but the spatial attention effect occurred in the form of a PN rather than as an enhancement of any exogenous component.

These across-modality spatial-attention effects were much weaker than the corresponding intramodal effects (for both modalities), however. Thus, if a stimulus does not belong to the attended modality, the ERP effect of the attended stimulus location is attenuated. Consequently, these data suggest that stimulus location and modality might be cues of similar priority level in attentional selection when the relevant and irrelevant stimulus loci are far apart.

Consequences of Visual-Spatial Attention as Indicated by Early ERP Effects. In the foregoing, ERP effects of visual-spatial attention were reviewed. The perceptual and behavioral consequences of this attentional selection function that is indexed by ERP modulation may be summarized as follows:

1. Improved detection (d') of stimuli presented at this location, as illustrated in Figs. 6.40 and 6.43 (for reviews, see Mangun & Hillyard, 1990a, 1990b; Mangun et al., in press).

2. A faster RT response to target stimuli presented at the attended location (see Fig. 6.43) (Mangun & Hillyard, 1990b).

3. Termination of further processing in unattended locations, as indicated by the absence of later ERP waves elicited by stimuli presented at these locations (Mangun & Hillyard, 1988, 1990a). A prime example is provided by the N2 wave, which is only elicited when the stimulus occurs at the attended location (see Heinze, Luck, et al., 1990). This wave is not elicited by stimuli occurring in nearby locations, although these stimuli may elicit some P1 and/or N1 enhancement, which suggests that stimulus selection is sharpened between the latencies of the P1 (or N1) and N2 generator processes. In addition, in Hillyard and Münte (1984), the processing of stimuli for color was prematurely terminated when these stimuli were presented outside the attended location, even though stimulus relevance was defined on the basis of both color and location attributes.

An ERP Test of the Feature-Integration Theory

One of the predictions of the feature-integration theory (Section 2.5) is that the speed of detecting feature-present targets does not depend on set size, whereas that of feature-absent targets does (Treisman & Souther, 1985).[4]

This prediction was recently tested by Luck and Hillyard (1990). They found that the P3 latency (for targets and distractors) did not depend on set size when feature-present targets were used but did depend on set-size when feature-absent targets were used. These data were interpreted as supporting the feature-integration theory; they seemed to indicate that the search for feature presence was conducted in parallel for all items in the display, whereas feature-absent targets had to be searched for in a serial manner.

The P3 amplitude also supported the feature-integration theory in that the set-size effect on this amplitude was clearly smaller when the feature-present targets were used than when the feature-absent targets were used. Furthermore, target-detection ERPs were qualitatively somewhat different in the two conditions, which suggests that different modes of processing accompany the detection of the two types of targets.

All aspects of Luck and Hillyard's (1990) results did not support the feature-integration theory, however. Namely, it was also found that in the

[4]Feature-present targets differ from distractors by having a feature (e.g., a vertical line) that is absent from the distractors, whereas feature-absent targets differ from distractors by not having a feature that is present in the distractors.

feature-present conditions, targets elicited an N2 that was larger at scalp sites contralateral than ipsilateral to the location of the target. This location-specific scalp distribution implied, apparently, that information about target location was available at some level of the nervous system. This result was therefore taken by the authors as suggesting, contrary to the feature-integration theory, that localization may be necessary for feature identification.

ERPs and NonSpatial Visual Attention

As reviewed previously, only visual-spatial attention appears to be associated with enhanced exogenous ERP components (and even that not always). In contrast, when relevant and irrelevant stimuli occur in the same spatial locus (or cannot be discriminated on the basis of the spatial cue), attentional selection is predominantly associated with slow negativities, perhaps equivalent to the auditory processing negativity. Pioneering work in clarifying these negativities in vision has been conducted by the late M. R. Harter and his colleagues, who called them "selection negativities." This research was initiated by R. G. Eason and colleagues in the late 1960s (see Eason, Harter, & White, 1969) and mainly continued by Harter and his associates (Aine & Harter, 1984a, 1984b, 1986; Harter & Anllo-Vento, 1990, 1991; Harter & Guido, 1980; Harter & Previc, 1978; Harter & Salmon, 1972; Harter et al., 1982; Harter, Anllo-Vento, & Wood, 1989; Harter, Millter, et al., 1989; Previc & Harter, 1982). Selection negativities are, according to Harter and Aine (1984), due to the efferent facilitation of neuronal populations that represent the attended stimulus dimension.

Attention to Stimulus Size. In a particularly important study, Harter and Previc (1978) presented a random sequence of eight equiprobable visual stimuli that consisted of a diffuse flash and flashed checkerboards having seven different check sizes. In each run, one of the flashes was designated as the target, requiring a fast motor response or simply counting. In both tasks, a sizable occipital (only Oz electrode was used) slow negativity, as revealed by subtraction, emerged. The onset latency was reported to be 100–150 msec and peak latency 240–280 msec.

The most interesting result was the narrowing of the bandwidth of the selective-attention effect during its time course (see Fig. 6.45). As early as 160 msec from stimulus onset, some attentional selectivity was evident, with stimuli having check sizes very different from the target size apparently eliciting less PN than more similar stimuli. This selectivity became much narrower at 200 msec from stimulus onset and was further narrowed by 260 msec, at which time the attentional negativity reached its maximum

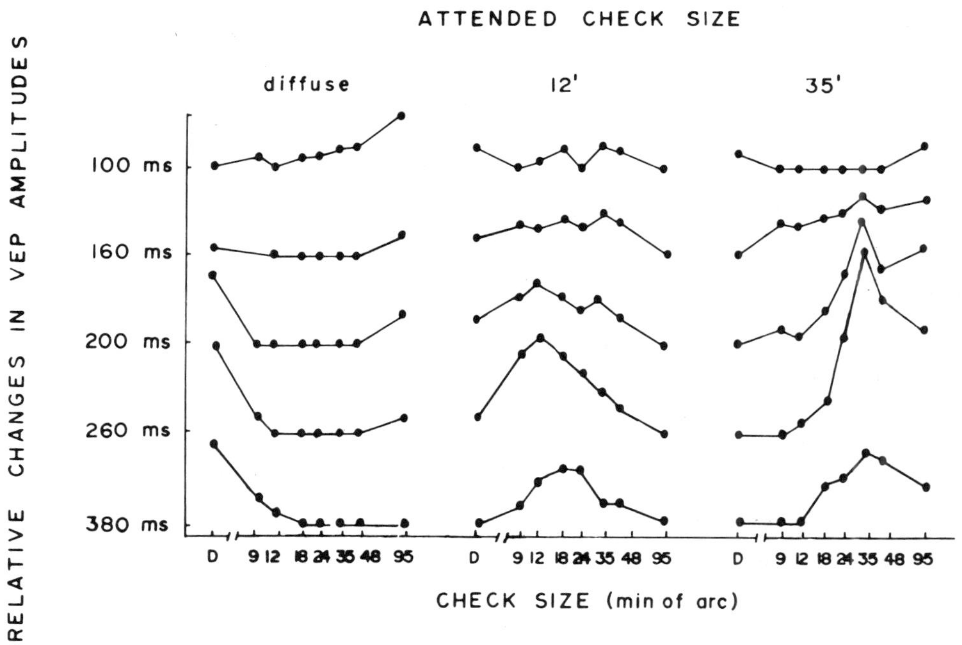

FIG. 6.45 The effect of selective attention to diffuse light, 12′ checks, or 35′ checks on the grand-average occipital (Oz) ERP amplitude to the 8 stimuli as indicated on the abscissa (with the main effects of flashed and attended check size statistically removed). ERP amplitudes were measured at 100, 160, 200, 260, and 380 msec after flash onset. Negativity up except for the 380-msec measure for which polarity was inverted (positive up). (From Harter & Previc, 1978. Copyright © 1978 by Elsevier Science Publishers, Ireland. Reprinted with permission.)

amplitude. Even here, the adjacent-sized stimuli generally elicited a large PN approaching the size of that to target stimuli.

The next measurement latency was 380 msec, at which point the attentional negativity could no longer be observed. Rather, the target ERP was more positive than ERPs to the other stimuli (the P3 target effect). P3 also showed stimulus generalization, but this was somewhat wider than that shown by PN at its most tuned phase (at 260 msec).

Interestingly, that narrowest bandwidth of the negative attention effect corresponded quite well to that reflected by errors in motor responses, which were almost totally limited to stimuli adjacent in size to the targets. Even a good temporal correspondence was found, in that from RTs (median 322 msec) it could be inferred that response decision tended to occur at the latency of the maximal PN tuning. Moreover, this final and narrowest PN bandwidth roughly corresponded to the bandwidth of the cortical size-specific channels revealed by psychophysical (Blake & Levinson, 1977; Blakemore & Campbell, 1969) and electrophysiological (Campbell & Maffei, 1970; Harter, Towle, & Musso, 1976) studies.

The observed latencies of the ERP attention effects are consistent with this interpretation, as it is known that activation of central, cortical, size-specific channels occurs at approximately 140–160 msec from stimulus onset (Harter et al., 1976), which corresponds to the onset of Harter and Previc's (1978) widely generalized selection negativity. Consequently, the authors made the far-reaching suggestion that the selective-attention mechanism might act by selectively modulating the excitability of these functional cortical sensory systems (see later).

A slow attentional negativity has also been observed when subjects attended to a grating stimulus of a designated spatial frequency, ignoring a concurrent grating stimulus of another frequency (Previc & Harter, 1982).

Attention to Stimulus Orientation. Harter and Guido (1980) presented three equiprobable visual stimuli in random order. One of the stimuli, a diffuse flash, was very different from the remaining two stimuli, which were somewhat similar to each other, one being a patterned flash with horizontal, the other with vertical, gratings. The subject's task was to press a button as quickly as possible to the one of the three stimuli designated as the target.

It was found that when the diffuse stimulus was the target, the occipital ERP for this stimulus included a negative displacement relative to this ERP when one of the gratings was the target. This displacement was continuous between approximately 150 and 280 msec and peaked at 235 msec. When one of these gratings was the target, this elicited a similarly timed attentional negativity relative to the ERP to this stimulus when the diffuse stimulus was the target. This effect also started at 150 msec. A smaller and later negativity was obtained when the non-target grating ERP was subtracted from the target-grating ERP; the onset of the negativity was now at 180 msec.

This study therefore suggested that the attentional negativity reflects elementary discriminations, for instance, whether the stimulus is patterned or unpatterned, at a shorter latency than it reflects more demanding discriminations (e.g., whether gratings are vertical vs. horizontal). The study also demonstrated that the attentional negativity can reflect these two discriminations in succession when they are required to the same stimulus. When the diffuse stimulus was the target, it sufficed to decide whether the stimulus had gratings or not; when one of the grating stimuli was the target, the negativity reflected both the decision about the presence versus absence of gratings and, if the stimulus had gratings, whether their orientation was correct.

This study also suggested that the earlier component of the visual attentional negativity is modality-specifically distributed. Further, this component was followed by a second, frontocentral component at about 260 msec. The latter component, however, reflected only rough discriminations despite its long latency; it was elicited when the target and evoking stimuli both were diffuse or when they both had a grating of any orientation. This negativity appears to be equivalent to N2b (see Wijers, 1989).

Rugg et al. (1987) also found an ERP correlate of attention to stimulus orientation. This was a late fronto-central negativity at about 200–400 msec. (See also Previc & Harter, 1982, to be discussed in a later section.)

Attention to Color. Harter and Salmon (1972) were the first to describe ERP effects of attention to stimulus color. This effect was a slow, late occipital negativity peaking at about 220–250 msec from stimulus onset. A somewhat similar color effect was also observed by Harter et al. (1982), who defined relevant stimuli on the basis of their location and color + shape (either a white ring or a solid green circle; therefore, it is not clear whether the color effect reported was only due to color). This negativity was larger over the left than the right posterior hemisphere regardless of the hemifield attended, thus differing in distribution from the negativity associated with spatial selection that was initially contralateral to the hemifield attended.

Later studies have shown that the color-selection negativity over the occiput is accompanied by a positivity at more anterior electrodes (Aine & Harter, 1986; Hillyard & Münte, 1984; Wijers, Lamain, et al., 1989; Wijers, Mulder, Okita, & Mulder, 1989; Wijers, Mulder, Okita, Mulder, & Scheffers, 1989; Wijers, Mulder, Otten, Feenstra, & Mulder, 1989). For an illustration, see Fig. 6.46, which presents data from the study of Wijers, Mulder, Okita, Mulder, and Scheffers (1989). This negative–positive color-attention effect does not seem to be simply due to an attentional modulation of a single generator: For instance, as illustrated in Fig. 6.46, the positive and negative effects differ in onset latency (Wijers, Mulder, Okita, & Mulder, 1989; Wijers, Mulder, Okita, Mulder, & Scheffers, 1989). In addition, with wide spatial separation, Hillyard and Münte's (1984) occipital color-attention effect was clearly contralateralized, whereas the anterior attention effect of positive polarity did not show this asymmetry.

The contralateralization of the color-attention effect, found also by Wijers, Lamain, et al. (1989), has not been a consistent finding, however, as Hillyard and Münte's (1984) symmetrical color-attention effect with small spatial separation indicates. Aine and Harter (1984a) also found a symmetrical effect, whereas Aine and Harter (1986) reported a right-hemisphere dominance.

The onset latency (about 150 msec) of the color-attention effect is shorter than for most other nonspatial forms of attention but clearly longer than

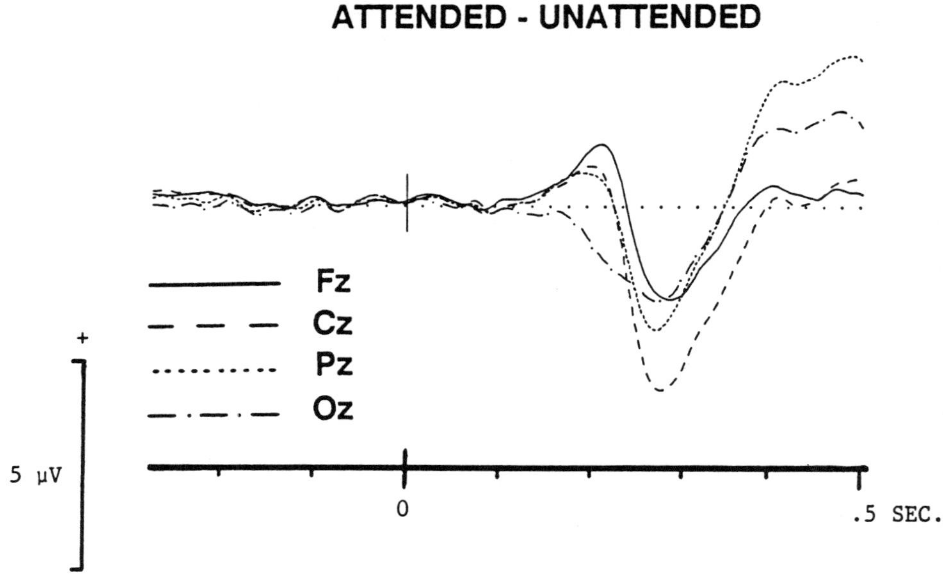

FIG. 6.46 Grand-average frontal (Fz), vertex (Cz), parietal (Pz), and occipital (Oz) difference waves (ERPs to unattended-color stimuli subtracted from the ERPs to attended-color stimuli). (From Wijers, Mulder, Okita, Mulder, & Scheffers, 1989. Copyright © 1989 The Society for Psychophysiological Research. Reprinted with permission.)

for spatial attention when attended and unattended locations are widely separated (see Hillyard & Münte, 1984). The early onset of the color-selection negativity is illustrated in Fig. 6.46. In this figure, the effect starts as an occipital negativity at about 160 msec from stimulus onset, whereas the accompanying anterior positivity commences even earlier, at about 120–130 msec.

This figure also reveals a later attention effect, which was found in other studies as well (Okita et al., 1985; Scheffers et al., 1991; Wijers, Mulder, Okita, & Mulder, 1989; Wijers, Mulder, Otten, et al., 1989). Starting at about 230 msec and peaking at 270–290 msec, the attention effect was negative at all leads and was largest at Cz. Hence, this effect was biphasic in all electrodes anterior to Oz. The authors interpreted this later attention effect in terms of N2b, suggesting that it was associated with "the covert orienting of attention, after an earlier identification process has determined that the stimulus has to be attended" (Wijers, Mulder, Okita, Mulder, & Scheffers, 1989, p. 99).

The N2b interpretation was supported by the enhancement of this effect when preceding stimuli were of the irrelevant color (for an analogical auditory result, see Sams et al., 1983), whereas the early effect was not affected. The N2b effect is not specific to color selection but occurs with other selection cues as well, such as attended diagonal (Okita et al., 1985), letter size (Wijers, Mulder, Okita, & Mulder, 1989), or location (Scheffers et al., 1991).

Several studies have defined stimuli to be attended via a conjunction of location and color (for instance, attend to red stimuli on the left). The results obtained suggest the primacy of location selection over color selection when relevant and irrelevant stimulus locations are widely separated (Harter et al., 1982; Hillyard & Münte, 1984; Wijers, Lamain, et al., 1989). In these studies, ERP signs of color selection were considerably attenuated in the irrelevant location when compared with those in the relevant location (see Fig. 6.47). In contrast, ERP signs of location selection were largely unaffected by the relevance versus irrelevance of the color of the stimulus falling on the attended location.

This primacy of location selection over color selection is probably based on location selection occurring at a lower level than color selection in the visual processing system, as evidenced by the nature (exogenous vs. endogenous) and latency of the effects (Hillyard & Münte, 1984). As a consequence, the color-selection mechanism might receive reduced sensory input from stimuli falling on an unattended location, or the attentional processing of color is prematurely terminated because of the failure of the stimulus to fulfill the faster, spatial criterion of the attended stimulus (Hansen & Hillyard, 1983; Hawkins, 1969; Hillyard & Münte, 1984; Näätänen, 1975, 1982, 1990; Snodgrass & Townsend, 1980; see also "reactive inhibition," Näätänen, 1990, p. 270).

On the other hand, when the relevant and irrelevant stimulus locations are situated close together, the precedence of location selection over color selection, as reflected by ERPs, appears to vanish. With small spatial separation, Hillyard and Münte (1984) observed ERP signs of selection for color rather to precede those for location: "Thus, the timing and pattern of the attention-sensitive ERPs were entirely dependent upon the discriminability of the task-relevant cues" (p. 194). It was also found that these ERP signs for either attribute were stronger when the other attribute also matched with that of the stimulus to be attended. Spatial selection even seemed to be more affected by the outcome of color selection than vice versa.

This turning point, as location separation is gradually diminished, might be separation at which spatial attention ceases to enhance exogenous components and begins to add an endogenous component, the selection or processing negativity. This negativity, maximal at the frontal sites, was significant between 225 and 400 msec for Hillyard and Münte's (1984) small separation.

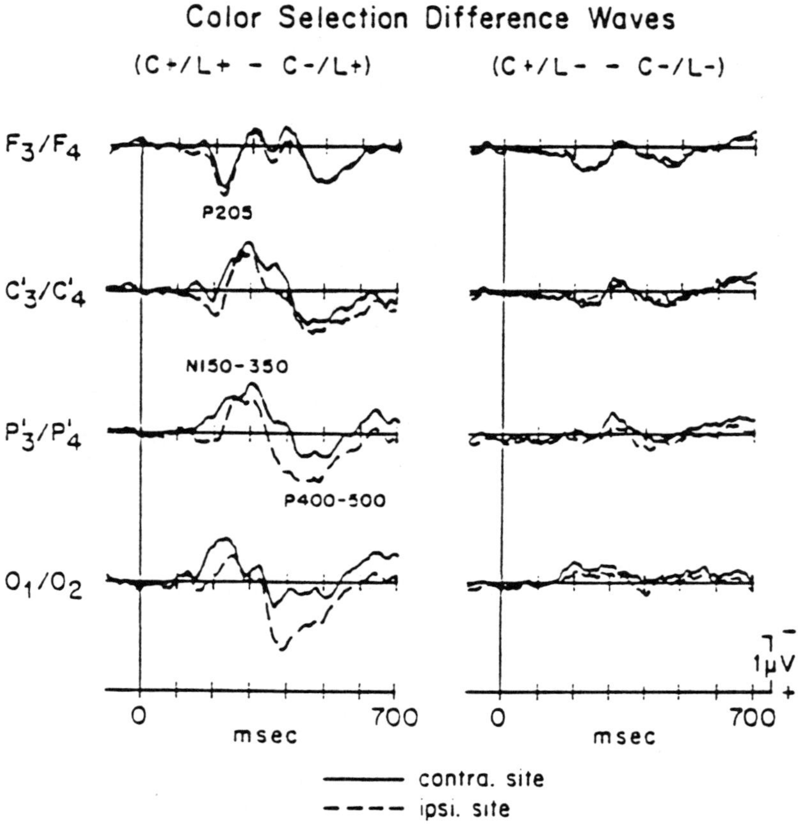

FIG. 6.47 Grand-average ERP difference waves for stimuli of attended versus unattended color at different electrode locations as indicated on the left. The left column presents difference waves reflecting selection of color at the attended location, and the right column presents difference waves associated with color selection at the unattended location. Solid lines indicate difference waves for ERPs recorded over sites contralateral to the attended visual field, dashed lines those for ERPs recorded ipsilaterally to the attended visual field. (From Hillyard & Münte, 1984. Copyright © 1984 by The Psychonomic Society, Inc. Reprinted with permission.)

Wijers, Lamain, et al.'s (1989) color-attention effect seemed to depend hierarchically on the preceding spatial attention effect. Furthermore, the two effects generalized to irrelevant stimulus locations rather similarly. The later color-attention effect, N2b, did not follow the generalization of the spatial effect in that it generalized only to the adjacent location. P3b was only elicited by stimuli of the relevant color appearing in the relevant location, thus disclosing no generalization.

In Wijers, Lamain, et al.'s (1989) divided-attention conditions, the early color effect was elicited in each of the four locations of the hemifield to be attended. Interestingly, N2b was elicited by all stimuli of the relevant hemifield but also by stimuli of the irrelevant hemifield closest to the midline. The authors concluded that the N2b component reflects an orienting of attention that is relatively independent of the earlier stages of selective processing.

When color is combined with some other stimulus attribute than location, it seems to dominate as an attentional cue in selection of conjunction stimuli. Wijers, Mulder, Okita, and Mulder's (1989) ERP effect of attending to letter size was contingent on the relevance of color. Interestingly, N2b showed a more independent pattern of results: The relevance of letter size resulted in an N2b enhancement independently of the relevance of the color, and vice versa.

Attentional Negativity to Stimulus Conjunction. Previc and Harter (1982) presented four equiprobable grating stimuli in the same display location. The gratings comprised either 9- or 36-min bars and were oriented either horizontally or vertically: 9V, 9H, 36V, 36H. The subject was required to respond to one of the gratings at a time, for instance to 9H, and to ignore the other three gratings. A large Nd was obtained by subtracting the 36V ERP (neither feature common with the target) from the 9H ERP. The authors also subtracted the 36V ERP separately from the 36H and 9V ERPs (both sharing one feature with the target) and obtained a small Nd for each. When these individual Nds were summed, the resulting Nd was somewhat earlier and clearly smaller than the target (9H) Nd.

Previc and Harter (1982) interpreted that the remaining, additional Nd, with a delayed time-course in relation to those of the "feature-specific" attention effects (the sum Nd), as reflecting the conjunction of features defining the target. There is also an alternative interpretation for this result, however: When the stimulus shares only one relevant feature with the target, the Nd resulting from the match in this feature may be reduced and prematurely terminated because of the failure of the stimulus to match with the other target feature (cf. Hansen & Hillyard, 1983; Hillyard & Münte, 1984). That is, PN generated by a match in this feature is smaller and shorter in duration when the stimulus does not match than when it matches the relevant stimulus in the other feature.

This might apply to the Nd associated with the orientation match in particular, insofar as this Nd had a longer latency than Nd for spatial frequency. Consistently with this, Nd for orientation was very small when the stimulus differed from the target in spatial frequency (Previc & Harter, 1982, Fig. 4). Consequently, the negativity (sum Nd) obtained by summing the two individual Nds, each obtained when the stimulus matched the target in one but not in the other feature defining the relevant stimulus, underestimates the sum of these feature-specific Nds elicited by a stimulus meeting both criteria of a target. Therefore, no separate Nd for a conjunction of relevant stimulus features seems, in fact, to have been demonstrated.

Hillyard and Münte (1984), too, interpreted their results as demonstrating, in addition to the individual Nds for the two features, a separate Nd for feature conjunction. However, this additional negativity, too, might be an artifact of a premature termination of the matching process for the slower feature (color) when the faster feature (spatial position) did not match with the stimulus to be attended. This explanation, however, is not quite consistent with the topographical aspects of their data.

ERP Signs of Further Processing of Attended Stimuli

Experiments conducted in Mulder's laboratory in Groningen, The Netherlands, have been highly informative with regard to further processing performed for visual stimuli passing the stage of initial selection. For instance, Okita et al. (1985), Wijers, Mulder, Okita, & Mulder (1989) and Wijers et al. (1987) described a "search negativity," a late, slow negativity with a broad midline distribution and a vertex maximum. This negativity is elicited when a subject has to decide whether any of the letters of a visual display belongs to a memory set of letters shown in advance. Stimuli to be ignored, for instance those appearing in an irrelevant location or having an irrelevant color, do not elicit this negativity or elicit only its initial phase (Wijers, Mulder, Okita, & Mulder, 1989).

The best evidence for this negativity being related to memory search is its enhancement with an increased memory-set size (Fig. 6.48). This negativity is followed, although with some temporal overlap, by a large, posterior P3b-type of positivity if a target is found in the search process. The amplitude of this positivity decreases and its latency increases as a function of memory and display load, that is, with the duration of the preceding memory- or visual-search negativities.

Mental rotation of a stimulus belonging to a relevant stimulus category was also associated with a late, slow negativity that was not elicited by stimuli belonging to the irrelevant category (Wijers, Mulder, Otten, et al., 1989). The amplitude of this negativity, with a midline distribution posterior to that of the search negativity, increased as a function of the angle with which stimuli departed from their normal upright position.

Neural-Specificity Theory of Visual Attention

As the studies reviewed thus far have clearly established, selective attention either enhances exogenous components or causes endogenous components.

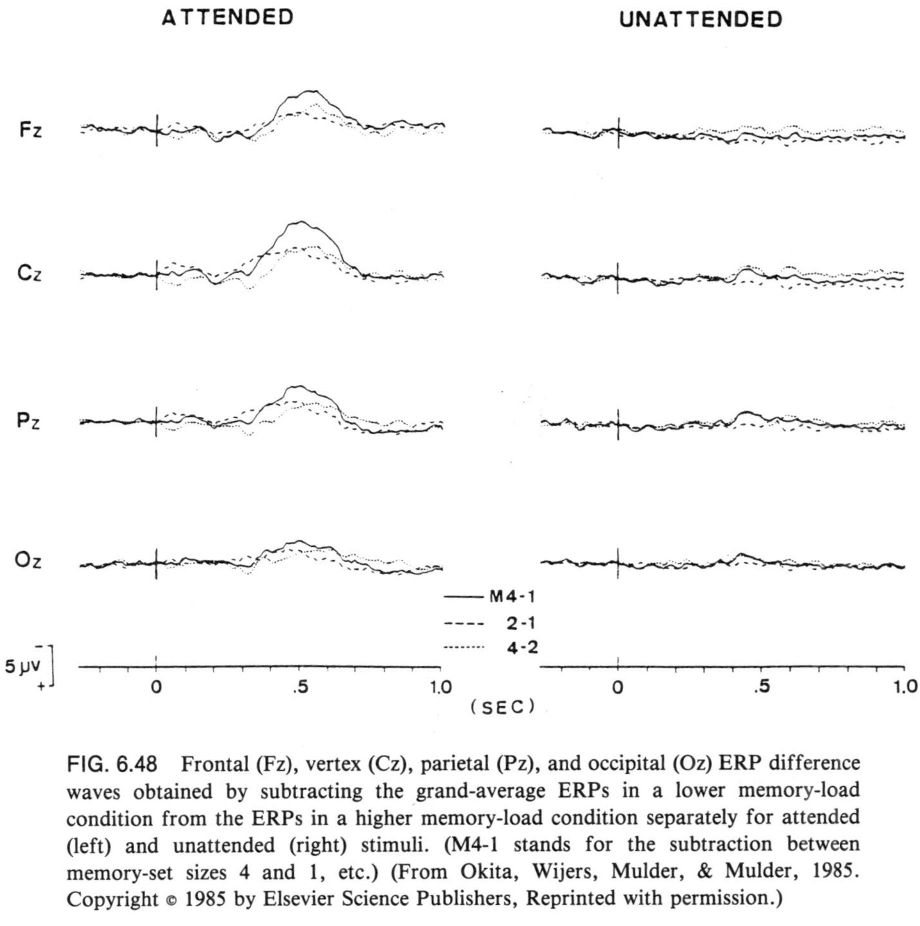

FIG. 6.48 Frontal (Fz), vertex (Cz), parietal (Pz), and occipital (Oz) ERP difference waves obtained by subtracting the grand-average ERPs in a lower memory-load condition from the ERPs in a higher memory-load condition separately for attended (left) and unattended (right) stimuli. (M4-1 stands for the subtraction between memory-set sizes 4 and 1, etc.) (From Okita, Wijers, Mulder, & Mulder, 1985. Copyright © 1985 by Elsevier Science Publishers, Reprinted with permission.)

The endogenous slow negativities associated with stimulus selection can probably be accounted for by the matching process postulated by the attentional-trace theory (Näätänen, 1982, 1990). On the other hand, exogenous effects suggest quite a different type of theory, which holds that attention can affect even earlier stages of stimulus processing. This type of theory is represented by Harter and Aine's (1984) "neural-specificity theory," which was developed on the basis of ERP and single-unit data. This theory proposes that visual selective attention is accomplished by efferent pre-stimulus facilitation (and/or inhibition) of the different feature-specific neuronal populations participating in sensory analysis of visual stimuli. Thus, the very same mechanisms that are responsible for representing the different attributes of our visual percepts, such as location, shape, orientation, color, and so on, are efferently facilitated (and/or inhibited) in accordance with experimental instructions to selectively attend to certain stimuli. For instance, if the subject is requested to attend to stimuli delivered to the left visual field and to ignore those to the right visual field, the neuronal populations coding the left visual field, or perhaps the relevant location within it, would be facilitated (and the neuronal population for the right visual field perhaps inhibited) by efferent influences. A stimulus corresponding to the facilitated neuronal population (in this case, a left-field stimulus) would elicit a selection negativity. As stated by Harter and Aine (1984):

> Selection negativity is a measure of the relative increase in the neural response to a stimulus when it does versus when it does not have specified features in common with the relevant stimulus. It presumably reflects the enhanced response of aggregates of neurons with similar receptive field properties (sensory channels) due to efferent modulation by higher mechanisms involved in directing attention prior to stimulus presentation. It may reflect enhanced responsiveness to the relevant information and/or suppressed responsiveness to irrelevant information.
>
> The data presented indicate that selection negativity does not reflect a single underlying process but many functionally different processes in different projection systems. . . . The time of onset and overlapping nature of selection negativities to different stimulus features suggests the different types of channels are activated in series; but once activated, such activations continue in parallel. The overall amplitude and duration of the negativity presumably will be determined by the summation of the selection negativities associated with processing the different features and conjunctions of features defining the relevant stimulus. The relative order of the onset of the various types of neural channel selection discussed was the selection of location, contour, color, spatial frequency, orientation, conjunction of features, and/or the relevant stimulus per se. (pp. 313–314)

In addition, Harter and Aine (1984) proposed that spatial stimulus selection involves the tectopulvinar-parietal pathway, whereas selection based on non-spatial attributes is performed in the geniculostriate-inferotemporal pathway.

Next, criticism (Hillyard & Mangun, 1986; Näätänen, 1986e) directed against the neural-specificity theory is reviewed.

1. **Selective Facilitation of the Sensory Systems Should Enhance Exogenous Components in Response to Corresponding Stimuli Rather Than Elicit Endogenous Slow Negativities.** If a neuronal population for a certain stimulus feature in the sensory projection system is facilitated, why should this facilitation cause a slow negativity, an entirely new component, in response to the corresponding stimulus rather than an enhancement of the

obligatory, much faster, components (Hillyard & Mangun, 1986; Näätänen, 1986e)? Unlike the exogenous components, those slower shifts do not represent typical responses of the afferent neuronal populations involved; these types of responses are not elicited by visual stimuli without an attention-demanding task (Näätänen, 1986e).

2. **Onset Latencies of the Selection Negativities Are Too Long.** Harter and Aine (1984) assumed that the onset latency of a selection negativity (that is, Nd onset) indicates the moment at which the corresponding feature analysis is initiated. This implicates, among other things, that the different attributes of visual percepts would emerge rather late. Moreover, in this case, it might be somewhat problematic to find a role for all the shorter-latency activity in the central visual projection system.

3. **The Onset Latency of a Selection Negativity Depends on Discriminability.** It is unlikely that the onset latency of a selection negativity indicates the moment of initiation of the corresponding feature analysis, insofar as the onset latency of this *difference* negativity (Nd) depends strictly on the physical difference between relevant and irrelevant stimuli (Hillyard & Mangun, 1986; Näätänen, 1986e). Larger differences are associated with earlier onsets of the selection negativity (Hillyard & Münte, 1984; see also Hansen & Hillyard, 1980). As already discussed (Section 6.2), this result can be accounted for by the fact that even to-be-ignored stimuli elicit some attentional negativity, with the same onset latency as that elicited by to-be-attended stimuli, which is larger and/or lasts longer for smaller physical separations (Section 6.2). Thus, the early attentional negativity common to attended and ignored stimuli is subtracted out from the difference negativity (Nd). Consequently, contrary to the neural-specificity theory, the onset of the selection negativity does not indicate the *onset* of processing of the stimulus feature in question (see also Harter & Aine, 1986).

Moreover, for the same reason, the onsets of the different feature-analysis processes cannot be arranged in a strict temporal order on the basis of the onset latencies of the different selection negativities. As noted earlier, Hillyard and Münte (1984) showed that with a large spatial separation the ERP signs of spatial selection preceded those of color selection but did not when spatial separation was small (see also Hillyard & Mangun, 1986).

4. **The Theory Cannot Explain ERP Data on Multidimensional Selective Attention.** As already reviewed, in several visual (Hillyard & Münte, 1984; Previc & Harter, 1982; Wijers, Lamain, et al., 1989) and auditory (Section 6.2) studies defining the relevant stimulus by two attributes, processing of the "more difficult" attribute was prematurely terminated when the "easier" attribute did not match with the relevant stimulus. This cannot be readily accounted for by the neural-specificity theory, which predicts that the processing system of even the more difficult attribute should generate a

selection negativity that is similar irrespective of whether the stimulus corresponds to the relevant stimulus in the "easier" attribute or not.

5. **The Distinction to the TectoPulvinar and GeniculoStriate Processing Systems of Visual Selective Attention Proposed by the Theory is Not Supported by Topographical Data.** The scalp distribution of the selection negativities provides no clear support to this distinction (Hillyard & Mangun, 1986):

> We do not feel that the available scalp data fit neatly into the scheme of separate tectopulvinar-parietal and geniculostriate-inferotemporal systems for inter- and intralocation selections, respectively. Instead, we think that present evidence tends to favor a geniculostriate participation in both inter- and intralocation selections, although the inherent limitations of scalp data for inferring generator locations makes this conclusion somewhat speculative. In line with this view are the recent findings of Moran and Desimone (1985) that the activity of neurons in the geniculostriate-inferotemporal projection (i.e. extrastriate regions V4 and the inferotemporal cortex) are modulated during spatial selective attention. (p. 276)

The foregoing criticism of the neural-specificity theory by Hillyard and Mangun (1986) and Näätänen (1986e) was responded to by Harter and Aine (1986). For a useful discussion on the neural-specificity theory, see Wijers (1989), who succeeded, perhaps better than the aforementioned authors, in pointing out the strong aspects of this influential theory. Wijers (1989) concluded that: "in vision, the type of selection cue appears a more important factor in selective attention than discriminability" (p. 232).

6.4 SELECTIVE ATTENTION AND SOMATOSENSORY ERPS

Desmedt, with his group, pioneered research on ERP effects of selective attention in the somatosensory modality. In one of the early studies, Desmedt and Robertson (1977) presented electrical stimuli equiprobably to four fingers (the second and third finger of each hand) with 400-msec mean ISIs. The subject was instructed to count silently target-finger stimuli and to ignore the other stimuli.

It was found that attention enhanced the amplitude of the negative deflection peaking at about 140–150 msec called the N140, whereas the early components (N20 and P45) were not affected (Fig. 6.49). The N140 enhancement occurred for both the target and nontarget (adjacent) fingers, whereas a late positivity peaking at about 400 msec was only found in the target-finger ERPs. The N140 enhancement was larger, and its onset latency

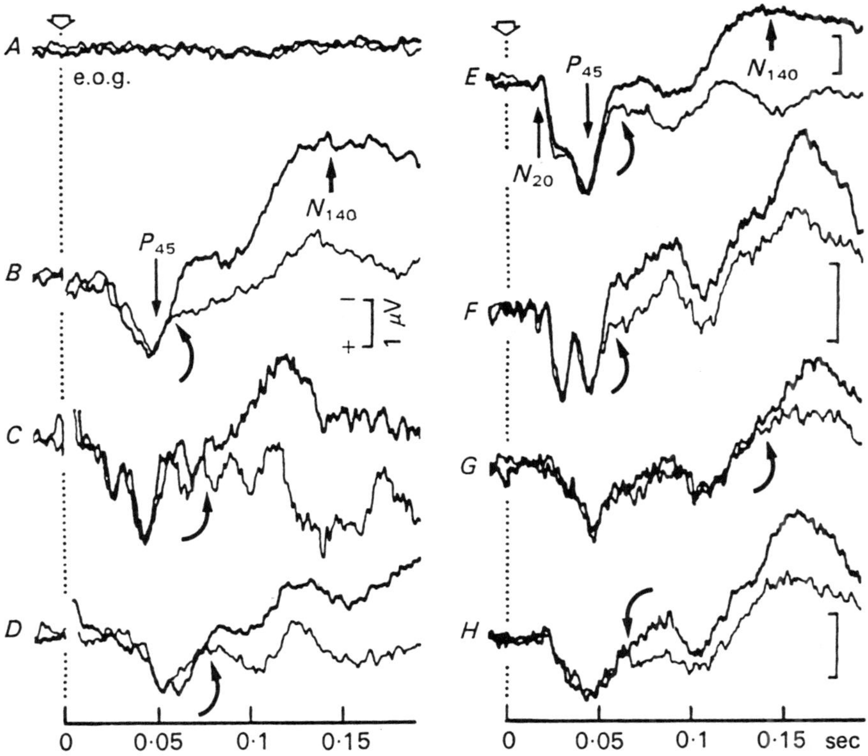

FIG. 6.49 Somatosensory ERPS of individual subjects to identical finger stimuli when this finger was attended (thicker trace) or when the subject attended either target clicks in B-D (overall delivery rate of clicks and shocks 40/min) or, in other experiments, target-finger stimuli in the opposite hand in E-H (overall delivery rate of shocks to four fingers 130/min). The curved arrows point to the divergence of the two traces. Data of 6 different subjects are illustrated. Records G and H from the same subject represent somatosensory ERPs to stimulation of the second finger of either the right (G) or the left (H) hand. Calibration 1 μV. (From Desmedt & Robertson, 1977. Reprinted with the permission of The Physiological Society.)

shorter, at the contralateral parietal electrode (where the primary components were present) than at the ipsilateral electrode. The mean onset latency of the N140 enhancement was 78 msec, but the effect occasionally began as early as at 55 msec, almost 100 msec before the N140 peak.

Figure 6.49 suggests that the N140 enhancement is a part of a long-duration negative displacement of ERPs for attended stimuli relative to those for unattended stimuli, which may begin as early as at 55 msec and persist beyond 200 msec. This negativity, resembling typical auditory attention effects at the N1 latency zone, therefore appears to be a somatosensory PN (Näätänen & Michie, 1979a).

In a small number of subjects, target stimuli did not elicit this negativity but instead an increased positivity with a peak latency of approximately 100 msec. Desmedt and Robertson (1977) suggested that this "P100 enhancement" to targets may represent a major individual difference in brain electrogenesis in processing of target and non-target stimuli.

In achieving their N140 attention effect, the authors pointed, among other things, to the rapid stimulus rate. That the effect indeed cannot be produced with slow stimulus rates was shown by Desmedt, Robertson, Brunko, and Debecker (1977), who delivered stimuli at random intervals between 500 and 4000 msec (mean 1500 msec). The task and procedure were otherwise quite similar to those of Desmedt and Robertson (1977). No systematic N140 attention effect was observed at this slower stimulus rate, although a clear P400 was elicited by target stimuli. The P400, though a smaller one, was also elicited by nontarget stimuli, especially by those delivered to the "attended hand," in the strong-intensity condition.

With such a slow stimulus rate, the negative attentional displacement of the somatosensory ERP occurs, however, in intermodal tasks. Desmedt and Robertson's (1977) subjects received, in one of the conditions, electrical shocks to either one of two adjacent fingers of one hand and binaural clicks in random order, and were instructed to respond either to shock stimuli given on a designated finger or to clicks of a slightly different intensity. The negative attention effect to stimuli in the attended modality was found even though the mean ISI was as long as 1500 msec. Moreover, the onset latency of the negative attention effect for target-finger stimuli was much the same as in Desmedt and Robertson's (1977) comparable intramodal task with much shorter ISIs (mean 400 msec).

Subsequent studies have considerably altered the picture of attention effects on the somatosensory ERP by demonstrating (a) very early attention effects that may be of exogenous nature and (b) endogenous attention effects that appear in the form of slow positivities rather than negativities. In one of these studies, Josiassen, Shagass, Roemer, Ercegovac, and Straumanis (1982) demonstrated a "P45" attention effect, an effect on a positivity peaking at about 45 msec from stimulus onset. These authors delivered shock stimuli in random order to four fingers, two adjacent ones in each hand, the mean ISI being as long as 2.8 sec. Stimuli delivered to a designated finger were to be counted. In addition to the P45 enhancement, counting also increased the P100, P190, N230, and P400 amplitudes. Whereas the P45, P100, and P190 effects were also observed in response to the finger adjacent to the target finger, the late P400 effect (and possibly the N230 effect) was limited to the target finger.

Michie (1984), however, using a somewhat similar paradigm but with considerably shorter ISIs and occasional infrequent stimuli within each stimulus channel, obtained no earlier attention effects than a slow negative displacement that commenced between the N1 and P2 peak latencies. This effect, interpreted in terms of a somatosensory PN, was larger contra- than ipsilaterally to the "attended hand," and larger for targets than standards delivered to this hand. Conversely, Michie, Bearpark, Crawford, and Glue (1987) found no clear attentional negativity but rather a slow positivity. A short-duration PN preceding this slow positivity might have been present in their data, however.

Papanicolaou, Moore, and Gary (1989) also failed to observe any very early selective-attention effects in the somatosensory modality. Desmedt, Nguyen, and Bourguet (1983), however, reported such effects, the "cognitive P40" over the contralateral parietal area between about 25–45 msec from stimulus onset, and the "cognitive N60" over the contralateral prerolandic region at a somewhat longer latency. (N20, the earliest cortical response to somatosensory stimuli [Desmedt & Cheron, 1981], and P22 were not affected.) However, because the to-be-attended stimuli of this study were also infrequent stimuli, the early effects reported might be, at least in part, due to the low stimulus probability.

Desmedt and Tomberg (1989), however, seem to have succeeded in demonstrating that the P40 effect is indeed associated with selective attention. In addition, they described a still earlier positive attention effect, the "cognitive P30," which was also parietal but could be dissociated from the P40 effect. Some of these data are illustrated in Fig. 6.50. On the basis of topographical evidence, the authors suggested that both effects are due to enhancements of exogenous components at these latencies, rather than to an elicitation of endogenous components.

The authors observe that the processes generating the P30 effect were initiated only a few milliseconds after the arrival of the somatosensory volley in the parietal cortex, as indexed by the N20 exogenous component generated in area 3B of somatosensory primary cortex (Desmedt & Cheron, 1981). The authors concluded that "the cognitive P30 and P40 reflect selective attention-related enhancements of the neural generators in receiving somatosensory cortex" (Desmedt & Tomberg, 1989, p. 321). These early attention effects were followed by P100 and N140 effects.

The very early onset of an attention effect of positive polarity in the somatosensory modality was very recently confirmed by García-Larrea, Bastuji, and Mauguière (1991). On the basis of their topographical evidence, these authors interpreted the effect as an attentional enhancement of an exogenous type of early component.

In conclusion, selective attention appears to enhance early, or relatively early, exogenous components of the somatosensory ERP under some conditions. Even the earliest of the effects observed, however, occurred later than the earliest stimulus effects in the contralateral receiving cortex, therefore providing no evidence for subcortical attentional modulation of

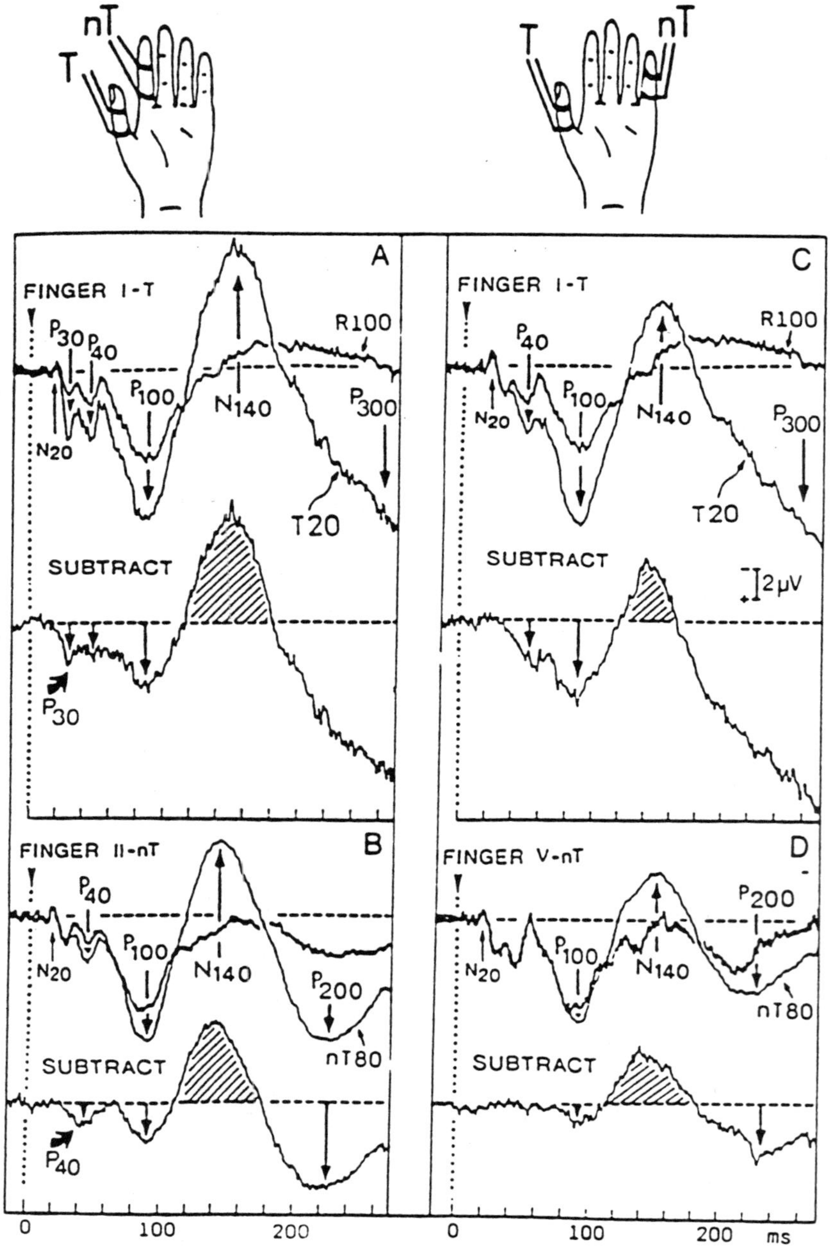
T
nT
A
FINGER I-T
R100
P30
P40
P100
N140
P300
N20
T20
SUBTRACT
P30
B
FINGER II-nT
P40
P100
N140
P200
N20
nT80
SUBTRACT
P40
C
FINGER I-T
R100
P40
P100
N140
P300
N20
T20
SUBTRACT
2 μV
D
FINGER V-nT
P200
P100
N140
N20
nT80
SUBTRACT
0
100
200
ms

FIG. 6.50

the afferent inflow in somesthesis. Some slower attention effects also occur, but it is not clear whether these effects are of exogenous/endogenous nature. An enhancement of the somatosensory analogue of the auditory (supratemporal) N1 might be among these later effects. Some clearly endogenous effects have also been observed. These have emerged in the form of either slow negativities (somatosensory processing negativities; cf. García-Larrea et al., 1991; Michie, 1984) or similar slow positivities (Michie et al., 1987).

6.5. ERPS AND RESOURCE THEORIES OF ATTENTION

ERPs, initially the N1 wave and subsequently the P3 wave, have been used for testing resource- or capacity-allocation theories of attention such as those proposed by Kahneman (1973), Kantowitz and Knight (1976), Norman and Bobrow (1975), and Wickens (1980, 1984). As already reviewed in Section 2.4, these models assume that processing resources are limited in quantity and can be shared between concurrently performed tasks. More recent formulations of such theories tend to emphasize the existence of different kinds of resources rather than just one resource pool; they hold that different processing units have their own supply of resources that can be shared between several ongoing cognitive operations (Kinsbourne & Hicks, 1978; Navon & Gopher, 1979; Sanders, 1983; Wickens, 1980) (see Section 2.4).

Hink, van Voorhis, Hillyard, and Smith (1977) were, apparently, the first to investigate the limited-resource notion with ERPs. The dichotic-listening paradigm was used. In their divided-attention condition, the subject was requested to search for targets in both ears at the same time. In the focused-attention condition, targets were searched in the input to a designated ear.

It was found that the divided-attention N1 was halfway in amplitude

---

FIG. 6.50 Effects of difficulty of discrimination task on somatosensory ERPs from parietal scalp contralateral to hand stimulated in an individual subject. Left thumb received T-20 (targets, probability .20) throughout. nT-80 stimuli (non-targets, probability .80) were delivered either to the left index finger (A + B; a difficult discrimination task) or to the left fifth finger (C + D; an easy discrimination task). r100 denotes ERPs recorded in response to repetition (100%) of the nT-80 stimulus while the subject was reading. The two upper "SUBTRACT" curves indicate difference waves obtained by subtracting the r100 response from that elicited by targets (T) in the difficult (nontargets to the adjacent finger; left) and in the easy (nontargets to the most distant finger; right) discrimination task. The two lower "SUBTRACT" curves indicate the respective difference waves for the two nontargets. (From Desmedt & Tomberg, 1989. Copyright © 1989 by Elsevier Science Publishers, Ireland. Reprinted with permission.)

between the N1s to attended and ignored stimuli in focused attention. Further, the total N1 output was larger in these active conditions than in a passive, control condition. Hink et al. (1977) suggested that "the amplitude of the N1 wave reflects the relative distribution of attention among competing input channels . . . If N1 amplitude is an index of the amount of processing resources committed to a channel, then Kahneman's capacity model would predict the observed pattern of data" (p. 603). Corroborating results were obtained by Parasuraman (1978).

It is somewhat difficult to evaluate these results, because both studies measured attention effects as possible changes in the "exogenous N1 component." (See also Näätänen & Michie, 1979a.) Also, an inherent problem in these studies using short ISIs might be the resolution of the slow attentional negativity probably emerging under these conditions (Näätänen, 1988a; see also Woldorff, in press). During divided attention, all stimuli being relevant, this negativity may still be resolving at the onset of the next stimulus and might therefore cancel some of the negativity that this stimulus elicits. With focused attention, the situation is different. In the case of two equiprobable stimulus categories, for example, only a half of that resolution would cancel attentional negativity, insofar as that resolution overlaps in time with the ERP to relevant stimuli only on a half of the trials (see also Näätänen, 1975).

More recently, the P3 wave has been employed as a physiological measure in testing different formulations of resource-allocation theories of attention. The results of these studies, initiated by Donchin and his colleagues (for reviews, see Donchin, Kramer, & Wickens, 1986; Gopher & Donchin, 1986; Kramer & Spinks, 1991), seem, in general, to support the P3 amplitude as a measure of limited-capacity perceptual or perceptual-cognitive resources and therefore this type of attention theory.

The central idea was to use the amplitude of P3 elicited by secondary-task deviants (targets) as an inverted measure of capacity allocated to the primary task. This was based on the well-established finding that the elicitation of P3 by deviants in an oddball paradigm depends on attention (Donchin et al., 1978; see Section 6.1.). It was therefore assumed that the P3 amplitude in a secondary task would gradually attenuate as more and more resources are allocated to the primary task, and vice versa. The oddball task appeared to provide a nonintrusive secondary task, inasmuch as the target tones occur relatively infrequently, are easily discriminable, and do not require an overt response. Another advantage would be that the oddball task could be inserted into virtually any operational setting without requiring modifications in the system associated with the primary task (Gopher & Donchin, 1986).

This approach is illustrated by Wickens, Isreal, and Donchin (1977), who used a tracking task as the primary task. The subject was instructed to cancel computer-generated cursor movements (with a joystick), so that the cursor remained superimposed on a target in the center of a CRT display. The difficulty of this primary task was varied by requiring the subject to track in either one or two dimensions (horizontal and/or vertical). In addition to the tracking, subjects were also instructed to count occasional pitch-deviant tones in a concurrent tone sequence (the secondary task).

It was found that the introduction of the tracking task drastically diminished the P3 amplitude to the pitch-deviant tones. However, the P3 amplitude was not further reduced as tracking difficulty increased by requiring tracking to be performed in two dimensions rather than only in one.

Isreal, Chesney, Wickens, and Donchin (1980) also required subjects to perform a compensatory tracking task concurrently with a counting task but manipulated task difficulty by varying the bandwidth of the random forcing function rather than the number of dimensions of the tracking task. With the increase in bandwidth, the tracking task became progressively more demanding. The bandwidth was gradually increased until the cursor's speed reached the highest level the subject could tolerate without exceeding a preset error criterion.

Again, the P3 amplitude was diminished by the introduction of the tracking task, but increases in the bandwidth did not further diminish this amplitude. According to Gopher and Donchin (1986), "these results cannot be explained easily within the framework of an undifferentiated-capacity theory if we assume that P300 amplitude indexes the demands placed on the subject by the primary task" (p. 41–36).

The results can, however, be accounted for by the multiple-resource theory reviewed in Section 2.4. If the manipulation of the dimensionality and bandwidth of the tracking task affects the need of resources associated largely with response selection and execution processes, then the P300 amplitude should not be affected because it is mainly determined by relatively early stimulus-evaluation processes (Gopher & Donchin, 1986). On the other hand, if the perceptual demands of a task were manipulated, then the P3 amplitude of the secondary task should covary with primary-task difficulty.

This hypothesis was tested by Isreal, Wickens, Chesney, and Donchin (1980) by combining the oddball secondary task (either with RT or counting instructions) with visual monitoring as the primary task in which subjects monitored a simulated air-traffic control display for course changes. The difficulty of the primary task was increased by increasing the number of elements on the display.

It was found that the RT in the secondary task monotonically increased from the control condition to the condition in which subjects were monitoring eight elements simultaneously for course changes.

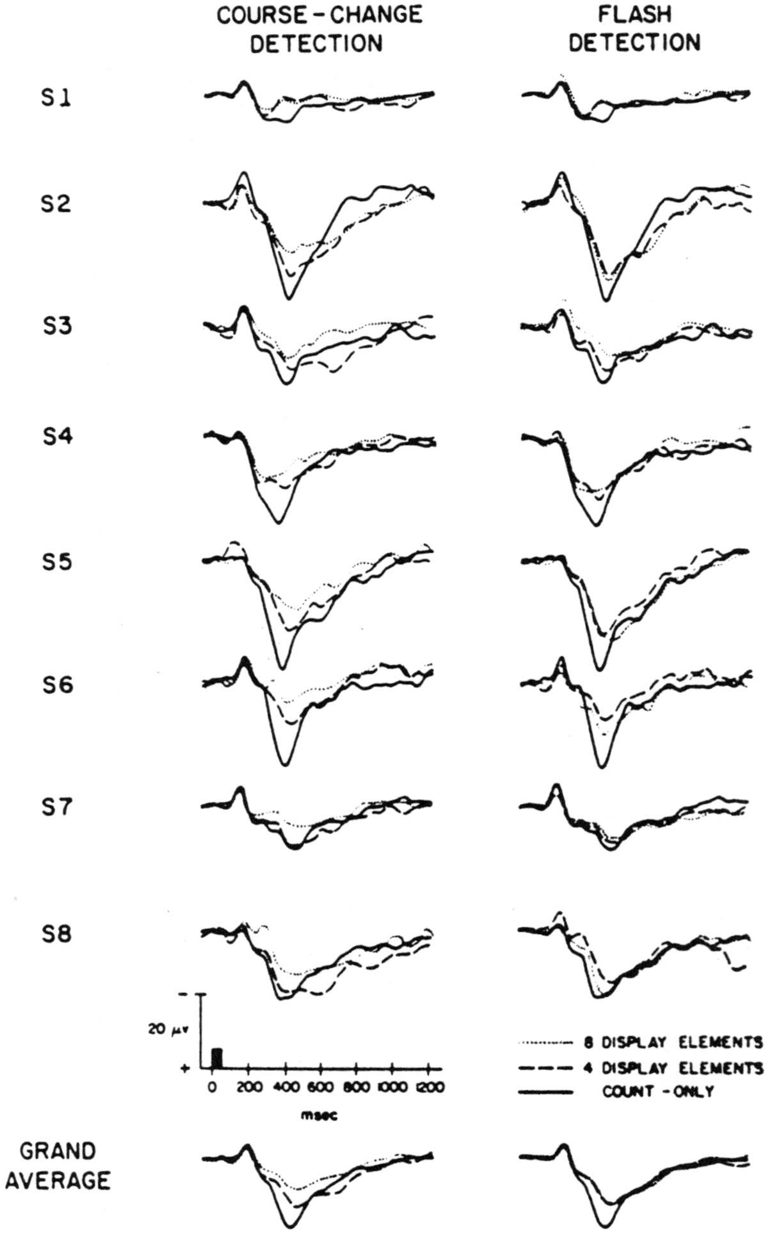
COURSE - CHANGE DETECTION
FLASH DETECTION
S1
S2
S3
S4
S5
S6
S7
S8
20 µv
0 200 400 600 800 1000 1200
msec
8 DISPLAY ELEMENTS
4 DISPLAY ELEMENTS
COUNT - ONLY
GRAND AVERAGE

In addition, as shown in Fig. 6.51, the P3 amplitude for counted infrequent tones of the secondary task was attenuated with the introduction of the course-change detection task and was further decreased with the number of elements displayed in the latter task.

These data were interpreted as suggesting that the P3 amplitude of the secondary task is sensitive to the perceptual demands of the primary task. Corroborating results were provided by Kramer et al. (1986), Kramer, Sirevaag, and Braune (1987), Kramer, Sirevaag, and Hughes (1988), Kramer and Strayer (1988), Kramer, Wickens, and Donchin (1983), Kramer, Wickens, and Donchin (1985), and Wickens, Mountford, and Schneider (1981).

P300 and Resource Reciprocity. The studies reviewed herein have demonstrated that the secondary-task P3 decreases in amplitude with increases in the perceptual/central processing difficulty or resource demand of the primary task. Thus, within the framework of the resource theory, this result is taken as indicating that there is a reciprocal relationship between the resources allocated to the primary and secondary tasks. If this interpretation is correct, then the amplitude of P3 elicited by task-relevant discrete events embedded within the primary task should be enhanced with increasing primary-task difficulty.

This prediction was confirmed by Kramer, Wickens, Vanasse, and Donchin (1981; see also Hoffman et al., 1985; Horst, Munson, & Ruchkin, 1984; Kramer et al., 1985; Sirevaag, Kramer, Coles, & Donchin, 1984; Wickens et al., 1983). These authors found that P3 elicited by task-relevant events embedded within a tracking task increased in amplitude as this task was made more demanding. Donchin et al. (1986) regarded this result as "particularly encouraging to the utility of the ERP as a measure of workload in extra-laboratory environments" (p. 716), because, according to them, the P3-eliciting oddball task as a secondary task cannot be regarded as entirely unobtrusive.

FIG. 6.51 Parietal (Pz) ERPs of 8 individual subjects (S1-S8) and the corresponding grand-averaged ERPs (bottom) to occasional, counted higher-pitched tones in a sequence of lower-pitched tones (a secondary task) when the subjects were monitoring a display in which numerous targets were moving (primary task). On occasion, one of the targets could briefly intensify. On other occasions, the target could change course. Task difficulty was varied by varying the number of elements in the monitored display. Note that when the subjects only performing the counting task (solid lines) started to monitor the display for course changes, the P300 amplitude was reduced (dashed lines). The amplitude was further reduced when the number of elements in the display was increased (dotted lines). The effect was specific to the course-detection task (the left panel). When the subject was monitoring the display for flashes (the right panel), the effect was much diminished. (From Isreal, Wickens, Chesney, & Donchin, 1980. Copyright © 1980 by The Human Factors Society, Inc. Reprinted with permission.)

Hoffman et al. (1985) combined consistent-mapping search task with a discrimination task and varied the relative importance of each task. They reported that the P3 amplitude in each task was a function of "the relative amount of attention allocated to that task," and that this trade-off in the P3 amplitude was closely related to the accuracy in performing that task. Reductions in the P3 amplitude resulted in linear reductions in accuracy (d'), and the same linear relationship between d' and the P3 amplitude held for both tasks, "further confirming the presence of a single resource required by both tasks. This resource clearly plays a pivotal role in the accuracy of performance" (Hoffman et al., 1985, pp. 59–60).

Basically similar results, although with the visual P1 component, were obtained by Mangun and Hillyard (1990b), reviewed in Section 6.3 (Figs. 6.42 and 6.43).

Strayer and Kramer (1990), in their dual-task study discussed in Section 4.7, also found evidence for the reciprocity of allocation of attention. In different conditions, subjects were instructed to maximize their performance on either the Sternberg memory search or the recognition running-memory task, or to perform as well as possible simultaneously in both tasks. Stimuli belonging to each task were presented in an alternating order at constant ISIs of about 1.5 sec.

Processing priority, as defined by instructions, was found to have a large effect on performance and the P3 amplitude when the variable-mapping condition of the memory-search task was paired with the running-memory task. Thus, when the running-memory task was heavily emphasized, the memory-search performance was poor, and only small P3s were elicited by stimuli belonging to the latter task. In contrast, as already reviewed (Section 4.7), when the consistent-mapping version of the memory-search task was paired with the running-memory task, the memory-search performance was relatively unaffected by task priority. In addition, large P3s were elicited in the memory-search task that were insensitive to task priority. These P3s were interpreted by Strayer and Kramer (1990) as reflecting an obligatory allocation of attention to the consistent-mapping probes (see Section 2.2).

In conclusion, the studies reviewed herein appear to support the conceptualization of attention in terms of allocatable and sharable limited resources (Wickens, 1980; Section 2.4)—before automaticity has developed so far as to override the subject's attentional control, of course.

7

MEG Studies of Attention

7.1. MEG EFFECTS OF AUDITORY ATTENTION

The MEG methodology has, quite recently, also been applied in research of brain mechanisms of attention. Most of these studies have addressed the persistent issue of the possible selective-attention enhancement of the exogenous N1 in audition—in this case, its supratemporal component visible to the MEG. It was hoped that, due to the better localizability of (certain) cerebral sources with magnetic than electric measurements (chapters 3 and 5), one could determine whether or not the selective-attention effect and the supratemporal component of N1 emanate from the same locus in the auditory cortex. In addition, MEG studies have also tried to clarify the issue of the attentional sensitivity/insensitivity of MMN, the advantage being that N2b usually overlapping MMN in electrical recordings is not visible in the MEG.

To start with the studies mentioned most recently, Kaukoranta et al. (1989) and Lounasmaa, Hari, Joutsiniemi, and Hämäläinen (1989) recorded MEG responses in the oddball paradigm by comparing MMNm to deviant stimuli in attend and ignore conditions. (For effects of attention on ERPs recorded in the oddball paradigm, see Sections 4.4. and 6.1.) Kaukoranta et al. (1989) investigated MEG responses to duration decrements and Lounasmaa et al. (1989) to intensity decrements. Both studies found a very similar MMNm under target-discrimination and reading conditions, providing evidence for attentional insensitivity of MMN in the oddball paradigm. For an illustration of these results, see Fig. 7.1.

Kaufman and Williamson (1987, 1988) and Curtis, Kaufman, and

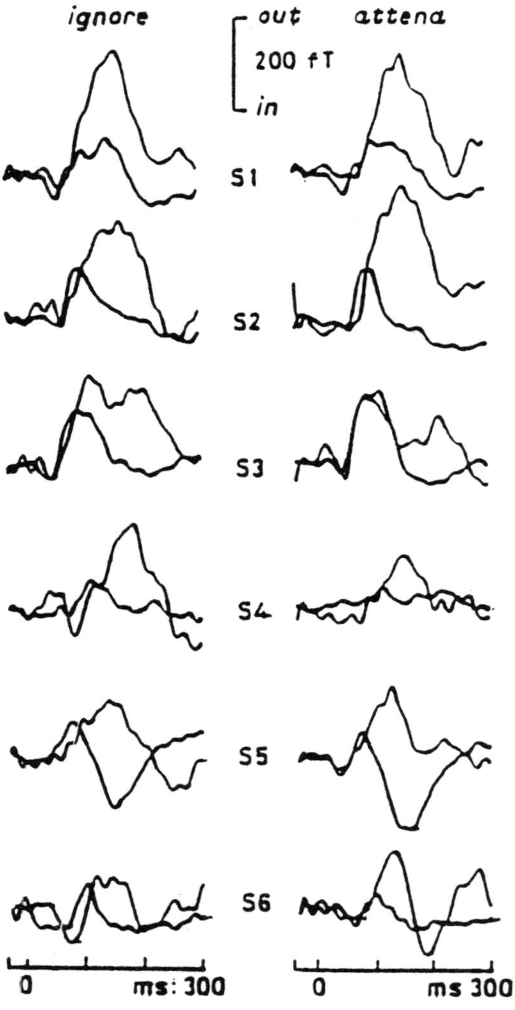

FIG. 7.1 Magnetoencephalographic (MEG) responses of six individual subjects (S1-S6) to standard (thick lines) and deviant (thin lines) tones when the subject either ignored the stimuli by reading (left) or was paying attention to them by counting the deviants (right). The recordings are from the anterior field extremum over the right temple. (Unpublished figure from Kaukoranta, Sams, Hari, Hämäläinen, & Näätänen, 1989.)

Williamson (1988) were the first to report MEG responses during selective attention. These authors interpreted their results, obtained with dichotic stimuli delivered at a very fast rate, as evidence for an attentional modulation of the exogenous N1 and P2 components. A close examination of their data, however, suggests that these effects might in fact be endogenous, for the peak latencies and durations of the attend N1m and

P2m tend to be longer than those in response to ignored stimuli (Fig. 7.2). Curtis et al. (1988), however, presented some evidence for a very similar locus of generation of the attention effect and the exogenous N1m and P2m components.

Curtis et al. (1988) also reported a MEG attention effect with a monaural presentation of relevant and irrelevant tone bursts differing in pitch. This effect was comparable to that found in their dichotic conditions.

Arthur, Hillyard, Flynn, and Smidt (1989) and Hari, Hämäläinen,

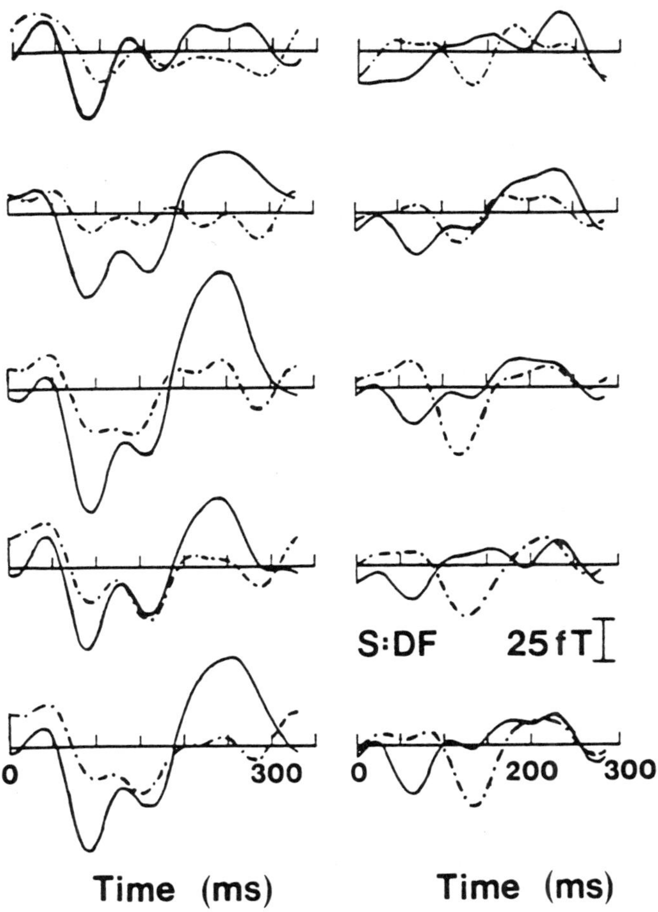

FIG. 7.2 Magnetoencephalographic (MEG) responses of an individual subject recorded over the anterior extremum of the left hemisphere for the sequences of tones presented at 3 Hz (left) and at 3.5 Hz (right). The solid tracings show responses when the 3-Hz sequence was attended, and the dashed tracings when the 3.5-Hz sequence was attended. The 5 pairs of waveforms in each column are the responses simultaneously recorded by the individual sensors of the probe. (From Kaufman & Williamson, 1987. Copyright © 1987 by Butterworths. Reprinted with permission.)

Kaukoranta, Mäkelä, Joutsiniemi, and Tiihonen (1989) reported the first MEG analogue of Nd (Ndm). Arthur and her colleagues used a dichotic paradigm with short, random ISIs varying from 200 to 400 msec. They found an MEG attention effect over the left temporal cortex that occurred in two consecutive phases. The first phase coincided with N1m peaking at 120–150 msec from stimulus onset, whereas the second phase appeared as a slow, protracted displacement in the latency range of 200–500 msec. Simultaneously recorded electric responses were essentially identical in waveform.

The equivalent current dipole for the late MEG attention effect clearly differed from that for N1m to unattended stimuli. For the early attention effect, however, in five out of six observations, the equivalent current dipole could not be statistically significantly distinguished from the equivalent current dipole for N1m elicited by unattended stimuli. (For very recent corroborating results, see Rif, Hari, Hämäläinen, & Sams, 1991.) Arthur et al. (1989), however, observed a tendency for the early Ndm centroid "to be slightly shifted (1 cm or less) from the N1m centroid" (p. 115).

Arthur et al. (1991) presented their stimuli dichotically at rather long, constant ISIs of 800 msec, as did Näätänen et al. (1978). The MEG selective-attention effect was a slow displacement of the attended-stimulus response relative to that to ignored stimuli, corresponding to ERP findings in similar conditions (Section 6.2). Magnetic resonance imaging (MRI) showed that the equivalent current dipoles for both N1m and Ndm were located in auditory cortex along the posterior regions of the Sylvian fissure. Error estimates based on the "Monte Carlo method" (Medvick, Lewis, Aine, & Flynn, 1989) indicated that the equivalent current dipole for Ndm is near but significantly anterior to that for N1m. Because of the long latency of their MEG attention effect (approximately 150 msec), the authors proposed that the ERP equivalent of the effect might be the late rather than the early PN component.

Hari, Hämäläinen, Kaukoranta, Mäkelä, Joutsiniemi, and Tiihonen (1989), too, found a slow, protracted MEG attention effect in their dichotic study with rather long (1 sec), constant ISIs (Fig. 7.3). The field pattern of the effect suggested that it originated from supratemporal auditory cortex. It remained unclear, however, whether the attention effect and the supratemporal N1m component were generated from the same or adjacent loci, but Arthur et al.'s (1991) and Rif et al.'s (1991) very recent results seem to indicate that these loci are different when ISIs are not very short.

The results of Hari and her colleagues are illustrated in Fig. 7.3. Interestingly, even the to-be-ignored stimuli elicited some "magnetic PN," judging from a comparison of these responses with those elicited by identical stimuli in a reading condition. This irrelevant-stimulus Ndm is, however, shorter in duration and lower in amplitude than Ndm for the relevant stimulus. This data pattern consequently provides converging

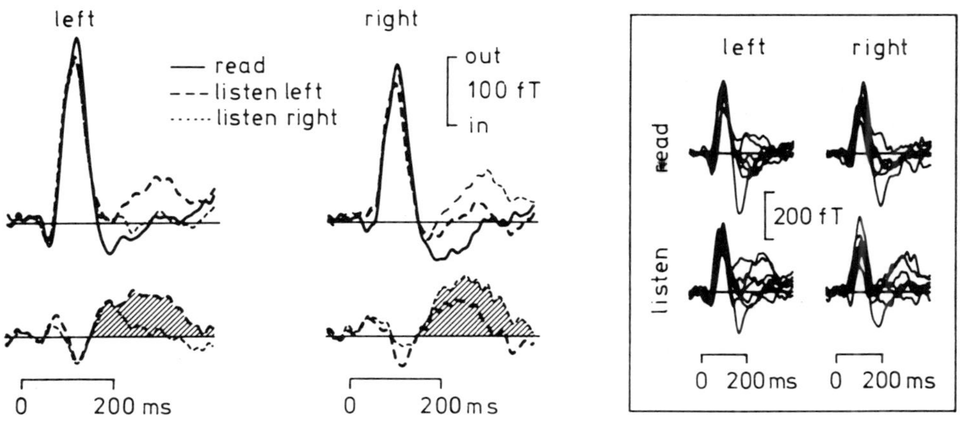

FIG. 7.3 Grand-average magnetoencephalographic (MEG) responses recorded over the right fronto-temporal area to the left- and right-ear tone pips when the subject was either reading (Read) or counting (Listen left and Listen right) the stimuli. The difference curves (Listen-Read) are shown below the grand averages; the shadowed areas illustrate the magnetic counterpart of the "processing negativity" (the whole shadowed area for counted stimuli and the early part of the shadowed area for uncounted stimuli while the subject was counting stimuli presented to the opposite ear). The insert on the right shows the individual waveforms for 7 subjects. (From Hari et al., 1989. Copyright © 1989 by Springer-Verlag. Reprinted with permission.)

evidence for one of the basic claims of the attentional-trace theory that even irrelevant stimuli elicit some PN during selective attention (Section 6.2).

7.2. MEG EFFECTS OF VISUAL ATTENTION

Luber, Kaufman, and Williamson (1989) employed a paradigm that closely resembled those used in ERP studies of visual-spatial selective attention (Section 6.3). These authors presented their stimuli in random order either 5° to the left or 5° to the right of a central fixation cross with irregular ISIs (mean 1100 msec). The subject was instructed to maintain his or her gaze throughout the block on a fixation cross and to attend to a designated visual field in order to detect an occasional, somewhat different pattern.

It was found that selective attention modulated MEG responses (both to standards and targets) but, more notably, not earlier than until about 150–210 msec after stimulus onset, well after the first major component of the response. This attention effect was consequently quite late in comparison with the P1 effects of visual-spatial attention in ERP studies (Section 6.3). However, a small attention effect at a latency corresponding to that of the P1 effect in electrical recordings might be present in their occipital data (see their Fig. 1).

Aine, George, Oakley, Medvick, and Flynn (1990) found distinct MEG effects of visual-spatial attention that occurred at a latency comparable to ERP effects recorded in the same study and in previous studies (Section 6.3). These MEG effects appeared as an attentional enhancement of activity recorded contralaterally to the stimulus between 100–130 msec and ipsilaterally between 120–160 msec. These data are illustrated in Figs. 7.4 and 7.5. Equivalent current dipoles for attend and non-attend responses calcu-

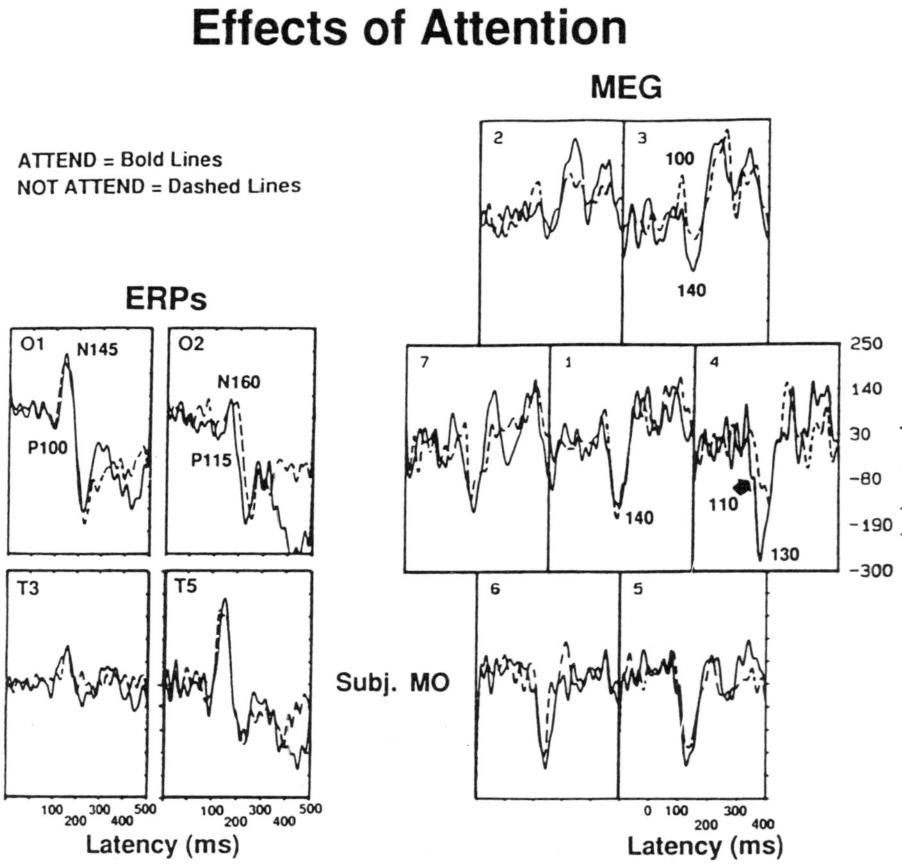

FIG. 7.4 ERP (left) and MEG (right) waveforms for one subject in response to a grating stimulus presented 2 degrees in the lower right quadrant when the stimulus was attended (bold lines) and when it was not attended (dashed lines), the target stimulus being located in the lower left quadrant. ERPs were recorded from occipital (O1 and O2) and temporal (T3 and T5) regions. MEG waveforms were recorded over left occipital cortex. (From Aine, George, Oakley, Medvick, & Flynn, 1990. Copyright © 1990 by Tilburg University Press. Reprinted with permission.)

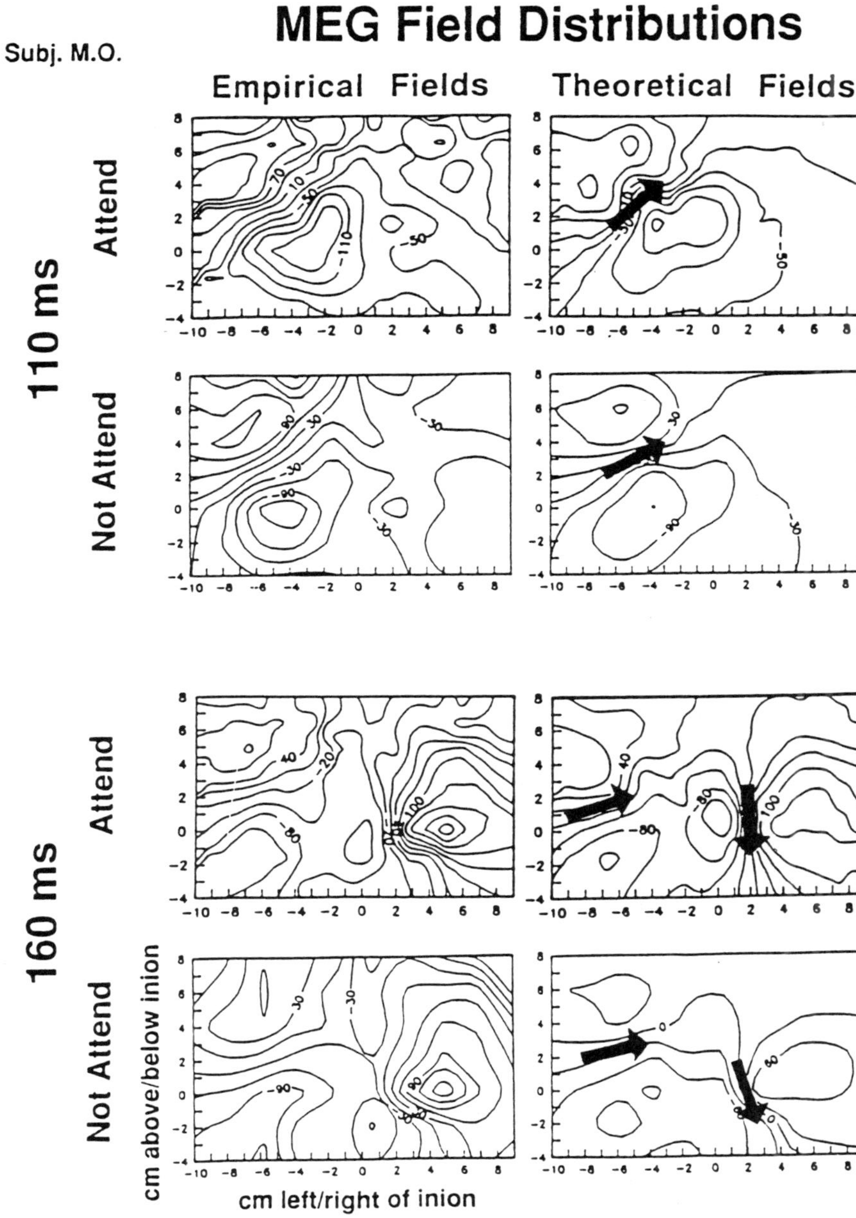

FIG. 7.5 *Left:* MEG field distributions at latencies of 110 msec (top) and 160 msec (bottom) for the right visual-field stimulus when it was attended versus not attended for the subject whose data are presented in Fig. 7.4. The origin ($x = 0$, $y = 0$) of these head-surface maps is at the inion. *Right:* Corresponding theoretical field distributions derived using the parameters of the best-fitting equivalent current dipole (ECD) model. (From Aine, George, Oakley, Medvick, & Flynn, 1990. Copyright © 1990 by Tilburg University Press. Reprinted with permission.)

lated for this interval were very similar with regard to the location and orientation parameters, whereas the dipole strength was considerably greater for attend responses. The authors therefore concluded that selective attention enhances responses of neuronal populations that normally respond to specific types of afferent information, thus supporting gain theories of visual-spatial attention such as that of Harter and Aine (1984) (see section 6.3).

8

Regional Cerebral Blood-Flow (rCBF) and Metabolic Studies of Selective Attention

This chapter begins with the early studies on selective attention that used nontomographic rCBF methods (Section 3.6.). These methods permitted rCBF determination only at the cortical level. Related PET and SPECT work, which made it possible to measure rCBF and regional metabolic changes (PET) in the entire brain, is reviewed thereafter.

8.1. NONTOMOGRAPHIC rCBF MEASUREMENTS DURING ATTENTION

As discussed in Section 3.6., the regional distribution of the cerebral blood-flow during task performance indicates cerebral regions participating in task performance, because there is a monotonic relation between rCBF and regional energy metabolism.

The normal rCBF resting pattern is "hyperfrontal" (Ingvar, 1979). The prefrontal and frontal regions, as well as the posterior Sylvian region, appear to be relatively active, whereas the temporal, parietal, and postcentral Rolandic regions are less active. This resting hyperfrontal pattern is diffused during anaesthesia and spontaneous sleep (Ingvar, 1979).

The resting hyperfrontal rCBF pattern in a group of anxious patients (Johanson, 1991) is illustrated on the left side of Fig. 8.1. (A similar pattern can also be recorded with normal subjects.) The right side of the figure shows the rCBF pattern of the same patients during anxiety provocation. Increased anxiety caused no change in the hemispheric mean flow level but considerably modified the regional flow distribution, as shown by the difference map in the bottom of the figure. The principal change was an rCBF increase in the frontotemporal areas, especially in the fronto-orbital region of the left hemisphere. (See also Hagstadius, 1989; Johanson, Gustafson, & Risberg, 1986; Reiman, Fusselman, Fox, & Raichle, 1989.) It appears that the hyperfrontality of even the resting rCBF pattern (also in normal subjects) is, at least in part, due to stress and anxiety caused by the measurement situation (Johanson et al., 1986; Reivich, Gur, & Alavi, 1983; Risberg, Maximilian, & Prohovnik, 1977).

In an early study on task-specific rCBF, Risberg and Ingvar (1973) found that in problem solving using Raven matrices or a backward digit-span memory test, the flow increased in premotor and frontal regions. In addition, the Raven test, which involves visual input, activated parieto-

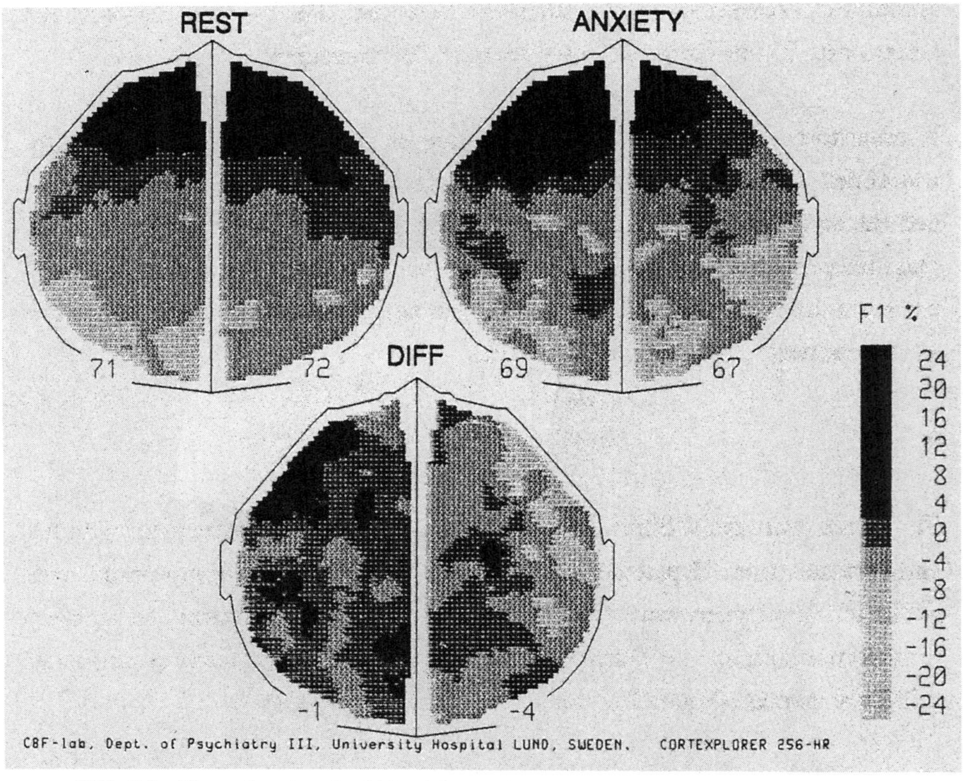

FIG. 8.1 The regional cerebral blood-flow (rCBF) distribution during rest (upper left) and anxiety (upper right). The bottom map shows the difference in rCBF between anxiety and rest. Regional values are given in percent of the hemispheric mean. In the scale to the right, the hemispheric mean is represented by the grey shade at point 0. (From Johanson, 1991. Reprinted with permission.)

occipital regions. Ingvar (1979) concluded that abstract thinking, memorizing, and problem solving especially involve frontal and parietal association cortices of the dominant hemisphere.

Somatosensory Attention. In his pioneering work on rCBF changes associated with attention, Roland (1981) measured rCBF in 254 cortical loci of the same hemisphere while the subject focused his or her attention on the tip of the index finger for a possible very weak touch stimulus. During focused attention of a period of 40 sec (no stimulus was actually given), the rCBF increased by 25% from resting state in the contralateral somatosensory finger area. This rCBF increase was somatotopical: The rCBF in the rest of the Rolandic strip was unaffected, though some somatosensory association areas were also activated. Smaller increases occurred in the superior prefrontal and midfrontal regions, and even smaller, statistically nonsignificant increases occurred in the middle part of the posterior parietal region. In addition, there was a diffuse rCBF increase in the frontal and parietal association areas. When attention was directed toward the upper lip instead of the finger, the rCBF increase followed the same pattern as just described, but the contralateral somatosensory mouth area rather than the finger area was now activated.

The magnitude of the focal rCBF increase was considerable. A similar increase occurs when different objects are intensely and quickly pressed against the fingers to discriminate object shapes (Roland, 1981). Further, strong mechanical stimuli applied to the tip of the index finger elicit a smaller rCBF increase in the sensory finger area than does selective attention (Roland, 1981; Roland, Larsen, & Lassen, 1980).

Roland (1981) concluded that preparatory differential tuning of the relevant somatotopical postcentral area occurs when attention is focused on a spot of the skin surface. He proposed that this tuning mainly resulted from the local sum of many EPSPs (excitatory post-synaptic potentials) integrated during the attention period of 40 sec and, further, that this tuning reflected increased local excitability, which might improve detection. Roland regarded the tuning of the sensory area as being most probably controlled by the superior and midfrontal cortical areas, which, he assumed, probably did not participate in the analysis of somatosensory signals.

Hence, selective attention increased the rCBF most in the frontal and in the modality-specific areas of the brain, both increases showing a well-defined spatial pattern, the frontal actually two separate activation patterns. Unfortunately, the poor temporal resolution of the method (Section 3.6) does not permit the determination of the temporal order of the different rCBF increases, which would indicate the order of emergence of the underlying increases in neuronal activity. One might, however, assume that the increase in frontal activity, essential to voluntarily directed attention (Luria & Homskaya, 1970; Pribram & Luria, 1973), occurred first, producing and commanding the sensory-specific selective activity.

As to the two frontal patterns, the superior, medial one presumably emerged first, expressing executive activity. This region is activated in a wide variety of tasks, their common aspect being that the subject follows a plan of action or processes sensory information according to a prior instruction (Roland, 1981). On the other hand, the area of the midfrontal region activated appears to serve as a functional link between the executive frontal activity and the performing sensory-specific activity. This was suggested by the fact that the activation of this midfrontal region seemed to be specific to somatosensory tasks: The same region was also activated in two other types of somatosensory tasks in previous studies (Roland & Larsen, 1976; Roland, Skinhøj, Larsen, & Endo, 1977), whereas a somewhat different midfrontal region was activated during visual and auditory tasks (Roland, Skinhøj, & Lassen, 1981; Roland & Skinhøj, 1981).

Attention in a MultiModal Situation. In a subsequent study, Roland (1982) delivered sequences of concurrent visual, auditory, and somatosensory stimuli. The subject was instructed to perform a discrimination task in one modality at a time and to ignore the stimuli of the two other modalities. In the visual task, rCBF in (a part of) visual association cortex was increased, compared with activity recorded when auditory or somatosensory stimuli were attended (which was above rest levels even then).

The auditory task increased rCBF in auditory cortex (a measure combining activity of both primary and immediate association cortices) from the level prevailing during attention to the other modalities. On the other hand, no attention effect was found in somatosensory association cortex (in the part of it monitorable with the methodology used). Many other areas showed an rCBF increase irrespective of the attended modality, whereas a consistent fall in rCBF occurred in no region.

The primary projection area could be monitored directly only in the somatosensory modality. In the contralateral somatosensory hand area, there was an increase from the rest level of the same magnitude regardless of the direction of attention. The same was true for the perisensory hand area. Because the rCBF increase in the somatosensory hand area even when another modality was attended was larger than when subjects performed the same somatosensory task in another study (Roland & Larsen, 1976) in which no other stimuli were presented, Roland (1982) inferred that "there was no significant subcortical inhibition of this sensory input no matter to what modality the subjects turned their attention" (p. 1074) and that "*a priori* irrelevant signals were processed, at least preliminarily, by the cortex" (p. 1060).

Thus, Roland (1982) found two main sources of rCBF increase in the sensory regions: the increase due to sensory stimulation and that due to attention, with both modality-specific and -nonspecific components. Again, the author concluded that this specific component was induced by differential tuning, which he regarded as the physiological manifestation of modality-specific attention. This differential tuning expresses "a mechanism that is anticipatory, task dependent, independent of stimulus intensity and stimulus rate, that differentially enhances and inhibits the metabolism in cortical areas" (Roland, 1982, p. 1076).

Roland (1982) assumed that the superior, anterior prefrontal cortex participated in the control of this differential tuning. This same region was activated during each selective-attention task, and much more strongly than in otherwise similar attention tasks but with no concurrent stimuli of other modalities. According to Roland (1985), it is probably the midsection of the superior prefrontal cortex that has the highest flow values during selective attention.

On the other hand, the posterior, superior, lateral frontal region modulated its rCBF according to the attended sensory modality in Roland's (1982) study. Consistently with this, this region showed, as already mentioned, a modality-specific pattern of rCBF increase in separate unisensory discrimination tasks involving each of the three modalities.

Hemispheric Asymmetries. Risberg and Prohovnik's (1983) rCBF data suggest that the right frontal lobe is more important than the left in the control of selective attention. In addition, there was a notable diffuse rCBF increase in the whole frontal lobe superimposed on a more specific rCBF pattern. The parietal rCBF was also increased by attention. Risberg, Maximilian, and Prohovnik (1977), too, found nonspecific frontal activation during mental activity. This diffuse rCBF component of selective attention, which was also observed by Roland (1981, 1982), supports attention theories proposing both nonspecific and specific components of attention (Posner & Boies, 1971; Posner & Petersen, 1990).

Hemispheric asymmetries related to linguistic processing were observed by Maximilian (1982). He found a higher rCBF in the left- than right-hemisphere temporo-parietal region during processing of verbal stimulus material requiring discrimination (cf. Risberg et al., 1975). This effect occurred independently of the ear stimulated. Carmon, Lavy, Gordon, and Portnoy (1975) found that during listening to verbal material, flow increase was greater in the left hemisphere, whereas listening to music induced larger increases in the right hemisphere.

8.2. POSITRON EMISSION TOMOGRAPHY (PET) STUDIES OF ATTENTION

Auditory Studies

Early PET studies (Alavi et al., 1981; Reivich et al., 1979) with monaural presentation of meaningful stimulus material (a story to be remembered) found that glucose metabolism was, in particular, increased in the right temporal lobe irrespective of the ear stimulated. In contrast, Mazziotta, Phelps, Carson, and Kuhl (1982; see also Reivich, Gur, & Alavi, 1983) found that verbal stimuli caused larger increases in glucose utilization in the left than the right hemisphere (in right-handed subjects). A small but significant activation was also found in the left thalamus. On the other hand, nonverbal stimuli (e.g., musical chords) primarily activated right-hemispheric, particularly inferior frontal, parietal, and superior, temporal regions. In addition, the hemispheric asymmetry of glucose utilization depended, according to the authors, on the subject's strategy in listening to sequences of musical notes in order to determine whether notes in a sequence differed from those of the previous sequence. An analytical strategy, followed by musically sophisticated subjects, was predominantly associated with a larger left-hemisphere glucose consumption that was specially strong in the posterior temporal region. Musically less sophisticated subjects, using a less analytical strategy, had strongest activations in the right hemisphere, mainly in the inferior parietal and temporo-occipital regions.

Mazziotta et al. (1982) also found that frontal cortical regions were, in general, more activated during task performance than in passive listening. In addition, in subjects instructed to recall certain specific aspects of auditory stimuli, the medial temporal lobe (hippocampus, parahippocampus) showed increased glucose consumption, which was never observed in other auditory tasks (for a review, see Phelps & Mazziotta, 1985).

Reivich et al. (1983) found an rCBF increase in the right inferior parietal lobule both in auditory and visual attention (discrimination) tasks. The authors interpreted this finding as possibly suggesting right parietal predominance in directed attention.

Visual Studies

In an early study, Phelps, Mazziotta, Engel, and Kuhl (1981) found that glucose consumption of visual cortex was increased with increasing complexity of visual stimulation and, further, that this increase was larger in visual association (Areas 18 and 19) than primary (Area 17) cortex.

The Posterior Visual Spatial-Attention System. Evidence for a posterior visual spatial-attention system was obtained by Posner, Petersen, Fox, and Raichle (1988), who found increased rCBF in a certain region of posterior parietal cortex during visual spatial attention. No part of the assumed posterior visual-spatial attentional system seems to be activated by mere presentation of single words, but simple tasks that require monitoring of visual input or using visual imagery do activate this parietal system (Posner et al., 1988).

From these and some lesion results, Posner et al. (1988; see also Posner, Sandson, Dhawan, & Shulman, 1989) concluded that "visual word reading is automatic in that it does not require activation of the visual spatial attention system" (p. 1630). This is further supported by PET data showing that the ventral occipital lobe is similarly activated irrespective of whether the subject responds actively to the word presented or remains passive (Posner et al., 1989).

The Anterior and Posterior Attention Systems. In addition, Posner et al. (1988) reviewed some PET (Petersen, Fox, Posner, Mintun, & Raichle, 1988, and Petersen, Fox, Posner, Mintun, & Raichle, 1989) and other evidence for participation of the anterior cingular gyrus of the medial frontal lobe in "attention for action" (Allport, 1980; Duncan, 1980; Näätänen, 1988a; see also chapter 1). Posner et al. (1988) wrote:

> . . . selective attention appears to use neural systems separate from those involved in passively collecting information about a stimulus. In the posterior part of the brain, the ventral occipital lobe appears to develop the visual word form. If active selection or visual search is required, this is done by a spatial system that is deficient in patients with lesions of the parietal lobe. . . . Similarly, in the anterior brain the lateral left frontal lobe is involved in the semantic network for coding word associations. Local areas within the anterior cingulate become increasingly involved when the output of the computations within the semantic network is to be selected as a relevant target. Thus the anterior cingulate is involved in the computations in selecting language or other forms of information for action. This separation of anterior and posterior attention systems helps clarify how attention can be involved both in early visual processing and in the selection of information for output. (p. 1630)

Posner et al. (1989) hypothesized that a simultaneous performance of two operations using the same, or closely interconnected, brain regions would produce specific interference. One of the tasks employed by the authors was shadowing (repeating back) auditory words as quickly as possible. This task was found to interfere with shifts of visual attention in the direction of peripheral cues. According to the authors, the two tasks require common attentional operations localized to the medial frontal lobe.

In contrast, shadowing did not interfere with operations involving priming of a visual word form, which engages certain occipital areas not activated during shadowing, but interfered with semantic priming which involves, as does shadowing, both anterior semantic and attentional areas. Posner and his colleagues concluded that the interference in question involves operations performed by the anterior attention system and, more generally, that their findings support the notion that mental operations will produce no interference when they use anatomically separate neural systems.

The attention system, with both anterior and posterior components, proposed by Posner et al. (1988, 1989), is illustrated in Fig. 8.2.

Similarly, Posner (1988) concluded that the system of visual spatial attention is not an independent module but shares operation with a more general attention system that is also involved in processing of language: "Even if the basic visual spatial attention system is posterior, . . . its control system may lie within the frontal lobes and affect both language and spatial function" (p. 194).

Pardo, Pardo, Janer, and Raichle (1990) measured rCBF in the Stroop conflict situation (Section 2.2). They found that the Stroop interference effect was, in particular, associated with a strong activation of the anterior cingulate cortex, suggesting that "this cortical region may be a component of an anterior attentional system" (Pardo et al., 1990, p. 258). Also several other regions showed stronger activation in Stroop than control conditions, which led the authors to conclude that the Stroop task seems to cause "some alterations in the high-level sensory encoding of the visual information" (p. 259) and, further, that "the Stroop interference effect cannot be explained simply in terms of stimulus encoding or response interference" (p. 256).

In contrast to several other brain regions, the left medial extrastriate cortex showed no difference between the Stroop and non-Stroop conditions. This accords with Posner et al.'s (1988) suggestion that this area is "uniquely concerned with the visual word form" (p. 238), for there were no word-form differences between the two conditions.

The Role of the Pulvinar in Visual Attention. LaBerge (1990) reviewed PET studies providing evidence for the participation of the pulvinar in visual attentional selection. This is the largest thalamic nucleus, containing high-resolution maps of the contralateral visual field. In one of these studies, LaBerge and Buchsbaum (1990) investigated glucose uptake in the pulvinar in a filtering task, which involved detection of a target letter in the middle locus surrounded by resembling irrelevant, "flanker" letters. They reported that glucose uptake was greater in the pulvinar contralateral to the side of the filtering task than in the pulvinar contralateral to a nonfiltering task. Because this difference mainly involved the upper part of the pulvinar,

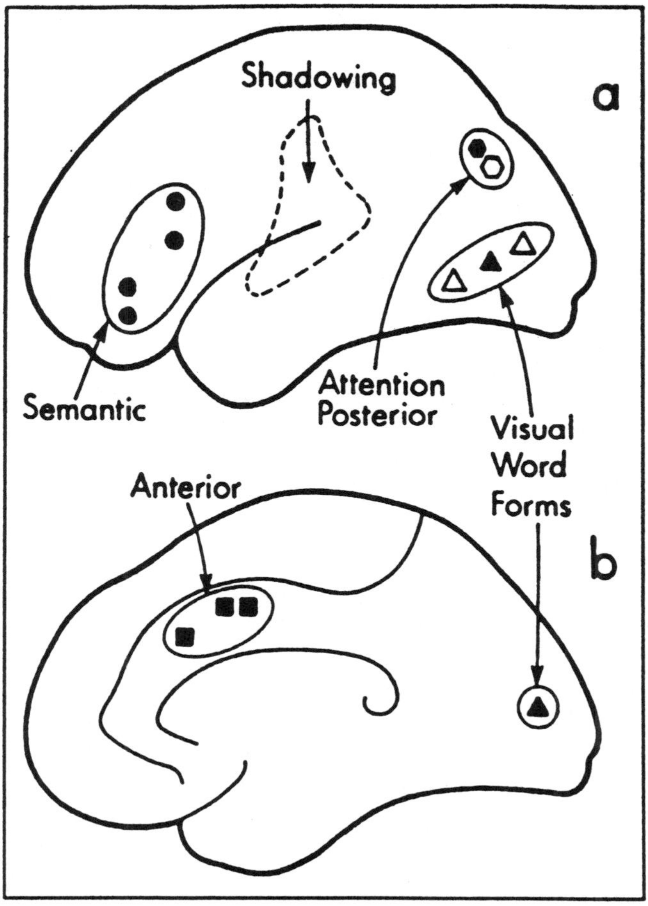

FIG. 8.2 A summary of data from PET studies of visual and auditory words. The areas on the lateral portions of the cortex (a) and on the medial portion (b) that are involved in visual word forms (triangles), semantic analysis (circles), anterior attention (squares), or posterior attention (hexagons). For lateralized activation, solid indicates left hemisphere and open indicates right hemisphere. The hemisphere of midline activations is not known. The areas suggested as being activated in shadowing (repeating auditory words) are surrounded by a dotted area. (From Posner, Sandson, Dhawan, & Shulman, 1989. Copyright © 1989 by the Massachusetts Institute of Technology. Reprinted with permission.)

LaBerge (1990) concluded that "any differential activity in the superior colliculus and lateral geniculate due to type of task was not influencing the pulvinar effects measured here" (p. 361).

LaBerge and Buchsbaum (1990) tentatively proposed that visual identification of an object in a precued locus in a cluttered field involves a filtering process in the subcortical pulvinar that operates in interaction with cortical structures underlying shape identification but, according to LaBerge (1990), probably is not the site of the initial selection operation in such an identification task:

> Some process upstream of the pulvinar, in higher-order processes, would seem to be responsible for the initial selection of the center item of a display as the target to be identified. What the filter does is to transform a selection signal that it receives from higher order processes into a form that can operate effectively on complex cortical processing, such as the filtering of one part of the array of information flowing from V1 to the areas where shape identification or other judgments about the shape are carried out. (p. 362)

Feature-Specific Activation Foci During Attention. Recent PET studies (e.g., Corbetta, Miezin, Dobmeyer, Shulman, & Petersen, 1990) have also provided evidence for feature-specific activation foci when different features of visual stimuli were to be attended. These different rCBF foci were found in extrastriate visual cortex when targets to be detected among a sequence of visual stimuli were defined either by their color, shape, or movement velocity. These attention-dependent rCBF foci corresponded to regions of extrastriate visual cortex that appear to be specialized for processing sensory information corresponding to the attended attribute. Attention to movement velocity activated a region in the left inferior parietal module and attention to color a region in the collateral sulcus and dorsolateral occipital cortex. (See also Lueck et al., 1989.) The same region in the collateral sulcus was also activated by attention to shape which in addition activated fusiform, parahippocampal gyri, as well as some regions of temporal cortex.

Regions that were uniformly active when attention was directed to any one of the three features were the posterior thalamus/colliculus, caudate nucleus, lateral orbitofrontal cortex, globus pallidus, and insular-premotor regions (Corbetta, Miezin, Dobmeyer, Shulman, & Petersen, 1991). Further, dividing attention between the three stimulus features activated, in contrast to focused attention, the anterior cingulate cortex and dorsolateral prefrontal cortex (Corbetta et al., 1991).

According to the theory of visual attention proposed by LaBerge (1990), activation foci related to the direction of attention revealed by PET are due to feature-specific expectations ("expectant attention"). These local activity increases were described as "peaked activity distributions" in these loci, which would, according to LaBerge (1990), increase the accuracy and speed of perceiving the corresponding feature, with generalization to similar stimuli. He tentatively assumed that these distributions of increased neuronal activity are generated and maintained by a thalamic enhancement mechanism in an appropriate thalamic nucleus, proposing that the thalamic (pulvinar) mechanism is "a particular type of circuit that reciprocally connects thalamic relay cells to cortical cells. This circuit, which is characteristic of thalamic nuclei in general, appears to embody an algorithm that enhances firing in a target set of cells while inhibiting firing in the surrounding set of cells" (LaBerge, 1990, p. 358). According to LaBerge, the thalamic enhancement mechanism is, in turn, commanded by a higher mechanism apparently located in the anterior cingulate cortex.

Brain Mechanisms of Sustained Attention. This form of attention, also called vigilance, is usually studied by presenting occasional threshold-level signals over a longer period of time and measuring performance decrement developing during this time (chapter 1). Cerebral mechanisms of sustained attention were studied by Pardo, Fox, and Raichle (1991). These authors measured rCBF with PET in two different conditions, each lasting for 40 sec: (a) In a somatosensory vigilance task, subjects monitored their left (right) great toe for brief pauses in a volley of suprathreshold touches with a von Frey hair; (b) subjects monitored near-threshold luminance changes of a dim central fixation mark.

It was found that the prefrontal and superior parietal cortices primarily in the right hemisphere were activated in both tasks. Both activations consisted of clusters of activation foci. The right-hemispheric preponderance could be observed regardless of the modality or laterality of sensory input. In the somatosensory task there seemed to be an additional, temporal right-hemispheric activation focus that did not occur in the visual task. (In addition, the somatosensory task of course activated certain somatosensory areas and the visual task certain visual areas.)

Pardo et al. (1991) interpreted their results as revealing a cerebral system of vigilance:

> These data identify and localize in healthy humans an anatomically distinct and asymmetric neural system mediating sustained attention to sensory stimuli. Vigilance, then, is one cognitive component of human attention that is right-lateralized. The vigilance system encompasses both right prefrontal and right superior parietal cortices and can operate independently of midline anterior attentional systems. (p. 63)

8.3. CLASSIFICATION OF ACTIVATION PATTERNS AS REFLECTED BY REGIONAL BLOOD-FLOW AND METABOLIC MEASURES

The results reviewed earlier in this chapter seem to illustrate the point made in chapter 1: Attention might be best understood in terms of *task-dependent central activation patterns.* Task performance is, internally, a rapid sequence of activations/inhibitions of different interlinked functional mechanisms of the brain. The aspect of selectivity is, as stressed in chapter 1, present almost everywhere, in any task-dependent sequence of processes. Consequently, isolating "attention" from these sequences of highly specific activation patterns is not easy and might at times appear arbitrary. It seems, however, that a meaningful use for the attention construct must be searched from the most central, control, elements of these task-dependent activation patterns (chapter 1). Activation patterns may be classified as follows.

Activation Patterns Related to Sensory Stimuli

In addition to task-dependent patterns, there is also an exogenous activation pattern: that related to external stimuli, of course. This pattern usually provides a base on which task-dependent patterns are formed. Exogenous activation patterns can be examined in considerable detail by recording ERPs and their MEG equivalents, as reviewed in the previous chapters. In addition, some exogenous rCBF and regional metabolic patterns caused by stimulation (e.g., Alavi et al., 1981; Mazziotta et al., 1982; Phelps et al., 1981; Posner et al., 1988, 1989; Reivich et al., 1979; Roland, 1982) were already reviewed in this chapter.

The high spatial localization accuracy of PET is illustrated by a PET demonstration of a tonotopic organization of primary auditory cortex. Lauter, Herschovitch, Formby, and Raichle (1985) found that the rCBF foci for pure tones of 500 Hz and 4000 Hz are differently located. In the same vein, Fox, Miezin, Allman, Van Essen, and Raichle's (1987) and Fox, Mintun, Raichle, Miezin, and Allman's (1986) PET measurements of rCBF have demonstrated a retinotopic organization of primary visual cortex. Fox et al. (1986) estimated that the anatomical precision of the map obtained with PET measurements exceeds those previously obtained with other methodologies in man. Fox et al.'s (1986) data also provided "the first direct, noninvasive measurements" of the cortical magnification factor (Rovamo & Virsu, 1979) in humans.

In addition to exogenous patterns, sensory systems may also have purely endogenous activation patterns. Such a pattern was illustrated by Roland's (1981) aforementioned rCBF focus, which developed in somatosensory cortex in anticipation of a weak touch stimulus before any stimulus was presented.

Visual presentation of words activates certain areas in the left, medial extrastriate visual cortex (Petersen, Fox, Snyder, & Raichle, 1990; see also Petersen, Fox, Posner, Mintun, & Raichle, 1988). The same areas were, however, also activated by pseudowords obeying English spelling rules but not by nonsense strings of letters or letter-like phonemes. Petersen et al. (1990) therefore concluded that visual word-form computations are based on learned distinctions between words and nonwords. In addition, passively presented words activated a left frontal area that was thought to be related to semantic processing, judging from the fact that pseudowords did not cause this activation.

Petersen et al.'s (1988) PET measurements during processing of individual auditory and visual words provided support for different, widely separated areas for sensory-specific, phonological, articulatory, and semantic coding. Furthermore, these results also suggested that separate brain regions are involved in visual and auditory coding of words, each with an independent access to supramodal articulatory and semantic systems.

The authors consequently interpreted their results as supporting multiple, parallel routes between localized sensory-specific, phonological, articulatory, and semantic-coding areas (see Coltheart, 1985) and, therefore, as arguing against obligatory visual-to-auditory recoding and serial types of models. (See also Petersen et al., 1990; Posner & Petersen, 1990.)

Activation Patterns Related to Motor Behavior

Complex cerebral activation patterns are associated with motor action. Roland, Larsen, and Lassen (1980) studied rCBF changes related to cerebral organization of voluntary movements. rCBF increases were exclusively found in both supplementary motor areas (SMA), while subjects were "programming" (imaging or mentally executing) a well-practiced complex sequence of fast movements involving different fingers without actually executing them. During execution of this motor sequence, both contra- and ipsilateral SMAs were again equivalently activated, but now also primary motor cortex was activated. This activation was contralateral to the fingers involved in the movement. The left superior frontal region was also activated.

Conversely, when the movement was made simple and repetitive (fast flexions of the same finger), or the muscular contraction was sustained, the contralateral primary motor area was activated without SMA activation. Some other focal activations, as well as a diffuse activation increase, were also observed during the different tasks.

Roland, Larsen, and Lassen (1980) concluded that the primary motor area (and the part of the motor system it projects to) can control ongoing simple ballistic movements, whereas more complex motor sequences require SMA programming. Further, the SMAs program motor subroutines and form a "queue" of time-ordered motor commands before voluntary movements are executed with the participation of the contralateral primary motor area not involved in the programming (cf. chapter 1).

These rCBF results are paralleled by electric data on a slow premovement negativity that initially is bilateral but becomes contralateralized closer to the actual movement onset. The first phase of this negativity appears to be generated by a bilateral SMA activation, whereas the second phase originates from the primary motor cortex contralateral to the moving hand. For a review, see Deecke, Heise, Kornhuber, Lang, and Lang (1984).

In a subsequent study, Roland, Skinhøj, Lassen, and Larsen (1980) compared rCBF changes occurring when subjects moved in extrapersonal space (that is, relative to the external world) and when they moved in intrapersonal space (relative to their own body). Movements in extrapersonal space were associated with a bilateral rCBF increase in the superior and inferior parietal regions. Otherwise, the areas activated were the same for the two types of movements: the SMAs were bilaterally activated, whereas the premotor areas, as well as the primary sensory and motor hand–arm areas, showed a contralateral rCBF increase. The authors proposed that the parietal regions "provide information to the motor programming neurons about the demanded direction of motion in extrapersonal space in relation to proprioceptive reference systems" (Roland, Skinhøj, et al., 1980, p. 137). In addition, it was found that certain specific parts of the premotor areas were activated when a motor program was learned or a previously learned program was modulated.

In a recent study, Seitz, Roland, Bohm, Greitz, and Stone-Elander (1990) investigated rCBF changes occurring during the course of learning of a complex sequence of right-hand finger movements. PET measurements of rCBF were first performed during the phase of initial learning when (blindfolded) subjects knew exactly what to do, but were slow because of deficient practice ("Initial Learning"). The last rCBF measurement ("Skilled Performance") occurred after a long practice period, which dramatically increased the performance speed.

In comparison with rest, rCBF increased during Initial Learning in structures participating in: (a) *voluntary motor activity:* the premotor areas, the SMAs, the primary motor hand area, the basal ganglia, the ventrolateral thalamus, the red nucleus and the substantia-nigra region, the pontine-nuclei region, and the cerebellum; (b) *analysis of somatosensory information* from the skin, joints, muscles, and tendons of the hand: the left ventral posteriolateral thalamus, the left somatosensory hand area in the postcentral gyrus, certain somatosensory association areas, SMA, and the cortex in the intraparietal sulcus; and (c) *the production of internal language:* the left and right inferior frontal gyri.

Interestingly, decreases from the resting level were found in the mid-sectors of the putamen-globus pallidus, the red-nucleus region, and the pontine region.

As learning progressed, the initially strong activation of the somatosensory association cortices gradually diminished both in extent and intensity.

This activation drop was most dramatic in the hemisphere (right) ipsilateral to the finger movements. In addition, the rCBF foci in the inferior frontal gyrus disappeared. This was paralleled by subjects reporting that they no longer needed to count silently the number of times the fingers should touch the thumb. All the limbic and paralimbic structures, too, showed decreased activation.

In contrast, the contralateral primary motor hand area became increasingly activated, which appeared to be related to the increased speed of finger movements and to the higher frequency of EMG bursts. On the other hand, improved performance did not change rCBF observed during Initial Learning in the contralateral somatosensory hand area, ventrolateral, postlateral, and mediodorsal thalamus, and the right anterior lobe of the cerebellum. The rCBF decrease below the resting-state level found during Initial Learning in the mid-sector of putamen, the external globus pallidus, and the brainstem at the site of the red nucleus was markedly reduced as learning progressed.

This complex pattern of rCBF changes associated with learning seems to indicate changes in the pattern of cerebral activation, which explain the improved, usually faster and more precise, performance. These changes, typically a drop-off of unnecessary mechanisms and phases, as proposed by Näätänen (1973), result in a more adequate, differentiated ("sharper"), and economical, in view of the performance at hand, patterning of activation.

Lang and colleagues (1988) studied rCBF changes associated with learning of a visuomotor task by using SPECT (Section 3.6). The task to be learned was inverted tracking of a visual target moving on a screen. For example, target movements to the right were to be tracked with hand movements to the left. Compared with a normal, non-inverted tracking task, rCBF increased in several regions including the middle frontal gyri, frontomedial cortex (including SMA), right basal ganglia, and the left cerebellum.

The simultaneously recorded slow negative DC-potential shifts were larger in the inverted than in the normal tracking, especially in frontal regions. (For comparable results obtained by varying task complexity, see McCallum et al., 1989.) This additional frontal negativity was found to covary with the degree of success in learning. Similar results have been obtained by Lang, Lang, Kornhuber, Deecke, and Kornhuber (1983, 1986).

Lang et al. (1988) concluded that the frontal lobe plays an important role in visuomotor learning. Their previous studies (Deecke et al., 1984; Lang, Lang, Kornhuber, Deecke, & Kornhuber, 1984) had suggested that slow negative potential shifts recorded during task performance contain task-dependent patterns expressing task-specific distribution of cerebral activation. Also, the Bereitschaftspotential (Kornhuber & Deecke, 1965) has been shown to reflect task-specific anticipatory activation patterns (Benecke, Dick, Rothwell, Day, & Marsden, 1985; Lang et al., 1984; Schreiber et al., 1983).

Activation Patterns Associated With Pure Central Activity (Thinking)

rCBF measurements have also revealed activation patterns associated with pure central activity, occurring in the absence of sensory, at least external, stimuli and motor movements. Roland and Friberg (1985, see also Roland, 1987) studied rCBF nontomographically during three different thinking tasks: (a) a continuous silent subtraction of 3, starting from 50 ("50 − 3 Thinking"); (b) thinking every second word in a 9-word circular jingle ("Jingle Thinking"); and (c) imagining a route starting from the front door of the subject's home with alternating left–right turns at every second corner ("Route Thinking").

It was found that thinking was associated with activation of multiple homotypical cortical fields, that is, areas outside the primary and immediate sensory association areas as well as motor areas. All three types of thinking tasks activated areas in superior prefrontal cortex equivalently, which was attributed to the "organization of thinking." Elsewhere in the prefrontal cortex, multifocal rCBF increases were observed, whose loci and intensities depended on the type of thinking. For an illustration of these results, see Fig. 8.3.

During 50 − 3 Thinking, the angular cortex was bilaterally activated, which was attributed to "the retrieval of the numerical memory and memory for subtractions" (p. 1219). Jingle Thinking increased rCBF in right midtemporal cortex (an intermediate auditory association area), which did not occur during the other thinking tasks. This activation was attributed to the rhythmic structure of the task; the same area is activated when subjects discriminate tone rhythms (Roland, 1982; Roland et al., 1981).

During Route Thinking, rCBF increased in the intermediate and remote visual association areas. Additional rCBF increases in this task occurred in the superior occipital, posterior inferior temporal, and posterior superior parietal cortex, which were attributed to "the retrieval of the visual and spatial memory" (Roland & Friberg, 1985, p. 1219). In previous studies, exactly the same areas were activated when subjects discriminated shapes of visually presented ellipses (Roland & Skinhøj, 1981) or when they were looking at familiar surroundings (Mazziotta, Phelps, & Halgren, 1983).

Each rCBF increase covered an area of a few square centimeters of cortical surface. In addition, no rCBF decreases were found during any thinking task. Roland and Friberg (1985) estimated that cortical energy consumption during thinking was of the same magnitude as, or even larger

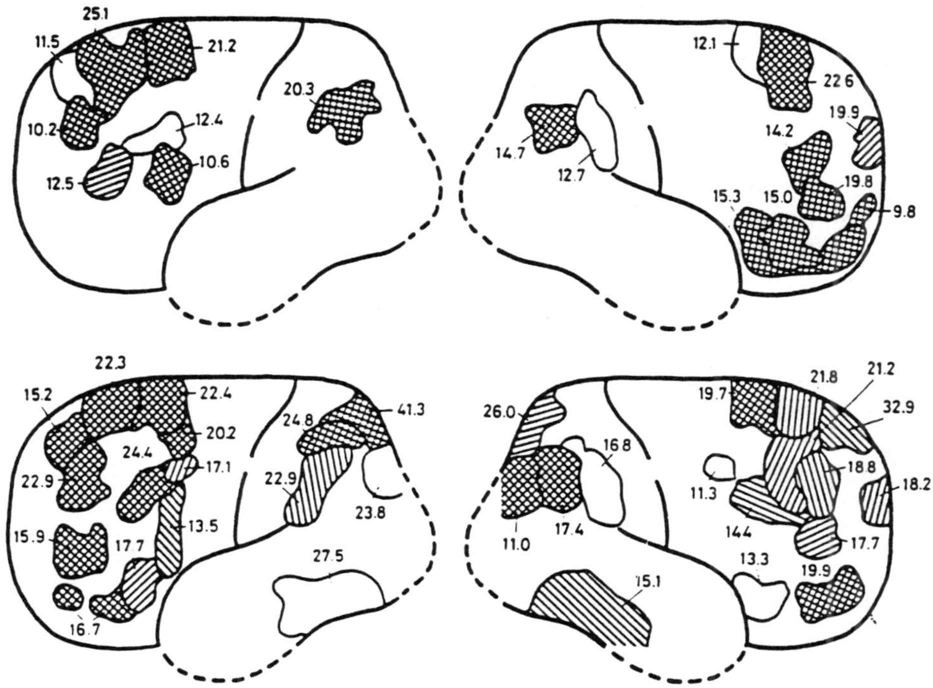

FIG. 8.3 Across-subject increases of regional cerebral blood flow (rCBF) in percent and their average distribution in cortex while subjects were performing two different types of thinking tasks. The two upper diagrams represent a subtraction task; the two lower diagrams represent visually imagined walking of a specific route in a familiar surrounding. LEFT: the left hemisphere. RIGHT: the right hemisphere. All subjects had hatched areas activated. Cross-hatched areas: rCBF increases significant at 0.005 level; hatched areas: $p < .01$; other areas: $p < .05$. (Adapted from Roland and Friberg, 1985. Copyright © 1985 by the American Physiological Society. Reprinted with permission.)

than, during intense voluntary movements or intense processing of external sensory information.

Notably, all rCBF increases observed during the different thinking tasks always occurred outside the motor cortices as well as the primary sensory areas and their immediate association areas. This resulted, apparently, from the fact that subjects neither made voluntary movements nor received any external sensory stimuli. Consistently with this, when Roland's (1982) subjects attended to visual stimuli in his three-modality study, rCBF was enhanced in the intermediate and remote visual association areas. This enhancement occurred despite the fact that stimulation was not changed. "This means that the target areas for the retrieval of visual images from memory were the same as the target areas for the direction of attention toward visual spatial signals. The difference between reception and discrimination of external visual information is that the primary visual area and the immediate visual association cortex is activated when the information comes from the external world but not when it is retrieved from visual-spatial memory" (Roland & Friberg, 1985, p. 1242).

Goldenberg, Podreka, Steiner, and Willmes (1987) presented their subjects with an auditory word list, instructing one group of subjects to try to remember them and the other to try to remember them by visualizing the referents of the words. The latter group showed a more intense rCBF, measured with SPECT, in the occipital lobes, particularly in the left inferior occipital area. Similar results were obtained when subjects were asked questions requiring visual imagery (e.g., "Is the green of pine trees darker than the green of grass?") than when questions did not require visual imagery. The technique used in this study, however, did not permit one to determine whether primary visual cortex was activated by imagery, but Farah (1989), after reviewing related ERP results, regarded this as unlikely.

Imagery using episodic-memory contents activated lateral inferior temporal regions that were not activated in semantic-memory tasks. The latter tasks, in turn, specifically activated the left inferior parietal lobe not activated in the episodic-memory task.

The available rCBF data suggest that visual imagery is predominantly associated with left-hemisphere activity (for a review, see Farah, 1989). In a study on split-brain patients, Kosslyn, Berndt, and Doyle (1985) found that the isolated left hemisphere is capable of complex visual imagery, whereas the isolated right hemisphere is not. On the other hand, mental rotation induces a larger rCBF increase in the right than the left hemisphere, in particular in the right parietal region (Papanicolaou et al., 1987). Consistently with this, probe ERPs to flashes presented during mental rotation in that study were more suppressed over the right than left hemisphere relative to ERPs during passive viewing of the flashes. This hemispheric asymmetry probably resulted from a larger proportion of the right- than left-hemisphere neurons being engaged in activity related to mental rotation.

9

Concluding Discussion

9.1. A MODEL OF AUTOMATIC AND ATTENTIVE STIMULUS PROCESSING IN AUDITION

A central aspect in any theory of attention in stimulus processing is how this theory defines the borderline between automatic and nonautomatic processing. That is, how far up, according to the theory, is the chain of processes triggered by an auditory stimulus independent of attention? In trying to outline the role of attention in stimulus processing, a major problem has been the lack of a reliable measure for automaticity of sensory processing. In reviewing physiological literature, however, we came across an ERP component that appeared to be unique among the current physiological, at least ERP, measures of automatic sensory processing in that this component can measure sensory processing in terms of actual extraction and flow of sensory information (Section 4.4). This component was the mismatch negativity (MMN).

Automatic Sensory Processing

It is essential in this regard that MMN, at least to frequency change, is elicited even in the absence of attention, as suggested by a multitude of converging results from different experimental paradigms. The occurrence of MMN to slight frequency deviations in the unattended input indicates that sensory stimulus features are fully or extensively processed (encoded) independently of attention: A sensitive response *specifically* to a deviation in the unattended input, one expressing the discrimination of that deviation, would be impossible, unless the representation of the standard stimulus had contained extensively processed sensory information (unless the deviant stimulus had been extensively processed). This information can, of course, enter the traces only from antecedent sensory processing. Thus, these unattended-channel MMNs provide strong evidence that auditory sensory information is extensively processed even in the absence of attention.

This is the starting point of the model of attention in audition proposed by Näätänen (1990), shown in Fig. 9.1. On this model, auditory stimuli receive complete processing (encoding) of all their physical features such as frequency, intensity, duration, rise time, and so forth, performed by the "Permanent Feature-Detector System". This is very rapid, "hard-wired" sensory processing, and a good deal of it occurs at the subcortical level. Näätänen (1990) proposed that this processing stage does not depend on attention, and characterized it as "automatic, parallel, and preconscious" (p. 229). Further, in the full absence of attention, the outcomes of this sensory analysis enter sensory memory (Arrow 4 in Fig. 9.1) but no higher forms of memory. The model consequently denied a *fully* automatic access of sensory stimuli to their semantic codes.

Conscious Perception

Consistently with this, the outcomes of these sensory processes do not in themselves, on the model, cause conscious perception but only provide its sensory-informational basis or contents. Whether a conscious percept also occurs would depend on the sensory attention-triggering characteristics of the stimulus: Besides the Permanent Feature-Detector System, sensory

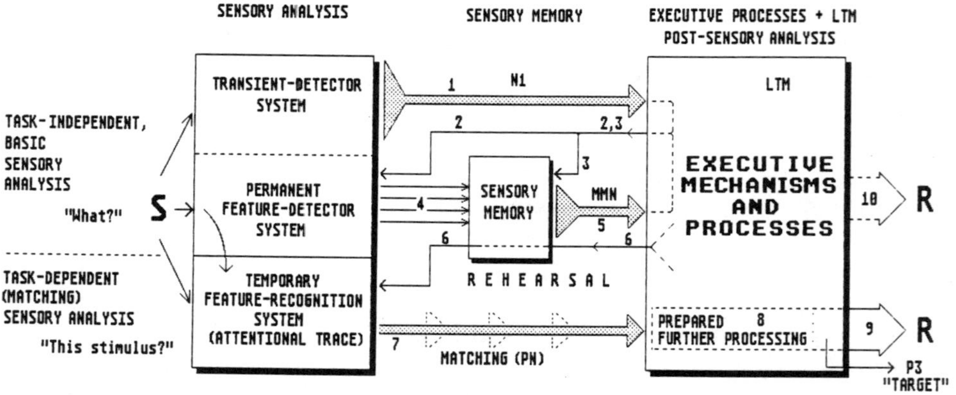

FIG. 9.1 A model illustrating the role of attention and automaticity in auditory processing. For explanation, see text. (Adapted from Näätänen, 1990. Copyright © 1990 Cambridge University Press. Reprinted with permission.)

input also activates, according to the model, a parallel system of sensory analysis, one sensitive only to onsets and offsets of stimulus energy. This is the "Transient-Detector System" in Fig. 9.1, detecting the occurrence of sensory events but not mediating qualitative aspects of these events. This system would trigger conscious perception of the subjectively "silent" sensory data when the response elicited by the stimulus in the Transient-Detector System, the "interrupt signal," exceeds some threshold.

Thus, conscious perception follows, on the model, when the Transient-Detector System is activated strongly enough to cause "Executive Mechanisms" to "look at" the output of the Permanent Feature-Detector System (Arrows 2 and 3). This means, the activation pattern of the Feature-Detector System encoded, according to the model, in the mechanism of Sensory Memory gets into contact with, activates, the semantic information stored in long-term memory (LTM) and may, consequently, enter conscious perception, for example, as a percept of a familiar time signal from the radio (Näätänen, 1990). This semantic activation might, however, even occur without causing conscious perception (cf. Öhman, in press; see, however, Holender, 1986). The existence of sensory and semantic activation thresholds that are lower than that of conscious perception might explain results that suggest priming caused by behaviorally undetected stimuli (cf. Underwood, 1990). Similarly, these differential thresholds might also provide an account for the finding that certain brain-lesion patients can have sensory information, as revealed by their forced-choice performance, without being consciously aware of this information (the "Blindsight"; Weiskrantz, 1986).

Perception and Sensory Memory

Hence, the stage of sensory-specific processing from which sensory information is "read" to conscious perception is, according to Näätänen (1990), the short phase of sensory memory lasting only 200-300 msec. Cowan (1984, 1988) proposed a distinction within sensory memory to this short phase and to one with a considerably longer duration, on the order of 10–20 sec. In the short phase, the stimulus-caused activation pattern of the Permanent Feature-Detector System is, on the model, mapped onto, encoded in, Sensory Memory (Näätänen, 1990).

In this phase, the outputs from the different feature-specific analyzers and their combinations are probably integrated into unitary stimulus representations, providing conditions for unitary auditory percepts. In addition, the integration of the feature-detector outputs might take place also in the time domain. This could explain why the "perceptual presence" seems to consist of acoustic events over a certain range of time rather than strictly of the same instant. This is particularly clear in perception of music and speech. In addition, stimuli of very brief duration are experienced as lasting considerably longer (Cowan, 1988; Efron, 1970; Plomp, 1964; Scharf & Houtsma, 1986), which might also be related to the suggested temporal window of integration. Another related phenomenon might be the occurrence of loudness integration over a period of about 200 msec (Scharf & Houtsma, 1986).

On the grounds of this type of evidence, Näätänen (1990) proposed that Cowan's shorter phase of sensory memory might form the "background" of perceptual experience when stimuli follow one another in close succession. This temporal integration "might considerably expand the window of the 'psychological presence' in audition relative to the timeless 'cutting edge' of physical presence that continuously turns the future into the past." (Näätänen, 1990, p. 275). Consequently, this shorter phase of sensory memory should not be regarded as a "pure" memory but rather as an intermediate phase between perception and memory (Näätänen, 1990).

Winkler, Reinikainen, and Näätänen's (1991) results on backward masking might bear on these time estimates. These authors found that a masking stimulus must follow a test stimulus within approximately 100–150 msec in order to deteriorate memory of this stimulus and to reduce or eliminate MMN to deviants in these stimulus blocks (see Section 4.4). Consequently, this might be the duration needed for the development of the sensory-memory trace; an appropriate sensory input to the system during this time, may, presumably, deteriorate or eliminate the trace while it is still in the developmental phase. Similar time estimates for the development of the sensory-memory trace might be derived from behavioral literature on backward masking (see, for example, Hawkins & Presson, 1986).

The time course of the post-stimulus facilitation, as indicated by the enhanced N1m, the magnetic N1, of Loveless et al. (1989; see Section 5.1) in response to a subsequent stimulus, and the related physiological (reviewed by Rohrbaugh et al., 1990) and behavioral (reviewed by Loveless et al., 1989) findings, also is comparable to the shorter phase of sensory memory. These data suggest that during a short post-stimulus time period, the responsiveness of the organism to further sensory input is enhanced. This facilitation might be an expression of a brief post-stimulus time window of activation of the aforementioned temporal-integration mechanism, one integrating coincident and nearly coincident sensory events on temporal basis and thus subserving the integrity of auditory event perception. Possibly the previously discussed post-stimulus period of vulnerability to masking reflects the same mechanism.

In addition, the 40-Hz transient, oscillatory response, apparently triggered by any auditory stimulus and lasting some 100–200 msec (Section 4.2), might also express this post-stimulus period of integration (see also

Llinas, Grace, & Yarom, 1991). As already mentioned, an analogous phenomenon also occurs in the visual and somatosensory modalities.

Attention-Trigger Signal Generated by Transient-Detector Mechanisms

In the preceding, a route for preconscious sensory data to conscious perception was surmised to proceed through an attention switch to sensory memory. Further, the attention-trigger signal generated by the transient-detector mechanism must, according to the model, exceed some threshold, varying from moment to moment, in order for an attention switch to occur. The strength of this signal would depend on (a) the dynamogenic properties of the stimulus (see Graham, 1979; Loveless, 1983; Loveless & Brunia, 1990; MacMillan, 1973) such as intensity and rise time; and (b) the momentary degree of excitability of the transient-detector mechanism.

It has been proposed (Näätänen, 1986a, 1990; Näätänen & Picton, 1987) that the supratemporal component of N1, at least a good deal of it, might be generated by this attention-trigger mechanism. In this case, the midline-N1 amplitude would provide a measure of the strength of the attention-trigger signal generated by the transient-detector mechanism. It was further suggested that the generator mechanism of the nonspecific N1 component might also be involved in this attention-trigger function (see also Kenemans et al., 1989; Verbaten, 1990). This is supported by the fact that the amplitude of these two components, that of the nonspecific component in particular, strongly depends on the stimulus rate (Fig. 4.14). The excitability of the generator mechanisms of these two components is relatively low with short ISIs but high when the preceding silent interval has lasted several seconds. General state factors also exert an influence on the excitability in particular of the nonspecific-N1 mechanism (Section 4.3).

The attention-trigger threshold is, in turn, probably mainly controlled by the direction and strength of attention at the stimulus moment, that is, the nature and demand of the task performed. Thus, when attention is anticipatorily directed to a stimulus, this threshold is low. In addition, the attention-trigger signal is then probably facilitated, judging from an attentional enhancement of the N1 amplitude in active relative to passive conditions (Section 4.3). The lowered attention-trigger threshold and the enhanced attention-trigger signal might contribute to the fact that even a very weak stimulus is consciously detected during attention to these stimuli.

The excitability increase caused by attention in the mechanisms generating the attention-trigger signal is probably stimulus-nonspecific, as N1s both to relevant and irrelevant stimuli seem to be similarly enhanced during the period of increased excitability (for a review, see Näätänen & Picton,

1987). As already discussed, it is not excluded, however, that N1 (some subcomponent of the supratemporal N1) could be stimulus-specifically enhanced under conditions of a very strong attentional focus (Giard, 1990; Hillyard et al., 1973; Scharf, 1990).

The very recent data of Giard, Perrin, and Echallier (submitted) seem to reveal that the supratemporal N1 is paralleled by a frontal N1 component at a similar latency. In this case, it might be, as proposed by the authors, the frontal rather than supratemporal component of N1 that is associated with the attention-trigger function suggested. It is also possible that the two generator mechanisms jointly serve this vital function and that the supratemporal generator possibly acts as an initiator.

As to the external stimulus events activating the attention-trigger mechanism discussed, they occur frequently in acoustic input stream. These events include abrupt or relatively abrupt onsets of discrete stimuli and offsets of longer-duration stimuli. In addition, when the stimulus is continuous, the mechanism is also activated by increases or decreases in stimulus energy from one level to another, even by a purely qualitative change, such as a frequency change with no intensity change (see Fig. 4.9). The sensitivity of the transient-detector system even to merely qualitative changes in a continuous stimulus probably results from this system being, to a certain extent, organized in a stimulus-specific manner (Section 4.3); therefore a merely qualitative change produces an input to a "fresh" neuronal population of the N1 generator.

It is also possible that the 40-Hz transient, oscillatory response triggered by stimulus onset is related to the conscious-perception/attention-trigger function discussed. This is in particular suggested by the rate sensitivity of the effect: the size of this response with long ISIs such as 10 sec is about 10 times that with very short ISIs (Section 4.2). In addition, the event-related perturbations in the steady-state response (SSR) to 40-Hz stimulation (Makeig & Galambos, 1989b; Rohrbaugh et al., 1989, 1990, 1991) might be related to attention-switching because, as reviewed in Section 4.2, these SSR perturbations have several features that suggest an affinity to attention switching. In view of the extended time course of the SSR effect, it might indicate a transient arousal response associated with an attention switch.

Attention Switch Caused by Stimulus Change. The model also suggested a second, memory-dependent route to attention switch. This is via the MMN-generation mechanism, which is activated by a change in a sequence of discrete stimuli. On the model, the stimulus-elicited activation pattern of the Permanent Feature-Detector System is mapped onto the mechanism of Sensory Memory. This precise neural representation encodes all physical stimulus features, even temporal or highly complex ones, judging from MMN elicitation with any kind of suprathreshold stimulus change (Section 4.4). This presumably attention-independent memory system keeps in an accessible form a precise record of the whole auditory past spanning the last few seconds. This explains how the semantic processing of initially unattended sounds can occur when attention is switched to the sound even a few seconds after its offset.

It appears that stimulus change (against this neural representation) is initially and preconsciously detected by a sensory-specific mechanism of auditory cortex, the generator of the sensory-specific MMN subcomponent, which in turn triggers the frontal process that generates the frontal MMN subcomponent (Giard et al., 1990; Näätänen & Michie, 1979a; Paavilainen et al., 1991). This predominantly right-hemispheric frontal process might underlie the attention-triggering function postulated. If MMN is followed by a P3a, then that attention-trigger process has probably succeeded in causing attention switch to the eliciting stimulus (see Section 4.5).

When stimuli are attended, the MMN generator processes seem to trigger, in addition to the mechanism of P3a, those of many other endogenous components, most notably those of N2b and the slow parietal positivity (Section 6.1). Attention in oddball conditions seems to be expressed by a temporary link of facilitation between the MMN process and the subsequent endogenous processes, so that these endogenous processes are triggered even by a very weak MMN process. This further sequence is not quite the same under attend and ignore conditions, however, judging from the fact that the slow parietal positivity is probably not at all elicited in ignore conditions even when the stimulus deviation is consciously perceived (Sams, Paavilainen, et al., 1985). Furthermore, the threshold of N2b elicitation is considerably higher in ignore than attend conditions, whereas P3a does not show a similarly strong attentional dependence (Näätänen et al., 1982).

Organization of Sensory Memory

Sensory memory in audition might be located in auditory cortex, possibly in the vicinity of the primary cortex, judging from the estimated locus of the generation of the sensory-specific component of MMN (Section 4.4) and of its MEG equivalent MMNm (Section 5.1). This is in particular suggested by the possible feature-specific loci of generation of the sensory-specific MMN subcomponent (Paavilainen et al., 1991; Giard, Lavikainen, Reinikainen, Perrin, Bertrand, & Näätänen, in preparation). The most parsimonious account for such data appears to be that the neural stimulus representation involved in the mismatch response is located where this response is generated (Näätänen, 1984). In this case, the stimulus representation would, in fact, be distributed to the different feature-specific regions of auditory cortex which would then jointly accommodate the sensory-memory trace for this stimulus (Näätänen, 1990).

The neural traces for short-term and long-term storing of sensory information should not be understood as involving two anatomically separate cerebral systems, however. As reviewed in Section 4.4, some very recent results (Cowan et al., 1991; Näätänen et al., 1991) suggest that with MMN, even *long-term* effects of sensory stimulation could be probed. Further, these results also suggest that those long-term sensory traces of the standard stimulus facilitate MMN elicitation by a deviant stimulus, as predicted by Banquet et al. (1990), Grossberg (1990), Karmos and Csépe (1990), and Verleger (1990).

These data consequently implicate that:

1. There is a long-term system for storing of apparently merely sensory stimulus information.
2. This trace system forms the neuroanatomical basis of not only long-term but also short-term sensory memory (echoic memory).
3. Echoic memory is based on a development and/or activation of a trace in the long-term trace system rather than in a separate short-term storing system (Cowan, 1988; see also Norman, 1968). Therefore, the separation of Sensory Memory from long-term memory (LTM) in the model should be understood in functional rather than anatomical terms.
4. Access of stimuli also to the long-term storing system of sensory data is automatic.
5. If sensory stimuli do not automatically activate their semantic codes, as claimed by the model, then the long-term storing mechanisms of sensory and semantic stimulus information are probably at least to some extent separate (see Kahneman & Treisman, 1984, for a distinction to sensory and semantic stimulus representations).

These suggestions divide sensory memory, in fact, into three different, consecutive phases (but implicate their occurrence in the same system):

1. *A very short phase* during which sensory stimulus information is being encoded in the mechanism of sensory memory. This phase is, according to the present hypothesis, associated with stimulus perception, providing its sensory-specific contents (which may remain subjectively silent or be consciously perceived, depending on other factors, as explained previously.)
2. *A short phase* following encoding during which the encoded sensory information remains in an activated state. During this period, corresponding to echoic memory, MMN elicitation by a

deviant stimulus, as well as the use of this sensory information in stimulus selection (the development of the attentional trace), is possible if the momentary strength of the trace is sufficient.

3. *A long, or permanent, phase* that corresponds to the passive, inactivated system for long-term storing of sensory information.

Attention Switch and Semantic Analysis

As already explained, the present model suggests that preconscious sensory analysis of auditory stimuli automatically elicits cerebral attention-trigger processes in response to different types of common events in auditory input, including stimulus onsets, offsets of long-duration stimuli, and stimulus changes, both in discrete and continuous stimuli. Further, these types of sensory events automatically cause attention switching by the attention-trigger process if some threshold is exceeded. These sensory events preceding, and possibly leading to, an attention switch are, on the model, preconscious and involuntary, and do not occupy the central limited-capacity system (until attention switch occurs, of course).

These involuntary attention switches make the limited-capacity system evaluate the portion of sensory data that are likely to have the greatest biological urgency or informational significance to the organism. Depending on the outcome of this passively elicited evaluation, that is, passive attention, active attention may also be initiated.

These brief, completely involuntary attention switches might, at least in part, account for the behavioral data of selective-attention studies interpreted in terms of "the breakthrough of the unattended" (Section 4.5). These data do not, therefore, unequivocally support the late-selection theories of selective attention and automaticity of semantic processing. These findings might be explained, at least in part, by (a) an efficient attention-switching mechanism, one driven by certain common physical characteristics of auditory stimulation which therefore causes frequent attention switches to (b) the fully elaborated representations of sensory stimulus features. These extensively processed sensory data enter, presumably, the limited-capacity system even during a very brief attentional "glimpse" of the to-be-ignored input (Cowan, Lichty, & Grove, 1990; Dawson & Schell, 1982; Holender, 1986; Näätänen, 1990; Öhman, in press).

The present explanation was not however meant to account for all auditory data interpreted in terms of the breakthrough of the unattended.

The rest might be explained by submaximal voluntary focusing of attention, because of less than maximal task loads for example, and temporary problems in voluntarily focusing attention (e.g., "attention wandering"). There is no

> reason to doubt that during periods when attention is not fully focused, the sensory codes of the to-be-ignored input usually activate the corresponding semantic codes. The model, however, was for the processing during *full* focused attention. I wonder how much semantic processing of the unattended channel still occurs under those spells of selective listening in high-load conditions when attention is really *maximally* focused and attention switching because of sensory stimulus events does not occur. According to the present model, even very brief contacts provided by attention switching between sensory information and the semantic-code system stored in long-term memory can activate complex semantic codes and the associated network. . . . (Recall also that although an attention-triggering sensory event can occur only in ongoing sensory processing, sensory information reaching the semantic analyzers in attention switching may include, as suggested by the model, the immediate acoustic past of several seconds.) This may give an impression of fully automatic semantic processing although it is still unclear whether sensory codes of audition have an automatic access to semantic analyzers. (Näätänen, 1990, p. 263)

Furthermore, as remarked Kahneman and Treisman (1984), the evidence for breakthrough does not suggest that this occurs every time. For example, Moray (1959), in his frequently cited study, found that subjects became aware of the occurrence of their names in the unattended channel in only about a third of the trials.

> Admittedly, problems of measurement (e.g., memory decay) should be taken into account, but a tempting alternative interpretation suggests itself: When semantic information was obtained from the to-be-ignored channel, attention was not maximally focused or, as the model suggests, attention switching caused by physical events in this channel occurred when sensory data carrying that semantic information were present either in ongoing sensory analysis or in sensory storage. (Näätänen, 1990, p. 263)

The previously-discussed mechanisms of attention switching, or passive attention (James, 1890), thus appear to provide for powerful environmental control over the attentional focus of an individual. They frequently cause the organism to attend to and consciously perceive ongoing stimuli and the environmental situation by interrupting, though usually only very briefly, an attentional focus directed to task performance (Näätänen, 1990). This mechanism of vital significance is shared by lower species besides humans, as indicated by an analogous phenomenon in animals (Section 4.4).

In sum, *task-independent* sensory analysis is based on: (a) rigid, hard-wired, partially subcortical, neuronal mechanisms with very brief refractory periods that extract information about specific physical stimulus features for perception and sensory memory but do not necessarily lead to semantic analysis or conscious percept; (b) storage of these sensory data in the mechanism of sensory memory; (c) transient-detector mechanisms, activated by onsets, offsets, and modulations of stimulus energy (N1 and/or the transient, 40-Hz oscillatory response), as well as change-detector mechanisms, activated by changes in a repeating stimulus (MMN). The attention-switch signals cause semantic processing and conscious perception of the subjectively silent, specific stimulus information if a momentary threshold is exceeded.

Functions of Automatic Processing

These suggestions implicate, consequently, that automatic processing in audition has three different functions:

1. To produce *sensory stimulus representations* containing extensively processed sensory information which provide the specific sensory contents for percepts (but do not per se result in the emergence of conscious percepts);
2. To cause *attention switching and hence conscious perception* via the operation of the parallel mechanism sensitive to the transients and changes but not to the specific stimulus contents;
3. To provide *arousal* via the operation of the stimulus-triggered arousal mechanisms of the brain that are especially sensitive to auditory stimuli.

Task-Dependent Sensory Processing. The model proposed in Fig. 9.1 suggests that there are two fundamentally different modes of sensory processing: In addition to the task-independent sensory analysis already discussed, there is also a task-dependent mode of sensory analysis. Further, although the task-independent processing is going on all the time, the task-dependent processing only occurs, of course, in the presence of a task that calls the task-dependent mechanisms of sensory processing into action. The model further suggests that the two processing modes can operate in part in parallel, in a cascading manner.

The role of the task-independent sensory processing is to "report" in an unbiased manner on everything going on in the external world ("What?"), whereas the task-dependent sensory processing seeks for stimuli with a certain kind(s) of physical feature(s): "Is the incoming stimulus the type of stimulus searched for?"

The underlying mechanisms of the two processing systems are, evidently, functionally separate but, at the macro level of examination, overlap neuroanatomically at least to some extent. The task-independent processing of specific stimulus features probably mainly involves lower levels of the auditory processing system than does task-dependent processing, which is likely to occur mostly at levels higher than primary cortex. These suggestions derive some support from monkey single-unit data bearing on the locus of attentionally sensitive and insensitive neurons (for a review, see Woods, 1990).

The task-dependent sensory processing is based on sensory mechanisms of early stimulus selection. This means that the organism can voluntarily "tune" its sensory systems so that certain kinds of stimuli become automatically selected for further processing, while the other stimuli are rejected. So, only the setting up, or tuning, of the selection mechanism is, on the model, a controlled process, whereas the subsequent stimulus selection is an automatic consequence of the selection mechanism being "on."

Consequently, this selection mechanism subserves fast recognition and selection of acoustic input meeting certain preset sensory criteria, those defined by the task. This selection occurs as a sensory-level matching process in which each sensory input is very rapidly compared with a representation of the physical stimulus feature or features defining the relevant stimulus (the Temporary Feature-Recognition System, Attentional Trace, in Fig. 9.1). The high speed and accuracy of this selection mechanism, as evidenced by performance and ERP data (Section 6.2), arises, presumably, because the mechanism operates at an early stage of sensory processing (cf. intrasensory selection of Johnston & Dark, 1982). Consistently with this, ERP effects associated with the operation of this selection mechanism occur at short latencies and are generated in or near the primary auditory cortex. Consequently, the mechanism is, obviously, reached by sensory input very shortly after stimulus onset. Therefore the matching process involved occurs, the model suggests, in part in parallel with the task-independent, "basic," sensory processing and the matching process uses early outcomes of the task-independent processing.

In addition, according to the model, the sensory-specific PN component is an on-line expression of the matching or comparison process (Arrow 7). Further, this self-terminating process, and thus PN generation, is initiated by each auditory input when an attentional trace exists, and is continued longer the more similar the input is to the stimulus represented by the attentional trace. The largest and longest-duration PN is generated when the stimulus is identical to that represented by the attentional trace (match).

When a match occurs, the stimulus gains access to the further processing or response belonging to the task. The match triggers the prepared further-processing chain of events, held by the Executive Mechanism in readiness, to be released by the occurrence of a match with the attentional trace (Arrow 8). In addition, when a target is found in this further processing, the designated response is released (Arrow 9). ERPs to the target usually contain a large P3 wave, often also an N2b and some slower activity, such as a late, slow frontal negativity (Loveless, 1979) (separable from the late, usually frontal, or frontocentral, PN component).

The further-processing chain of brain events may be characterized as a "prepared reflex" (Woodworth, 1938), to be released immediately when a certain antecedent condition is met, in this case, a match with the attentional trace occurs. Normally, when there is no preprogrammed further-processing sequence ready to be released, the response systems are under the direct control of the Executive Mechanisms (Arrow 10). The response is then slow—long-term memory search and evaluation is often involved—but highly flexible (Näätänen, 1990).

On the other hand, when the input fails to match the attentional trace, this input does not gain entry to further processing. Nevertheless, the task-independent processing of this stimulus runs its full course, the model suggests. This would result in the development of a sensory-memory trace accurately representing this stimulus but if no attention-switching mechanism is sufficiently activated by the stimulus or subsequent ones in close succession, then no semantic processing or conscious perception would occur.

In order to set up the highly stimulus-specific representation, the Attentional Trace, the Executive Mechanism, must, the model further proposes, use the corresponding stimulus representation of sensory memory ("Rehearsal"; Arrow 6). In addition, this representation must be recently activated by a corresponding sensory input. These assumptions are supported by Hansen and Hillyard's (1988) results that a few exemplars of the stimulus to be attended are needed in the beginning of a session before Nd can be obtained, that is, presumably, before the attentional trace can be developed to the stage permitting an efficient stimulus selection (Näätänen, 1982, 1990).

The rCBF data reviewed in chapter 8 might be interpreted as suggesting that during the existence of the attentional trace, there is a temporary functional link between the executive frontal-lobe activity and the sensory-specific mechanisms of stimulus selection (Näätänen, 1990; Näätänen & Picton, 1987). The existence of this temporary link is also consistent with the PN component structure with its sensory-specific and frontal subcomponents (Näätänen & Picton, 1987). It is possible, however, that the frontal PN component is not associated with the focusing of attention but rather with an orienting or arousal response triggered by the attended stimulus (Näätänen, 1987, 1990; Näätänen & Michie, 1979a). This possibility is supported by several features of the frontal component such as its habituability, elicitation mainly by auditory stimuli, and enhancement with long ISIs (see Section 6.2). Another expression of this orienting or arousal response might be found in the previously discussed event-related SSR perturbations (Makeig & Galambos, 1989b; Rohrbaugh et al., 1989, 1990, 1991).

The attentional trace only exists while maintained by the executive mechanism, that is, when the subject, during gaps between relevant stimuli, rehearses or imagines the feature defining these stimuli, or, when relevant stimulation is more or less continuous (such as speech), simply "listens" to it (Näätänen, 1990).

The maintenance activity does not always succeed, however. The subject may be exhausted by the long experimental session and may therefore be unable to concentrate on task performance. In addition, occasional distracting thoughts for reasons external to the task, such as a bill to be paid, might intrude in his or her mind. Probably more frequently, however, the attentional trace is lost, for brief periods of time, because the N1 or MMN generator processes are activated by corresponding stimulus events, such as the occurrence of a discrete stimulus after a silent period in the "unattended ear" (N1), and cause involuntary attention switches to the irrelevant input (Näätänen, 1985, 1990; Woods, 1990).

The attentional trace is, consequently, assumed to depend on (a) the existence of the corresponding, sufficiently activated, sensory stimulus representation in the mechanism of sensory memory; and (b) voluntary "tuning" and maintenance activity (Näätänen, 1990). This activity in turn depends on the subject's motivation and momentary ability to concentrate on task performance, probably also on temporal expectancies with regard to the occurrence of the relevant stimulus (Niemi & Näätänen, 1981).

9.2. WHAT IS ATTENTION?

Selection of Sensory Information. In the preceding section, a mechanism of selective attention underlying stimulus selection in audition was discussed. The mechanism described could account for stimulus-set type of attention of Broadbent (1970) dealt with in Section 2.3. Stimulus selection was suggested to follow the matching principle: Each input is compared with the representation of the to-be-attended stimulus and is admitted to further processing or response only if it corresponds to this representation, whereas other stimuli are rejected. The rejected stimulus nevertheless receives, the model proposes, complete processing of its physical features, which are encoded in the mechanism of sensory memory. On the other hand, this stimulus would not activate its semantic code if attention really remains strongly focused, that is, the attentional trace is maximally maintained irrespective of the attention-trigger signals elicited by the irrelevant stimulus.

The present theory of auditory attention thus assumed that attention does not affect initial stimulus representations. This is supported by auditory PN data reviewed in chapter 6 suggesting that attentional stimulus selection is, at least mainly, realized by means of a matching process rather than selective facilitation/inhibition of stimulus-elicited obligatory processes. Complementary evidence is provided by the fact that exogenous components, including the supratemporal N1 component, as well as MMN, at least to frequency change, do not seem to be enhanced by attention.

The opposite type of attention theory can be called gain theory (Näätänen, 1986e). According to this type of theory, attention can modify initial stimulus representations. This means that only attended stimuli result in fully processed initial stimulus representations, whereas unattended stimuli receive suppressed processing and therefore result in deficient sensory representations. This type of theory is illustrated by Harter and Aine's (1984) neural-specificity theory of visual attention, which was examined in Section 6.3.

Strong evidence for an attentional gain mechanism in vision can be found in the enhancement caused by visual spatial attention in the exogenous P1 and N1 components of the visual ERP and the correlation of these effects with the level of perceptual performance (Section 6.3). Consistently with this, behavioral literature suggests a special status for spatial location in visual attention (Section 2.5). This special status appears to be further supported by PET and other evidence (chapter 8) for the existence of a special posterior system for focusing attention on a certain location in the visual field (Posner et al., 1988, 1989).

On the other hand, selective attention to visual stimuli defined by some other, nonspatial attribute, such as color or shape, appears to result in stimulus selection operating at a stage in which initial stimulus representations have already been developed: This selection is associated with processing or selection negativities (Harter & Aine, 1984) rather than enhancements of exogenous components (Section 6.3).

So, both in vision and audition, selective attention can affect sensory processes. At least in vision, possibly also in somesthesis, selective attention can affect even those processes that result in the formation of initial stimulus representations (spatial attention). In contrast, physiological data do not enable one to decide with full certainty whether or not selective attention in audition can, when strongly focused, operate by selectively redistributing the gain (excitability) in the system of different feature-specific obligatory sensory analyzers. If not, then auditory selective attention is exclusively based on a separate, fully endogenous stimulus-selection system, one not at all involved in stimulus analysis in the absence of attention. Scharf, Quigley, Aoki, Peachey, and Reeves (1987; see also Scharf, 1990), however, provided behavioral data that might be interpreted as supporting selective facilitation of obligatory sensory analyzers.

On the other hand, if attention to a spatial location does not in fact increase the magnitude of the response when examined at the level of single-trial data but synchronizes the response better to stimulus onset, a possibility suggested previously, then the P1 effect observed does not qualify as evidence for attentionally increased sensory gain (but does not of course contradict it, however).

If there is a separate attentional selection system in audition, then this would permit fully developed initial stimulus representations even in the full absence of attention. The automatic development of these representations would be of vital biological significance as a prerequisite for the operation of the suggested alarm mechanism activated by changes in unattended stimuli (Section 4.5). These automatically developed and maintained high-quality representations would enable the higher mechanisms to evaluate auditory stimuli without sacrificing attention but only intermittently from the forms of information processing and action which depend on a more continuous attentional support.

Automatic processing up to initial stimulus representations appears, in general, to be important in auditory perception, because a good deal of sounds are, presumably, initially received in the absence of attention. This is due to their unpredictable occurrence and type and to the fact that attention is, as suggested earlier, long periods of time focused on visual stimuli or engaged in other activities such as motor control (chapters 1 and 8). If only deficient sensory data were available when passive-attention mechanisms of audition are activated, then initially unattended sounds could not be heard, or further processed from memory, accurately and correctly. This is because the sensory analysis of the specific stimulus features occurs, on the model, much earlier than attention can be switched to the stimulus. Auditory stimulus representations must, presumably, often even "queue" for access to higher mechanisms when they are engaged with other activities, that is, attention is focused on elsewhere, and enter these mechanisms as "chunks" composed of the whole activated part of sensory memory at the moment of an attention switch. This would in part explain the longer duration of echoic memory for stimulus sequences than that of comparable memories of the other sensory modalities (Cowan, 1988).

Automatic sensory analysis in audition is, on the model, of significance also to voluntary selective attention to auditory stimuli. If this attentional selection mechanism indeed uses sensory memory, then this sensory information must be available at the moment of the intended focusing of attention, that is, sensory data must have been extensively processed during the preceding period of absence of attention.

Commanding and Performing Mechanisms in Attentional Stimulus Selection. Mechanisms of sensory attention in each modality appear to be composed of two hierarchically organized systems: (a) the sensory mechanisms of stimulus selection, that is, the performing mechanisms; and (b) the higher mechanisms commanding and controlling these sensory performing mechanisms (Näätänen, 1988a). A similar division was implicated by Posner and Petersen (1990) and Posner et al. (1988, 1989) when they proposed a distinction to anterior and posterior attention systems.

The performing mechanisms were already discussed—the attentional trace in audition as well as in nonspatial selection in vision, and the selective gain modulation of the feature-processing system in visual spatial attention. This gain modulation is manifested by a facilitation of a part of the visual-spatial processing system that corresponds to the attended location of the visual field.

As to the commanding and controlling mechanisms, at least the frontal lobes are involved. Perhaps the most illustrative evidence comes from rCBF studies describing an activation pattern in the midsection of the superior prefrontal cortex, which appears to be the same irrespective of the sensory modality attended or the nature of the attention-demanding performance involved (see Roland, 1985).

This pattern probably reflects the earliest cerebral events in the initiation of selective attention (though the rCBF methodology does not enable one to determine the order of emergence of the different activation foci; see chapter 3). In addition, as already reviewed (Section 8.1), during selective attention, a second frontal region is also activated, whose exact location varies with the modality attended. It is therefore tempting to assume that the neural processes causing this modality-dependent frontal activation focus provide a functional link from the commanding (initiating) frontal mechanisms to the performing sensory-specific mechanisms (Section 8.1).

Deecke, Asenbaum, and Lang's (1990) very recent data on slow negative shifts during selective attention suggest that the right and left hemispheres might have somewhat different roles in the assumed frontal control function.

In visual-spatial attention, the parietal lobe appears to be involved in stimulus selection, judging from ERP (Section 6.3) and PET results (Section 8.2), as well as from observations in patients with parietal injuries (Critchley, 1953; Posner, Cohen, Choate, Hockey, & Maylor, 1984). Furthermore, a multitude of monkey data show an increase in the firing of single cells in posterior parietal cortex, in a certain region of the pulvinar, and in midbrain areas related to eye movements during attention to a certain spatial locus (Hyvärinen, 1982; Hyvärinen, Poranen, Jokinen, Näätänen, & Linnankoski, 1975; Mountcastle, Andersen, & Motter, 1981; Wurtz, Goldberg, & Robinson, 1980).

Posner et al. (1988, 1989) proposed that visual-spatial attention is based on a hierarchical organization of two systems, the anterior and posterior ones. Consistently with this, there are strong anatomical connections between the two regions (Goldman-Rakic, 1988). The anterior one is a more general, higher, control system, commanding the posterior attention system, the actual performing mechanism for the spatial selection of visual stimuli (Posner, Sandson, Dhawan, & Shulman, 1989).

Corbetta et al.'s (1990, in press; see also Lueck et al., 1989) PET data suggest that selective attention to different visual stimulus features is associated with different feature-specific activation foci in extrastriate cortex, expressing an extrastriate stimulus-selection mechanism for these nonspatial features. LaBerge's (1990) theory, reviewed in chapter 8, also suggested feature-specific activation foci as the performing mechanism of stimulus selection in visual attention. He further proposed that these activation foci are commanded and maintained, through a "thalamic enhancement mechanism," by a higher mechanism apparently located in the anterior cingulate cortex.

Somatosensory attention seems to be based on a similar hierarchical organization, reviewed in chapter 8, in which frontal executive mechanisms maintain and control sensory-specific selection mechanisms of the contralateral somatosensory cortex (Roland, 1981).

Consequently, selective attention in sensory processing could be identified with a prestimulus activation of mechanisms of stimulus selection. Thus, what we in fact select in selective attention is, strictly speaking, not certain stimuli but rather certain specific sensory systems of stimulus selection. Selection of a given stimulus takes place by selectively tuning the stimulus-selection mechanisms according to this stimulus prior to its occurrence. This stimulus-selective activation of the selection mechanism then results in corresponding attentional selection of sensory stimuli in which stimuli matching with that represented by the selection mechanism are accepted for further processing, while the others are rejected. Selective sensory processing can therefore be understood as a direct consequence of the voluntary turn-on and maintenance of the sensory stimulus-selection mechanism. This is selective attention in sensory processing.

Understanding attention in stimulus processing in terms of activation of a mechanism for stimulus selection, rather than directly as stimulus selection, dispels some of the mysticity surrounding the attention concept (see Johnston & Dark, 1986). It is only our body that is under our direct control: Via developing selective sensory states (Näätänen, 1975), we can control, select, external stimuli impinging on the receptor organs. Attention in sensory processing could, therefore, be understood as one form of selective action, the production and maintenance of a stimulus-selective state.

As already reviewed, rCBF measurements provide quite a detailed picture of these selective prestimulus states in different modalities. In addition, ERP recordings of Harter, Millter, et al. (1989; Harter & Anllo-Vento, 1991) have revealed prestimulus slow shifts with a topography suggestive of the development of a selective sensory state (Section 6.3). See also Deecke et al. (1984).

Attention and Action. Selective activation, namely, production and maintenance of task-dependent spatiotemporal activation patterns, seems to be essential in human action in general (chapter 8). Because of this, it was proposed in chapter 1 (see also Allport, 1980; Duncan, 1980; Evarts et al., 1984; Requin, 1985) that the attention concept should not be limited to stimulus processing but that it is equally relevant to motor and "purely central" behavior.

In difficult, not yet "automatized," motor performance, for example, the aspect of focusing of attention is evident. We concentrate on the production and release of the spatiotemporal motor activation pattern optimal to the task. Here again, according to the physiological data reviewed (Section 8.3), two cerebral, hierarchically organized activation patterns can be distinguished: (a) the performing pattern of motor areas, causing the muscular contractions producing the externally observable motor behavior, and (b) the control element. The cerebral executive, mainly frontal-lobe, systems (Näätänen & Picton, 1987) probably have in motor behavior a command and control function analogous to that in sensory processing: to select, program, initiate, maintain, and modify spatiotemporal activation patterns of the appropriate central performing systems.

This rapidly fluctuating sequence of executive processes of frontal cortex in motor behavior can now to a certain extent be reconstructed by recording ERPs preceding voluntary movements (Deecke et al., 1984). Among other things, slow negative potentials that precede voluntary movements suggest that SMAs (supplementary motor areas) act as a timing mechanism in control of motor behavior (Deecke, Kornhuber, Lang, Lang, & Schreiber, 1985). In addition, as reviewed in chapter 8, Roland, Larsen, and Lassen (1980) found converging rCBF evidence for an involvement of both SMAs in this control element of motor action. These authors interpreted their rCBF results as suggesting that "the supplementary motor areas are programming areas for motor subroutines and that these areas form a queue of time-ordered motor commands before voluntary movements are executed by way of the primary motor area" (Roland, Larsen, & Lassen, 1980, p. 118). In addition, there is physiological evidence for the role of certain additional frontal regions in control of motor behavior (Lang et al., 1988; Roland, Larsen, & Lassen, 1980).

Furthermore, a certain part of the premotor area is activated when a motor program is learned or modified (Roland, Skinhøj, et al., 1980; see also Seitz et al., 1990). Consistently with this, when only very simple motor movements are performed, SMAs and premotor areas are not significantly activated (Roland, 1985).

The performing cerebral mechanism in a motor task involves the motor-specific system whose spatiotemporal activation–inhibition patterns are moment-by-moment mapped onto muscles, thereby producing the overt behavior involved. Roland (1985) concluded that if overt behavior is required, fields in the motor areas are activated but that otherwise the cerebral organization of overt behavior does not, in principle, differ from other brain work.

In purely mental performance, such as in imagining a scene according to instructions or in problem solving, the cerebral organization of action appears to be much the same as when the performance situation involves stimulus input or motor output (chapter 8). Thus, thinking is also based on cerebral activation patterns, extremely specific ones, of course. Although thought sequences are, admittedly, often composed of free associations—one mental representation, memory, or node activating the next—much of the time our thinking has a definite goal. This is the case in goal-directed or selective thinking such as problem solving. When the chain of thoughts slips away from the task to an irrelevant "track"—due for example to free associations or distracting stimuli—it is promptly returned to the relevant tract. Evidently, the ongoing mental process is monitored in relation to, and guided toward, its goal stored in memory (Näätänen, 1988a; see also Ingvar, 1985). This mechanism apparently commands and controls the performing cerebral mechanisms determined by the specific nature of the thinking task.

Thus, even in thinking, the executive, control element seems to be, as in input or output selection, separable from the performing elements. Consistently with this, Roland and Friberg (1985) found that different thinking tasks induced very different task-dependent rCBF patterns elsewhere (Section 8.3) but in the superior prefrontal cortex where the rCBF increased equivalently during the different tasks which was attributed to "the organization of thinking." This superior prefrontal activation appears to express the executive mechanism in goal-directed thinking.

Consequently, selective sensory, motor, and central action, and any of their combinations, are based on specific spatiotemporal activation–inhibition patterns in the brain. In each case, an executive mechanism expressed by complex, mainly frontal, activation patterns commands and controls the performing, task-specific brain mechanism. Consistently with this, Kristeva and Cheyne (1990) proposed the concept of an "intentional trace" which, according to them, would form a central element in the presumably predominantly frontal-lobe control of all action. Furthermore, Roland (1985) proposed a division of the superior prefrontal cortex into three functionally separable command systems. In addition, Ingvar (1983) concluded that action programs for speech and language, like other serial programs of the brain, are specifically controlled by the prefrontal cortex.

In keeping with this, Pribram and Luria (1973) suggested that the activation of the anterior parts of the brain are associated with programming of goal-directed, intentional behavior.

Roland (1985) concluded from his rCBF results that the midsection of the superior prefrontal cortex is most intensely activated when (a) the subject has to maintain, or protect, selective processing of relevant stimuli in the presence of concurrent, competing stimulation; and (b) when "the differential tuning has to be switched from one group of cortical fields and areas to another group" (Roland, 1985, p. 164), that is, the attentional focus has to be changed. Furthermore, the Stroop-interference effect is associated in particular with the activation of the anterior cingulate cortex, apparently because of the increased load to the control system due to the presence of the conflicting stimulus element (Pardo et al., 1990). Also, an increased attentional load when subjects have to divide attention between several stimulus aspects rather than focusing it on one of them activates this structure not activated in focused attention (Section 8.2).

Consequently, maintaining and controlling the direction of behavior, be it overt or covert, that is, a certain spatiotemporal pattern of activation of the performing mechanisms, and changing it when needed, is, evidently, the task of the frontal executive mechanism. This mechanism has to choose one among the possible alternative activation patterns and has to defend this pattern against competing activation patterns such as those associated with erroneous movements or those elicited by distracting stimuli (Näätänen, 1973). Evidently, the better in line with the performance required and the more specific the performing activation pattern is, that is, only the relevant mechanisms are activated, the higher is the level of performance (Haier et al., 1988; Näätänen, 1973). In addition to attention, the adequacy of the activation pattern depends, of course, on the degree of practice (Näätänen, 1973; Seitz et al., 1990).

As to the performing central-level elements in a sensory task, these involve sensory-specific regions that correspond to the sensory selection required. In a motor task, the performing cerebral mechanism involves the motor-specific system whose spatiotemporal activation pattern is moment-by-moment mapped onto muscles that produce overt behavior. In a central task ("thinking"), the performing elements are reflected by complex cerebral activation patterns, as indicated by the rCBF findings reviewed (chapter 8), that correspond to the specific thinking performance required, and do not involve the primary sensory and immediate association areas or motor areas (Roland, 1985). Roland and Friberg (1985) estimated that the cortical energy consumption during thinking is equivalent, or even larger, than that during intense voluntary movements or intense processing of external sensory information.

Näätänen (1988a) stressed that selective attention, in its traditional input sense, is just "one form of selective doing or performance" (p. 152), similar in principle to other goal-directed action, a conclusion supported by the regional blood-flow and metabolic studies reviewed in chapter 8. (This holds true irrespective of whether the task requires selection among continuous stimulation or the maintenance of selective-set type of preparation preceding stimulation, Posner, 1978; the two situations invoke very similar rCBF activation patterns, Roland, 1985). Therefore he even expressed some doubt as to the usefulness of the very concept: "The attention concept appears, therefore, unnecessary, even confusing and could be replaced with the appropriate specific concept expressing the selective doing or performance (e.g., listen to this voice; search for this visual stimulus) required in a given situation. The borderlines between the sensory, central, and motor domains thus are largely artificial, at least from the point of view of a brain scientist, who should focus on brain processes rather than on their peripheral expressions in an attempt at a meaningful conceptualization of the problem area investigated" (Näätänen, 1988a, p. 153).

References

Aaltonen, O., Niemi, P., Nyrke, T., & Tuhkanen, J.M. (1987). Event-related brain potentials and the perception of a phonetic continuum. *Biological Psychology, 24,* 197–207.

Aaltonen, O., Tuomainen, J., Laine, M., & Niemi, P. (in press). Discrimination of speech and non-speech sounds by brain-damaged subjects: Electrophysiological evidence for distinct sensory processes. *Brain and Language.*

Achim, A., Richer, F., & Saint-Hilaire (1988). Methods for separating temporally overlapping sources of neuroelectric data. *Brain Topography,* 1, 22–28.

Achor, L.J., & Starr, A. (1980). Auditory brainstem responses in the cat. II. Intracranial and extracranial recordings. *Electroencephalography and Clinical Neurophysiology, 48,* 154–173.

Adrian, E.D. (1954). The physiological basis of perception. In J.F. Delafresnay (Ed.), *Brain mechanisms and consciousness* (pp. 237–248). Oxford: Blackwell.

Ahlfors, S.P., Ilmoniemi, R.J., & Hämäläinen, M.S. (1992). Estimates of visually evoked cortical currents. *Electroencephalography and Clinical Neurophysiology, 82,* 225–236.

Aine, C.J., George, J.S., Medvick, P.A., Supek, S., Flynn, E.R., & Bodis-Wollner, I. (1989). Identification of multiple sources in transient visual evoked neuromagnetic responses. In S.J. Williamson, M. Hoke, G. Stroink, & M. Kotani (Eds.), *Advances in Biomagnetism* (pp. 193–196). New York: Plenum Press.

Aine, C.J., George, J.S., Oakley, M.T., Medvick, P.A., & Flynn, E.R. (1990). Effects of spatial attention on visual-evoked neuromagnetic responses. In C.H.M. Brunia, A.W.K. Gaillard & A. Kok (Eds.), *Psychophysiological Brain Research* (Vol. 1, 3–11). Tilburg University Press, Tilburg, The Netherlands.

Aine, C.J., & Harter, M.R. (1984a). Event-related potentials to Stroop stimuli: Color and word processing. In R. Karrer, J. Cohen, & P. Tueting (Eds.), *Brain and information: Event-related potentials. Annals of the New York Academy of Sciences* (Vol. 425, pp. 152–153). The New York Academy of Sciences.

Aine, C.J., & Harter, M.R. (1984b). Hemispheric differences in event-related potentials to Stroop stimuli: Attention and color/word processing. In R. Karrer, J. Cohen & P. Tueting

(Eds.), *Brain and information:* Event-related potentials. *Annals of the New York Academy of Sciences,* (Vol. 425, pp. 154–156). NY: The New York Academy of Sciences.

Aine, C.J., & Harter, M.R. (1986). Visual event-related potentials to colored patterns and color names: Attention to features and dimensions. *Electroencephalography and Clinical Neurophysiology, 64,* 228–245.

Alavi, A., Reivich, M., Greenberg, J., Hand, P., Rosenquist, A., Rintelmann, W., Christman, D., Fowler, J., Goldman, A., MacGregor, B., & Wolf, A. (1981). Mapping of functional activity in brain with 18-F-fluoro-deoxyglucose. *Seminars Nuclear Medicine, 11,* 24–31.

Alho, K. (1987). Mechanisms of selective listening reflected by event-related brain potentials in humans. *Annales Academiae Scientiarum Fennicae, Dissertationes Humanarum Litterarum, 46,* 86.

Alho, K. (in press). Selective attention in auditory processing as reflected by event-related brain potentials. *Psychophysiology.*

Alho, K., Donauer, N., Paavilainen, P., Reinikainen, K., Sams, M., & Näätänen, R. (1987). Stimulus selection during auditory spatial attention as expressed by event-related potentials. *Biological Psychology, 24,* 153–162.

Alho, K., Lavikainen, J., Reinikainen, K., Sams, M., & Näätänen, R. (1990). Event-related brain potentials in selective listening to frequent and rare stimuli. *Psychophysiology, 27,* 73–86.

Alho, K., Niittyvuopio, T., Paavilainen, P., Summala, H., & Näätänen, R. (1992). Selective-attention effect on the auditory event-related potential in early blind human subjects. Submitted for publication.

Alho, K., Paavilainen, P., Reinikainen, K., Sams, M., & Näätänen, R. (1986). Separability of different negative components of the event-related potential associated with auditory stimulus processing. *Psychophysiology, 23,* 613–623.

Alho, K., Sainio, K., Sajaniemi, N., Reinikainen, K., & Näätänen, R. (1990). Event-related brain potential of human newborns to pitch change of an acoustic stimulus. *Electroencephalography and Clinical Neurophysiology, 77,* 151–155.

Alho, K., Sams, M., Paavilainen, P., & Näätänen, R. (1986). Small pitch separation and the selective-attention effect on the ERP. *Psychophysiology, 23,* 189–197.

Alho, K., Sams, M., Paavilainen, P., Reinikainen, K., & Näätänen, R. (1989). Event-related brain potentials reflecting processing of relevant and irrelevant stimuli during selective listening. *Psychophysiology, 26,* 514–528.

Alho, K., Töttölä, K., Reinikainen, K., Sams, M., & Näätänen, R. (1987). Brain mechanism of selective listening reflected by event-related potentials. *Electroencephalography and Clinical Neurophysiology, 68,* 458–470.

Alho, K., Woods, D.L., Algazi, A., Knight, R.T., & Näätänen, R. (1991). Lesions of frontal cortex diminish the auditory mismatch negativity in humans. *Society for Neuroscience* (Vol. 17, p. 655). Abstract No. 258.5

Alho, K., Woods, D.L., Algazi, A., & Näätänen, R. (in press). Intermodal selective attention II: Effects of attentional load on processing of auditory and visual stimuli in central space. *Electroencephalography and Clinical Neurophysiology.*

Allison, T. (1962). Recovery functions of somatosensory evoked responses in man. *Electroencephalography and Clinical Neurophysiology, 42,* 185–197.

Allison, T., Matsumiya, Y., Goff, G.D., & Goff, W.R. (1977). The scalp topography of human visual evoked potentials. *Electroencephalography and Clinical Neurophysiology, 42,* 185–197.

Allport, D.A. (1977). On knowing the meaning of words we are unable to report: The effects of visual masking. In S. Dornic (Ed.), Attention and performance (Vol. 6., pp. 505–533). Hillsdale NJ: Lawrence Erlbaum Associates.

Allport, D.A. (1980). Attention and performance. In G. Claxton (Ed.), *Cognitive psychology, new directions* (pp. 112-153). London: Routledge & Kegan Paul.

Allport, D.A., Antonis, B., & Reynolds, P. (1972). On the division of attention: A disproof of the single channel hypothesis. *Quarterly Journal of Experimental Psychology, 24,* 225-235.

Amadeo, M., & Shagass, C. (1973). Brief latency click-evoked potentials during waking and sleep in man. *Psychophysiology, 10,* 244-250.

Anch, M. (1977). The auditory evoked brain response during adult human sleep. *Waking and Sleeping, 1,* 189-194.

Anthony, B.J. (1985). In the blink of an eye: Implications of reflex modification for information processing. In P.K. Ackles, J.R. Jennings, & M.G.H. Coles (Eds.), *Advances in Psychophysiology* (Vol. 1, pp. 167-218). Greenwich, CT: JAI Press Inc.

Arezzo, J., Pickoff, A., & Vaughan, H.G., Jr. (1975). The sources and intracerebral distribution of auditory evoked potentials in the alert rhesus monkey. *Brain Research, 90,* 57-73.

Arlinger, S., Elberling, C., Bak, C., Kofoed, B., Lebech, J., & Saermark, K. (1982). Cortical magnetic fields evoked by frequency glides of a continuous tone. *Electroencephalography and Clinical Neurophysiology, 54,* 642-653.

Arnsten, A.F.T., Segal, D.S., Neville, H.J., Hillyard, S.A., Janowsky, D.S., Judd, L.L., & Bloom, F.E. (1983). Naloxone augments electrophysiological signs of selective attention in man. *Nature, 304,* 725-727.

Arthur, D.L., Flynn, E.R., & Williamson, S.J. (1987). Source localization of long-latency auditory evoked magnetic fields in human temporal cortex. In R. Johnson, Jr., J.W. Rohrbaugh, & R. Parasuraman (Eds.), Current Trends in Event-Related Research. *Electroencephalography and Clinical Neurophysiology.* (Suppl. 40, pp. 429-439). Amsterdam: Elsevier.

Arthur, D., Hillyard, S., Flynn, E., & Smidt, A. (1989). Neural mechanisms of selective auditory attention. In L. Kaufman, M. Hoke, G. Stroink, & M. Kotani (Eds.), *Advances in Biomagnetism* (pp. 113-116). New York: Plenum Press.

Arthur, D.L., Lewis, P.S., Medvick, P.A., & Flynn, E.R. (1991). A neuromagnetic study of selective auditory attention. *Electroencephalography & Clinical Neurophysiology, 78,* 348-360.

Atkinson, R.C., Holmgren, J.E., & Juola, J.F. (1969). Processing time as influenced by the number of elements in a visual display. *Perception and Psychophysics, 6,* 321-326.

Averbach, E., & Coriell, A.S. (1961). Short term memory in vision. Bell System Technical Journal, 40, 309-328.

Averbach, E., & Sperling, G. (1961). Short term storage of information in vision. In E.C. Cherry (Ed.), *Information theory* (pp. 196-211). London: Butterworths.

Baddeley, A.D. (1986). *Working memory.* Oxford Psychological Series N. 11. Oxford: Oxford University Press.

Baddeley, A.D., & Lieberman, K. (1980). Spatial working memory and imagery mnemonics. In R. Nickerson (Ed.), *Attention and performance VIII* (pp. 521-539). Hillsdale, NJ: Lawrence Erlbaum Associates.

Bak, C.K., Lebech, J., & Saermark, K. (1985). Dependence of the auditory evoked magnetic field (100 ms signal) of the human brain on the intensity of the stimulus. *Electroencephalography and Clinical Neurophysiology, 61,* 141-149.

Balaban, M.T., Anthony, B.J., & Graham, F.K. (1985). Modality-repetition and attentional effects on reflex blinking in infants and adults. *Infant Behavior & Development, 8,* 443-457.

Balota, D.A. (1983). Automatic semantic activation and episodic memory encoding. *Journal of Verbal Learning and Verbal Behavior, 22,* 88-104.

Banquet, J.P., Smith, M.J., & Renault, B. (1990). Bottom-up versus top-down: An alternative to the automatic-attended dilemma? *Behavioral and Brain Sciences, 13,* 233-234.

Başar, E. (1980). *EEG-Brain dynamics. Relation between EEG and brain evoked potentials.* Elsevier: Amsterdam.

Başar, E. (Ed.). (1988). *Dynamics of sensory and cognitive processing by the brain.* Berlin: Springer.

Bashore, T. (1990). Age-related changes in mental processing. In J.W. Rohrbaugh, R. Parasuraman, & R. Johnson, Jr. (Eds.), *Event-related brain potentials: Basic issues and applications* (pp. 242–275). New York: Oxford University Press.

Baule, G.M., & McFee, R. (1963). Detection of the magnetic field of the heart. *American Heart Journal, 66,* 95–96.

Beagley, H.A., & Knight, J.J. (1967). Changes in the auditory evoked response with intensity. *The Journal of Laryngology, 81,* 881–873.

Beaton, R., & Miller, J.M. (1975). Single cell activity in the auditory cortex of the unanesthetized, behaving monkey: Correlation with stimulus controlled behavior. *Brain Research, 100,* 543–562.

Beatty, J., Barth, D.S., Richer, F., & Johnson, R.A. (1986). Neuromagnetometry. In M.G.H. Coles, E. Donchin, & S.W. Porges (Eds.), *Psychophysiology: Systems, processes, and applications* (pp. 26–40). New York: Guilford Press.

Beaumont, G.J. (1983). The EEG and task performance: A tutorial review. In A.W.K. Gaillard & W. Ritter (Eds.), *Tutorials in ERP research: Endogenous components* (pp. 385–406). Amsterdam: North-Holland Publishing Company.

Belliveau, J.W., Kennedy, D.N., McKinstry, R.C., Buchbinder, B.R., Weisskoff, R.M., Cohen, M.S., Vevea, J.M., Brady, T.J., & Rosen, B.R. (1991). Functional mapping of the human visual cortex by magnetic resonance imaging. *Science, 254,* 716–719.

Benecke, R., Dick, J.P.R., Rothwell, J.C., Day, B.L., & Marsden, C.D. (1985). Increase in the Bereitschaftspotential in simultaneous and sequential movements. *Neuroscience Letters, 62,* 347–352.

Benson, D.A., & Hienz, R.D. (1978). Single unit activity in the auditory cortex of monkeys selectively attending left vs. right ear stimuli. *Brain, 159,* 307–320.

Berger, H. (1929). Über das Elektroenkephalogramm des Menschen. [On the electroencephalogram in man] Archives für Psychiatrie, 87, 527–570.

Berman, S., Friedman, D., & Cramer, M. (1990). Age-related changes in processing negativity during selective attention to speech sounds and pure tones. In C.H.M. Brunia, A.W.K. Gaillard & A. Kok (Eds.), *Psychophysiological Brain Research,* Vol. 2, pp. 147–151. Tilburg, The Netherlands: Tilburg University Press.

Berman, S.M., Heilweil, R., Ritter, W., & Rosen, J. (1989). Channel probability and Nd: An event-related potential sign of attention strategies. *Biological Psychology, 29,* 107–124.

Bernstein, A.S. (1969). To what does the orienting response respond? *Psychophysiology, 6,* 338–350.

Bernstein, A.S. (1979). The orienting response as novelty *and* significance detector: Reply to O'Gorman. *Psychophysiology, 16,* 263–273.

Bernstein, A.S. (1981). The orienting response and stimulus significance: Further comments. *Biological Psychology, 12,* 171–185.

Bertrand, O., Perrin, F., Echallier, J., & Pernier, J. (1988). Topography and model analysis of auditory evoked potentials: tonotopic aspects. In G. Pfurtscheller & F.H. Lopes da Silva (Eds.), *Functional Brain Imaging* (pp. 75–82) Toronto: Hans Huber Publishers.

Bickford, R.G., Jacobson, J.L., & Cody, R.T. (1964). Nature of average evoked potentials to sound and other stimuli in man. In H.E. Whipple (Ed.), *Sensory Evoked Response in Man.* Annals of the New York Academy of Sciences (Vol. 112, pp. 204–218). NY: The New York Academy of Sciences.

Blake, R., & Levinson, E. (1977). Spatial properties of binocular neurones in the human visual system. *Vision Research, 27,* 221–232.

Blakemore, C., & Campbell, F.W. (1969). On the existence of neurones in the human visual system selectively sensitive to the orientation and size of retinal images. *Journal of Physiology (London), 203,* 237–260.

Bohlin, G., & Kjellberg, A. (1979). Orienting activity in two-stimulus paradigms as reflected in heart rate. In H.D. Kimmel, E.H. van Olst, & J.F. Orlebeke (Eds.), *The orienting reflex in humans* (pp. 169–198). Hillsdale, NJ: Lawrence Erlbaum Associates.

Bonfils, P., Remond, M.D., & Pujol, R. (1986). Efferent tracts and cochlear frequency selectivity. *Hearing Research, 24,* 277–283.

Bookbinder, J., & Osman, E. (1979). Attentional strategies in dichotic listening. *Memory and Cognition, 7,* 511–520.

Boring, E.G. (1942). *Sensation and perception in the history of experimental psychology.* New York: Appleton-Century-Crofts.

Born, J., Bothor, R., Pietrowsky, G., Fehm-Wolfsdorf, G., Pauschinger, R., & Fehm, H.L. (1987). Influences of vasopressin and oxytocin on human event-related brain potentials in an attention task. *Journal of Psychophysiology, 4,* 351–360.

Born, J., Brüninger, W., Fehm-Wolfsdorf, G., Voigt, K.H., Pauschinger, P., & Fehm, H.L. (1987). Dose-dependent influences on electrophysiological signs of attention in humans after neuropeptide ACTH 4–10. *Experimental Brain Research, 67,* 85–92.

Born, J., Fehm-Wolfsdorf, G., Lutzenberger, W., Voigt, K.H., & Fehm, H.L. (1986). Vasopressin and electrophysiological signs of attention in man. *Peptides, 7,* 189–193.

Born, J., Kern, W., Fehm-Wolfsdorf, G., & Fehm, H.L. (1987). Cortisol effects on attentional processes in man as indicated by event-related potentials. *Psychophysiology, 24,* 286–292.

Born, J., Kern, W., Pietrowsky, R., Sittig, W., & Fehm, H.L. (1989). Fragments of ACTH affect electrophysiological signs of controlled stimulus processing in humans. *Psychopharmacology, 99,* 439–444.

Böttcher-Gandor, C., & Ullsperger, P. (in press) Mismatch negativity in ERPs to auditory stimuli as a function of varying interstimulus interval. *Psychophysiology.*

Brenner, D., Lipton, J., Kaufman, L., & Williamson, S.J. (1978). Somatically evoked magnetic fields of the human brain. *Science, 199,* 81.

Brenner, D., Okada, Y.C., Maclin, E.L., Williamson, S.J., & Kaufman, L. (1981). Evoked magnetic fields reveal different visual areas in human cortex. In S.N. Erne, H.D. Hahlbohm, & H. Lubbig (Eds.), *Biomagnetism* (pp. 431–444). Berlin: de Gruyter.

Brenner, D., Williamson, S.J., & Kaufman, L. (1975). Visually evoked magnetic fields of the human brain. *Science, 190,* 480–482.

Bressler, S.L. (1990). The gamma wave: a cortical information carrier? *Trends in Neurosciences, 13,* 161–162.

Brix, R. (1984). The influence of attention on the auditory brain stem evoked response. *Acta Otolaryngology (Stockholm), 98,* 89–92.

Broadbent, D.E. (1958). *Perception and communication.* New York: Pergamon.

Broadbent, D.E. (1970). Stimulus set and response set: Two kinds of selective attention. In D.I. Mostofsky (Ed.), *Attention: contemporary theory and analysis* (pp. 51–60). New York: Appleton-Century-Crofts.

Broadbent, D.E. (1971). *Decision and stress.* New York: Academic Press.

Broadbent, D.E. (1982). Task combination and selective intake of information. *Acta Psychologica, 50,* 253–290.

Broadbent, D.E. (1984). The maltese cross, A new simplistic model for memory. *The Behavioral and Brain Sciences, 7,* 55–94.

Broadbent, D.E., & Gregory, M. (1964). Stimulus set and response set, The alternation of attention. *Quarterly Journal of Experimental Psychology, 16,* 309–317.

Brookhuis, K.A., Mulder, G., Mulder, L.J.M., Gloerich, A.B.M., Van Dellen, H.J., Van Den

Meere, J.J., & Ellerman, H. (1981). Late positive components and stimulus evaluation time. *Biological Psychology, 13,* 107–123.

Brooks, L.R. (1968). Spatial and verbal components of the act of recall. *Canadian Journal of Psychology, 22,* 349–368.

Brownell, W.E., Bader, C.R., Bertrand, D., & de Ribeaupierre, V. (1985). Evoked mechanical responses of isolated cochlear outer hair cells. *Science,* 227, 194–196.

Brugge, J.F., & Merzenich, M.M. (1973). Patterns of activity of single neurons of the auditory cortex in monkey. In A. Møller (Ed.), *Basic mechanisms in hearing* (pp. 745–767). New York: Academic Press.

Brugge, J.F., & Reale, R.A. (1985). Auditory cortex. In A. Peters & E.G. Jones (Eds.), *Cerebral cortex, Vol. 4. Association and auditory cortices* (pp. 229–271). New York: Plenum.

Brunia, C.H.M., & Boelhouwer, A.J.W (1988). Reflexes as a tool: A window in the central nervous system. *Advances in Psychophysiology, 3,* 1–67.

Brunia, C.H.M., Möcks, J., Berg-Lenssen, M.M.C. van den, Coelho, M., Coles, M.G.H., Elbert, T., Gasser, T., Gratton, G., Ifeachor, E.C., Jervis, B.W., Lutzenberger, W., Sroka, L., Blokland-Vogelsang, A.W. van, Driel, G. van, Woestenburg, J.C., Berg, P., McCallum, W.C., Tuan, P.D., Pocock, P.V., & Roth, W.T. (1989). Correction of ocular artifacts in the EEG—a comparison of several methods. *Journal of Psychophysiology, 3,* 1–50.

Buchsbaum, M. (1976). Self-regulation of stimulus intensity, Augmenting/reducing and the average evoked response. In G.E. Schwartz & D.Shapiro (Eds.), *Consciousness and self-regulation* (pp. 101–135). New York: Plenum.

Butler, R.A. (1968). Effect of changes in stimulus frequency and intensity on habituation of the human vertex potential. *Journal of the Acoustical Society of America, 44,* 945–950.

Butler, R.A. (1972). The auditory evoked response to stimuli producing periodicity pitch. *Psychophysiology, 9,* 233–237.

Butler, R.A., Diamond, I.T., & Neff, W.D. (1957). Role of the auditory cortex in discrimination of changes in frequency. *Journal of Neurophysiology, 20,* 108–120.

Butler, R.A., Keidel, W.D., & Spreng, M. (1969). An investigation of the human cortical evoked potential under conditions of monaural and binaural stimulation. *Acta Oto-Laryngologica, 68,* 317–326.

Cammann, R. (1990). Is there a mismatch negativity (MMN) in the visual modality? *Behavioral and Brain Sciences, 13,* 234–235.

Campbell, F.W., Atkinson, J., Francis, M.R., & Green, D.M. (1977). Estimation of auditory thresholds using evoked potentials. In J.E. Desmedt (Ed.), Auditory Evoked Potentials in Man: New Developments (Vol. 2, pp. 68–78). Basel: Karger.

Campbell, F.W., & Maffei, L. (1970). Electrophysiological evidence for the existence of orientation and size detectors in the human visual system. *Journal of Physiology (London), 207,* 635–652.

Campbell, K.B., & Bartoli, E.A. (1986). Human auditory evoked potentials during natural sleep: The early components. *Electroencephalography and Clinical Neurophysiology, 65,* 142–149.

Campbell, K, Bell, I, & Bastien, C. (1991). Evoked potential measures of information processing during natural sleep. In R. Broughton & R. Ogilvie (Eds.), *Sleep, arousal and performance* (pp. 88–116). Cambridge, MA: Birkhauser, Boston.

Carelli, P., Del Cratta, C., Foglietti, V., Modena, I., Parquerelli, A., Pizzella, V., Pullano, M., Romani, G.L., & Torrioli, G. (1989). A nine channel DC SQUID system for biomagnetism. In S.J. Williamson, M. Hoke, G. Stroink, & M. Kotani (Eds.), *Advances in Biomagnetism* (pp. 669–672). New York: Plenum.

Carmon, A., Lavy, S., Gordon, H., & Portnoy, Z. (1975). Hemispheric differences in rCBF during verbal and nonverbal tasks. In D.H. Ingvar & N.A. Lassen (Eds.), *Brain work: The coupling of function, metabolism and blood flow in the brain* (pp. 414–423). Copenhagen: Munksgaard.

Celesia, G.G. (1976). Organization of auditory cortical areas in man. *Brain, 99,* 403–414.

Celesia, G.G., & Puletti, F. (1969). Auditory cortical areas of man. *Neurology, 19,* 211–220.

Celesia, G.G., & Puletti, F. (1971). Auditory input to the human cortex during states of drowsiness and surgical anaesthesia. *Electroencephalography and Clinical Neurophysiology, 31,* 603–609.

Chapman, R.M. (1965). Evoked responses to relevant and irrelevant visual stimuli while problem solving. *Proceedings of the 73rd Annual Convention on the American Psychological Association* (pp. 177–178).

Chapman, R.M., & Bragdon, H.R. (1964). Evoked responses to numerical and nonnumerical visual stimuli while problem solving. *Nature, 203,* 1155–1157.

Cherry, E.C. (1953). Some experiments on the recognition of speech with one and with two ears. *Journal of the Acoustical Society of America, 25,* 975–979.

Ciesielski, K.T., Courchesne, E., & Elmasian, R. (1990). Focused selective attention in normal and autistic subjects: Dissociation between ERPs and behavior. In: C.H.M. Brunia, A.W.K. Gaillard, & A. Kok (Eds.), *Psychophysiological Brain Research* (Vol. 1, pp. 166–172) Tilburg: Tilburg University Press.

Ciganek, L. (1964). Excitability cycle of the visual cortex in man. In: H.E. Whipple (Ed.), Sensory evoked responses in man. *Annals of the New York Academy of Sciences* (Vol. 112, pp. 241–253). NY: The New York Academy of Sciences.

Clynes, M. (1969). Dynamics of vertex evoked potentials: The R–M brain function. In E. Donchin & D.B. Lindsley (Eds.), *Average evoked potentials: Methods, results and evaluations* (NASA SP–191, pp. 363–374). Washington: U.S. Government Printing Office.

Cohen, D. (1968). Magnetoencephalography: Evidence of magnetic fields produced by alpha rhythm currents. *Science, 161,* 784–786.

Cohen, M.M. (1977). Effects of stimulus repetition rate and sensation level upon the EEG following response of awake human subjects. Unpublished doctoral dissertation, New York University, New York.

Cohen, M.M. (1982). Coronal topography of the middle latency auditory evoked potentials (MLAEPs) in man. *Electroencephalography and Clinical Neurophysiology, 53,* 231–236.

Collet, L., & Duclaux, R. (1986). Auditory brainstem evoked responses and attention: Contribution to a controversial subject. *Acta Otolaryngology (Stockholm), 101,* 439–441.

Collet, L., Hellal, H., Chanal, J.M., & Morgon, A. (1988). Are BAEP and MLR suited for the study of a hypothetical peripheral selective attention effect? *International Journal of Neuroscience, 41,* 97–102.

Coltheart, M. (1985). Cognitive neuropsychology and the study of reading. In M.I. Posner & O.S.M. Marin (Eds.), Attention and Performance XI (pp. 3–37). Hillsdale, NJ: Lawrence Erlbaum Associates.

Connolly, J.F., Aubry, K., McGillivary, N., & Scott, D.W. (1989). Human brainstem auditory evoked potentials, fail to provide evidence of efferent modulation of auditory input during attentional tasks. *Psychophysiology, 26,* 292–303.

Conrad, C. (1974). Context effects in sentence comprehension: A study of the subjective lexicon. *Memory and Cognition, 1,* 63–72.

Corbetta, M., Miezin, F.M., Dobmeyer, S., Shulman, G.L., & Petersen, S.E. (1990). Attentional modulation of neural processing of shape, color, and velocity in humans. *Science, 248,* 1556–1559.

Corbetta, M., Miezin, F.M., Dobmeyer, S., Shulman, G.L., & Petersen, S.E. (1991). Selective and divided attention during visual discriminations of shape, color, and speed: Functional anatomy by positron emission tomography. *The Journal of Neuroscience, 11,* 2383–2402.

Corby, J.C., & Kopell, B.S. (1973). The effect of predictability on evoked response enhancement in intramodal selective attention. *Psychophysiology, 10,* 335–346.

Corteen, R.S., & Dunn, D. (1974). Shock-associated words in a nonattended message: A test for momentary awareness. *Journal of Experimental Psychology, 102,* 1143–1144.

Corteen, R.S., & Wood, B. (1972). Autonomic responses for shock-associated words in an unattended channel. *Journal of Experimental Psychology, 94,* 308–313.

Courchesne, E., Courchesne, R.Y., & Hillyard, S.A. (1978). The effect of stimulus deviation on P3 waves to easily recognized stimuli. *Neuropsychologia, 16,* 189–199.

Courchesne, E., Ganz, L., & Nocia, A.M. (1981). Event-related potentials to human faces in infants. *Child Development, 52,* 804–811.

Courchesne, E., Hillyard, S.A., & Courchesne, R.Y. (1977). P3 waves to the discrimination of targets in homogeneous and heterogeneous stimulus sequences. *Psychophysiology, 14,* 590–597.

Courchesne, E., Hillyard, S.A. & Galambos, R. (1975). Stimulus novelty, task relevance and the visual evoked potential in man. *Electroencephalography and Clinical Neurophysiology, 39,* 131–143.

Cowan, N. (1984). On short and long auditory stores. *Psychological Bulletin, 96,* 341–370.

Cowan, N. (1988). Evolving concepts of memory storage, selective attention, and their mutual constraints within the human information-processing system. *Psychological Bulletin, 104,* 163–191.

Cowan, N., Lichty, W., & Grove, T.R. (1990). Properties of memory for unattended spoken syllables. *Journal of Experimental Psychology: Learning, Memory & Cognition, 16,* 258–269.

Cowan, N., Winkler, I., Teder, W., & Näätänen, R. (1991). Short- and long-term memory prerequisites of the auditory mismatch negativity in the event-related brain potentials. Submitted for publication.

Critchley, M. (1953). *The parietal lobes.* London: Edward Arnold.

Csépe, V., Karmos, G., & Molnár, M. (1987). Evoked potential correlates of stimulus deviance during wakefulness and sleep in cat: Animal model of mismatch negativity. *Electroencephalography and Clinical Neurophysiology, 66,* 571–578.

Csépe, V., Karmos, G., & Molnár, M. (1988a). Evoked potential correlates of sensory mismatch process during sleep in cats. In W.P. Koella, F. Obal, H. Schulz, & P. Visser (Eds.), *Sleep '86* (pp. 281–283). Stuttgart: Gustav Fisher Verlag.

Csépe, V., Karmos, G., & Molnár, M. (1988b). Subcortical evoked potential correlates of sensory mismatch process in cats. In M. Bajic (Ed.), *Neuron, Brain and Behaviour* (pp. 43–46). Oxford: Pergamon Press.

Csépe, V., Karmos, G., & Molnár, M. (1989). Subcortical evoked potential correlates of early information processing: Mismatch negativity in cats. In E. Basar & T.H. Bullock (Eds.), *Springer Series in Brain Dynamics 2* (pp. 279–289). Berlin: Springer Verlag.

Csépe, V., Molnár, M., Karmos, G., & Winkler, I. (1989). Effect of changes in stimulus frequency on auditory evoked potentials in awake and anaesthetised cats. In J. Horne & P. Lovie (Eds.) *Sleep '88* (pp. 210–211). Stuttgart-New York: Gustav Fischer Verlag.

Cuffin, B.N., & Cohen, D. (1977). Magnetic fields of a dipole in special volume conductor shapes. *IEEE Transactions on Biomedical Engineering-24,* 372–381.

Curry, S.H., Cooper, R., McCallum, W.C., Pocock, P.V., Papakostopoulos, D., Skidmore, S., & Newton, P. (1983). The principal components of auditory target detection. In A.W.K. Gaillard & W. Ritter (Eds.), *Tutorials in ERP research: Endogenous components* (pp. 79–117). Amsterdam: North-Holland.

Curtis, S., Kaufman, L., & Williamson, S.J. (1988). Divided attention revisited: Selection based on location or pitch. In K. Atsumi, M. Kotani, S. Ueno, T. Katila, & S.J. Williamson (Eds.), *Biomagnetism '87* (pp. 138–141). Tokyo: Tokyo University Press.

Czigler, I. (1983). Pattern-specific visual evoked potentials: Relations to subjective experience at suprathreshold level and the effect of attention. In R. Sinz & M.R. Rosenzweig, (Eds.), *Psychophysiology 1980* (pp. 371–378). Jena (GDR): VEB Gustav Fischer Verlag.

Czigler, I., & Csibra, G. (1990). Event-related potentials in a visual discrimination task:

Negative waves related to detection and attention. *Psychophysiology, 27,* 669–676.

Dallos, P. (1981). Cochlear physiology. *Annual Review of Psychology, 32,* 153–190.

Darcey, T.M., Ary, J.P., & Fender, D.H. (1980). Methods for the localization of electrical sources in the human brain. In H.H. Kornhuber & L. Deecke (Eds.), *Motivation, motor and sensory processes in the human brain. Progress in brain research, Vol. 54 (pp. 128–134).* Amsterdam: Elsevier.

David, E., Finkenzeller, P., Kallert, S., & Keidel, W.D. (1969). Akustischen Reizen zugeordnete Gleichspannungsänderungen am intakten Schädel des Menschen [DC-changes associated with auditory stimuli obtained from the intact human skull.] *Pflügers Archiv, 309,* 362–367.

Davis, A., & Beagley, H. (1985). Acoustic brainstem responses for clinical use: The effect of attention. *Clinical Otolaryngology, 10,* 311–314.

Davis, H. (1964). Enhancement of evoked cortical potentials in humans related to a task requiring a decision. *Science, 145,* 182–183.

Davis, H., Davis, P.A., Loomis, A.L., Harvey, R.N., & Hobart, G. (1939). Electrical reactions of the human brain to auditory stimulation during sleep. *Journal of Neurophysiology, 2,* 500–514.

Davis, H., Mast, T., Yoshie, N., & Zerlin, S. (1966). The slow response of the human cortex to auditory stimuli: Recovery process. *Electroencephalography and Clinical Neurophysiology, 21,* 105–113.

Davis, H., Osterhammel, P.A., Wier, C.C., & Gjerdingen, D.B. (1972). Slow vertex potentials: Interactions among auditory, tactile, electric and visual stimuli. *Electroencephalography and Clinical Neurophysiology, 33,* 537–545.

Davis, H., & Zerlin, S. (1966). Acoustic relations of the human vertex potential. *Journal of the Acoustical Society of America, 39,* 109–116.

Davis, J.C., & Smith, M.C. (1972). Memory for unattended input. *Journal of Experimental Psychology, 96,* 380–388.

Davis, P.A. (1939). Effects of acoustic stimuli on the waking human brain. *The Journal of Neurophysiology, 2,* 494–499.

Dawson, G.D. (1951). A summation technique for detecting small signals in a large irregular background. *Journal of Physiology (London), 115,* 2P–3P.

Dawson, M.E., & Schell, A.M. (1982). Electrodermal responses to attended and unattended significant stimuli during dichotic listening. *Journal of Experimental Psychology: Human Perception and Performance, 8,* 315–324.

Dawson, M.E., & Schell, A.M. (1983). Lateral asymmetries in electrodermal responses to nonattended stimuli: A reply to Walker and Ceci. *Journal of Experimental Psychology: Human Perception and Performance, 9,* 148–150.

Debecker, J., & Desmedt, J.E. (1971). Cerebral evoked potential correlates in forced-paired tasks. *Nature New Biology, 234,* 118–120.

Deecke, L., Asenbaum, S., & Lang, W. (1990). "Context-related" brain DC activity during selective attention. *Behavioral and Brain Sciences, 13,* 239–240.

Deecke, L., Heise, B., Kornhuber, H.H., Lang, M., & Lang, W. (1984). Brain potentials associated with voluntary manual tracking: Bereitschaftspotential, conditioned pre-motor positivity, directed attention potential, and relaxation potential. Anticipatory activity in the limbic and frontal cortex. In R. Karrer, J. Cohen, & P. Tueting (Eds.), *Brain and information: Event-related potentials. Annals of the New York Academy of Sciences,* (Vol. 425, pp. 450–464). New York: The New York Academy of Sciences.

Deecke, L., Kornhuber, H.H., Lang, W., Lang, M., & Schreiber, H. (1985). Timing function of the frontal cortex in sequential motor and learning tasks. *Human Neurobiology, 4,* 143–154.

Dellen, H.J. van, Brookhuis, K.A., Mulder, G., Okita, T., & Mulder, L.J.M. (1985). Evoked potential correlates of practice in a visual search task. In D. Papakostopoulos (Ed.), *Clinical and experimental neuropsychology* (pp. 132–155). Beckenham: Croom Helms.

DelPezzo, E.M., & Hoffman, H.S. (1980). Attentional factors in the inhibition of a reflex by a visual stimulus. *Science, 210,* 673–674.

Dennis, I. (1977). Component problems in dichotic listening. *Quarterly Journal of Experimental Psychology, 29,* 437–450.

Desimone, R., & Ungerleider, L.G. (1989). Neural mechanisms of visual processing in monkeys. In F. Boller & J. Grafman (Eds.), *Handbook of neurophysiology* (Vol. 2, pp. 267–299). Amsterdam: Elsevier Science Pub. V.B.

Desmedt, J.E. (1975). Physiological studies of the efferent recurrent auditory system. In W. Keidel & W.D. Neff (Eds.), *Handbook of Sensory Physiology* (Vol. 5, pp. 219–246). Berlin: Springer-Verlag.

Desmedt, J.E. (1988). Somatosensory evoked potentials. In T.W. Picton (Ed.), *Human event-related potentials. Handbook of electroencephalography and clinical neurophysiology* (Vol. 3, pp. 245–360). Amsterdam: Elsevier.

Desmedt, J.E., & Cheron, G. (1981). Non-cephalic reference recording of early somatosensory potentials to finger stimulation in adult or aging normal man: Differentiation of widespread N18 and contralateral N20 from the prerolandic P22 and N30 components. *Electroencephalography and Clinical Neurophysiology, 52,* 553–570.

Desmedt, J.E., Nguyen, T.H., & Bourguet, M. (1983). The cognitive P40, N60 and P100 components of somatosensory evoked potentials and the earliest electrical signs of sensory processing in man. *Electroencephalography and Clinical Neurophysiology, 56,* 272–282.

Desmedt, J.E., & Robertson, D. (1977). Differential enhancement of early and late components of the cerebral somatosensory evoked potentials during forced-paced cognitive tasks in man. *Journal of Physiology, (London), 271,* 761–782.

Desmedt, J.E., Robertson, D., Brunko, E., & Debecker, J. (1977). Somatosensory decision tasks in man: Early and late components of the cerebral potentials evoked by stimulation of different fingers in random sequences. *Electroencephalography and Clinical Neurophysiology, 43,* 404–415.

Desmedt, J.E., & Tomberg, C. (1989). Mapping early somatosensory evoked potentials in selective attention: Critical evaluation of control conditions used for titrating by difference the cognitive P30, P40, P100 and N140. *Electroencephalography and Clinical Neurophysiology, 74,* 321–346.

Deutsch, D. (1975). The organisation of short-term memory for a single acoustic attribute. In D. Deutsch, & J.A. Deutsch (Eds.), *Short-term memory* (pp. 107–149). New York: Academic Press.

Deutsch, J.A. (1977). On the category effect in visual search. *Perception and Psychophysics, 21,* 590–592.

Deutsch, J.A., & Deutsch, D. (1963). Attention: Some theoretical considerations. *Psychological Review, 70,* 80–90.

Diamond, D.M., & Weinberger, N.M. (1984). Physiological plasticity of single neurons in auditory cortex of cat during acquisition of the pupillary conditioned response: II, Secondary field (AII). *Behavioral Neuroscience, 98,* 189–210.

DiChiro, G. (1987). Neuroimaging. In G. Adelman (Ed.), *Encyclopedia of Neuroscience, Vol II.* (pp. 796–797) Boston: Birkhäuser.

Dimberg, U. (1990). Facial electromyography and emotional reactions. *Psychophysiology, 27,* 481–494.

Dixon, N.F. (1971). *Subliminal perception.* London: McGraw-Hill.

Dixon, N. (1981). *Preconscious processing.* New York: Wiley.

Dobie, R.A., & Norton S.J. (1980). Binaural interaction in human auditory evoked potentials. *Electroencephalography and Clinical Neurophysiology, 49,* 303–313.

Donald, M.W. (1976). Topography of evoked potential amplitude fluctuations. In W.C. McCallum & J.R. Knott (Eds.), *Responsive brain* (pp. 10–14). Bristol: John Wright & Sons.

Donald, M.W. (1979). Limits on current theories of transient evoked potentials. In J. Desmedt (Ed.), *Cognitive components in cerebral event-related potentials and selective attention. Progress in clinical Neurophysiology, Vol. 6.* (pp. 187–199). Basel, Switzerland: Karger.

Donald, M.W. (1983). Neural selectivity in auditory attention: Sketch of a theory. In A.W.K. Gaillard & W. Ritter (Eds.), *Tutorials in ERP research: Endogenous components* (pp. 37–77). Amsterdam: North-Holland.

Donald, M.W., & Goff, W.R. (1973). Contingent negative variation and sensory evoked responses: Their interaction and relationship to auditory discrimination. In W.C. McCallum & J.R. Knott (Eds.), *Event-related slow potentials of the brain: Their relations to behavior* (pp. 109–117). (Supplement 33 to Electroencephalography and clinical Neurophysiology). Amsterdam: Elsevier.

Donald, M.W., & Little, R. (1981). The analysis of stimulus probability inside and outside the focus of attention, as reflected by the auditory N1 and P3 components. *Canadian Journal of Psychology, 35,* 175–187.

Donald, M.W., & Nugent, P.M. (1986). Attentional tuning of a spatially specific auditory component. In W.C. McCallum, R. Zappoli, & F. Denoth (Eds.), *Cerebral Psychophysiology: Studies in Event-Related Potentials* (pp. 38–42). (Supplement 38 to Electroencephalography and Clinical Neurophysiology). Amsterdam: Elsevier.

Donald, M.W., & Young, M.J. (1982). The time course of selective neural tuning in auditory attention. *Experimental Brain Research, 46,* 357–367.

Donchin, E., & Coles, M.G.H. (1988). Is the P300 component a manifestation of context updating? *The Behavioral and Brain Sciences, 11,* 357–374.

Donchin, E., & Heffley, E.F. (1978). Multivariate analysis of event related potential data: A tutorial review. In D.A. Otto (Ed.), *Multidisciplinary perspectives in event-related brain potential research* (pp. 555–572). Washington, DC: U.S. Environmental Protection Agency.

Donchin, E., Kramer, A.F., & Wickens, C. (1986). Applications of brain event-related potentials to problems in engineering psychology. In M.G.H. Coles, E. Donchin, & S.W. Porges (Eds.), *Psychophysiology: Systems, processes, and applications* (pp. 702–778). New York: Guilford Press.

Donchin, E., Ritter, W., & McCallum, W.C. (1978). Cognitive psychophysiology: The endogenous components of the ERP. In E. Callaway, P. Tueting, & S.H. Koslow (Eds.), *Event-related brain potentials in man* (pp. 349–441). New York: Academic Press.

Donchin, E., & Smith, D.B.D. (1970). The contingent negative variation and the late positive wave of the average evoked potential. *Electroencephalography and Clinical Neurophysiology, 29,* 201–203.

Downing, C.J. (1988). Expectancy and visual-spatial attention: Effects on perceptual quality. *Journal of Experimental Psychology: Human Perception and Performance, 14,* 188–202.

Downing, C.J., & Pinker, S. (1985). The spatial structure of visual attention. In M.I. Posner & O.S.M. Marin (Eds.), *Attention and performance XI* (pp. 171–187). Hillsdale, NJ: Lawrence Erlbaum Associates.

Duffy, E. (1962). *Activation and behavior.* New York: Wiley.

Duncan, J. (1980). The demonstration of capacity limitation. *Cognitive Psychology, 12,* 75–96.

Duncan, C.C., & Kaye, W.H. (1987). Effects of clonidine on event-related potential measures of information processing. In R. Johnson, Jr., J.W. Rohrbaugh, & R. Parasuraman (Eds.), *Current trends in event-related potential research* (pp. 527–531). (Supplement 40 to Electroencephalography and Clinical Neurophysiology). Amsterdam: Elsevier.

Duncan-Johnson, C.C., & Donchin, E. (1977). On quantifying surprise: The variation of event-related potentials with subjective probability. *Psychophysiology, 14,* 456–467.

Duncan-Johnson, C.C., & Donchin, E. (1982). The P300 component of the event-related brain potential as an index of information processing. *Biological Psychology, 14,* 1-52.

Eason, R.G. (1981). Visual evoked potential correlates of early neural filtering during selective attention. *Bulletin of the Psychonomic Society, 18,* 203-206.

Eason, R.G., Harter, M.R., & White, C.T. (1969). Effects of attention and arousal on visually evoked cortical potentials and reaction time in man. *Physiology and Behavior, 4,* 283-289.

Eason, R.G., Oakley, M., & Flowers, L. (1983). Central and neural influences on the human retina during selective attention. *Physiological Psychology, 11,* 18-28.

Easterbrook, J.A. (1959). The effect of emotion on cue utilization and the organization of behavior. *Psychological Review, 66,* 183-201.

Efron, R. (1970). The relationship between the duration of a stimulus and the duration of a perception. *Neuropsychologia, 8,* 37-55.

Egeth, H.E., Virzi, R.A., & Garbart, H. (1984). Searching for conjunctively defined targets. *Journal of Experimental Psychology: Human Perception and Performance, 10,* 32-39.

Egly, R., & Homa, D. (1984). Sensitization of the visual field. *Journal of Experimental Psychology: Human Perception and Performance, 10,* 778-793.

Eich, E. (1984). Memory for unattended events: Remembering with and without awareness. *Memory Cognition, 12,* 105-111.

Elberling, C., Bak, C., Kofoed, B., Lebech, J., & Saermark, K. (1980). Magnetic auditory responses from the human brain. *Scandinavian Audiology, 9,* 185-190.

Elberling, C., Bak, C., Kofoed, B., Lebech, J., & Saermark, K. (1981). Auditory magnetic fields from the human cortex. Influence of stimulus intensity. *Scandinavian Audiology, 10,* 203-207.

Elberling, C., Bak, C., Kofoed, B., Lebech, J., & Saermark, K. (1982). Auditory magnetic fields. Source location and "tonotopic organization" in the right hemisphere of the human brain. *Scandinavian Audiology, 11,* 61-65.

Emmerson, R.Y., Dustman, R.E., Shearer, D.E., & Turner, C.W. (1989). P3 latency and symbol digit performance correlations in aging. *Experimental Aging Research, 15,* 151-159.

Epstein, S. (1973). Expectancy and magnitude of reaction to a noxious UCS. *Psychophysiology, 10,* 100-107.

Eriksen, C.W., & Hoffman, J.E. (1973). The extent of processing of noise elements during selective encoding from visual displays. *Perception and Psychophysics, 14,* 155-160.

Eriksen, C.W., & Schultz, D.W. (1979). Information processing in visual search: A continuous flow model and experimental results. *Perception and Psychophysics, 25,* 249-263.

Eriksen, C.W., & Yeh, Y.Y. (1985). Allocation of attention in the visual field. *Journal of Experimental Psychology: Human Perception and Performance, 11,* 583-597.

Erné, S.N., Scheer, H.-J., Hoke, M., Pantev, C., & Lütkenhöner, B. (1987). Brainstem auditory magnetic fields in response to stimulation with brief tone pulses. *International Journal of Neuroscience, 37,* 115-125.

Evans, E.F. (1982). Functional anatomy of the auditory system. In H.B. Barlow & J.D. Mollon (Eds.) *The Senses* (pp. 251-305). Cambridge, MA: Cambridge University Press.

Evarts, E.V., Shinoda, Y., & Wise, S.P. (1984). *Neurophysiological approaches to higher brain functions.* New York: Wiley.

Eysenck, M.W. (1982). *Attention and arousal: Cognition and performance.* Berlin: Springer-Verlag.

Farah, M.J. (1989). The neural basis of mental image. *Trends in Neuroscience, 12,* 395-399.

Farwell, L.A., & Donchin, E. (1986). The "brain detector": P300 in the detection of deception. *Psychophysiology, 23,* 435.

Farwell, L.A., & Donchin, E. (1991). The truth will out: Interrogative polygraphy ("Lie detection") with event-related brain potentials. *Psychophysiology, 28,* 531-547.

Feltz, D.L., & Landers, D.M. (1983). The effects of mental practice on motor skill learning and performance: A meta-analysis. *Journal of Sport Psychology, 5,* 25–57.

Fieandt, K. von, & Moustgaard, I.K. (1977). *The perceptual world.* London: Academic Press.

Fitzgerald, P.G., & Picton, T.W. (1981). Temporal and sequential probability in evoked potential studies. *Canadian Journal of Psychology, 35,* 188–200.

Fitzgerald, P.G. & Picton, T.W. (1983). Event-related potentials recorded during the discrimination of improbable stimuli. *Biological Psychology, 17,* 241–276.

Ford, J.M., & Hillyard, S.A. (1981). Event related potentials, ERPs, to interruptions of steady rhythm. *Psychophysiology, 18,* 322–330.

Ford, J.M., & Pfefferbaum, A. (1985). The utility of brain potentials in determining age-related changes in central nervous system and cognitive functioning. In L.W. Poon (Ed.), *Aging in the 1980s* (pp. 115–124). Washington, DC: American Psychological Association.

Ford, J.M., Roth, W.T., Dirks, S.J., & Kopell, B.S. (1973). Evoked potential correlates of signal recognition between and within modalities. *Science, 181,* 465–466.

Ford, J.M., Roth, W.T., & Kopell, B.S. (1976a). Auditory evoked potentials to unpredictable shifts in pitch. *Psychophysiology, 13,* 32–39.

Ford, J.M., Roth, W.T., & Kopell, B.S. (1976b). Attention effects on auditory evoked potentials to infrequent events. *Biological Psychology, 4,* 65–77.

Forster, P.M., & Govier, E. (1978). Discrimination without awareness. *Quarterly Journal of Experimental Psychology, 30,* 282–295.

Fox, J. (1978). Continuity, concealment and visual attention. In G. Underwood (Ed.), *Strategies of information processing* (pp. 23–66). New York: Academic Press.

Fox, P.T., Miezin, F.M., Allman, J.M., Van Essen, D.C., & Raichle, M.E. (1987). Retinotopic organization of human visual cortex mapped with positron emission tomography. *Journal of Neuroscience, 7,* 913–922.

Fox, P.T., Mintun, M.A., Raichle, M.E., Miezin, F.M., & Allman, J.M. (1986). Mapping human visual cortex with positron emission tomography. *Nature, 323,* 806–809.

Fox, P.T., & Raichle, M.E. (1986). Focal physiological uncoupling of cerebral blood flow and oxidative metabolism during somatosensory stimulation in human subjects. *Proceedings of the National Academy of Sciences of the USA, 83,* 1140–1144.

Friedman, A., Polson, M.C., & Dafoe, C.G. (1988). Dividing attention between the hands and the head: Performance trade-offs between rapid finger tapping and verbal memory. *Journal of Experimental Psychology: Human Perception and Performance, 14,* 60–68.

Friedman, A., Polson, M.C., Dafoe, C.G., & Gaskill, S.J. (1982). Dividing attention within and between hemispheres: Testing a multiple resources approach to limited-capacity information processing. *Journal of Experimental Psychology: Human Perception and Performance, 8,* 625–650.

Froehlich, P., Collet, L., Chanal, J.M., & Morgon, A. (1990). Variability of the influence of a visual task on the active micromechanical properties of the cochlea. *Brain Research, 508,* 286–288.

Fruhstorfer, H. (1971). Habituation and dishabituation of the human vertex response. *Electroencephalography and Clinical Neurophysiology, 30,* 306–312.

Fruhstorfer, H., & Bergström, R.M. (1969). Human vigilance and auditory evoked responses. *Electroencephalography and Clinical Neurophysiology, 27,* 346–355.

Fruhstorfer, H., Järvilehto, T., Lumio, J., & Soveri, P. (1970). Changes in spinal excitability during an auditory vertex response in man. *Acta Physiologica Scandinavica, 80,* 42A.

Fruhstorfer, H., & Soveri, P. (1968). Alcohol and auditory evoked responses in man. *Acta Physiologica Scandinavica, 74,* 26A–27A.

Fruhstorfer, H., Soveri, P., & Järvilehto, T. (1970). Short-term habituation of the auditory evoked response in man. *Electroencephalography and Clinical Neurophysiology, 28,* 153–161.

Gaillard, A.W.K. (1976). Effects of warning-signal modality on the contingent negative variation, CNV. *Biological Psychology, 4,* 139–154.

Gaillard, A.W.K. (1978). *Slow brain potentials preceding task performance.* Amsterdam: Academische Press B.V.

Gaillard, A.W.K., & Arkel, A.E. van (1986). Learning effects on ERPs in a memory comparison task. In W.C. McCallum, R. Zappoli, & F. Denoth (Eds.), *Cerebral psychophysiology: Studies in event-related potentials* (pp. 115–117). (Suppl. 38 to Electroencephalography and Clinical Neurophysiology) Amsterdam: Elsevier.

Gaillard, A.W.K., & Lawson, E.A. (1984). Evoked potentials to consonant-vowel syllables in a memory-scanning task. In R. Karrer, J. Cohen, & P. Tueting (Eds.), *Brain and information: Event-related potentials. Annals of the New York Academy of Sciences,* (Vol. 425, pp. 204–209). NY: The New York Academy of Sciences.

Gaillard, A.W.K. & Näätänen, R. (1973). Slow potential changes and choice reaction time as a function of interstimulus interval. *Acta Psychologica, 377,* 173–186.

Gaillard, A.W.K., & Verduin, C.J. (1985). Comparisons across paradigms: An ERP study. In M.I. Posner & O.S.M. Marin (Eds.), *Attention and performance XI* (pp. 275–388). Hillsdale, NJ: Lawrence Erlbaum Associates.

Galaburda, A.M., Sanides, F., & Geschwind, N. (1978). Human brain-cytoarchitectonic left-right asymmetries in the temporal speech region. *Archives of Neurology, 35,* 812–817.

Galambos, R. (1982). Tactile and auditory stimuli repeated at high rates (30–50 per sec) produce similar event-related potentials. In: I. Bodis-Wollner (Ed.), *Evoked Potentials. Annals of the New York Academy of Sciences* (vol. 388, pp. 722–728). NY: New York Academy of Sciences.

Galambos, R., Makeig, S., & Talmachoff, P.J. (1981). A 40-Hz auditory potential recorded from the human scalp. *Proceedings of the National Academy of Sciences, 78,* 2643–2647.

García-Larrea, L., Bastuji, H., & Mauguière, F. (1991). Mapping study of somatosensory evoked potentials during selective spatial attention. *Electroencephalography and Clinical Neurophysiology, 80,* 201–214.

Gastaut, H., Regis, H., Lyagoubi, S., Mano, T., & Simon, L. (1967). Comparison of the potentials recorded from the occipital, temporal and central regions of the human scalp, evoked by visual, auditory and somatosensory stimuli. *Electroencephalography and Clinical Neurophysiology, 26 (Supplement),* 19–28.

Gatti, S.W., & Egeth, H.E. (1978). Failure of spatial selectivity in vision. *Bulletin of the Psychonomic Society, 11,* 181–184.

George, J.S., Aine, C.J., & Flynn, E.R. (1988). Visual evoked responses to sinusoidal gratings presented in central and right visual fields. In K. Atsumi, M. Kotani, S. Ueno, T. Katila, & S.J. Williamson (Eds.), *Biomagnetism '87.* (pp. 238–241). Tokyo: Tokyo University Press.

Gersuni, G.V. (1971). Temporal organization of the auditory function. In G.V. Gersuni (Ed.), *Sensory processes at the neuronal and behavioral levels* (pp. 85–114). New York: Academic Press.

Geschwind, H., & Levitsky, W. (1968). Human brain: Left asymmetries in temporal speech region. *Science, 161,* 186–187.

Gevins, A.S. (1986). Quantitative human neurophysiology. In H.J. Hannay (Ed.), *Experimental techniques in human neuropsychology* (pp. 419–456). New York: Oxford University Press.

Gevins, A.S., & Schaffer, R.E. (1980, October). A critical review of electroencephalographic (EEG) correlates of higher cortical functions. *CRC Critical Reviews in Bioengineering,* pp. 113–164.

Giard, M.-H. (1990). More in the early selection process than the attentional-trace mechanism? *Behavioral and Brain Sciences, 13,* 240–241.

Giard, M.-H. (1991, June). *Scalp potential and current density mapping: Application for the analysis of long-latency auditory ERPs.* Paper presented at The First European Psychophysiology Conference, Tilburg, The Netherlands.

Giard, M.-H., Collet, L., Bouchet, P., & Pernier, J. (1991). Cochlear tuning: A selective auditory attention effect. Manuscript submitted for publication.

Giard, M.-H., Lavikainen, J., Reinikainen, K., Perrin, F., Bertrand, O., & Näätänen, R. (in preparation). Separation of intracranial generators for frequency, intensity, and duration mismatch negativities.

Giard, M.-H., Perrin, F., & Echallier, J.F. (1991). *Dissociation of temporal and frontal activities during the human auditory N1 wave: A scalp current density and dipole model analysis.* Manuscript submitted for publication.

Giard, M.-H., Perrin, F., Pernier, J., & Bouchet, P. (1990). Brain generators implicated in processing of auditory stimulus deviance: A topographic event-related potential study. *Psychophysiology, 27,* 627–640.

Giard, M.-H., Perrin, F., Pernier, J., & Peronnet, F. (1988). Several attention-related waveforms in auditory areas: a topographic study. *Electroencephalography and Clinical Neurophysiology, 69,* 371–384.

Giese-Davis, J.E., Miller, G.A., & Knight, R.A. (1991). *Stimulus mismatch effects in anhedonia and dysthymia.* Manuscript submitted for publication.

Gille, H.G., Böttcher, C., & Ullsperger, P. (1986). Einfluss der Intensität belästigender Schallereignisse während geistiger Arbeit auf die P300 des evozierten Hirnpotentials. [Influence of the intensity of disturbing auditory events during mental tasks on the P300 wave of the auditory event-related brain potential.] *Zeitschrift Gesamte Hygienie, 32,* 566–568.

Glaser, E.M., & Ruchkin, D.S. (Eds.). (1976). *Principles of neurobiological signal analysis.* New York: Academic Press.

Glenn, J.F., & Oatman, L.C. (1977). Effects of visual attention on the latency of auditory evoked potentials. *Experimental Neurology, 57,* 34–40.

Glucksberg, S., & Cowen, G.N.J. (1970). Memory for nonattended auditory material. *Cognitive Psychology, 1,* 149–156.

Goff, W.R., Allison, T., & Vaughan, H.G. Jr. (1978). The functional neuroanatomy of event-related potentials. In E. Callaway, P. Tueting, & S.H. Koslow (Eds.), *Event-related brain potentials in man* (pp. 1–79). New York: Academic Press.

Goff, W.R., Matsumiya, Y., Allison, T., & Goff, G.D. (1969). Cross-modality comparisons of averaged evoked potentials. In E. Donchin & D.B. Lindsley (Eds.), Average evoked potentials (pp. 95–141). Washington, DC: NASA.

Goff, G.D., Matsumiya, Y., Allison, T., & Goff, W.R. (1977). The scalp topography of human somatosensory and auditory evoked potentials. *Electroencephalography and Clinical Neurophysiology, 42,* 57–76.

Goff, W.R., Rosner, B.S., & Allison, T. (1962). Distribution of cerebral somatosensory evoked responses in normal man. *Electroencephalography and Clinical Neurophysiology, 14,* 697–713.

Goldenberg, G., Podreka, I., Steiner, M., & Willmes, K. (1987). Patterns of regional cerebral blood flow related to meaningfulness and imaginability of words—An emission computer tomography study. *Neuropsychologia, 25,* 473–485.

Goldman-Rakic, P.S. (1988). Topography of cognition: Parallel distributed networks in primate association cortex. *Annual Review of Neuroscience, 11,* 137–156.

Goldstein, M.H., Hall J.L., & Butterfield, B.O. (1968). Single-unit activity in the primary auditory cortex of unanesthetized cats. *The Journal of the Acoustical Society of America, 43,* 444–456.

Goodin, D.S., Squires, K.C., Henderson, B.H., & Starr, A. (1978a). Age-related variations in evoked potentials to auditory stimuli in normal human subjects. *Electroencephalography and Clinical Neurophysiology, 44,* 447–458.

Goodin, D.S., Squires, K.C., Henderson, B.H., & Starr, A. (1978b). An early event-related cortical potential. *Psychophysiology, 15,* 360-365.

Goodin, D.S., Squires, K.C., & Starr, A. (1983). Variations in early and late event-related components of the auditory evoked potential with task difficulty. *Electroencephalography and Clinical Neurophysiology, 55,* 680-686.

Gopher, D., & Donchin, E. (1986). Workload – An examination of the concept. In K.R. Boff, L. Kaufman, & J.P. Thomas (Eds.), *Handbook of perception and human performance, Vol. 2: Cognitive Processes & Performance.* (pp. 41-1 – 41-49). New York: Wiley.

Gorbach, A.M., Tsicalov, E.N., Kuznetsova, G.D., & Shevelev, I.A. (1989). Infrared mapping of the cerebral cortex. *Thermology, 3,* 108-112.

Gordon, E., Kraiuhin, C., & Meares, R.A. (1986). Images of the brain in psychiatry. *Australian and New Zealand Journal of Psychiatry, 20,* 122-133.

Graham, F.K. (1973). Habituation and dishabituation of responses innervated by the autonomic nervous system. In H.V.S. Peeke & M.J.Hertz (Eds.), *Habituation: Vol. I. Behavioral studies* (pp. 163-218). London: Academic Press.

Graham, F.K. (1979). Distinguishing among orienting, defence and startle reflexes. In H.D. Kimmel, E.H. van Olst, & J.F. Orlebeke (Eds.), *The orienting reflex in humans* (pp. 137-167). Hillsdale, NJ: Lawrence Erlbaum Associates.

Graham, F.K. (1984). An affair of the heart. In M.G.H. Coles, J.R. Jennings, & J.A. Stern (Eds.), *Psychophysiological Perspectives: Festschrift for Beatrice and John Lacey* (pp. 171-187). New York: Van Nostrand Reinhold Company.

Graham, F.K., & Clifton, R.K. (1966). Heart rate changes as a component of the orienting response. *Psychological Bulletin, 65,* 305-320.

Greenberg, J., Hand, P., Sylvestro, A., & Reivich, M. (1979). Localized metabolic-flow couple during functional activity. *Acta Neurologica Scandinavica, 50 (Supplement 72),* 12-13.

Gregory, S.D., Heath, S.A., & Rosenberg, M.E. (1989). Does selective attention influence the brain-stem auditory evoked potentials? *Electroencephalography and Clinical Neurophysiology, 73,* 557-560.

Grings, W.W. (1973). Cognitive factors in electrodermal conditioning. *Psychological Bulletin, 79,* 200-210.

Gross, M.M., Begleiter, H., Tobin, M., & Kissin, B. (1966). Changes in auditory evoked response induced by alcohol. *Journal of Nervous and Mental Disease, 143,* 152-156.

Grossberg, S. (1982). The processing of expected and unexpected events during conditioning and attention: A psychophysiological theory. *Psychological Review, 89,* 529-572.

Grossberg, S. (1984). Some psychophysiological and pharmacological correlates of a developmental, cognitive and motivational theory. Brain and information: In R. Karrer, J. Cohen, & P. Tueting (Eds.), *Event-related potentials. Annals of the New York Academy of Sciences,* (Vol. 425, pp. 58-151). NY: The New York Academy of Sciences.

Grossberg, S. (1990). Attention and recognition learning by adaptive resonance. *Behavioral and Brain Sciences, 13,* 241-242.

Guinan, J.J., Jr., & Gifford, M.L. (1988a). Effects of electrical stimulation of efferent olivocochlear neurons on cat auditory-nerve fibres. I. Rate-level functions. *Hearing Research, 33,* 97-114.

Guinan, J.J., Jr., & Gifford, M.L. (1988b). Effects of electrical stimulation of efferent olivocochlear neurons on cat auditory-nerve fibres. II. Spontaneous rate-level. *Hearing Research, 33,* 115-127.

Hackley, S.A., & Graham, F.K. (1983). Early selective attention effects on cutaneous and acoustic blink reflexes. *Physiological Psychology, 11,* 235-242.

Hackley, S.A., & Graham, F.K. (1987). Effects of attending selectively to the spatial position of reflex-eliciting and reflex-modulating stimuli. *Journal of Experimental Psychology: Human Perception and Performance, 13,* 411–424.

Hackley, S.A., Woldorff, M., & Hillyard, S.A. (1987). Combined use of microreflexes and event-related brain potentials as measures of auditory selective attention. *Psychophysiology, 24,* 632–647.

Hackley, S.A., Woldorff, M., & Hillyard, S.A. (1990). Cross-modal selective attention effects on retinal, myogenic, brainstem and cerebral evoked potentials. *Psychophysiology, 27,* 195–208.

Hagstadius, S. (1989). Brain function and dysfunction. Academic thesis. Lund: Lund University.

Haier, R.J., Siegel, B.V., Jr., Nuechterlein, K.H., Hazlett, E., Wu, J.C., Paek, J., Browning, H.L., & Buchsbaum, M.S. (1988). Cortical glucose metabolic rate correlates of abstract reasoning and attention studied with positron emission tomography. Intelligence, 12, 199–217.

Halliday, A.M. (1982). *Evoked potentials in clinical testing.* London: Churchill Livingstone.

Hämäläinen, H., Kekoni, J., Saarinen, M., Lähteenmäki, A., Reinikainen, K., & Näätänen, R. (in preparation). *Somatosensory ERPs evoked by occasional changes in stimulus parameters.*

Hämäläinen, H., Kekoni, J., Sams, M., Reinikainen, K., Hämäläinen, M., & Näätänen, R. (1990). Human somatosensory evoked potentials to mechanical pulses and vibration: Contributions of SI and SII somatosensory cortices to P50 and P100 components. *Electroencephalography and Clinical Neurophysiology, 75,* 13–21.

Hansen, J.C., Dickstein, P.W., Berka, C., & Hillyard, S.A. (1983). Event-related potentials during selective attention to speech sounds. *Biological Psychology, 16,* 211–224.

Hansen, J.C., & Hillyard, S.A. (1980). Endogenous brain potentials associated with selective auditory attention. *Electroencephalography and Clinical Neurophysiology, 49,* 277–290.

Hansen, J.C., & Hillyard, S.A. (1983). Selective attention to multidimensional auditory stimuli. *Journal of Experimental Psychology: Human Perception and Performance, 9,* 1–19.

Hansen, J.C., & Hillyard, S.A. (1984). Effects of stimulation rate and attribute cuing on event-related potentials during selective auditory attention. *Psychophysiology, 21,* 394–405.

Hansen, J.C., & Hillyard, S.A. (1988). Temporal dynamics of human auditory selective attention. *Psychology, 25,* 316–329.

Hari, R. (1980). Evoked potentials elicited by long vibrotactile stimuli in the human EEG. *Pflügers Archiv, 384,* 167–170.

Hari, R. (1988). Interpretation of cerebral magnetic fields elicited by somatosensory stimuli. In E. Basar (Ed.), *Springer Series in Brain Dynamics 1,* (pp. 305–310). Berlin: Springer-Verlag.

Hari, R. (1990). The neuromagnetic method in the study of the human auditory cortex. In F. Grandori, M. Hoke, & G.L. Romani (Eds.), *Auditory evoked magnetic fields and electric potentials. Advances in audiology* (Vol. 6. pp. 222–282). Basel: Karger.

Hari, R., Aittoniemi, K., Järvinen, M.L., Katila, T., & Varpula, T. (1980). Auditory transient and sustained magnetic fields of the human brain. Localization of neural generators. *Experimental Brain Research, 40,* 237–240.

Hari, R., Hämäläinen, H., Hämäläinen, M., Kekoni, J., Sams, M., & Tiihonen, J. (1990). Separate finger representations at the human second somatosensory cortex. *Neuroscience, 37,* 245–249.

Hari, R., Hämäläinen, M., Ilmoniemi, R., Kaukoranta, E., Reinikainen, K., Salminen, J., Alho, K., Näätänen, R., & Sams, M. (1984). Responses of the primary auditory cortex to pitch changes in a sequence of tone pips: neuromagnetic recordings in man. *Neuroscience Letters, 50,* 127–132.

Hari, R., Hämäläinen, M., & Joutsiniemi, S.-L. (1989). Neuromagnetic steady-state responses to auditory stimuli. *Journal of the Acoustic Society of America, 86,* 1033–1039.

Hari, R., Hämäläinen, M., Kaukoranta, E., Mäkelä, J., Joutsiniemi, S.-L., & Tiihonen, J. (1989). Selective listening modifies activity of the human auditory cortex. *Experimental Brain Research, 74,* 463–470.

Hari, R., Hämäläinen, M., Kaukoranta, E., Reinikainen, K., & Teszner, T. (1983). Neuromagnetic responses from the second somatosensory cortex in man. *Acta Neurologica Scandinavica, 68,* 207–212.

Hari, R., & Ilmoniemi, R.J. (1986). Cerebral magnetic fields. *CRC Critical Reviews in Biomedical Engineering, 14,* 93–126.

Hari, R., Joutsiniemi, S.-L., Hämäläinen, M., & Vilkman, V. (1989). Responses of human auditory cortex to change in temporal stimulation patterns. *Neuroscience Letters, 99,* 164–168.

Hari, R., Joutsiniemi, S.-L., & Sarvas, J. (1988). Spatial resolution of neuromagnetic records: Theoretical calculations in a spherical model. *Electroencephalography and Clinical Neurophysiology, 71,* 64–72.

Hari, R., Kaila, K., Katila, T., Tuomisto, T., & Varpula, T. (1982). Interstimulus interval dependence of the auditory vertex response and its magnetic counterpart: Implications for their neural generation. *Electroencephalography and Clinical Neurophysiology, 54,* 561–569.

Hari, R., & Kaukoranta, E. (1985). Neuromagnetic studies of the somatosensory system. *Progress in Neurobiology, 24,* 233–256.

Hari, R., Kaukoranta, E., Reinikainen, K., Huopaniemi, T., & Mauno, J. (1983). Neuromagnetic localization of cortical activity evoked by painful dental stimulation in man. *Neuroscience Letters, 42,* 77–82.

Hari, R., & Lounasmaa, O.V. (1989). Recording and interpretation of cerebral magnetic fields. *Science, 244,* 432–436.

Hari, R., Lu, S.T., & Sams, M. (1991). *Effects of infrequent changes of spectral and periodicity pitch on the activity of human auditory cortex.* Manuscript submitted for publication.

Hari, R., & Mäkelä, J.P. (1986). Neuromagnetic responses to frequency modulation of a continuous tone. *Acta Otolaryngology,* Suppl. 432, 26–32.

Hari, R., & Mäkelä, J.P. (1988). Modification of neuromagnetic responses of the human auditory cortex by masking sounds. *Experimental Brain Research, 71,* 87–92.

Hari, R., Pelizzone, M., Mäkelä, J.P., Hällström, J., Leinonen, L., & Lounasmaa, O.V. (1987). Neuromagnetic responses of the human auditory cortex to on- and offsets of noise bursts. *Audiology, 26,* 31–43.

Hari, R., Reinikainen, K., Kaukoranta, E., Hämäläinen, M., Ilmoniemi, R., Penttinen, A., Salminen, J., & Teszner, D. (1984). Somatosensory evoked cerebral magnetic fields from SI and SII in man. *Electroencephalography and Clinical Neurophysiology, 57,* 254–263.

Hari, R., Rif, J., Tiihonen, J. & Sams, M., (1992). Auditory mismatch fields to single and paired tones. *Electroencephalography and Clinical Neurophysiology, 82,* 152–154.

Harter, M.R., & Aine, C.J. (1984). Brain mechanisms of visual selective attention. In R. Parasuraman & R. Davies (Eds.), *Varieties of attention* (pp. 293–321). London: Academic Press.

Harter, M.R., & Aine, C.J. (1986). Discussion of neural-specificity model of selective attention: A response to Hillyard and Mangun and to Näätänen. *Biological Psychology, 23,* 297–312.

Harter, M.R., & Aine, C., & Schroeder, C. (1982). Hemispheric differences in the neural processing of stimulus location and type: Effects of selective attention on visual evoked potentials. *Neuropsychologia, 20,* 421–436.

Harter, M.R., & Anllo-Vento, L. (1990). Modality differences: Memory trace development or efferent cortical priming? *Behavioral and Brain Sciences, 13,* 243–244.

Harter, M.R., & Anllo-Vento, L. (1991). Visual-spatial attention: preparation and selection in children and adults. In C.H.M. Brunia, G. Mulder, & M.N. Verbaten (Eds.), *Event-related potentials of the brain.* (pp. 183–194). (Suppl. 42 to Electroencephalography and Clinical Neurophysiology). Amsterdam: Elsevier.

Harter, M.R., Anllo-Vento, L., & Wood, F.B. (1989). Event-related potentials, spatial orienting, and reading disabilities. *Psychophysiology, 26,* 404–421.

Harter, M.R., & Guido, W. (1980). Attention to pattern orientation: Negative cortical potentials, reaction time, and the selection process. *Electroencephalography and Clinical Neurophysiology, 49,* 461–475.

Harter, M.R., Millter, S.L., Price, N.J., LaLonde, M.E., & Keyes, A.L. (1989). Neural processes involved in directing attention. *Journal of Cognitive Neuroscience, 1,* 223–237.

Harter, M.R., & Previc, F.H. (1978). Size-specific information channels and selective attention: Visual evoked potential and behavioral measures. *Electroencephalography and Clinical Neurophysiology, 45,* 628–640.

Harter, M.R., & Salmon, L.E. (1972). Intra-modality selective attention and evoked cortical potentials to randomly presented patterns. *Electroencephalography and Clinical Neurophysiology, 32,* 605–613.

Harter, M.R., Towle, V.L., & Musso, M.F. (1976). Size specificity and interocular suppression: Monocular evoked potentials and reaction times. *Vision Research, 16,* 1111–1117.

Hartley, I.R. (1970). The effect of stimulus relevance on the cortical evoked potentials. *Quarterly Journal of Experimental Psychology, 22,* 531–546.

Hawkins, H.L. (1969). Parallel processes in complex visual discrimination. *Perception and Psychophysics, 5,* 56–64.

Hawkins, H.L., & Presson, J.C. (1986). Auditory information processing. In K.R. Boff, L. Kaufman, & J.P. Thomas (Eds.), *Handbook of Perception and Human Performance* (pp. 26.1–64). New York: Wiley.

Hecox, K., Squires, N., & Galambos, R. (1976). Brainstem auditory evoked responses in man. I. Effect of stimulus rise–fall time and duration. *Journal of the Acoustical Society of America, 60,* 1187–1192.

Hede, A.J. (1981). Perceptual selection in dichotic listening. *Acta Psychologica, 49,* 189–200.

Heilman, K.A. (1979). Neglect and related disorders. In K.A. Heilman & E. Valenstein (Eds.), *Clinical Neuropsychology* (pp. 268–307). New York: Oxford University Press.

Heilman, K.A., & Abell, T. van den (1980). Right hemisphere dominance for attention: The mechanism underlying hemisphere asymmetries of inattention (neglect). *Neurology, 30,* 327–330.

Heinze, H.J., Künkel, H., & Scholtz, M. (1988). Iterative estimation of single-trial evoked potentials. In E. Başar (Ed.), *Dynamics of Sensory and Cognitive Processing by the Brain* (pp. 321–332). Berlin: Springer.

Heinze, H.J., Luck, S.J., Mangun, G.R., & Hillyard, S.A. (1990). Visual event-related potentials index focused attention within bilateral stimulus arrays. I. Evidence for early selection. *Electroencephalography and Clinical Neurophysiology, 75,* 511–527.

Heinze, H.J., Mangun, G.R., & Hillyard, S.A. (1990). Visual event-related potentials index perceptual accuracy during spatial attention to bilateral stimuli. In C.H.M. Brunia, A.W.K. Gaillard, & A. Kok (Eds.), *Psychophysiological brain research* (pp. 196–202). Tilburg: Tilburg University Press.

Helmholtz, H. von (1896). *Handbuch der physiologischen Optik* (2nd ed.) [Handbook of Physiological Optics]. Hamburg: Voss.

Hernández-Peón, R. (1955). Central mechanism controlling conduction along central sensory pathways. *Acta Neurologica Latinoamericana, 1,* 256–264.

Hernández-Peón, R. (1961). Reticular mechanisms of sensory control. In W.A. Rosenblith (Ed.), *Sensory communication.* (pp. 497–520). Cambridge, Mass: MIT. Press.

Hernández-Peón, R. (1966). Physiological mechanisms in attention. In R.W. Russell (Ed.), *Frontiers in physiological psychology* (pp. 121–147). New York: Academic Press.

Hernández-Peón, R., Scherrer, H., & Jouvet, M. (1956). Modification of electrical activity in the cochlear nucleus during attention in unanesthetized cats. *Science, 123,* 331–332.

Hillyard, S.A. (1973). The CNV and human behavior. A review. *Electroencephalography and Clinical Neurophysiology, Suppl. 33,* 161–171.

Hillyard, S.A. (1981). Selective auditory attention and early event-related potentials: A rejoinder. *Canadian Journal of Psychology, 35,* 85–100.

Hillyard, S.A., Hink, R.F., Schwent, V.L., & Picton, T.W. (1973). Electrical signs of selective attention in the human brain. *Science, 182,* 177–180.

Hillyard, S.A., & Mangun, G.R. (1986). The neural basis of visual selective attention: A commentary on Harter and Aine. *Biological Psychology, 23,* 265–279.

Hillyard, S.A., & Mangun, G.R. (1987). Commentary: Sensory gating as a physiological mechanism for visual selective attention. In R. Johnson, Jr., R. Parasuraman, & J.W. Rohrbaugh (Eds.), *Current trends in event-related potential research* (pp. 61–67). (Suppl. 40 to Electroencephalography and Clinical Neurophysiology). Amsterdam: Elsevier.

Hillyard, S.A., & Münte, T.F. (1984). Selective attention to color and location: An analysis with event-related brain potentials. *Perception and Psychophysics, 36,* 185–198.

Hillyard, S.A., Münte, T.F., & Neville, H.J. (1985). Visual-spatial attention, orienting and brain physiology. In M.I. Posner & O.S.M. Marin (Eds.), *Attention and performance XI* (pp. 63–84). Hillsdale, NJ: Lawrence Erlbaum Associates.

Hillyard, S.A., & Picton, T.W. (1978). ON and OFF components in the auditory evoked potential. *Perception and Psychophysics, 24,* 391–398.

Hillyard, S.A., & Picton, T.W. (1979). Event-related brain potentials and selective information processing in man. In J. Desmedt (Ed.), *Cognitive components in cerebral event-related potentials and selective attention. Progress in Clinical Neurophysiology 6* (pp. 1–52). Basel: Karger.

Hillyard, S.A., Simpson, G.V., Woods, D.L., Voorhis, S. van, & Münte, T. (1984). Event-related brain potentials and selective attention to different modalities. In F. Reinoso-Suarez & C. Ajmone-Marsan (Eds.), *Cortical integration* (pp. 395–414). New York: Raven Press.

Hillyard, S.A., Woldorff, M., Mangun, G.R., & Hansen, J.C. (1987). Mechanisms of early selective attention in auditory and visual modalities. In R.J. Ellingson, N.M.F. Murray, & A.M. Halliday (Eds.), *The London Symposia* (pp. 317–324) Suppl. 39 to Electroencephalography and Clinical Neurophysiology. Amsterdam: Elsevier.

Hink, R.F., Fenton, W.H., Jr., Pfefferbaum, A., Tinklenberg, J.R., & Kopell, B.S. (1978). The distribution of attention across auditory input channels: An assessment using the human evoked potential. *Psychophysiology, 15,* 466–473.

Hink, R.F., Hillyard, S.A., & Benson, P.J. (1978). Event-related brain potentials and selective attention to acoustic and phonetic cues. *Biological Psychology, 6,* 1–16.

Hink, R.F., Voorhis, S.T. van, Hillyard, S.A., & Smith, T. (1977). The division of attention and the human auditory evoked potentials. *Neuropsychologia, 15,* 597–605.

Hintzman, D.L., Carre, F.A., Eskridge, V.L., Owens, A.M., Shaff, S.S., & Sparks, E.M. (1972). "Stroop" effect: Input or output phenomenon. *Journal of Experimental Psychology, 95,* 458–459.

Hirschhorn, T.N., & Michie, P.T. (1990). Brainstem auditory evoked potentials (BAEPS) and selective attention revisited. *Psychophysiology, 27,* 495–512.

Hocherman, S., Benson, D.A., Goldstein, M.H., Heffner, H.E., & Hienz, R.D. (1976). Evoked unit activity in auditory cortex of monkeys performing a selective attention task. *Brain Research, 117,* 51–68.

Hockey, G.R.J., Coles, M.G.H., & Gaillard, A.W.K. (1986). Energetical issues in research on human information processing. In R.G.J. Hockey, A.W.K. Gaillard, & M.G.H. Coles (Eds.), *Energetics and human information processing* (pp. 3–23). Dordrecht: Martinus Nijhoff Publishers.

Hoffman, J.E. (1979). A two-stage model of visual search. *Perception and Psychophysics, 25,* 319–327.

Hoffman, J.E. (1986). Spatial attention in vision: Evidence for early selection. *Psychological Research, 48,* 221–229.

Hoffman, J.E., Houck, M.R., MacMillan, F.W., Simons, R.F., & Oatman, L.C. (1985). Event-related potentials elicited by automatic targets: A dual-task analysis. *Journal of Experimental Psychology: Human Perception and Performance, 11,* 50–61.

Hoffman, J.E., & MacMillan, F.W. (1985). Is semantic priming automatic? In M.I. Posner & O.S.M. Marin (Eds.), *Attention and performance XI* (pp. 585–599). Hillsdale, NJ: Lawrence Erlbaum Associates.

Hoffman, J.E., Nelson, B., & Houck, M.R. (1983). The role of attentional resources in automatic detection. *Cognitive Psychology, 15,* 379–410.

Hoffman, J.E., Simons, R.F., & Houck, M.R. (1983). Event-related potentials during controlled and automatic target detection. *Psychophysiology, 20,* 625–632.

Hoffmann, E.J., & Phelps, M.E. (1986). Positron emission tomography: Principles and quantification. In M.E. Phelps, J.C. Mazziotta, & H.R. Schelbert (Eds.), *Positron emission tomography and autoradiography.* (pp. 237–286). New York: Raven Press.

Hoke, M. (1988). SQUID-based measuring techniques—A challenge for the functional diagnostics in medicine. In B. Kramer (Ed.), *The art of precise measurement in physics and medicine* (pp. 287–335). Weinheim: Verlag Chemie.

Hoke, M., Feldmann, H., Pantev, C., Lütkenhöner, B., Lehnertz, K. (1989). Objective evidence of tinnitus in auditory evoked magnetic fields. *Hearing Research, 37,* 281–286.

Hoke, M., Lehnertz, K., Lütkenhöner, B., & Pantev, C. (1989). Cortical auditory evoked magnetic fields: Mapping of time and frequency domain aspects. In K. Maurer (Ed.), *Topographic brain mapping of EEG and evoked potentials.* (pp. 537–564). Berlin: Springer-Verlag.

Holender, D. (1986). Semantic activation without conscious identification in dichotic listening, parafoveal vision, and visual masking: A survey and appraisal. *The Behavioral and Brain Sciences, 9,* 1–66.

Holtzman, J.D., Sidtis, J.J., Volpe, B.T., Wilson, D.H., & Gazzaniga, M.S. (1984). Dissociation of spatial information for stimulus localization and the control of attention. *Brain, 104,* 861–872.

Holtzman, J.D., Volpe, B.T., & Gazzaniga, M.S. (1984). Spatial orientation following commissural section. In R. Parasuraman & D.R. Davies (Eds.), *Varieties of attention* (pp. 375–394). London: Academic Press.

Horn, G. (1952). The neurological basis of thought. *Mermaid, 18,* 17–25.

Horn, G. (1965). Physiological and psychological aspects of selective perception. In D.S. Lehrmann & R.A. Hinde (Eds.), *Advances in animal behavior 1.* (pp. 155–215). New York: Academic Press.

Horst, R., Munson, R., & Ruchkin, D. (1984). Event-related potential indices of workload in a single task paradigm. In M.L. Alluisi, S. DeGroot, & E.A. Alluisi (Eds.), *Proceedings of the Human Factors Society, 28th Annual Meeting* (pp. 727–731). San Antonio, TX: Human Factors Society.

Houck, M.R., & Hoffman, J.E. (1986). Conjunction of color and form without attention: Evidence from an orientation-contingent color aftereffect. *Journal of Experimental Psychology: Human Perception and Performance, 12,* 186–199.

Howe, S.W., & Decker, T.N. (1984). Monaural and binaural auditory brainstem responses in relation to the psychophysical loudness growth function. *Journal of the Acoustical Society of America, 76,* 787–793.

Hughes, H.L., & Zimba, L.D. (1987). Natural boundaries for the spatial spread of directed visual attention. *Neuropsychologia, 25,* 5–18.

Hulbert, S.F. (1957). Drivers' GSRs in traffic. *Perceptual and Motor Skills, 7,* 305–315.

Humphreys, G.W. (1981). Direct vs. indirect tests of the information available from masked displays: What visual masking does and does not prevent. *British Journal of Psychology, 72,* 323–330.

Huttunen, J., Hari, R., & Leinonen, L. (1987). Cerebral magnetic responses to stimulation of ulnar and median nerves. *Electroencephalography and Clinical Neurophysiology, 66,* 391–400.

Huttunen, J., Hari, R., & Vanni, S. (1987). Crossmodal interaction is reflected in vertex potentials but not in evoked magnetic fields. *Acta Neurologica Scandinavica, 75,* 410–416.

Hyvärinen, J. (1982). *The parietal cortex of monkey and man.* New York: Springer-Verlag.

Hyvärinen, J., Poranen, A., Jokinen, Y., Näätänen, R., & Linnankoski, I. (1975). Observations on unit activity in the primary somesthetic cortex of behaving monkeys. In H.H. Kornhuber (Ed.), *The somatosensory system.* (pp. 241–249). Stuttgart: Thieme.

Ilmoniemi, R. (1991). Estimates of neuronal current distributions. *Acta Otolaryngology* (Stockh), Suppl. *491,* 80–87.

Ilmoniemi, R., Hari, R., & Reinikainen, K. (1984). A four-channel SQUID-magnetometer for brain research. *Electroencephalography & Clinical Neurophysiology, 58,* 467–473.

Ingvar, D.H. (1979). Brain activation patterns revealed by measurements of regional cerebral blood flow. In J.E. Desmedt (Ed.), *Cognitive components in cerebral event-related potential and selective attention: Progress in clinical neurophysiology,* (Vol. 6, pp. 200–215). Basel: Karger.

Ingvar, D.H. (1983). Serial aspects of language and speech related to prefrontal cortical activity. A selective review. *Human Neurobiology, 2,* 177–189.

Ingvar, D.H. (1985). "Memory of the future": An essay on the temporal organization of conscious awareness. *Human Neurobiology, 4,* 127–136.

Inhoff, A.W. (1982). Parafoveal word perception: A further case against semantic preprocessing. *Journal of Experimental Psychology: Human Perception and Performance, 8,* 137–145.

Isreal, J.B., Chesney, G.L., Wickens, C.D., & Donchin, E. (1980). P300 and tracking difficulty: Evidence for multiple resources in dual-task performance. *Psychophysiology, 17,* 259–273.

Isreal, J.B., Wickens, C.D., Chesney, G.L., & Donchin, E. (1980). The event-related brain potential as an index of display-monitoring workload. *Human Factors, 22,* 211–224.

James, W. (1890). *The principles of psychology.* New York: Holt.

Janday, B.S., Swithenby, S.J., & Thomas, I.M. (1988). Combined magnetic field and electrical potential investigation of the visual pattern reversal response. In K. Atsumi, M. Kotani, S. Ueno, T. Katila, & S.J. Williamson (Eds.), *Biomagnetism '87* (pp. 246–249). Tokyo: Tokyo Denki University Press.

Järvilehto, T., Hari, R., & Sams, M. (1978). Effect of stimulus repetition on negative sustained potentials associated with motor and mental acts in man. *Biological Psychology, 7,* 1–12.

Järvilehto, T., Laakso, M.L., & Virsu, V. (1975). Human auditory evoked responses during hangover. *Psychopharmacologia, 42,* 173–177.

Javitt, D.C., Schroeder, C.E., Arezzo, J., & Vaughan, H.G., Jr. (1991). Selective inhibition of "processing-contingent" auditory event-related potentials by the phencyclidine (PCP)-like agent MK-801. *Electroencephalography and Clinical Neurophysiology, 79,* 65P.

Javitt, D., Schroeder, C.E., Steinschneider, M., Arezzo, J.C., & Vaughan, H.G., Jr. (in press). Demonstration of mismatch negativity in the monkey. Electroencephalography and Clinical Neurophysiology.

Jeffreys, D.A. (1971). Cortical source locations of pattern-related visual evoked potentials recorded from the human scalp. *Nature, 229,* 502–504.

Jeffreys, D.A., & Axford, J.G. (1972a). Source locations of pattern-specific components of human visual evoked potentials. I. Component of striate cortical origin. *Experimental Brain Research, 16,* 1–21.

Jeffreys, D.A., & Axford, J.G. (1972b). Source locations of pattern-specific components of human visual evoked potentials. II. Component of extrastriate cortical origin. *Experimental Brain Research, 16,* 22–40.

Jewett, D.L., & Williston, J.S. (1971). Auditory-evoked far fields averaged from the scalp of humans. *Brain, 94,* 681–696.

Johanson, A., Gustafson, L., & Risberg, J. (1986). Behavioural observations during performance of the WAIS Block Design Test related to abnormalities of regional cerebral blood flow in organic dementia. *Journal of Clinical Experimental Neuropsychology, 8,* 201–209.

Johanson, A. (1991). Neuropsychological Studies of Dementia and Anxiety. Relations between psychological and neurophysiological aspects of cognition and emotional adaptation in patients with organic dementia and anxiety neurosis. Lund: BTJ Tryck.

Johnson, R., Jr., (1988). The amplitude of the P300 component of the event-related potential: Review and synthesis. *Advances in Psychophysiology, 3,* 69–137.

Johnston, W.A., & Dark, V.J. (1982). In defence of intraperceptual theories of attention. *Journal of Experimental Psychology: Human Perception and Performance, 8,* 407–421.

Johnston, W.A., & Dark, V.J. (1985). Dissociable domains of selective processing. In M.I. Posner & O.S.M. Marin (Eds.), *Attention and performance XI* (pp. 567–583). Hillsdale, NJ: Lawrence Erlbaum Associates.

Johnston, W.A., & Dark, V.J. (1986). Selective attention. *Annual Review of Psychology, 37,* 43–75.

Johnston, W.A., & Hawley, K.J. (1990). Novel popout in vision. *Behavioral and Brain Sciences, 13,* 244–245.

Johnston, W.A., & Heinz, S.P. (1978). Flexibility and capacity demands of attention. *Journal of Experimental Psychology: General, 107,* 420–435.

Johnston, W.A., & Heinz, S.P. (1979). Depths of nontarget processing in an attention task. *Journal of Experimental Psychology: Human Perception and Performance, 5,* 168–175.

Johnston, W.A., & Wilson, J. (1980). Perceptual processing of nontargets in an attentional task. *Memory and Cognition, 8,* 372–377.

Jonides, J. (1981). Voluntary versus automatic control over the mind's eye's movements. In J. Long & A. Baddeley (Eds.), *Attention and performance IX.* (pp. 187-203). Hillsdale, NJ: Lawrence Erlbaum Associates.

Josiassen, R.C., Shagass, C., Roemer, R.A., Ercegovac, D.V., & Straumanis, J.J. (1982). Somatosensory evoked potential changes with a selective attention task. *Psychophysiology, 19,* 146–159.

Joutsiniemi, S.-L. (1988). Comparison between electric field potentials, source dipole components and magnetic evoked fields elicited by noise/square-wave stimuli. *Acta Neurologica Scandinavica, 78,* 337–343.

Joutsiniemi, S.-L., & Hari, R. (1989). Omissions of auditory stimuli may activate frontal cortex. *European Journal of Neuroscience, 1,* 524–528.

Joutsiniemi, S.-L., Hari, R., & Vilkman, V. (1989). Cerebral magnetic responses to noise bursts and pauses of different durations. *Audiology, 28,* 325–333.

Jouvet, M., & Courjon, J. (1958). Variation of the subcortical visual responses during attention in man. *Electroencephalography and Clinical Neurophysiology, 10,* 344.

Julesz, B. (1975). Experiments in the visual perception of texture. *Scientific American, 232,* 34–43.

Julesz, B., & Bergen, J.R. (1983). Textons, the fundamental elements in preattentive vision and perception of textures. *Bell System Technical Journal, 62,* 1619–1645.

Kahneman, D. (1973). *Attention and effort.* Englewood Cliffs, NJ: Prentice-Hall.

Kahneman, D., & Henik, A. (1981). Perceptual organization and attention. In M. Kubovy & J.R. Pomerantz (Eds.), *Perceptual organization* (pp. 181–211). Hillsdale, NJ: Lawrence Erlbaum Associates.

Kahneman, D., & Treisman, A. (1984). Changing views of attention and automaticity. In R. Parasuraman & D.R. Davies (Eds.), *Varieties of attention* (pp. 29–61). New York: Academic Press.

Kahneman, D., Treisman, A., & Burkell, J. (1983). The cost of visual filtering. *Journal of Experimental Psychology: Human Perception and Performance, 9,* 510–522.

Kajola, M., Ahlfors, S., Ehnholm, G.J., Hällström, J., Hämäläinen, M.S., Ilmoniemi, R.J., Kiviranta, M., Knuutila, J., Lounasmaa, O.V., Tesche, C.D., & Vilkman, V. (1989). A 24-channel magnetometer for brain research. In S.J. Williamson, M. Hoke, G. Stroink, & M. Kotani (Eds.), *Advances in Biomagnetism* (pp. 669–672). New York: Plenum Press.

Kantowitz, B.H., & Knight, J.L. (1976). Testing tapping time-sharing, Part 2: Auditory secondary task. *Acta Psychologica, 40,* 343–362.

Karhu, J., Hari, R., Lu, S.-T., Paetau, R., & Rif, J. (1991). Cerebral magnetic fields to lingual stimulation. *Electroencephalography and Clinical Neurophysiology, 80,* 459–468.

Karlin, L. (1959). Reaction time as a function of foreperiod duration and variability. *Journal of Experimental Psychology, 58,* 185–191.

Karlin, L. (1970). Cognition, preparation, and sensory-evoked potentials. *Psychological Bulletin, 73,* 122–136.

Karmos, G., & Csépe, V. (1990). Is ERP the right key to open the "black box"? *Behavioral and Brain Sciences, 13,* 245–246.

Kaufman, L., Okada, Y., Brenner, D., & Williamson, S.J. (1981). On the relation between somatic fields and potentials. *International Journal of Neuroscience, 15,* 223–239.

Kaufman, L., Okada, Y., Tripp, J., & Weinberg, H. (1984). Evoked neuromagnetic fields. In R. Karrer, J. Cohen, & P. Tueting (Eds.), *Brain and information: Event-related potentials. Annals of New York Academy of Sciences* (Vol. 425, pp. 722–742). NY: The New York Academy of Sciences.

Kaufman, L., Schwartz, B., Salustri, C., & Williamson, S.J. (1990). Modulation of spontaneous brain activity during mental imagery. *Journal of Cognitive Neuroscience, 2,* 124–132.

Kaufman, L., & Williamson, S.J. (1982). Magnetic location of cortical activity. In I. Bodis-Wollner (Ed.), *Evoked Potentials. Annals of the New York Academy of Sciences,* (Vol. 388, 197–213). NY: The New York Academy of Sciences.

Kaufman, L., & Williamson, S.J. (1986). The neuromagnetic field. In R.Q. Cracco & I. Bodis-Wollner (Eds.), Frontiers of Clinical Neuroscience, *Evoked potentials,* (*Vol. 3,* pp. 85–98). New York: Alan R. Liss, Inc.

Kaufman, L., & Williamson, S.J. (1987). Recent developments in neuromagnetism. In C. Barber & T. Blum (Eds.), *Evoked potentials III* (pp. 100–113). London: Butterworths.

Kaufman, L., & Williamson, S.J. (1989). Neuromagnetic localization of neuronal activity in visual and extra-visual cortex. In B. Cohen & I. Bodis-Wollner (Eds.) *Vision and the brain: The organization of the central visual systems* (Vol. 67, pp. 271–287). Research Publications: Association for Research in Nervous and Mental Disease.

Kaufman, L., & Williamson, S.J. (1988b). Recent developments in neuromagnetism: Implications for imaging. In G. Pfurtscheller & F.H. Lopes da Silva (Eds.), *Functional brain imaging* (pp. 11–29). Bern: Hans Huber Publishers.

Kaufman, L., & Williamson, S.J. (1991). Neuromagnetic studies of sensory functions and mental imagery. In C.H.M. Brunia, G. Mulder, & M.N. Verbaten (Eds.), *Event-Related*

Potentials of the Brain (pp. 13-23). (Suppl. 42 to Electroencephalography and Clinical Neurophysiology). Amsterdam: Elsevier.

Kaukoranta, E., Hari, R., Hämäläinen, M., & Huttunen, J. (1986). Cerebral magnetic fields evoked by peroneal nerve stimulation. *Somatosensory Research, 3,* 309-321.

Kaukoranta, E., Hari, R., & Lounasmaa, O.V. (1987). Responses of the human auditory cortex to vowel onset after fricative consonants. *Experimental Brain Research, 69,* 19-23.

Kaukoranta, E., & Reinikainen, K. (1985). *Somatosensory evoked magnetic fields from SI: An interpretation of the spatiotemporal field pattern and effects of stimulus repetition rate* (p. 10). Helsinki University of Technology, Low Temperature Laboratory, Report TKK-F-A581.

Kaukoranta, E., Sams, M., Hari, R., Hämäläinen, M., & Näätänen, R. (1989). Reactions of human auditory cortex to a change in tone duration. *Hearing Research, 41,* 15-22.

Keele, S.W. (1973). Attention and human performance. Pacific Palisades, California: Goodyear.

Keidel, W.D. (1971). D.C.-potentials in the auditory evoked response in man. *Acta Otolaryngology, 71,* 242-248.

Keidel, W.D. (1976). The physiological background of evoked response audiometry. In W.D. Keidel & W.D. Neff (Eds.), *Handbook of Sensory Physiology* (Vol. V/3. pp. 105-231). Berlin: Springer-Verlag.

Kemp, D.T. (1978). Stimulated acoustic emissions from the human auditory system. *The Journal of the Acoustical Society of America, 64,* 1386-1391.

Kenemans, J.L., Verbaten, M.N., Roelofs, J.W., & Slangen, J.L. (1989). Initial- and change-orienting reactions: An analysis based on single-trial event-related potentials. *Biological Psychology, 28,* 199-226.

Kerr, B. (1973). Processing demands during mental operations. *Memory and Cognition, 1,* 401-412.

Kety, S.S., & Schmidt, C.F. (1948). Nitrous oxide method for the quantitative determination of the cerebral blood flow in man: Theory, procedure, and normal values. *The Journal of Clinical Investigation, 27,* 476-483.

Kevanishvili, Z.S., & Specht, H. von (1979). Human slow auditory evoked potentials during natural and drug-induced sleep. *Electroencephalography and Clinical Neurophysiology, 47,* 280-288.

Kimmel, H.D., Olst, F.H. van, & Orlebeke, J.F. (Eds.). (1979). The orienting reflex in humans. Hillsdale, NJ: Lawrence Erlbaum Associates.

Kinchla, R.A. (1980). The measurement of attention. In R.S. Nickerson (Ed.), *Attention and performance VIII* (pp. 215-238). Hillsdale, NJ: Lawrence Erlbaum Associates.

King, A.J., & Moore, D.R. (1991). Plasticity of auditory maps in the brain. *Trends in Neurosciences, 14,* 31-37.

Kinsbourne, M., & Hicks, R.E. (1978). Functional cerebral space: A model for overflow, transfer and interference effects in human performance. In J. Requin (Ed.), *Attention and performance VII.* (pp. 345-362). New York: Academic Press.

Kitajima, S., Morotomi, R., & Kanoh, M. (1975). Enhancement of averaged evoked responses to brief flashes after offset of preexposed light stimulation: A critical movement. *Vision Research, 15,* 1213-1216.

Klemmer, E.T. (1956). Time uncertainty in simple reaction time. *Journal of Experimental Psychology, 51,* 179-184.

Klimesch, W., Pfurtscheller, G., & Mohl, W. (1988). ERD mapping and long-term memory: The temporal and topographical pattern of cortical activation. In G. Pfurtscheller & F.H. Lopes da Silva (Eds.), *Functional brain imaging.* (pp. 131-141). Toronto: Hans Huber Publishers.

Klinke, R., Fruhstorfer, H., & Finkenzeller, P. (1968). Evoked responses as a function of external and stored information. *Electroencephalography and Clinical Neurophysiology, 25,* 119–122.

Knight, R.T. (1984). Decreased response to novel stimuli after prefrontal lesions in man. *Electroencephalography and Clinical Neurophysiology, 59,* 9–20.

Knight, R.T. (1985). Electrophysiology in behavioral neurology. In M. Marsel (Ed.), Principles of behavioral neurology (pp. 327-346). Philadelphia: F.A. Davis Co.

Knight, R.T. (1990). Neural mechanisms of event related potentials: Evidence from human lesion studies. In J.W. Rohrbaugh, R. Parasuraman, & R. Johnson, Jr. (Eds.), *Event-related brain potentials: Basic issues and applications* (pp. 3–18). New York: Oxford University Press.

Knight, R.T., Hillyard, S.A., Woods, D.L., & Neville, H.J. (1980). The effects of frontal and temporal-parietal lesions on the auditory evoked potential in man. *Electroencephalography and Clinical Neurophysiology, 50,* 112–124.

Knight, R.T., Hillyard, S.A., Woods, D.L., & Neville, H.J. (1981). The effects of frontal cortex lesions on event-related potentials during auditory selective attention. *Electroencephalography and Clinical Neurophysiology, 52,* 571–582.

Knowles, W.B. (1963). Operator loading tasks. *Human Factors, 5,* 151–161.

Kodera, K., Hink, R.F., Yamada, O., & Suzuki, J. (1979). Effects of rise time on simultaneously recorded auditory-evoked potentials from the early, middle and late ranges. *Audiology, 18,* 395–402.

Köhler, W., Held, R., & O'Connell, D.N. (1952). An investigation of cortical currents. *Proceedings of the American Philosophical Society, 96,* 290–330.

Köhler, W., Neff, W.D., & Wegener, J. (1955). Currents of the auditory cortex in the cat. *The Journal of Cellular and Comparative Physiology, 1,* 1–24.

Köhler, W., & O'Connell, D.N. (1957). Currents of the visual cortex in the cat. *The Journal of Cellular and Comparative Physiology, 49* (Suppl. 2) 1–43.

Köhler, W., & Wegener, J. (1955). Currents of the human auditory cortex. *The Journal of Cellular and Comparative Physiology, 1,* 25–54.

Kohn, M., Lifshitz, K., & Litchfield, D. (1978). Averaged evoked potentials and frequency modulation. *Electroencephalography and Clinical Neurophysiology, 45,* 236–243.

Kohn, M., Lifshitz, K., & Litchfield, D. (1980). Averaged evoked potentials and amplitude modulation. *Electroencephalography and Clinical Neurophysiology, 50,* 134–140.

Kolb, B., & Whishaw, I.Q. (1985). *Fundamentals of human neuropsychology* (2nd ed.). New York: Freeman.

Konorski, J.M. (1948). *Conditioned reflexes and neuron organization.* London: Cambridge University Press.

Kooi, K.A., Tipton, A.C., & Marshall, R.E. (1971). Polarities and field configurations of the vertex components of the human auditory evoked response: A reinterpretation. *Electroencephalography and Clinical Neurophysiology, 31,* 166–169.

Kornhuber, H.H., & Deecke, L. (1965). Hirnpotentialänderungen bei Willkürbewegungen und passiven Bewegungen des Menschen: Bereitschaftspotential und reafferente Potentiale. (Brain-potential changes associated with voluntary and passive movements in humans: The Bereitschaftspotential and reafferent potentials.) *Pflügers Archiv, 284,* 1–17.

Kosslyn, S.M., Berndt, R.S., & Doyle, T.J. (1985). Imagery and language processing: A Neurophysiological approach. In M.I. Posner & O.S.M. Marin (Eds.), *Attention and Performance XI* (pp. 319–334). Hillsdale, NJ: Lawrence Erlbaum Associates.

Kramer, A.F., & Spinks, J. (1991). Capacity views of human information processing. In R. Jennings & M.G.H. Coles (Eds.), Handbook of Cognitive Psychophysiology: Central and Autonomic Nervous Systems Approaches (pp. 179–249). London: John Wiley and Sons.

Kramer, A.F., Schneider, W., Fisk, A., & Donchin, E. (1986). The effects of practice and task structure on components of the event-related brain potential. *Psychophysiology, 23,* 33–47.

Kramer, A.F., Sirevaag, E., & Braune, R. (1987). A psychophysiological assessment of operator workload during simulated flight missions. *Human Factors, 29,* 145–160.

Kramer, A.F., Sirevaag, E.J., & Hughes, P.R. (1988). Effects of foveal task load on visual-spatial attention: Event-related brain potentials and performance. *Psychophysiology, 25,* 512–531.

Kramer, A.F., & Strayer, D.L. (1988). Assessing the development of automatic processing: An application of dual-task and event-related brain potential methodologies. *Biological Psychology, 26,* 231–267.

Kramer, A.F., Wickens, C.D., & Donchin, E. (1983). An analysis of the processing requirements of a complex perceptual-motor task. *Human Factors, 25,* 597–621.

Kramer, A.F., Wickens, C.D., & Donchin, E. (1985). Processing of stimulus properties: Evidence for dual-task integrality. *Journal of Experimental Psychology: Human Perception and Performance, 11,* 393–408.

Kramer, A.F., Wickens, C., Vanasse, L., & Donchin, E. (1981). Primary and secondary task analysis of step tracking: An event-related potentials approach. In R.C. Sugarman (Ed.), *Proceedings of the 25th Annual Meeting of the Human Factors Society* (pp. 43–47). Rochester, NY: Human Factors Society.

Krauskopf, J., Klemic, G., Lounasmaa, O.V., Travis, D., Kaufman, L., & Williamson, S.J. (1989). Neuromagnetic measurements of visual responses to chromaticity and luminance. In S.J. Williamson, M. Hoke, G. Stroink, & M. Kotani (Eds.), *Advances in Biomagnetism* (pp. 209–212). New York: Plenum Press.

Kristeva, R., & Cheyne, D. (1990). Similarities between attentional and preparatory states. *Behavioral and Brain Sciences, 13,* 247.

Kroll, N.E.A. (1975). Visual short-term memory. In D. Deutsch & J.A. Deutsch (Eds.), *Short-term memory* (pp. 108–151). New York: Academic Press.

Kuriki, S., & Murase, M. (1989). Neuromagnetic study of the auditory responses in right and left hemispheres of the human brain evoked by pure tones and speech sounds. *Experimental Brain Research, 77,* 127–134.

Kuriki, S., Isobe, Y., & Mizutani, Y. (1988). Measurements of auditory and somatically evoked magnetic fields and localization of their sources. *Frontiers in Medical and Biological Engineering, 1,* 107–118.

Kurtzberg, D. (1989). Cortical event-related potential assessment of auditory system function. *Seminars in Hearing, 10,* 252–261.

Kurtzberg, D., Stapells, D.R., & Wallace, I.F. (1988). Event-related potential assessment of auditory system integrity: Implications for language development. In P. Vietze & H.G. Vaughan, Jr. (Eds.), *Early identification of infants with developmental disabilities* (pp. 160–180). Philadelphia: Grune & Stratton.

Kurtzberg, D., Stone, C.L., & Vaughan, H.G., Jr. (1986). Cortical responses to speech sounds in the infant. In R.Q. Cracco & I. Bodis-Wollner (Eds.), *Evoked potentials* (pp. 513–520). New York: Alan R. Liss.

Kurtzberg, D., Vaughan, H.G., Jr., & Novak, G.P. (1986). Discriminative brain responses to speech sounds in the newborn high risk infant. In V. Gallai (Ed.), *Maturation of the CNS and evoked potentials* (pp. 253–259). Amsterdam: Elsevier.

LaBerge, D. (1973). Attention and the measurement of perceptual learning. *Memory and Cognition, 1,* 268–276.

LaBerge, D. (1975). Acquisition of automatic processing in perceptual and associative learning. In P.M.Å. Rabbitt & S. Vyas (Eds.), *Attention and performance V* (pp. 50–64). New York: Academic Press.

LaBerge, D. (1983). Spatial extent of attention to letters and words. *Journal of Experimental Psychology: Human Perception and Performance, 9,* 371–379.

LaBerge, D. (1990). Thalamic and cortical mechanisms of attention suggested by recent positron emission tomographic experiments. *Journal of Cognitive Neuroscience, 2,* 358–372.

LaBerge, D., & Buchsbaum, M.S. (1990). Positron emission tomographic measurements of pulvinar activity during an attention task. *The Journal of Neuroscience, 10,* 613–619.

LaBerge, D., & Samuels, J. (1974). Toward a theory of automatic information processing in reading. *Cognitive Psychology, 6,* 293–323.

Lacey, J.L. (1967). Somatic response patterning and stress: Some revisions of activation theory. In M. Appley & R. Trumbull (Eds.), *Psychological stress: Issues in research* (pp. 14–44). New York: Appleton-Century-Crofts.

Lackner, J.R., & Garrett, M.F. (1972). Resolving ambiguity: Effects of biasing context in the unattended ear. *Cognition, 1,* 359–372.

Lang, A.H., Nyrke, T., Ek, M., Aaltonen, O., Raimo, I., Näätänen, R. (1990). Pitch discrimination performance and auditory event-related potentials. In C.H.M. Brunia, A.W.K. Gaillard, & A. Kok (Eds.), Psychophysiological brain research (Vol. 1., pp. 294–298). Tilburg: Tilburg University Press.

Lang, A.H., Mikola, H., Rinne, J., & Eerola, O. (in preparation). *Interindividual variability of mismatch negativity* (MMN).

Lang, W., Lang, M., Kornhuber, A., Deecke, L., & Kornhuber, H.H. (1983). Human cerebral potentials and visuomotor learning. *Pflügers Archiv 284,* 1–17.

Lang, W., Lang, M., Kornhuber, A., Deecke, L., & Kornhuber, H.H. (1984). Brain potentials related to voluntary hand tracking: Motivation and attention. *Human Neurobiology, 3,* 235–240.

Lang, W., Lang, M., Kornhuber, A., Deecke, L., & Kornhuber, H.H. (1986). Electrophysiological evidence for right frontal lobe dominance in spatial visuomotor learning. *Archives of Italian Biology, 124,* 1–13.

Lang, W., Lang, M., Podreka, I., Steiner, M., Uhl, F., Suess, E., Müller, C., & Deecke, L. (1988). DC-potential shifts and regional cerebral blood flow reveal frontal cortex involvement in human visuomotor learning. *Experimental Brain Research, 71,* 353–354.

Larsson, L.E. (1956). The relation between the startle reaction and the nonspecific EEG response to sudden stimuli with a discussion on the mechanism of arousal. *Electroencephalography and Clinical Neurophysiology, 8,* 631–644.

Larsson, L.E. (1960a). Sensitization of the startle blink and nonspecific electroencephalographic response. *Electroencephalography and Clinical Neurophysiology, 12,* 727–733.

Larsson, L.E. (1960b). Correlation between the psychological significance of stimuli and the magnitudes of the startle blink and evoked EEG potentials in man. *Acta Physiologica Scandinavica, 48,* 276–294.

Lassen, N.A. (1966). The luxury perfusion syndrome and its possible relation to acute metabolic acidosis localized within the brain. *Lancet, 2,* 1112–1115.

Lassen, N.A., & Ingvar, D.H. (1961). The blood-flow of the cerebral cortex determined by radioactive krypton-85. *Experientia, 17,* 42–50.

Lauter, J.L., Herschovitch, P., Formby, C., & Raichle, M.E. (1985). Tonotopic organization in the human auditory cortex revealed by positron emission tomography. *Hearing Research, 20,* 199–205.

Lawson, E.A. (1966). Decisions concerning the rejected channel. *Quarterly Journal of Experimental Psychology, 18,* 260–265.

Legatt, A.D., Arezzo, J.C., & Vaughan, H.G., Jr. (1988). The anatomic and physiologic bases of brain stem auditory evoked potentials. *Neurology Clinics, 6,* 681–704.

Leenders, K.L. (1988). Positron emission tomographic studies of aging and dementia. In: G. Pfurtscheller & F.H. Lopes da Silva (Eds.), *Functional Brain Imaging* (pp. 201–211). Bern: Hans Huber Publishers.

Lehtonen, J.B. (1973). Functional differentiation between late components of visual evoked potentials recorded at occiput and vertex: Effect of stimulus interval and contour. *Electroencephalography and Clinical Neurophysiology, 35,* 75–82.

Lehtonen, J.B., & Koivikko, M.J. (1971). The use of a non-cephalic reference electrode in recording cerebral evoked potentials in man. *Electroencephalography and Clinical Neurophysiology, 31,* 154–156.

Leinonen, L., & Joutsiniemi, S-L. (1988). Auditory evoked potentials and magnetic fields in patients with lesions of the auditory cortex. *Acta Neurologica Scandinavica, 79,* 316–325.

Lewis, J. (1970). Semantic processing of unattended messages using dichotic listening. *Journal of Experimental Psychology, 85,* 225–228.

Liberman, M.C. (1988). Physiology of cochlear efferent and afferent neurons: Direct comparisons in the same animal. *Hearing Research, 34,* 179–192.

Liberman, M.C., & Brown, M.C. (1986). Physiology and anatomy of single olivocochlear neurons in the cat. *Hearing Research, 24,* 17–36.

Libet, B. (1990). Attentional theories and conscious perception. *Behavioral and Brain Sciences, 13,* 247–248.

Lickey, M.E., & Fox, S.S. (1966). Localization and habituation of sensory evoked DC responses in cat cortex. *Experimental Neurology, 15,* 437–454.

Linden, R.D., Campbell, K.B., Hamel, G., & Picton, T. (1985). Human auditory steady state evoked potentials during sleep. *Ear & Hearing, 6,* 167–173.

Linden, R.D., Picton, T.W., Hamel, G., & Campbell, K.B. (1987). Human auditory steady-state evoked potentials during selective attention. *Electroencephalography and Clinical Neurophysiology, 66,* 145–159.

Lindsley, D.B. (1960). Attention, consciousness, sleep and wakefulness. In J. Field, H.W. Magoun, & V.E. Hall (Eds.), *Handbook of physiology, neurophysiology III* (pp. 1553–1593). Washington DC: American Physiological Society.

Lindsley, D.B. (1961). The reticular activating system and perceptual integration. In D.E. Sheer (Ed.), *Electrical stimulation of the brain* (pp. 331–349). Austin, TX: University of Texas Press.

Lindsley, D.B. (1970). The role of nonspecific reticulo-thalamo-cortical systems in emotion. In P. Black (Ed.), *Physiological correlates of emotion.* (pp. 147–188). New York: Academic Press.

Livingstone, M., & Hubel, D. (1988). Segregation of form, color, movement, and depth: Anatomy, physiology, and perception. *Science, 240,* 740–749.

Llinás, R.R., Grace, A.A., & Yarom, Y. (1991). *In vitro* neurons in mammalian cortical layer 4 exhibit intrinsic oscillatory activity in the 10- to 50-Hz frequency range. *Proceedings of the National Academy of Sciences of the USA, 88,* 897–901.

Logan, G.D. (1979). On the use of a concurrent memory load to measure attention and automaticity. *Journal of Experimental Psychology: Human Perception and Performance, 5,* 189–207.

Lounasmaa, O.V., Hari, R., Joutsiniemi, S.-L., & Hämäläinen, M. (1989). Multi-SQUID recordings of human cerebral magnetic fields may give information about memory processes. *Europhysics Letters, 9,* 603–608.

Lounasmaa, O.V., Williamson, S.J., Kaufman, L., & Tanenbaum, R. (1985). Visually evoked responses from non-occipital areas of human cortex. In H. Weinberg, G. Stroink, & T. Katila (Eds.), *Biomagnetism: Applications & theory* (pp. 348–353). New York: Pergamon Press.

Loveless, N.E. (1979). Event-related slow potentials of the brain as expressions of orienting function. In H.D. Kimmel, E.H. van Olst, & J.F. Orlebeke (Eds.), *The orienting reflex in humans* (pp. 77–100). Hillsdale, NJ: Lawrence Erlbaum Associates.

Loveless, N.E. (1983). The orienting response and evoked potentials in man. In D. Siddle (Ed.), *Orienting and habituation: Perspectives in human research.* (pp. 71–108). New York: Wiley.

Loveless, N.E. (1986). Potentials evoked by temporal deviance. *Biological Psychology, 22,* 149–167.

Loveless, N.E., & Brunia, C.M.H. (1990). Effects of rise-time on late components of the auditory evoked potential. *Journal of Psychophysiology, 4,* 369–380.

Loveless, N.E., Hari, R., Hämäläinen, M., & Tiihonen, J. (1989). Evoked responses of human auditory cortex may be enhanced by preceding stimuli. *Electroencephalography and Clinical Neurophysiology, 74,* 217–227.

Loveless, N.E., & Sanford, A.J. (1974a). Effects of age on the contingent negative variation and preparatory set in a reaction-time task. *Journal of Gerontology, 29,* 52–63.

Loveless, N.E., & Sanford, A.J. (1974b). Slow potential correlates of preparatory set. *Biological Psychology, 1,* 303–314.

Loveless, N.E., Simpson, M., & Näätänen, R. (1987). Frontal negative and parietal positive components of the slow wave dissociated. *Psychophysiology, 24,* 340–345.

Lu, S.-T., Hari, R., Hämäläinen, M., Ilmoniemi, R.J., Lounasmaa, O.V., Sams, M., & Vilkman, V. (1991). Seeing faces activates three separate areas outside the occipital visual cortex in man. *Neuroscience, 43,* 287–290.

Luber, B., Kaufman, L., & Williamson, S.J. (1989). Brain activity related to spatial visual attention. In S.J. Williamson, M. Hoke, G. Stroink, & M. Kotani (Eds.), *Advances in Biomagnetism* (pp. 213–216). New York: Plenum Press.

Luck, S.J., Heinze, H.J., Mangun, G.R., & Hillyard, S.A. (1990). Visual event-related potentials index focused attention within bilateral stimulus arrays. II. Functional dissociation of P1 and N1 components. *Electroencephalography and Clinical Neurophysiology, 75,* 528–542.

Luck, S.J., & Hillyard, S.A. (1990). Electrophysiological evidence for parallel and serial processing during visual search. *Perception and Psychophysics, 48,* 603–617.

Lueck, C.J., Zeki, S., Friston, K.J., Deiber, M.P., Cope, P., Cunningham, V.J., Lammertsma, A.A., Kennard, C., & Frackowiak, R.S.J. (1989). The colour centre in the visual cortex of man. *Nature, 340,* 386–389.

Lukas, J.H. (1980). Human auditory attention: The olivocochlear bundle may function as a peripheral filter. *Psychophysiology, 17,* 444–452.

Lukas, J.H. (1981). The role of efferent inhibition in human auditory attention. An examination of the auditory brainstem potentials. *International Journal of Neuroscience, 12,* 137–145.

Luria, A.R., & Homskaya, E.D. (1970). Frontal lobes and the regulation of arousal processes. In D.I. Mostofsky (Ed.), *Attention: Contemporary theory and analysis* (pp. 303–330). New York: Appleton-Century-Crofts.

Luria, A.R., & Simernitskaya, E.G. (1977). Interhemispheric relations and the functions of the minor hemisphere. *Neuropsychologia, 15,* 175–178.

Lykken, D.T. (1981). *Tremor in the blood: Uses and abuses of the lie detector.* New York: McGraw-Hill.

Lykken, D.T., Macindoe, I., & Tellegen, A. (1972). Preception: Autonomic response to shock as a function of predictability in time and locus. *Psychophysiology, 9,* 318–333.

Lykken, D.T., & Tellegen, A. (1974). On the validity of the preception hypothesis. *Psychophysiology, 11,* 125–132.

Lynn, R. (1966). *Attention, arousal, and the orientation reaction.* Oxford: Pergamon Press.

Lyytinen, H. (1984). The psychophysiology of anticipation and arousal (Doctoral dissertation). *Jyväskylä studies in education, psychology and social research Vol. 52.* Jyväskylä: University of Jyväskylä.

Lyytinen, H., Blomberg, A.P., & Näätänen, R. (in press). Autonomic concomitants of event-related potentials in the auditory oddball paradigm. *Psychophysiology.*

Lyytinen, H., & Näätänen, R. (1987). Autonomic and ERP responses to deviant stimuli:

Analysis of covariation. In R. Johnson, Jr., R. Parasuraman, & J.W. Rohrbaugh (Eds.), Current trends in event-related potential research (pp. 108–117). (Suppl. 40 to Electroencephalography and Clinical Neurophysiology). Amsterdam: Elsevier.

MacKay, D.G. (1973). Aspects of a theory of comprehension, memory and attention. *Quarterly Journal of Experimental Psychology, 25,* 22–40.

Maclin, E., Okada, Y., Kaufman, L., & Williamson, S.J. (1983). Retinotopic map on the visual cortex for eccentrically placed patterns: First noninvasive measurements. *Il Nuovo Cimento, 2D,* 410–419.

MacLean, V., Öhman, A., & Lader, M. (1975). Effects of attention, activation, and stimulus regularity on short-term "habituation" of the averaged evoked response. *Biological Psychology, 3,* 57–69.

MacMillan, N.A. (1973). Detection and recognition of intensity changes in tone and noise: The detection–recognition disparity. *Perception and Psychophysics, 13,* 65–75.

Maiste, A.C., & Picton, T.W. (1987). Auditory evoked potentials during selective attention. In C. Barber & T. Blum (Eds.), *Evoked potentials III* (pp. 385–391). London: Butterworths.

Makeig, S. (1990). A dramatic increase in the auditory middle latency response at very slow rates. In C.H.M. Brunia, A.W.K. Gaillard, & A. Kok (Eds.), *Psychophysiological Brain Research* (Vol II, pp. 60–65). Tilburg: Tilburg University Press.

Makeig, S., & Galambos, R. (1989a). The CERP: Event-related perturbations in steady-state responses. In E. Basar & T. Bullock (Eds.), *Brain Dynamics: Progress and Perspectives* (pp. 375–400). Berlin: Springer Verlag.

Makeig, S., & Galambos, R. (1989b). The auditory 40 Hz-band evoked response lasts 150 ms and increases in size at slow rates. *Society for Neuroscience Abstracts, 15 (Part I),* 113.

Mäkelä, J.P. (1988). Auditory evoked magnetic fields in man. (Doctoral dissertation, Helsinki University of Technology and University of Helsinki. Espoo: TKK offset.

Mäkelä, J.P., & Hari, R. (1987). Evidence for cortical origin of the 40 Hz auditory evoked response in man. *Electroencephalography and Clinical Neurophysiology, 66,* 539–546.

Mäkelä, J.P., & Hari, R. (1990). Long-latency auditory evoked magnetic fields. In S. Sato (Ed.), *Advances in Neurology. Vol. 54: Magnetoencephalography.* (pp. 177–191). New York: Raven Press.

Mäkelä, J.P., Hari, R., & Leinonen, L. (1988). Magnetic responses of the human auditory cortex to noise/square wave transitions. *Electroencephalography and Clinical Neurophysiology, 69,* 423–430.

Mäkelä, J.P., Hari, R., & Linnankivi, A. (1987). Different analysis of frequency and amplitude modulations of a continuous tone in the human auditory cortex: A neuromagnetic study. *Hearing Research, 27,* 257–264.

Mäkelä, J.P., Hari, R., Valanne, L., & Ahonen, A. (1991). Auditory evoked magnetic fields after ischemic brain lesions. *Annals of Neurology, 30,* 76–82.

Malmo, R.B. (1959). Activation: A neuropsycological dimension. *Psychological Review, 66,* 367–386.

Maltzman, I. (1979). Orienting reflexes and significance: A reply to O'Gorman. *Psychophysiology, 16,* 274–282.

Mandler, G. (1975). *Mind and emotion.* New York: Wiley.

Mangun, G.R., Hansen, J.C., & Hillyard, S.A. (1986). Electroretinograms reveal no evidence for centrifugal modulation of retinal input during selective attention in man. *Psychophysiology, 23,* 156–165.

Mangun, G.R., Hansen, J.C., & Hillyard, S.A. (1987). The spatial orienting of attention: Sensory facilitation or response bias? In R. Johnson, Jr., J.W. Rohrbaugh, & R. Parasuraman (Eds.), *Current research in event-related brain potentials* (pp. 118–124). (Suppl. 40), to Electroencephalography and Clinical Neurophysiology, Amsterdam: Elsevier.

Mangun, G.R., & Hillyard, S.A. (1987). The spatial allocation of visual attention as indexed by event-related brain potentials. *Human Factors, 29,* 195–211.

Mangun, G.R., & Hillyard, S.A. (1988). Spatial gradients of visual attention: Behavioral and electrophysiological evidence. *Electroencephalography and Clinical Neurophysiology, 70,* 417–428.

Mangun, G.R., & Hillyard, S.A. (1990a). Electrophysiological studies of visual selective attention in humans. In A. Scheibel & A. Wechsler (Eds.), *The neurobiological foundations of higher cognitive function.* (pp. 271–294). New York: Guilford.

Mangun, G.R. & Hillyard, S.A. (1990b). Allocation of visual attention to spatial locations: Tradeoff functions for event-related brain potentials and detection performance. *Perception and Psychophysics, 47,* 532–550.

Mangun, G.R., Hillyard, S.A., & Luck, S.J. (in press). Electrocortical substrates of visual selective attention. In D. Meyer & S. Kornblum (Eds.), *Attention and Performance XIV.* Hillsdale, NJ: Lawrence Erlbaum Associates.

Mangun, G.R., Luck, S.J., Gazzaniga, M.S., & Hillyard, S.A. (1991). Electrophysiological measures of interhemispheric transfer of visual information: Studies in split-brain patients. *Society for Neuroscience* Abstracts (Vol. 17, Part 1, p. 866). Abstract # 340.4.

Mäntysalo, S., & Näätänen, R. (1987). The duration of a neuronal trace of an auditory stimulus as indicated by event-related potentials. *Biological Psychology, 24,* 183–195.

Marcel, A.J. (1983). Conscious and unconscious perception: An approach to the relation between phenomenal experience and perceptual processes. *Cognitive Psychology, 15,* 238–300.

Marcel, A.J., & Patterson, K.E. (1978). Word recognition and production: Reciprocity in clinical and normal studies. In J. Requin (Ed.), *Attention and performance VII.* Hillsdale, NJ: Erlbaum, pp. 209–226.

Marr, D. (1976). Early processing of visual information. *Philosophical Transactions of the Royal Society, London, B, 275,* 483–524.

Marshall, N.K., & Donchin, E. (1981). Circadian variation in the latency of brainstem responses and its relation to body temperature. *Science, 212,* 356–358.

Martin, M. (1980). Attention to words in different modalities: Four channel presentation with physical and semantic selection. *Acta Psychologica, 44,* 99–115.

Mast, T.E., & Watson, C.S. (1968). Attention and auditory evoked responses to low-detectability signals. *Perception and Psychophysics, 4,* 237–240.

Mauguière, F., & Desmedt, J.E. (1988). Thalamic pain syndrome of Dejérine-Roussy. Differentiation of four subtypes assisted by somatosensory evoked potentials data. *Archives of Neurology, 45,* 1312–1320.

Maximilian, V.A. (1982). Cortical blood flow asymmetries during monaural verbal stimulation. *Brain and Language, 15,* 1–11.

Mazziotta, J.C., Phelps, M.E., Carson, R.E., & Kuhl, D.E. (1982). Tomographic mapping of human cerebral metabolism: Auditory stimulation. *Neurology, 32,* 921–937.

Mazziotta, J.C., Phelps, M.E., & Halgren, E. (1983) Local cerebral glucose metabolic responses to audiovidual stimulation and deprivation: Studies in human subjects with positron CT. *Human Neurobiology, 2,* 11–23.

McCallum, W.C., Barrett, K., & Pocock, P.V. (1989). Late ERP components to eight equiprobable stimuli in an auditory target detection task. *Psychophysiology, 26,* 683–694.

McCallum, W.C., & Curry, S.H. (1979). Hemisphere differences in event related potentials and CNVs associated with monaural stimuli and lateralized motor responses. In D. Lehmann & E. Callaway (Eds.), *Human evoked potentials: Applications and problems* (pp. 235–250). New York: Plenum.

McCallum, W.C., & Curry, S.H. (1980). The form and distribution of auditory evoked potentials and CNVs when stimuli and responses are lateralized. In H.H. Kornhuber & L.

Deecke (Eds.), Motivation, motor and sensory processes of the brain: Electrical potentials, behaviour and clinical use. *Progress in Brain Research, Vol. 54.* (pp. 767–775). Amsterdam: Elsevier.

McCallum, W.C., Curry, S.H., Cooper, R., Pocock, P.V., & Papakostopoulos, D. (1983). Brain event-related potentials as indicators of early selective processes in auditory target localization. *Psychophysiology, 20,* 1–17.

McCauley, C., Permelee, C.M., Sperber, R.D., & Carr, T.H. (1980). Early extraction of meaning from pictures and its relation to conscious identification. *Journal of Experimental Psychology: Human Perception and Performance, 6,* 265–276.

McFarland, K., & Ashton, R. (1978). The influence of concurrent task difficulty on manual performance. *Neuropsychologia, 16,* 735–741.

McFarland, W.H., Vivion, M.C., & Goldstein, R. (1977). Middle components of the AER to tone-pips in normal-hearing and hearing-impaired subjects. *Journal of Speech and Hearing Research, 20,* 781–798.

McGurk, H., & MacDonald, J. (1976). Hearing lips and seeing voices. *Nature, 264,* 746–748.

McLeod, P. (1977). A dual task response modality effect: Support for multi-processor models of attention. *Quarterly Journal of Experimental Psychology, 29,* 651–667.

McLeod, P., Driver, J., & Crisp, J. (1988). Visual search for a conjunction of movement and form is parallel. *Nature, 332,* 154–155.

Medvick, P., Lewis, P.S., Aine, C.J., & Flynn, E.R. (1989). Monte Carlo Analysis of localization errors in magnetoencephalography. In S.J. Williamson, M. Hoke, G. Stroink, & M. Kotani (Eds.), *Advances in Biomagnetism* (pp. 543–546). New York: Plenum Press.

Mendel, M.I., Hosick, E.C., Windman, T.R., Davis, H., Hirsh, S.K., & Dinges, D.F. (1975). Audiometric comparison of the middle and late components of the adult auditory evoked potentials awake and asleep. *Electroencephalography and Clinical Neurophysiology, 38,* 27–33.

Mesulam, M.M. (1981). A cortical network for directed attention and unilateral neglect. *Annals Neurology, 10,* 309–325.

Mesulam, M.M. (1983). The functional anatomy and hemispheric specialization for directed attention. The role of parietal lobe and its connectivity. *Trends in Neurosciences, 6,* 384–387.

Michie, P.T. (1984). Selective attention effects on somatosensory event-related potentials. In R. Karrer, J. Cohen, & P. Tueting (Eds.), Brain and information: *Event-related potentials. Annals of the New York Academy of Sciences* (Vol. 425, pp. 250–255). New York: New York Academy of Sciences.

Michie, P.T., Bearpark, H.M., Crawford, J.M., & Glue, L.C.T. (1987). The effects of spatial selective attention on the somatosensory event-related potential. *Psychophysiology, 24,* 449–463.

Michie, P.T., Bearpark, H.M., Crawford, J.M., & Glue, L.C.T. (1990). The nature of selective attention effects on auditory event-related potentials. *Biological Psychology, 30,* 219–250.

Michie, P., Solowij, N., Crawford, J., & Glue, L. (1990). Auditory ERPs during auditory attention and a visual control task: Effects of auditory task difficulty. In C.H.M. Brunia, A.W.K. Gaillard, & A. Kok (Eds.), *Psychophysiological Brain Research* (pp. 208–211). Tilburg: Tilburg University Press.

Mikola, H., Lang, A.H., & Eerola, O. (in preparation) Mismatch negativity, reading speed and vigilance.

Mitzdorf, U. (1987). Properties of the evoked potential generators: Current source density analysis of the visually evoked potentials in the cat cortex. *International Journal of Neuroscience, 33,* 33–59.

Miyashita, Y. (1988). Neuronal correlate of visual associate long-term memory in the primate temporal cortex. *Nature, 335,* 817–820.

Möcks, J., Gasser, T.H., & Pham Dinh, T. (1984). Variability of single visual evoked potentials evaluated by two new statistical tests. *Electroencephalography and Clinical Neurophysiology, 57,* 571-580.

Møller, A.R. (1983). *Auditory physiology.* London: Academic Press.

Moran, J., & Desimone, R. (1985). Selective attention gates visual processing in the extrastriate cortex. *Science, 229,* 782-784.

Moray, N. (1959). Attention in dichotic listening: Affective cues and the influence of instructions. *Quarterly Journal of Experimental Psychology, 9,* 56-60.

Moray, N. (1967). Where is attention limited. A survey and a model. *Acta Psychologica, 27,* 84-92.

Moray, N. (1969). Attention: Selective processes in vision and hearing. London: Hutchinson.

Moray, N. (1975). A data base for theories of selective listening. In P.M.A. Rabbitt & S. Dornic (Eds.), *Attention and performance V* (pp. 119-135). London: Academic Press.

Moray, N., & O'Brien, T. (1967). Signal detection theory applied to selective listening. *Journal of the Acoustical Society of America, 42,* 765-772.

Moruzzi, G. & Magoun, H.W. (1949). Brain stem reticular formation and activation of the EEG. Electroencephalography and Clinical *Neurophysiology, 1,* 455-473.

Moscovitch, M., & Klein, D. (1980). Material-specific interference for visual words and faces: implications for models of capacity limitations, attention, and laterality. *Journal of Experimental Psychology: Human Perception and Performance, 6,* 590-604.

Mountcastle, V.B. (1978). Brain mechanisms for directed attention. *Journal of the Royal Society of Medicine, 71,* 14-28.

Mountcastle, V.B., Andersen, R.A., & Motter, B.C. (1981). The influence of attentive fixation upon the excitability of the light-sensitive neurons of the posterior parietal cortex. *The Journal of Neuroscience, 1,* 1218-1235.

Näätänen, R. (1967). Selective attention and evoked potentials. *Annales Academiae Scientiarum Fennicae B, 151,* 1-226.

Näätänen, R. (1970). Evoked potential, EEG and slow potential correlates of selective attention. In A.F. Sanders (Ed.), Attention and performance III. *Acta Psychologica, 33,* 178-192.

Näätänen, R. (1973). Inverted U-shaped relationship between activation and performance—A critical review. In S. Kornblum (Ed.), *Attention and performance IV* (pp. 155-174). New York: Academic Press.

Näätänen, R. (1975). Selective attention and evoked potentials in humans—A critical review. *Biological Psychology, 2,* 237-307.

Näätänen, R. (1979). Orienting and evoked potentials. In H.D. Kimmel, E.H. van Olst, & J.F. Orlebeke (Eds.), *The orienting reflex in humans* (pp. 61-75). Hillsdale, NJ: Lawrence Erlbaum Associates.

Näätänen, R. (1982). Processing negativity: An evoked-potential reflection of selective attention. *Psychological Bulletin, 92,* 605-640.

Näätänen, R. (1984). In search of a short-duration memory trace of a stimulus in the human brain. In L. Pulkkinen & P. Lyytinen (Eds.), *Human action and personality. Essays in honour of Martti Takala* (pp. 29-43). Jyväskylä: University of Jyväskylä.

Näätänen, R. (1985). Selective attention and stimulus processing: Reflections in event-related potentials, magnetoencephalogram and regional cerebral blood flow. In M.I. Posner & O.S.M. Marin (Eds.), *Attention and performance XI* (pp. 355-373). Hillsdale, NJ: Lawrence Erlbaum Associates.

Näätänen, R. (1986a). The orienting response theory: An integration of informational and energetical aspects of brain function. In R.G.J. Hockey, A.W.K. Gaillard, & M. Coles (Eds.), *Adaptation to stress and task demands: Energetical aspects of human information processing.* (pp. 91-111). Dordrecht: Martinus Nijhoff.

Näätänen, R. (1986b). Neurophysiological basis of the echoic memory as suggested by event-related potentials and magnetoencephalogram. In F. Klix & H. Hagendorf (Eds.), *Human memory and cognitive capabilities* (pp. 615-628). Amsterdam: Elsevier.

Näätänen, R. (1986c). Processing of the unattended message during selective dichotic listening. *Behavioral and Brain Sciences, 9,* 43-44.

Näätänen, R. (1986d). N2 and automatic versus controlled processes: A classification of N2 kinds of ERP components. In W.C. McCallum, R. Zappoli, & F. Denoth (Eds.), *Cerebral psychophysiology: Studies in event-related potentials* (pp. 169-172). (Suppl. 38 to Electroencephalography and Clinical Neurophysiology). Amsterdam: Elsevier.

Näätänen, R. (1986e). The neural-specificity theory of visual selective attention evaluated: A commentary on Harter and Aine. *Biological Psychology, 23,* 281-295.

Näätänen, R. (1987). Event-related brain potentials in research of cognitive processes—A classification of components. In E. van der Meer & J. Hoffmann (Eds.), *Knowledge aided information processing* (pp. 241-273). Amsterdam: Elsevier.

Näätänen, R. (1988a). Implications of ERP data for psychological theories of attention. *Biological Psychology, 26,* 117-163.

Näätänen, R. (1988b). Regional cerebral blood-flow studies supplementing information provided by event-related potentials on the brain mechanisms of selective attention. In G. Galbraith, E. Donchin, & M. Kietzman (Eds.), *Neurophysiology and psychology: Basic mechanisms and clinical applications* (pp. 144-156). Hillsdale, NJ: Lawrence Erlbaum Associates.

Näätänen, R. (1990). The role of attention in auditory information processing as revealed by event-related potentials and other brain measures of cognitive function. *Behavioral and Brain Sciences, 13,* 201-288.

Näätänen, R. (1991). Mismatch negativity (MMN) outside strong attentional focus: A commentary on Woldorff et al. Psychophysiology. 478-484.

Näätänen, R., & Gaillard, A.W.K. (1974). The relationship between the contingent negative variation and the reaction time under prolonged experimental conditions. *Biological Psychology, 1,* 277-291.

Näätänen, R., & Gaillard, A.W.K. (1983). The N2 deflection of ERP and the orienting reflex. In A.W.K. Gaillard & W. Ritter (Eds.), *EEG correlates of information processing: Theoretical issues* (pp. 119-141). Amsterdam: North Holland.

Näätänen, R., Gaillard, A.W.K., & Mäntysalo, S. (1978). Early selective attention effect on evoked potential reinterpreted. *Acta Psychologica, 42,* 313-329.

Näätänen, R., Gaillard, A.W.K., & Mäntysalo, S. (1980). Brain potential correlates of voluntary and involuntary attention. In H.H. Kornhuber & L. Deecke (Eds.), *Motivation, motor and sensory processes of the brain: Electrical potentials, behaviour and clinical use, Progress in Brain Research, 54* (pp. 343-348). Amsterdam: Elsevier.

Näätänen, R., Gaillard, A.W.K., & Varey, C.A. (1981). Early attention effect on evoked potential as a function of interstimulus interval. *Biological Psychology, 13,* 173-187.

Näätänen, R. & Lyytinen, H. (1989). Event-related potentials and the orienting response to nonsignal stimuli at fast stimulus rates. In N.W. Bond & D.A.T. Siddle (Eds.), *Psychobiology: Issues and Applications* (pp. 185-197). Amsterdam: Elsevier.

Näätänen, R., & Merisalo, A. (1977). Expectancy and preparation in simple reaction time. In S. Dornic (Ed.), *Attention and Performance VI* (pp. 115-138). Hillsdale, NJ: Lawrence Erlbaum Associates.

Näätänen, R., & Michie, P.T. (1979a). Early selective attention effects on the evoked potential. A critical review and reinterpretation. *Biological Psychology, 8,* 81-136.

Näätänen, R., & Michie, P.T. (1979b). Different variants of endogenous negative brain potentials in performance situations: A review and classification. In D. Lehmann & E. Callaway (Eds.), *Human Evoked Potentials* (pp. 251-267). New York: Plenum Publishing Corporation.

Näätänen, R., Muranen, V., & Merisalo, A. (1974). Timing of expectancy peak in simple reaction time situation. *Acta Psychologica, 38,* 461–470.

Näätänen, R., Paavilainen, P., Alho, K., Reinikainen, K., & Sams, M. (1987a). Inter-stimulus interval and the mismatch negativity. In C. Barber & T. Blum (Eds.), *Evoked potentials III* (pp. 392–397). London: Butterworths.

Näätänen, R., Paavilainen, P., Alho, K., Reinikainen, K., & Sams, M. (1987b). The mismatch negativity to intensity changes in an auditory stimulus sequence. In R. Johnson, Jr., J.W. Rohrbaugh, & R. Parasuraman (Eds.), *Current trends in event-related brain potential research* (pp. 125–131). (Suppl. 40 to Electroencephalography and Clinical Neurophysiology). Amsterdam: Elsevier.

Näätänen, R., Paavilainen, P., Alho, K., Reinikainen, K., & Sams, M. (1989). Do event-related potentials reveal the mechanism of the auditory sensory memory in the human brain? *Neuroscience Letters, 98,* 217–221.

Näätänen, R., Paavilainen, P., Lavikainen, J., Alho, K., Reinikainen, K., Teder, W., Sams, M., Strelets, V., & Rosenfeld, J. (in preparation). Mismatch negativity to auditory change and the memory-trace hypothesis.

Näätänen, R., Paavilainen, P., & Reinikainen, K. (1989). Do event-related potentials to infrequent decrements in duration of auditory stimuli demonstrate a memory trace in man? *Neuroscience Letters, 107,* 347–352.

Näätänen, R., Paavilainen, P., Tiitinen, H., Jiang, D., & Alho, K. (in press). Attention and mismatch negativity. *Psychophysiology.*

Näätänen, R., & Picton, T.W. (1987). The N1 wave of the human electric and magnetic response to sound: A review and an analysis of the component structure. *Psychophysiology, 24,* 375–425.

Näätänen, R., Sams, M. & Alho, K. (1986). Mismatch negativity: An ERP sign of a cerebral mismatch process. In: W.C. McCallum, R. Zappoli & F. Denoth (Eds.), *Cerebral psychophysiology: Studies in event-related potentials* (pp. 174–180). (Supplement 38 to Electroencephalography and clinical Neurophysiology). Amsterdam: Elsevier.

Näätänen, R., Sams, M., Alho, K., Paavilainen, P., Reinikainen, K., & Sokolov, E.N. (1988). Frequency and location specificity of the human vertex N1 wave. *Electroencephalography and Clinical Neurophysiology, 69,* 523–531.

Näätänen, R., Sams, M., Järvilehto, T., & Soininen, K. (1983). Probability of deviant stimulus and event-related brain potentials. In R. Sinz & M.R. Rosenzweig (Eds.), *Psychophysiology 1980* (pp. 397–405). Jena: VEB Gustav Fischer Verlag; and Amsterdam: Elsevier Biomedical Press, pp. 397–405.

Näätänen, R., Schröger, E., & Paavilainen, P. (1991). *Adaptive changes in neural mechanisms of auditory coding as reflected by the mismatch negativity.* Manuscript submitted for publication.

Näätänen, R., Simpson, M., & Loveless, N.E. (1982). Stimulus deviance and evoked potentials. *Biological Psychology, 14,* 53–98.

Näätänen, R., & Summala, H. (1976). *Road-user behavior and traffic accidents.* Amsterdam: North-Holland; and New York: American Elsevier.

Näätänen, R., & Teder, W. (1991). Attention effects on the auditory event-related potential. *Acta Otolaryngologica* (Stockh), Suppl. *491,* 161–167.

Näätänen, R., Teder, W., Alho, K., & Lavikainen, J. (1992) Dichotic listening and the auditory event-related potentials. Manuscript submitted for publication.

Nakayama, K., & Silverman, G.H. (1986). Serial and parallel processing of visual feature conjunctions. *Nature, 320,* 264–265.

Navon, D. (1985). Attention division or attention sharing? In M.I. Posner & O.S.M. Marin (Eds.), *Attention and performance XI* (pp. 133–146). Hillsdale, NJ: Lawrence Erlbaum Associates.

Navon, D., & Gopher, D. (1979). On the economy of the human processing system. *Psychological Review, 86,* 214–255.

Navon, D., & Gopher, D. (1980). Interpretations of task difficulty. In R. Nickerson (Ed.), *Attention and performance VIII.* (pp. 297-315). Hillsdale, NJ: Lawrence Erlbaum Associates.

Neisser, U. (1967). *Cognitive psychology.* New York: Appleton-Century-Crofts.

Nelson, D.A., & Lassman, F.M. (1973). Combined effects of recovery period and stimulus intensity on the human auditory evoked vertex response. *Journal of Speech and Hearing Research, 16,* 297–308.

Nelson, D.A., & Lassman, F.M. (1977). Re-examination of the effects of periodic and aperiodic stimulation on the auditory-evoked vertex response. *Audiology, 16,* 409–418.

Nelson, D.A., Lassman, F.M., & Hoel, R.L. (1969). The effects of variable-interval and fixed-interval signal presentation schedules on the auditory evoked response. *Journal of Speech and Hearing Research, 12,* 199–209.

Neville, H.J., & Lawson, D. (1987a). Attention to central and peripheral visual space in a movement detection task: An event-related potential and behavioral study. II. Congenitally deaf adults. *Brain Research, 405,* 268–283.

Neville, H.J., & Lawson, D. (1987b). Attention to central and peripheral visual space in a movement detection task. III. Separate effects of auditory deprivation and acquisition of visual language. *Brain Research, 405,* 284–294.

Neville, H.J., & Lawson, D. (1987c). Attention to central and peripheral visual space in a movement detection task: An event-related potential and behavioral study. I. Normal hearing adults. *Brain Research, 405,* 253–267.

Newstead, S.E., & Dennis, I. (1979). Lexical and grammatical processing of unshadowed messages: A re-examination of the Mackay effect. *Quarterly Journal of Experimental Psychology, 31,* 477–488.

Niemi, P., & Näätänen, R. (1981). Foreperiod and simple reaction time. *Psychological Bulletin, 89,* 133–162.

Nissen, M.J. (1985). Accessing features and objects: Is location special? In M.I. Posner & O.S.M. Marin (Eds.), *Attention and performance XI* (pp. 205–219). Hillsdale, NJ: Lawrence Erlbaum Associates.

Nordby, H., Hammerborg. D., Roth, W.T., & Hugdahl, K. (1991). ERPs to infrequent omissions and inclusions of stimulus elements. *Psychophysiology, 28,* S42.

Nordby, H., Roth, W.T., & Pfefferbaum, A. (1988a). Event-related potentials to time-deviant and pitch-deviant tones. *Psychophysiology, 25,* 249–261.

Nordby, H., Roth, W.T., & Pfefferbaum, A. (1988b). Event-related potentials to breaks in sequences of alternating pitches or interstimulus intervals. *Psychophysiology, 25,* 262–268.

Norman, D.A. (1968). Toward a theory of memory and attention. *Psychological Review, 75,* 522–536.

Norman, D.A., & Bobrow, D.B. (1975). On data-limited and resource-limited processes. *Cognitive Psychology, 7,* 44–64.

North, R.A. (1977). *Task components and demands as factors in dual-task performance* (Report No. ARL-77-2/AFOSE-77-2). Urbana, IL: University of Illinois at Urbana-Champaign, Aviation Research Laboratory.

Novak, G., Ritter, W., & Vaughan, H.G., Jr. (in press a). *Mismatch detection and the latency of temporal judgments. Psychophysiology.*

Novak, G., Ritter, W., & Vaughan, H.G., Jr. (in press b). *The chronometry of attention-modulated processing and automatic mismatch detection. Psychophysiology.*

Novak, G., Ritter, W., & Vaughan, H.G., Jr., & Wiznitzer, M.L. (1990). Differentiation of negative event-related potentials in an auditory discrimination task. *Electroencephalography and Clinical Neurophysiology, 75,* 255–275.

Nyman, G., Alho, K., Laurinen, P., Paavilainen, P., Radil, T., Reinikainen, K., Sams, M., & Näätänen, R. (1990). Mismatch negativity (MMN) for sequences of auditory and visual stimuli: Evidence for a mechanism specific to the auditory modality. *Electroencephalography and Clinical Neurophysiology, 77,* 436–444.

Oatman, L.C. (1971). Role of visual attention on auditory evoked potentials in unaesthetized cats. *Experimental Neurology, 32,* 341–356.

Oatman, L.C. (1976). Effects of visual attention on the intensity of auditory evoked potentials. *Experimental Neurology, 51,* 41–53.

Oatman, L.C., & Anderson, B.W. (1977). Effects of visual attention on tone burst evoked auditory potentials. *Experimental Neurology, 57,* 200–211.

Oatman, L.C., & Anderson, B.W. (1980). Suppression of the auditory frequency following response during visual attention. *Electroencephalography and Clinical Neurophysiology, 49,* 314–321.

Obrist, P.A., Howard, J.L., Lawler, J.E., Galosy, R.A., Meyers, K.A., & Gaebelein, C.J. (1974). The cardiac-somatic interaction. In P.A. Obrist, A.H. Black, J. Brener, & L.V. DiCara (Eds.), *Cardiovascular psychophysiology* (pp. 136–162). Chicago: Aldine-Atherton.

Obrist, W.D., Thompson, H.K., Jr., Wang, H.S., & Wilkinson, W.E. (1975). Regional cerebral blood flow estimated by 133-xenon inhalation. *Stroke, 6,* 245–256.

O'Gorman, J.G. (1979). The orienting reflex: Novelty or significance detector? *Psychophysiology, 16,* 253–262.

Öhman, A. (1979). The orienting response, attention and learning: An information-processing perspective. In H.D. Kimmel, E.H. van Olst, & J.F. Orlebeke (Eds.), *The orienting reflex in humans* (pp. 443–471). Hillsdale, NJ: Lawrence Erlbaum Associates.

Öhman, A. (in press). Orienting and attention: Preferred preattentive processing of potentially phobic stimuli. In B.A. Campbell, R. Richardson, & H. Hayne (Eds.), *Attention and information processing in infants and adults: Perspectives from human and animal research.* Hillsdale, NJ: Lawrence Erlbaum Associates.

Öhman, A., Kaye, J.J., & Lader, M. (1972). Regular interstimulus interval as a critical determinant of the short-term habituation of the auditory averaged evoked response. *Psychonomic Science, 27,* 275–278.

Öhman, A., & Lader, M. (1972). Selective attention and habituation of the auditory averaged evoked response in humans. *Physiology and Behavior, 8,* 79–85.

Öhman, A., & Lader, M. (1977). Short-term changes of the human auditory evoked potentials during repetitive stimulation. In J.E. Desmedt (Ed.), *Auditory evoked potentials in man. Psychopharmacology correlates of evoked potentials* (pp. 93–118). Basel: Karger.

Okada, Y.C. (1985). Discrimination of located and distributed current dipole source, and localized single and multiple sources. In H. Weinberg, G. Stroink, & T. Katila (Eds.), *Biomagnetism: Applications and theory* (pp. 266–272). New York: Pergamon.

Okada, Y.C., Kaufman, L., Brenner, D., & Williamson, S.J. (1981). Application of a SQUID to measurement of somatically evoked fields: Transient responses to electrical stimulation of the median nerve. In S. N. Erné, H.D. Hahlbohm, & H. Lubbig (Eds.), *Biomagnetism* (pp. 445–456). Berlin: Walter de Gruyter.

Okada, Y.C., Tanenbaum, R., Kaufman, L., & Williamson, S.J. (1984). Somatotopic organization of the human somatosensory cortex revealed by neuromagnetic techniques. *Experimental Brain Research, 56,* 197–205.

Okada, Y.C., Williamson, S.J., & Kaufman, L. (1982). Magnetic field of the human sensorimotor cortex. *International Journal of Neurophysiology, 17,* 33–38.

Okita, T. (1979). Event-related potentials and selective attention to auditory stimuli varying in pitch and localization. *Biological Psychology, 9,* 271–284.

Okita, T. (1981). Slow negative shifts of the human event-related potential associated with selective information processing. *Biological Psychology, 12,* 63–75.

Okita, T. (1987). Event-related potentials and selective attention to tones moving in location and pitch: An examination of movement velocity. *Biological Psychology, 24,* 225–237.

Okita, T. (1989). Within-channel selection and event-related potentials during selective auditory attention. *Psychophysiology, 26,* 127–139.

Okita, T., Konishi, K., & Inamori, R. (1983). Attention-related negative brain potential for speech words and pure tones. *Biological Psychology, 16,* 29–47.

Okita, T., Wijers, A.A., Mulder, G., & Mulder, L.J.M. (1985). Memory search and visual spatial attention: An event-related brain potential analysis. *Acta Psychologica, 60,* 263–292.

Onishi, S., & Davis, H. (1968). Effects of duration and rise time of tonebursts on evoked V-potentials. *Journal of the Acoustical Society of America, 44,* 582–591.

Osterhammel, P.A., Davis, H., Wier, C.C., & Hirsh, S.K. (1973). Adult auditory evoked vertex potentials in sleep. *Audiology, 12,* 116–128.

Osterhammel, P., Shallop, J., & Terkildsen, K. (1985). The effect of sleep on the auditory brainstem response (ABR) and the middle latency response (MLR). *Scandinavian Audiology, 14,* 47–50.

Paap, K.R., & Newsome, S.L. (1981). Parafoveal information is not sufficient to produce semantic or visual priming. *Perception and Psychophysics, 29,* 467–476.

Paavilainen, P., Alho, K., Reinikainen, K., Sams, M., & Näätänen, R. (1991). Right-hemisphere dominance of different mismatch negativities. *Electroencephalography and Clinical Neurophysiology, 78,* 466–479.

Paavilainen, P., Cammann, R., Alho, K., Reinikainen, K., Sams, M., & Näätänen, R. (1987). Event-related potentials to pitch change in an auditory stimulus sequence during sleep. In R. Johnson, Jr., R. Parasuraman & J.W. Rohrbaugh (Eds.), *Current trends in event-related potential research* (pp. 246–255). (Suppl 40 to Electroencephalography and Clinical Neurophysiology). Amsterdam: Elsevier.

Paavilainen, P., Karlsson, M.-L., Reinikainen, K., & Näätänen, R. (1989). Mismatch negativity to change in spatial location of an auditory stimulus. *Electroencephalography and Clinical Neurophysiology, 73,* 129–141.

Paetau, R., Kajola, M., & Hari, R. (1990). Magnetoencephalography in the study of epilepsy. *Neurophysiologique Clinique, 20,* 169–187.

Palestini, M., Davidovitch, A., & Hernández-Peón, R. (1959). Functional significance of centrifugal influences upon the retina. *Acta Neurologica Latinoamericana, 5,* 113–131.

Pandya, D.N., & Yeterian, A.H. (1985). Architecture and connections of cortical association areas. In A. Peters & E.G. Jones (Eds.), *Cerebral cortex: Vol. IV. Association and Auditory Cortices* (pp. 3–61). New York: Plenum Press.

Pantev, C., Gallen, C., Hampson, S., Buchanan, S., & Sobel, D. (in press). Reproducibility and validity of neuromagnetic source localization using a large array biometer. *Electroencephalography and Clinical Neurophysiology.*

Pantev, C., Hoke, M., Lehnertz, K. & Lütkenhöner, B. (1989). Neuromagnetic evidence of an amplitopic organization of the human auditory cortex. *Electroencephalography and Clinical Neurophysiology, 72,* 225–231.

Pantev, C., Hoke, M., Lehnertz, K., Lütkenhöner, B., Anogianakis, G., & Wittkowski, W. (1988). Tonotopic organization of the human auditory cortex revealed by transient auditory evoked magnetic fields. *Electroencephalography and Clinical Neurophysiology, 69,* 160–170.

Pantev, C., Hoke, M., Lehnertz, K., Lütkenhöner, B., Fahrendorf, G., & Stöber, U. (1990). Identification of sources of brain neuronal activity with high spatiotemporal resolution through combination of neuromagnetic source localization (MSL) and magnetic resonance imaging (MRI). *Electroencephalography and Clinical Neurophysiology, 75,* 173–184.

Pantev, C., Hoke, M., Lütkenhöner, B., & Lehnertz, K. (1989). Tonotopic organization of the auditory cortex: Pitch versus frequency representation. *Science, 246,* 486–488.

Pantev, C., Hoke, M., Lütkenhöner, B., Lehnertz, K., & Kumpf, W. (1989). Tinnitus remission objectified by neuromagnetic measurements. *Hearing Research, 40,* 261–266.

Pantev, C., Lütkenhöner, B., Hoke, M., & Lehnertz, K. (1986). Comparison between simultaneously recorded auditory-evoked magnetic fields and potentials elicited by ipsilateral, contralateral and binaural tone burst stimulation. *Audiology, 25,* 54–61.

Pantev, C., Makeig, S., Hoke, M., Galambos, R., Hampson, S., & Gallen, C. (1991). Human auditory evoked gamma band magnetic fields. Proceedings of the National Academy of Sciences, USA, *88,* 8996–9000.

Papanicolaou, A.C., Baumann, S., Rogers, R.L., Saudjari, C., Amparo, E.G., & Eisenberg, H.M. (1990). Localization of auditory response sources using magnetoencephalography and magnetic resonance imaging. *Archives of Neurology, 47,* 33–37.

Papanicolaou, A.C., Deutsch, G., Bourbon, W.T., Will, K.W., Loring, D.W., & Eisenberg, H.M. (1987). Convergent evoked potential and cerebral blood flow evidence of task-specific hemispheric differences. *Electroencephalography and Clinical Neurophysiology, 66,* 515–520.

Papanicolaou, A.C., Moore, B.D., & Gary, Jr., H.E. (1989). Selective attention effects on somatosensory evoked potentials. *International Journal of Neuroscience, 45,* 277–282.

Papanicolaou, A.C., Rogers, R.L., Baumann, S., Saudjari, S., & Eisenberg, H.M. (1990). Source localization of two evoked magnetic field components using two alternative procedures. *Experimental Brain Research, 80,* 44–48.

Parasuraman, R. (1978). Auditory evoked potentials and divided attention. *Psychophysiology, 15,* 460–465.

Parasuraman, R. (1980). Effects of information processing demands on slow negative shift latencies and N100 amplitude in selective and divided attention. *Biological Psychology, 11,* 217–233.

Parasuraman, R. (1984). The psychobiology of sustained attention. In J.S. Warm (Ed.), *Sustained attention in human performance* (pp. 61–101). London: Wiley.

Parasuraman, R., & Beatty, J. (1980). Brain events underlying detection and recognition of weak sensory signals. *Science, 210,* 80–83.

Parasuraman, R., Richer, F., & Beatty, J. (1982). Detection and recognition: Concurrent processes in perception. *Perception and Psychophysics, 31,* 1–12.

Pardo, J.V., Fox, P.T., & Raichle, M.E. (1991). Localization of a human system for sustained attention by positron emission tomography. *Nature, 349,* 61–64.

Pardo, J.V., Pardo, P.J., Janer, K.W., & Raichle, M.E. (1990). The anterior cingulate cortex mediates processing selection in the Stroop attentional conflict paradigm. *Proceedings of the National Academy of Science USA, 87,* 256–259.

Pashler, H. (1984). Evidence against late selection: Stimulus quality effects in previewed displays. *Journal of Experimental Psychology: Human Perception and Performance, 10,* 429–448.

Pashler, H. (1987). Detecting conjunctions of colour and form: Reassessing the serial search hypothesis. *Perception and Psychophysics, 41,* 191–201.

Pavlov, I.P. (1927). *Conditioned reflexes.* Oxford: Clarendon Press.

Pelizzone, M., Hari, R., Mäkelä, J.P., Huttunen, J., Ahlfors, S., & Hämäläinen, M. (1987). Cortical origin of middle-latency auditory evoked responses in man. *Neuroscience Letters, 82,* 303–307.

Pelizzone, M., Williamson, S.J., & Kaufman, L. (1985). Evidence for multiple areas in the human auditory cortex. In H. Weinberg, G. Stroink, & T. Katila (Eds.), *Biomagnetism: Applications and theory* (pp. 326–330). Pergamon: New York.

Penfield, W., & Jasper, H. (1954). *Epilepsy and the functional anatomy of the human brain.* Boston: Little & Brown.

Peronnet, F., Michel, F., Echallier, J.F., & Girod, J. (1974). Coronal topography of human auditory evoked responses. *Electroencephalography and Clinical Neurophysiology, 37,* 225–230.

Perrault, N., & Picton, T.W. (1984). Event-related potentials recorded from the scalp and nasopharynx. I. N1 and P2. *Electroencephalography and Clinical Neurophysiology, 59,* 177–194.

Perrin, F., Bertrand, O., Giard, M.H., & Echallier, J.F. (1987). Mapping of scalp potentials by surface spline interpolation. *Electroencephalography and Clinical Neurophysiology, 66,* 75–81.

Petersen, S.E., Fox, P.T., Posner, M.I., Mintun, M., & Raichle, M.E. (1988). Positron emission tomographic studies of the cortical anatomy of single-word processing. *Nature, 331,* 585–589.

Petersen, S.E., Fox, P.T., Posner, M.I., Mintun, M., & Raichle, M.E. (1989). Positron emission tomographic studies of the processing of single words. *Journal of Cognitive Neuroscience, 1,* 154–170.

Petersen, S.E., Fox, P.T., Snyder, A.Z., & Raichle, M.E. (1990). Activation of extrastriate and frontal cortical areas by visual words and word-like stimuli. *Science, 249,* 1041–1044.

Petsche, H., Lindner, K., Rappelsberger, P., & Gruber, G. (1988). The EEG—an adequate method to concretize brain processes elicited by music. *Music Perception, 6,* 133–159.

Petsche, H., Pockberger, H., & Rappelsberger, P. (1986). EEG topography and mental performance. In F.H. Duffy (Ed.), *Topographic mapping of the brain.* (pp. 63–98). Boston: Butterworths.

Petsche, H., Pockberger, H., & Rappelsberger, P. (1988). Cortical structure and electrogenesis. In E. Başar (Ed.), *Dynamics of sensory and cognitive processing of the brain.* (pp. 123–129). Berlin: Springer.

Pfefferbaum, A., Buchsbaum, M., & Gips, J. (1971). Enhancement of the average evoked response to tone onset and cessation. *Psychophysiology, 8,* 332–339.

Pfefferbaum, A., Ford, J.M., Wenegrat, B.G., Roth, W.T., & Kopell, B.S. (1984). Clinical application of the P3 component of event-related potentials. 1. Normal aging. *Electroencephalography and Clinical Neurophysiology, 59,* 85–103.

Pfurtscheller, G., & Klimesch, W. (1991). Event-related desynchronization during motor behavior and visual information processing. In C.H.M. Brunia, G. Mulder, & M.N. Verbaten (Eds.), *Event-Related Potentials of the Brain* (pp. 58–68). (Suppl. 42 to Electroencephalography and Clinical Neurophysiology). Amsterdam: Elsevier.

Pfurtscheller, G., Steffan, J., & Maresch, H. (1988). ERD mapping and functional topography: Temporal and spatial aspects. In G. Pfurtscheller & F.H. Lopes da Silva (Eds.), *Functional brain imaging* (pp. 117–130). Toronto: Hans Huber Publishers.

Phelps, M.E., & Mazziotta, J.C. (1985). Positron emission tomography: Human brain function and biochemistry. *Science, 228,* 799–809.

Phelps, M.E., Mazziotta, J.C., Engel, J., Jr., & Kuhl, E.D. (1981). Metabolic response of the brain to visual and auditory stimulation and deprivation. *Journal of Cerebral Blood Flow and Metabolism, 1* (Suppl. 1), S467–468.

Phillips, D.P., Orman, S.S., Musicant, A.D., & Wilson, G.F. (1985). Neurons in the cat's primary auditory cortex distinguished by their responses to tones and wide-spectrum noise. *Hearing Research, 18,* 73–86.

Picton, T.W. (1980). The use of human event-related potentials in psychology. In I. Martin & P.H. Venables (Eds.), *Techniques in psychophysiology.* (pp. 357–395). New York: Wiley.

Picton, T.W., Campbell, K.B., Baribeau-Braun, J., & Proulx, G.B. (1978). The neurophysiology of human attention. A tutorial review. In J. Requin (Ed.), *Attention and performance VII* (pp. 429–467). Hillsdale, NJ: Lawrence Erlbaum Associates.

Picton, T.W., Goodman, W.S., & Bryce, D.P. (1970). Amplitude of evoked responses to tones of high intensity. *Acta Otolaryngology, 70,* 77–82.

Picton, T.W., & Hillyard, S.A. (1974). Human auditory evoked potentials. II. Effects of attention. *Electroencephalography and Clinical Neurophysiology, 36,* 191–200.

Picton, T.W., Hillyard, S.A., Krausz, H.I., & Galambos, R. (1974). Human auditory evoked potentials. I. Evaluation of components. *Electroencephalography and Clinical Neurophysiology, 36,* 179–190.

Picton, T.W., Linden, R.D., Hamel, G., & Maru, J.T. (1983). Aspects of averaging. *Seminars in Hearing, 4,* 327–341.

Picton, T.W., Stapells, D.R., & Campbell, K.B. (1981). Auditory evoked potentials from the human cochlea and brainstem. *The Journal of Otolaryngology, 10,* 1–41.

Picton, T.W., Stuss, D.T., Champagne, S.C., & Nelson, R.F. (1984). The effects of age on human event-related potentials. *Psychophysiology, 21,* 312–325.

Picton, T.W., Stuss, D.T., & Marshall, K.C. (1986). Attention and the brain. In S.L. Friedman, K.A. Klivington, & R.W. Patterson (Eds.), *The brain, cognition, and education* (pp. 19–79). New York: Academic Press.

Picton, T.W., Woods, D.L., & Proulx, G.B. (1978a). Human auditory sustained potentials II. Stimulus relationships. *Electroencephalography and Clinical Neurophysiology, 45,* 198–210.

Picton, T.W., Woods, D.L., & Proulx, G.B. (1978b). Human auditory sustained potentials. I. The nature of the response. *Electroencephalography and Clinical Neurophysiology, 45,* 186–197.

Pietrowsky, R., Fehm, H.L., & Born, J. (1990). An analysis of the effects of corticotropin-releasing hormone (h-CRH), adrenocorticotropin (ACTH) and beta-endorphin on ERPs in humans. In C.M.H. Brunia, A.W.K. Gaillard, & A. Kok (Eds.), *Psychophysiological Brain Research* Vol II, (pp. 106–110). Tilburg: Tilburg University Press.

Plomp, R. (1964). Rate of decay of auditory sensation. *Journal of the Acoustical Society of America, 36,* 277–282.

Podgorny, P., & Shepard, R.N. (1983). Distribution of visual attention over space. *Journal of Experimental Psychology: Human Perception and Performance, 9,* 380–393.

Port, R.F. (in press). Can complex temporal patterns be automatized? *Behavioral and Brain Sciences.*

Posner, M.I. (1978). *Chronometric explorations of mind.* Hillsdale, NJ: Lawrence Erlbaum Associates.

Posner, M. (1980). Orienting of attention. *Quarterly Journal of Experimental Psychology, 32,* 3–25.

Posner, M. (1988). Structures and functions of selective attention. In T. Boll & B. Bryant (Eds.), *Clinical neuropsychology and brain function: Research, measurement, and practice* (pp. 169–202). Washington: American Psychological Association.

Posner, M.I., & Boies, S.J. (1971). Components of attention. *Psychological Review, 78,* 391–408.

Posner, M.I., Choate, L.S., Rafal, R.D., & Vaughn, J. (1985). Inhibition of return: Neural mechanisms and function. *Cognitive Neuropsychology, 2,* 211–228.

Posner, M.I., & Cohen, Y. (1984). Components of visual orienting. In H. Bouma & D. Bowhuis (Eds.), *Attention and performance X* (pp. 531–536). Hillsdale, NJ: Lawrence Erlbaum Associates.

Posner, M.I., Cohen, Y., Choate, L.S., Hockey, R., & Maylor, E. (1984). Sustained concentration: Passive filtering or active orienting? In S. Kornblum & J. Requin (Eds.), *Preparatory states and processes* (pp. 49–65). Hillsdale, NJ: Lawrence Erlbaum Associates.

Posner, M.I., Cohen, Y., & Rafal, R.D. (1982). Neural systems control over spatial orienting. *Philosophical Transaction Royal Society of London Series B, 2908,* 187–198.

Posner, M., Nissen, M.-J., & Klein, R. (1976). Visual dominance: An information-processing account of its origins and significance. *Psychological Review, 83,* 157–171.

Posner, M.I., & Petersen, S.E. (1990). The attention system of the human brain. *Annual Review of Neuroscience, 13,* 25–42.

Posner, M.I., Petersen, S.E., Fox, P.T., & Raichle, M.E. (1988). Localization of cognitive operations in the human brain. *Science, 240,* 1627–1631.

Posner, M.I., Sandson, J., Dhawan, M., & Shulman, G.L. (1989). Is word recognition automatic? A cognitive-anatomical approach. *Journal of Cognitive Neuroscience, 1,* 50–60.

Posner, M.I., & Snyder, C.R.R. (1975). Attention and cognitive control. In R.L. Solso (Ed.), *Information processing and cognition, The Loyola Symposium* (pp. 55–85). Hillsdale, NJ: Lawrence Erlbaum Associates.

Posner, M.I., Snyder, C.R.R., & Davidson, B.J. (1980). Attention and the detection of signals. *Journal of Experimental Psychology: General, 109,* 160–174.

Pratt, H., & Sohmer, H. (1977). Correlations between psychophysical magnitude estimates and simultaneously obtained auditory nerve, brain stem and cortical responses to click stimuli in man. *Electroencephalography and Clinical Neurophysiology, 43,* 802–812.

Pratt, H., & Sohmer, H. (1978). Comparison of hearing threshold determined by auditory pathway electric responses and behavioural responses. *Audiology, 17,* 285–292.

Prescott, J., Connolly, J.F., & Gruzelier, J.H. (1984). The augmenting/reducing phenomenon in the auditory evoked potential. *Biological Psychology, 19,* 31–44.

Previc, F.H., & Harter, M.R. (1982). Electrophysiological and behavioral indicants of selective attention to multifeature gratings. *Perception and Psychophysics, 32,* 465–472.

Pribram, K.H., & Luria, A.R. (1973). *Psychophysiology of the frontal lobes.* New York: Academic Press.

Prichard, J.W., & Shulman, R.G. (1986). NMR spectroscopy of brain metabolism in vivo. *Annual Review of Neuroscience, 9,* 61–85.

Prinzmetal, W. (1981). Principles of feature integration in visual perception. *Perception and Psychophysics, 30,* 330–340.

Pritchard, W.S. (1981). Psychophysiology of P300. *Psychological Bulletin, 89,* 506–540.

Puel, J., Bonfils, P., & Pujol, R. (1988). Selective attention modifies the active micromechanical properties of the cochlea. *Brain Research, 447,* 380–383.

Putnam, L. (1990). Great expectations: Anticipatory responses of the heart and brain. In J.W. Rohrbaugh, R. Parasuraman, & R. Johnson, Jr. (Eds.), *Event-related brain potentials: Basic issues and applications.* (pp. 109–129). Oxford: Oxford University Press.

Raichle, M.E. (1983). Positron emission tomography. *Annual Review of Neuroscience, 6,* 249–268.

Raichle, M.E. (1987). Circulatory and metabolic correlates of brain function in normal humans. In V.B. Mountcastle & F. Plum (Eds.), *Handbook of physiology: Section I. The nervous system V. Higher functions of the nervous system, Part 2* (pp. 643–674). Washington, DC: American Physiological Society.

Raichle, M.E., Grubb, R.L., Gado, M.H., Eichling, J.O., & Ter-Pogossian, M.T. (1976). Correlation between regional cerebral blood flow and oxidative metabolism. *Archives of Neurology (Chicago), 8,* 523–526.

Rapin, I., Schimmel, H., Tourk, L.M., Krasnegor, N.A., & Pollack, C. (1966). Evoked potentials to clicks and tones of varying intensity in waking adults. *Electroencephalography and Clinical Neurophysiology, 21,* 335–344.

Rayner, K., McConckie, G.W., & Ehrlich, S. (1978). Eye movements and integrating information across fixations. *Journal of Experimental Psychology: Human Perception and Performance, 4,* 529–544.

Rayner, K., McConckie, G.W., & Zola, D. (1980). Integrating information across eye movements. *Cognitive Psychology, 12,* 206–226.

Regan, D. (1981). Evoked potential studies of visual perception. *Canadian Journal of Psychology, 35,* 77–112.

Regan, D. (1988). *Human brain electrophysiology: Evoked potentials and evoked magnetic fields in science and medicine.* London: Chapman & Hall.

Reiman, E.M., Fusselman, M.J., Fox, P.T., & Raichle, M.E. (1989). Neuroanatomical correlates of anticipatory anxiety. *Science, 243,* 1071–1074.

Reite, M., Teale, P.D., Neumann, R., & Davis, K. (1987). Localization of a 50 msec latency auditory evoked field component. In R. Johnson, J.W. Rohrbaugh, & R. Parasuraman (Eds.), Current trends in event-related potential research (pp. 487–492). (Suppl. 40 to Electroencephalography and clinical Neurophysiology). Amsterdam: Elsevier.

Reite, M., Teale, P., Zimmerman, J., Davis, K., & Whalen, J. (1988). Source location of a 50 msec latency auditory evoked field component. *Electroencephalography and Clinical Neurophysiology, 70,* 490–498.

Reite, M., Zimmerman, J.E., Edrich, J., & Zimmerman, J.T. (1976). The human magnetoencephalogram: Some EEG and related correlations. *Electroencephalography and Clinical Neurophysiology, 40,* 59–66.

Reite, M., Zimmerman, J., Edrich, J., & Zimmerman, J.E. (1982). Auditory evoked magnetic fields: Response amplitude vs. stimulus intensity. *Electroencephalography and Clinical Neurophysiology, 54,* 147–152.

Reite, M., Zimmerman, J.T., & Zimmerman, J.E. (1981). Magnetic auditory evoked fields: Interhemispheric asymmetry. *Electroencephalography and Clinical Neurophysiology, 51,* 388–392.

Reivich, M., Greenberg, J., Alavi, A., Christman, D., Fowler, J., Hand, P., Rosenquist, A., Rintelmann, W., & Wolf, A. (1979). The use of the 18-F-fluorodeoxyglucose method for mapping of functional neural pathways in man. *Acta Neurologica Scandinavica Supplement, 72,* 198–199.

Reivich, M., Gur, R., & A. Alavi (1983). Positron emission tomographic studies of sensory stimuli, cognitive processes and anxiety. *Human Neurobiology, 2,* 25–33.

Remington, R., & Pierce, L. (1984). Moving attention: Evidence for time-invariant shifts of visual selective attention. *Perception and Psychophysics, 35,* 393–399.

Renault, B., Baribeau-Braun, J., Dalbokova, D., & El Massioui, F. (1986). Differential topographical analysis of auditory components in a selective attention task. In W.C. McCallum, R. Zappoli, & F. Denoth (Eds.), Cerebral psychophysiology: Studies in event-related potentials, (pp. 46–47). (Supplement 38 to Electroencephalography and Clinical Neurophysiology). Amsterdam: Elsevier.

Renault, B., & Lesévre, N. (1978). Topographical study of the emitted potential obtained after the omission of an expected visual stimulus. In D. Otto (Ed.), *Multidisciplinary perspectives in event-related brain potential research, EPA 600/9-77-043* (pp. 202–208). Washington: U.S. Government Printing Office.

Renault, B., & Lesévre, N. (1979). A trial-by-trial study of the visual omission response in reaction time situations. In D. Lehmann & E. Callaway (Eds.), *Human evoked potentials* (pp. 317–329). New York: Plenum Press.

Requin, J. (1985). Looking forward to moving soon: Ante factum selective processes in motor control. In M.I. Posner & O.S.M. Marin (Eds.), *Attention and performance XI* (pp. 147–167). Hillsdale, NJ: Lawrence Erlbaum Associates.

Richer, F., Barth, D.S., & Beatty, J. (1983). Neuromagnetic localization of two components of the transient visual evoked response to patterned stimulation. *Il Nuovo Cimento, 2d,* 420–428.

Rietveldt, W.J., Tordoir, W.E.M., & Hagenouw, J.R.B. (1967). The influence of alertness on the amplitude of the visual evoked response and on reaction time. *Acta Physiologica et Pharmacologica Neerlandica, 14,* 286–299.

Rif, J., Hari, R., Hämäläinen, M.S., & Sams, M. (1991). Auditory attention affects two different areas in the human supratemporal cortex. *Electroencephalography and*

Clinical Neurophysiology, 79, 464–472.

Risberg, J. (1987). Development of high-resolution two-dimensional measurement of regional cerebral blood flow. In J. Wade, S. Knezevic, V.A. Maximilian, Z. Mubrin, & I. Prohovnik (Eds.), *Impact of functional imaging in neurology and psychiatry* (pp. 35–43). London: Libbey & Co.

Risberg, J., Ali, Z., Wilson, E.M., Wills, E.L., & Halsey, J.H. (1975). Regional cerebral blood flow by 133-xenon inhalation. Preliminary evaluation of an initial slope index in patients with unstable flow compartments. *Stroke, 6,* 142–148.

Risberg, J., & Ingvar, D.H. (1973). Patterns of activation in the grey matter of the dominant hemisphere during memorizing and reasoning. A study of regional cerebral blood flow changes during psychological testing in a group of neurologically normal patients. *Brain, 96,* 737–756.

Risberg, J., Maximilian, A.V., & Prohovnik, I. (1977). Changes of cortical activity patterns during habituation to a reasoning test. A study with the 133Xe inhalation technique for measurement of regional cerebral blood flow. *Neuropsychologia, 15,* 793–798.

Risberg, J. & Prohovnik, I. (1983). Cortical processing of visual and tactile stimuli studied by non-invasive rCBF measurements. *Human Neurobiology, 2,* 5–10.

Ritter, W., Paavilainen, P., Lavikainen, J., Reinikainen, K., & Näätänen, R. (1991). Event-related potentials to repetition and change of auditory stimuli. Manuscript submitted for publication.

Ritter, W., Simson, R., & Vaughan, H.G., Jr. (1972). Association cortex potentials and reaction time in auditory discrimination. *Electroencephalography and Clinical Neurophysiology, 33,* 547–555.

Ritter, W., Simson, R., & Vaughan, H.G., Jr. (1983). Event-related potential correlates of two stages of information processing in physical and semantic discrimination tasks. *Psychophysiology, 20,* 168–179.

Ritter, W., Simson, R., Vaughan, H.G., Jr., & Friedman, D. (1979). A brain event related to the making of a sensory discrimination. *Science, 203,* 1358–1361.

Ritter, W., Vaughan, Jr., H.G., & Costa, L.D. (1968). Orienting and habituation to auditory stimuli: A study of short term changes in average evoked responses. *Electroencephalography and Clinical Neurophysiology, 25,* 550–556.

Rizzolatti, G., Riggio, L., Dascola, I., & Umilta, C. (1987). Reorienting attention across the horizontal and vertical meridians: Evidence for a premotor theory of attention. *Neuropsychologia, 25,* 31–40.

Robinson, D.L., & Rugg, M.D. (1988). Latencies of visually responsive neurons in various regions of the Rheins monkey brain and their relation to human visual responses. *Biological Psychology, 26,* 111–116.

Rodriguez, R., Picton, T., Linden, D., Hamel, G., & Laframboise, G. (1986). Human auditory steady state responses: Effects of intensity and frequency. *Ear & Hearing, 7,* 300–313.

Rohrbaugh, J.W. (1984). The orienting reflex: Performance and central nervous system manifestations. In R. Parasuraman & D.R. Davies (Eds.), *Varieties of attention.* (pp. 323–373). New York: Academic Press.

Rohrbaugh, J.W., & Gaillard, A.W.K. (1983). Sensory and motor aspects of the contingent negative variation. In A.W.K. Gaillard & W. Ritter (Eds.), *Tutorials in ERP research: Endogenous components* (pp. 269–310). Amsterdam: North Holland.

Rohrbaugh, J.W., Syndulko, K., & Lindsley, D.B. (1978). Cortical slow negative waves following non-paired stimuli: Effects of task factors. *Electroencephalography and Clinical Neurophysiology, 45,* 551–567.

Rohrbaugh, J.W., Syndulko, K., & Lindsley, D.B. (1979). Cortical slow negative waves following non-paired stimuli: Effects of modality, intensity, and rate of stimulation. *Electroencephalography and Clinical Neurophysiology, 46,* 416–427.

Rohrbaugh, J.W., Varner, J.L., Paige, S.R., Eckardt, M.J., & Ellingson, R.J. (1989). Event-related perturbations in an electrophysiological measure of auditory function: A measure of sensitivity during orienting. *Biological Psychology, 29,* 247–271.

Rohrbaugh, J.W., Varner, J.L., Paige, S.R., Eckardt, M.J., & Ellingson, R.J. (1990). Auditory and visual event-related perturbations in the 40 Hz auditory steady-state response. *Electroencephalography and Clinical Neurophysiology, 76,* 148–164.

Rohrbaugh, J.W., Varner, J.L., Paige, S.R., Eckardt, M.J., & Ellingson, R.J. (1991). Event-related perturbations in an electrophysiological measure of sensitivity: Effects of probability, intensity and repeated sessions. *International Journal of Psychophysiology, 10,* 17–32.

Roland, P.E. (1981). Somatotopical tuning of postcentral gyrus during focal attention in man. A regional cerebral blood flow study. *Journal of Neurophysiology, 46,* 744–754.

Roland, P.E. (1982). Cortical regulation of selective attention in man. A regional cerebral blood flow study. *Journal of Neurophysiology, 48,* 1059–1077.

Roland, P.E. (1985). Cortical organization of voluntary behavior in man. *Human Neurobiology, 4,* 155–167.

Roland, P.E. (1987). Changes in brain blood flow and oxidative metabolism during mental activity. *News in Physiological Sciences, 2,* 120–124.

Roland, P.E., Eriksson, L., Stone-Elander, S., & Widen, L. (1987). Does mental activity change the oxidative metabolism of the brain? *The Journal of Neuroscience, 7,* 2373–2389.

Roland, P.E., & Friberg, L. (1985). Localization of cortical areas activated by thinking. *Journal of Neurophysiology, 53,* 1219–1243.

Roland, P.E., & Larsen, B. (1976). Focal increase of cerebral blood flow during stereognostic testing in man. *Archives of Neurology, 33,* 551–558.

Roland, P.E., Larsen, B., & Lassen, N.A. (1980). Supplementary motor area and other cortical areas in organization of voluntary movements in man. *Journal of Neurophysiology, 43,* 118–136.

Roland, P.E., & Skinhøj, E. (1981). Focal activation of the cerebral cortex during visual discrimination in man. *Brain Research, 222,* 166–171.

Roland, P.E., Skinhøj, E., Larsen, B., & Endo, H. (1977). Perception and voluntary action: Localization of basic input and output functions as revealed by regional cerebral blood flow increases in human brain. In J.S. Meyer, H. Lechner, & M. Reivich (Eds.), *Cerebral Vascular Disease* (pp. 40–44). Amsterdam: Excerpta Medica.

Roland, P.E., Skinhøj, E., & Lassen, N.A. (1981). Focal activations of human cerebral cortex during auditory discrimination. *Journal of Neurophysiology, 45,* 1139–1151.

Roland, P.E., Skinhøj, E., Lassen, N.A., & Larsen, B. (1980). Different cortical areas in organization of voluntary movements in extrapersonal space. *Journal of Neurophysiology, 43,* 137–150.

Roland, P.E., & Widen, L. (1988). Quantitative measurements of brain metabolism during physiological stimulation. In G. Pfurtscheller & F.H. Lopes da Silva (Eds.), *Functional brain imaging* (pp. 213–228). Toronto: Hans Huber.

Romani, G.L., Williamson, S.J., & Kaufman, L. (1982). Tonotopic organization of the human auditory cortex. *Science, 216,* 1339–1340.

Romani, G.L., Williamson, S.J., Kaufman, L., & Brenner, D. (1982). Characterization of the human auditory cortex by the neuromagnetic method. *Experimental Brain Research, 47,* 381–393.

Rosenzweig, M.R. (1951). Representations of the two ears at the auditory cortex. *American Journal of Physiology, 167,* 147–158.

Rossignol, S., & Jones, G.M. (1976). Audio-spinal influence in man studied by the H-reflex and its possible role on rhythmic movements synchronized to sound. *Electroencephalography and Clinical Neurophysiology, 41,* 83–92.

Roth, W.T. (1973). Auditory evoked responses to unpredictable stimuli. *Psychophysiology, 10,* 125–137.

Roth, W.T. (1983). A comparison of P300 and skin conductance response. In A.W.K. Gaillard & W. Ritter (Eds.), *Tutorials in ERP research: Endogenous components* (pp. 177–199). Amsterdam: North-Holland.

Roth, W.T., Ford, J.T., & Kopell, B.S. (1978). Long-latency evoked potentials and reaction time. *Psychophysiology, 15,* 17–23.

Roth, W.T., & Kopell, B.S. (1969). The auditory evoked response to repeated stimuli during a vigilance task. *Psychophysiology, 6,* 301–309.

Rothman, H.H., Davis, H., & Hay, I.S. (1970). Slow evoked cortical potentials and temporal features of stimulation. *Electroencephalography and Clinical Neurophysiology, 29,* 225–232.

Rovamo, J., & Virsu, V. (1979). An estimation and application of the human cortical magnification factor. *Experimental Brain Research, 37,* 495–510.

Rubin, E. (1921). *Visuell wahrgenommene Figuren.* [Visual perception of figures] Berlin: Verlagsdrückerei Berlin.

Ruchkin, D.S., & Glaser, E.M. (1978). Some simple digital filters for examination of CNV and P300 waveforms on a single trial basis. In D. Otto (Ed.), *Multidiciplinary Perspectives in Event-Related Brain Potential (ERP) Research* (pp. 579–581). Washington: U.S. Government Printing Office.

Ruchkin, D.S., Johnson, R., Mahaffey, D., & Sutton, S. (1988). Toward a functional categorization of slow waves. *Psychophysiology, 25,* 339–353.

Ruchkin, D.S., & Sutton, S. (1983). Positive slow wave and P300: association and disassociation. In A.W.K. Gaillard & W. Ritter (Eds.), *Tutorials in event related potential research: Endogenous components.* (pp. 233–250). Amsterdam: North-Holland.

Ruchkin, D.S., Sutton, S., Mahaffey, D., & Glaser, J. (1986). Terminal CNV in the absence of motor response. *Electroencephalography and Clinical Neurophysiology, 63,* 445–463.

Rugg, M.D. (1991). ERPs and selective attention: Commentary. In C.H.M. Brunia, G. Mulder, & M.N. Verbaten (Eds.), *Event-Related Potentials of the Brain.* (pp. 222–227). (Suppl. 42 to Electroencephalography and Clinical Neurophysiology). Amsterdam: Elsevier.

Rugg, M.D., Milner, A.D., Lines, C.R., & Phalp, R. (1987). Modulation of visual event-related potentials by spatial and non-spatial visual selective attention. *Neuropsychologia, 25,* 85–96.

Sagi, D., & Julesz, B. (1985). Detection versus discrimination of visual orientation. *Perception, 14,* 619–628.

Salamy, A., & McKean, C.M. (1977). Habituation and dishabituation of cortical and brainstem evoked potentials. *International Journal of Neuroscience, 7,* 175–182.

Sams, M., Alho, K., & Näätänen, R. (1983). Sequential effects in the ERP in discriminating two stimuli. *Biological Psychology, 17,* 41–58.

Sams, M., Alho, K., & Näätänen, R. (1984). Short-term habituation and dishabituation of the mismatch negativity of the ERP. *Psychophysiology, 21,* 434–441.

Sams, M., Aulanko, R., Aaltonen, O., & Näätänen, R. (1990). Event-related potentials to infrequent changes in synthesized phonetic stimuli. *Journal of Cognitive Neuroscience, 2,* 344–357.

Sams, M., Aulanko, R., Hämäläinen, M., Hari, R., Lounasmaa, O.V., Lu, S.-T., & Simola, J. (1991). Seeing speech: Visual information from lip movements modifies activity in the human auditory cortex. *Neuroscience Letters, 127,* 141–145.

Sams, M., Hämäläinen, M., Antervo, A., Kaukoranta, E., Reinikainen, K., & Hari, R. (1985). Cerebral neuromagnetic responses evoked by short auditory stimuli. *Electroencephalography and Clinical Neurophysiology, 61,* 254–266.

Sams, M., Hari, R., Rif, J., & Knuutila, J. (in press). *The human auditory sensory memory trace persists about 10 s: Neuromagnetic evidence. Journal of Cognitive Neuroscience.*

Sams, M., Kaukoranta, E., Hämäläinen, M., & Näätänen, R. (1991). Cortical activity elicited by changes in auditory stimuli: Different sources for the magnetic N100m and mismatch responses. *Psychophysiology, 28,* 21–29.

Sams, M., & Näätänen, R. (1991). Neuromagnetic responses of the human auditory cortex to short frequency glides. *Neuroscience Letters, 121,* 43–46.

Sams, M., Paavilainen, P., Alho, K., & Näätänen, R. (1985). Auditory frequency discrimination and event-related potentials. *Electroencephalography and Clinical Neurophysiology, 62,* 437–448.

Sanders, A.F. (1966). Expectancy: application and measurement. *Acta Psychologica, 25,* 293–313.

Sanders, A.F. (1975). The foreperiod effect revisited. *Quarterly Journal of Experimental Psychology, 27,* 591–598.

Sanders, A.F. (1979). Some remarks on mental load. In N. Moray (Ed.), *Mental workload: Its theory and measurement* (pp. 41–71) New York: Plenum Press.

Sanders, A.F. (1983). Towards a model of stress and human performance. *Acta Psychologica, 53,* 61–97.

Satterfield, J.H. (1965). Evoked cortical response enhancement and attention in man. A study of responses to auditory and shock stimuli. *Electroencephalography and Clinical Neurophysiology, 19,* 470–475.

Satterfield, J.H., & Cheatum, D. (1964). Evoked cortical potential correlates of attention in human subjects. *Electroencephalography and Clinical Neurophysiology, 17,* 456.

Schafer, E.W.P. (1978). Brain responses while viewing television reflect program interest. *International Journal of Neuroscience, 8,* 71–77.

Schafer, E.W.P., & Marcus, M.M. (1973). Self-stimulation alters human sensory brain responses. *Science, 181,* 175–177.

Scharf, B. (1990). The case for preconscious effects of attention on auditory processing. *Behavioral and Brain Sciences, 13,* 252–253.

Scharf, B., & Houtsma, A.J. (1986). Audition II: Loudness, pitch, localization, aural distortion, pathology. In K.R. Boff, L. Kaufman, & J.P. Thomas (Eds.), *Handbook of perception and human performance: Volume I, Sensory processes and perception* (pp. 15.1–60). New York: Wiley.

Scharf, B., Quigley, S., Aoki, C., Peachey, N., & Reeves, H. (1987). Focused auditory attention and frequency selectivity. *Perception and Psychophysics, 42,* 215–223.

Scheffers, M.K., Wijers, A.A., & Mulder, G. (1991). Spatial selective attention: an ERP analysis of constant and variable cuing of location in a memory search task. Manuscript submitted for publication.

Scheibel, A.B. (1980). Session chairman's overview: Anatomical and physiological substrates of arousal. In J.A. Hobson & M.A.B. Brazier (Eds.), *The reticular formation* (pp. 129–134). New York: Raven Press.

Scherg, M. (1990). Fundamentals of dipole source potential analysis. In F. Grandori, M. Hoke, & G.L. Romani (Eds.), *Auditory evoked magnetic fields and electric potentials. Advances in audiology* (Vol. 6. pp. 40–69). Basel: Karger.

Scherg, M., & Cramon, D. von (1985a). Two bilateral sources of the late AEP as identified by a spatio-temporal dipole model. *Electroencephalography and Clinical Neurophysiology, 62,* 32–44.

Scherg, M., & Cramon, D. von (1985b). A new interpretation of the generators of BAEP waves I–V: Results of a spatio-temporal dipole model. *Electroencephalography and Clinical Neurophysiology, 62,* 290–299.

Scherg, M., & Cramon, D. von (1986). Evoked dipole source potentials of the human auditory cortex. *Electroencephalography and Clinical Neurophysiology, 65,* 344–360.

Scherg, M., Hari, R., & Hämäläinen, M.S. (1989). Frequency-specific sources of the auditory N19-P30 detected by a multiple source analysis of evoked magnetic fields and potentials. In S.J. Williamson, M. Hoke, G. Stroink, & M. Kotani (Eds.), *Advances in biomagnetism* (pp. 97–101). New York: Plenum Press.

Scherg, M., & Picton, T.W. (1990). Brain electric source analysis of the mismatch negativity. In C.M.H. Brunia, A.W.K. Gaillard, & A. Kok (Eds.), *Psychophysiological brain research* (Vol I, pp. 94–98). Tilburg: Tilburg University Press.

Scherg, M., & Picton, T.W. (1991). Separation and identification of event-related potential components by brain electric source analysis. In C.H.M. Brunia, G. Mulder, & M.N. Verbaten (Eds.), *Event-Related Potentials of the Brain.* (pp. 24–37). (Supplement 42 to Electroencephalography and Clinical Neurophysiology). Amsterdam: Elsevier.

Scherg, M., Vajsar, J., & Picton, T.W. (1989). A source analysis of the late human auditory evoked potentials. *Journal of Cognitive Neuroscience, 1,* 336–355.

Schiepers, C. (1980). Response latency and accuracy in visual word recognition. *Perception Psychophysics, 27,* 71–81.

Schneider, S., Abraham-Fuchs, K., Daalmans, G., Folberth, W., Hoenig, H.E., Reichenberger, H., Röhrlein, G., Seifert, H., & Wirth, A. (1989). Development and performance of a multichannel system for studies of biomagnetic signals of brain and heart. In S.J. Williamson, M. Hoke, G. Stroink, & M. Kotani (Eds.), *Advances in biomagnetism* (pp. 669–672). New York: Plenum Press.

Schneider, W. (1985). Toward a model of attention and the development of automatic processing. In M.I. Posner & O.S.M. Marin (Eds.), *Attention and performance XI* (pp. 475–492). Hillsdale, NJ: Lawrence Erlbaum Associates.

Schneider, W., Dumais, S.T., & Shiffrin, R.M. (1984). Automatic and control processing and attention. In R. Parasuraman & D.R. Davies (Eds.), *Varieties of attention.* (pp. 1–27). New York: Academic Press.

Schneider, W., & Fisk, A.D. (1982). Concurrent automatic and controlled visual search: Can processing occur without resource cost? *Journal of Experimental Psychology: Learning, Memory and Cognition, 8,* 261–278.

Schneider, W., & Shiffrin, R.M. (1977). Controlled and automatic human information processing: I. Detection, search, and attention. *Psychological Review, 84,* 1–66.

Schreiber, H., Lang, M., Lang, W., Kornhuber, A., Heise, B., Keidel, M., Deecke, L., & Kornhuber, H.H. (1983). Frontal hemispheric differences in the Bereitschaftspotential associated with writing and drawing. *Human Neurobiology, 2,* 197–202.

Schwent, V.L., & Hillyard, S.A. (1975). Evoked potential correlates of selective attention with multichannel auditory inputs. *Electroencephalography and Clinical Neurophysiology, 38,* 131–138.

Schwent, V.L., Hillyard, S.A., & Galambos, R. (1976). Selective attention and the auditory vertex potential. I. Effects of stimulus delivery rate. *Electroencephalography and Clinical Neurophysiology,* 40, 604–614.

Schwent, V.L., Snyder, E., & Hillyard, S.A. (1976). Auditory evoked potentials during multichannel selective listening: Role of pitch and localization cues. *Journal of Experimental Psychology: Human Perception and Performance, 2,* 313–325.

Seitz, R.J., Roland, P.E., Bohm, C., Greitz, T., & Stone-Elander, S. (1990). Motor learning in man: a positron emission tomographic study. *NeuroReport, 1,* 17–20.

Semjen, A., Bonnet, M., & Requin, J. (1973). Relation between the timecourse of Hoffman Reflexes and the foreperiod duration in a reaction-time task. *Physiology and Behaviour, 10,* 1041–1050.

Sereno, A.B. (1990). Searching for a neurophysiological view of ERP components. *Behavioral and Brain Sciences, 13,* 253–254.

Shaffer, H.L. (1975). Multiple attention in continuous verbal tasks. In P.M.A. Rabbitt & S. Dornic (Eds.), *Attention and performance V* (pp. 157–167). London: Academic Press.

Shaw, M. (1984). Division of attention among spatial locations: A fundamental difference between detection of letters and detection of luminance increments. In H. Bouma & D. Bouwhuis (Eds.), *Attention and performance X* (pp. 109–121). Hillsdale, NJ: Lawrence Erlbaum Associates.

Shaw, M., & Shaw, P. (1977). Optimal allocation of cognitive resources to spatial location. *Journal of Experimental Psychology: Human Perception and Performance, 3,* 201–211.

Sheatz, G.C., & Chapman, R.M. (1969). Task relevance and auditory evoked responses. *Electroencephalography and Clinical Neurophysiology, 26,* 468–475.

Shelley, A.M. (1991). *The neural substrate of selective attention: Electrophysiological correlates of catecholamine and endorphin modulation.* Academic Dissertation, University of New South Wales, Australia.

Shelley, A.M., Ward, P.B., Catts, S.V., Michie, P.T., Andrews, S., & McConaghy, N. (1991). Mismatch negativity: an index of a preattentive processing deficit in schizophrenia. *Biological Psychiatry, 30,* 1059–1062.

Shelley, A.M., Ward, P.B., Michie, P.T., Andrews, S., Catts, S.V., & McConaghy, N. (1991). The effect of repeated testing on ERP components during auditory selective attention. *Psychophysiology, 28,* 496–510.

Shevelev, I.A., Tsicalov, E.N., & Gorbach, A.M. (1988). Dynamic infra-red images of the brain. *IBRO News, 16,* 8–9.

Shiffrin, R.M. (1975). The locus and role of attention in memory systems. In P.M.A. Rabbitt & S. Dornic (Eds.), *Attention and performance V* (pp. 168–193). London: Academic Press.

Shiffrin, R.M., & Grantham, D.W. (1974). Can attention be allocated to sensory modalities? *Perception and Psychophysics, 15,* 460–474.

Shiffrin, R.M., McKay, D.P., & Shaffer, W.O. (1976). Attending to forty-nine spatial positions at once. *Journal of Experimental Psychology: Human Perception and Performance, 2,* 14–22.

Shiffrin, R.M., Pisoni, D.B., & Casteneda-Mendez, K. (1974). Is attention shared between the ears? *Cognitive Psychology, 6,* 190–215.

Shiffrin, R.M., & Schneider, W. (1977). Controlled and automatic information processing: II. Perceptual learning, automatic attending, and a general theory. *Psychological Review, 84,* 127–189.

Shulman, G.L., Remington, R.W., & McLean, J.P. (1979). Moving attention through visual space. *Journal of Experimental Psychology, 5,* 522–526.

Siddle, D.A.T. (1979). The orienting response and stimulus significance: Some comments. *Biological Psychology, 8,* 303–309.

Sidman, R.D., Giambalvo, V., Allison, T., & Bergey, P. (1978). A method for localization of sources of human cerebral potentials evoked by sensory stimuli. *Sensory Processes, 2,* 116–129.

Simson, R., Vaughan, Jr., H.G., & Ritter, W. (1976). The scalp topography of potentials associated with missing visual or auditory stimuli. *Electroencephalography and Clinical Neurophysiology, 40,* 33–42.

Simson, R., Vaughan, Jr., H.G., & Ritter, W. (1977a). The scalp topography of potentials in auditory and visual discrimination tasks. *Electroencephalography and Clinical Neurophysiology, 42,* 528–535.

Simson, R., Vaughan, Jr., H.G., & Ritter, W. (1977b). The scalp topography of potentials in auditory and visual GO/NO-GO tasks. *Electroencephalography and Clinical Neurophysiology, 43,* 864–875.

Sirevaag, E., Kramer, A.F., Coles, M.G.H., & Donchin, E. (1984). P300 amplitude and resource allocation. *Psychophysiology, 21,* 598–599.

Skinner, J.E., & Yingling, C.D. (1977). Central gating mechanisms that regulate event-related potentials and behavior. In J.E. Desmedt (Ed.), *Attention, voluntary contraction and event-related cerebral potentials: Progress in clinical neurophysiology* (Vol. 1, pp. 70–96). Basel, Switzerland: Karger.

Smith, M.C., & Burrows, D. (1974). Memory scanning: Effect of unattended input. *Journal of Experimental Psychology, 102,* 722–725.

Smith, M.C., & Groen, M. (1974). Evidence for semantic analysis of unattended verbal items. *Journal of Experimental Psychology: Learning, Memory, and Cognition, 9,* 697–712.

Snodgrass, J.G., & Townsend, J.T. (1980). Comparing parallel and serial models: Theory and implementation. *Journal of Experimental Psychology: Human Perception and Performance, 6,* 330–354.

Snyder, E., & Hillyard, S.A. (1976). Long-latency evoked potentials to irrelevant deviant stimuli. *Behavioural Biology, 16,* 319–331.

Sokoloff, L., Reivich, M., Kennedy, C., Des Rosiers, M.H., Patlak, C.S., Pettigrew, K.D., Sakurada, D., & Shinohara, M. (1977). The (14C) deoxyglucose method for the measurement of local cerebral glucose utilization: Theory, procedure, and normal values in the conscious and anesthetized albino rat. *Journal of Neurochemistry, 28,* 897.

Sokolov, E.N. (1960). Neuronal models and orienting reflex. In M.A.B. Brazier (Ed.), *The central nervous system and behaviour* (pp. 187–276). Madison, N.J.: Madison Printing.

Sokolov, E.N. (1963). Higher nervous functions: The orienting reflex. *Annual Review of Physiology, 25,* 545–580.

Sokolov, E.N. (1966). Orienting reflex as information regulator. In A. Leontiev, A. Luria, & S. Smirnov (Eds.), *Psychological research in the USSR.* (pp. 334–360) Moscow: Progress Publishers.

Sokolov, E.N. (1975). The neuronal mechanisms of the orienting reflex. In E.N. Sokolov & O.S. Vinogradova (Eds.), *Neuronal mechanisms of the orienting reflex* (pp. 217–235). Hillsdale, NJ: Lawrence Erlbaum Associates.

Solowij, N., Michie, P., Crawford, J., & Glue, L. (1990). Auditory ERPs during attention and a visual control task: Effects of visual task difficulty. In C.H.M. Brunia, A.W.K. Gaillard, & A. Kok (Eds.), *Psychophysiological brain research* (pp. 217–220). Tilburg: Tilburg University Press.

Sorkin, R.D., & Pohlmann, L.D. (1973). Some models of observer behavior in two-channel auditory signal detection. *Perception and Psychophysics, 14,* 101–109.

Sperling, G. (1960). The information available in brief visual presentations. *Psychological Monographs, 74,* (11, Whole No. 498).

Sperling, G. (1984). A unified theory of attention and signal detection. In R. Parasuraman & D.R. Davies (Eds.), *Varieties of attention* (pp. 103–181). New York: Academic Press.

Sperling, G., & Melchner, M.J. (1978). Visual search, visual attention, and the attention operating characteristic. In J. Requin (Ed.), *Attention and performance VII* (pp. 675–686). Hillsdale, NJ: Lawrence Erlbaum Associates.

Sperling, G. & Reeves, A. (1980). Measuring the reaction time of a shift of visual attention. In R.S. Nickerson (Ed.), *Attention and performance VIII* (pp. 347–360). Hillsdale, NJ: Lawrence Erlbaum Associates.

Spiegel, M.F., & Watson, C.S. (1981). Factors in the discrimination of tonal patterns. III. Frequency discrimination with components of well-learned patterns. *Journal of the Acoustical Society of America, 69,* 223–230.

Spong, P., Haider, M., & Lindsley, D.B. (1965). Selective attentiveness and cortical evoked responses to visual and auditory stimuli. *Science, 148,* 395–397.

Spoor, A., Timmer, F., & Odenthal, D.W. (1969). The evoked auditory response (ear) to intensity modulated and frequency modulated tones and tone bursts. *International Audiology, 8,* 410–415.

Spydell, J.D., Pattee, G., & Gouldie, W.D. (1985). The 40 Hz auditory event-related potential: Normal values and effects of lesions. *Electroencephalography and Clinical Neurophysiology, 62,* 193–202.

Squires, K.C., Donchin, E., Herning, R.I., & McCarthy, G. (1977). On the influence of task relevance and stimulus probability on event-related potential components. *Electroencephalography and Clinical Neurophysiology, 42,* 1–14.

Squires, K.C., Hillyard, S.A., & Lindsay, P.H. (1973). Vertex potentials evoked during auditory signal detection: Relation to decision criteria. *Perception and Psychophysics, 14,* 265–272.

Squires, K.C., Squires, N.K., & Hillyard, S.A. (1975). Decision-related cortical potentials during an auditory signal detection task with cued observation intervals. *Journal of Experimental Psychology: Human Perception and Performance, 1,* 268–279.

Squires, K.C., Wickens, C., Squires, N.K., & Donchin, E. (1976). The effect of stimulus sequence on the waveform of the cortical event-related potential. *Science, 193,* 1142–1146.

Squires, N.K., Squires, K.C., & Hillyard, S.A., (1975). Two varieties of long-latency positive waves evoked by unpredictable auditory stimuli in man. *Electroencephalography and Clinical Neurophysiology, 38,* 387–401.

Stapells, D.R., Linden, D., Suffield, J.B., Hamel, G., & Picton, T.W. (1984). Human auditory steady-state evoked potentials. *Ear & Hearing, 5,* 105–113.

Starr, A., & Achor, J. (1975). Auditory brain stem responses in neurological disease. *Archives on Neurology, 32,* 761–768.

Starr, A., & Don, M. (1988). Brain potentials evoked by acoustic stimuli. In T.W. Picton (Ed.), *Human event-related potentials. EEG handbook, Rev. series,* (vol. 3, pp. 97–157). Amsterdam: Elsevier.

Sternbach, R.A., (1966). *Principles of psychophysiology.* New York: Academic Press.

Sternberg, S. (1966). High speed scanning in human memory. *Science, 153,* 652–654.

Sternberg, S. (1969). The discovery and processing stages: Extension of Donders' method. *Acta Psychologica, 30,* 276–315.

Sternberg, S. (1975). Memory scanning: New findings and current controversies. *Quarterly Journal of Experimental Psychology, 27,* 1–32.

Sternberg, S., Monsell, S., Knoll, R.J., & Wright, C.E. (1978). The latency and duration of rapid movement sequences: Comparisons of speech and typewriting. In G.E. Stelmach (Ed.), *Information processing in motor control and learning* (pp. 117–152). New York: Academic Press.

Stevens, S.S. (1951). *Handbook of experimental psychology.* New York: Wiley.

Stok, C.J. (1987). The influence of model parameters on EEG/MEG single dipole source estimation. *IEEE Transactions in Biomedical Engineering, 34,* 289–296.

Strayer, D., & Kramer, A.F. (1990). Attentional requirements of automatic and controlled processing. *Journal of Experimental Psychology: Learning, Memory and Cognition, 16,* 67–82.

Stroop, J.R. (1935). Studies of interference in serial verbal reaction. *Journal of Experimental Psychology, 18,* 643–662.

Stuss, D.T., & Benson, D.F., (1986). *The frontal lobes.* New York: Raven Press.

Suga, N. (1977). Amplitude spectrum representation in the Doppler-shifted-CF processing area of the auditory cortex of the mustache bat. *Science, 196,* 64–67.

Sutton, S. (1979). P300—Thirteen years later. In H. Begleiter (Ed.), *Evoked brain potentials and behavior* (pp. 107–126). New York: Plenum Press.

Sutton, S., Braren, M., Zubin, J., & John, E.R. (1965). Evoked potential correlates of stimulus uncertainty. *Science, 150,* 1187–88.

Swinney, D.A. (1979). Lexical access during sentence comprehension: Reconsideration of context effects. *Journal of Verbal Learning and Verbal Behavior, 18,* 645–659.

Swinney, D.A. (1982). The structure and time-course of information interaction during speech comprehension: Lexical segmentation, access, and interpretation. In J. Mehler, E.C.T. Walker, & M. Garrett (Eds.), *Perspectives on mental representation.* (pp. 151–163). Hillsdale, NJ: Lawrence Erlbaum Associates.

Tassinari, G., Aglioti, S., Chelazzi, L., Marzi, C.A., & Berlucchi, G. (1987). Distribution in the visual field of the costs of voluntarily allocated attention and of the inhibitory aftereffects of covert orienting. *Neuropsychologia, 25,* 55–71.

Taylor, M.J. (1978). Bereitschaftspotential during the acquisition of a skilled motor task. *Electroencephalography and Clinical Neurophysiology, 83,* 161–191.

Taylor, M.J., Lindsay, P.M., & Forbes, S.M. (1967). Quantification of shared capacity processing in auditory and visual discrimination. *Acta Psychologica, 27,* 223–229.

Tecce, J.J. (1972). Contingent negative variation (CNV) and psychological processes in man. *Psychological Bulletin, 77,* 73–108.

Teder, W., Alho, K., Reinikainen, K., & Näätänen, R. (in press). Interstimulus interval and the selective attention effect on auditory ERPs: "N1 enhancement" vs. processing negativity. *Psychophysiology.*

Tello, F. (1904). Quoted by Horn, G., 1965. Physiological and psychological aspects of selective perception. In: D.S. Lehrmann & R.A. Hinde (Eds.), *Advances in animal behavior 1.* (pp. 155–215). New York: Academic Press.

Tervaniemi, M., Saarinen, J., Paavilainen, P., & Näätänen, R. (in preparation). Event-related potentials to changes in a paired stimulus.

Teszner, D., Hari, R., & Nicolas, P. (1983). Somatosensory evoked magnetic fields: Mappings and the influence of stimulus repetition rate. *Il Nuovo Cimento, Series D.* (429–437).

Teyler, T.J., Cuffin, B.N., & Cohen, D. (1975). The visual evoked magnetoencephalogram. *Life Sciences, 17,* 683–692.

Thompson, R.F., Berry, S.D., Rinaldi, P.C., & Berger, T.W. (1979). Habituation and the orienting reflex: The dual-process theory revisited. In H.D. Kimmel, E.H. van Olst, & J.F. Orlebeke (Eds.), *The orienting reflex in humans* (pp. 21–60). Hillsdale, NJ: Lawrence Erlbaum Associates.

Thompson, R.F., Groves, P.M., Teyler, T.J., & Roemer, R.A. (1973). A dual-process theory of habituation: Theory and behavior. In H.V.S. Peeke & M.J. Hertz (Eds.), *Habituation: Vol. I. Behavioral studies* (pp. 239–271). London: Academic Press.

Thompson, R.F., & Spencer, W.A. (1966). Habituation: A model phenomenon for the study of neuronal substrates of behavior. *Psychological Review, 173,* 16–43.

Thornton, A., Heneghan, C.P.H., James, M.F.M., & Jones, J.G. (1984). The effects of halothane and enflurane anesthesia on the early auditory evoked potentials in humans. In R.H. Nodar & C. Barber (Eds.), *Evoked potentials II.* (pp. 483–496). Boston: Butterworths.

Thornton, A., Mendel, M.I., & Anderson, C. (1977). Effects of stimulus frequency and intensity on the middle components of the averaged auditory EEG response. *Journal of Speech and Hearing Research, 20,* 81–94.

Tiihonen, J., Hari, R., & Hämäläinen, M. (1989). Early deflections of cerebral magnetic responses to median nerve stimulation. *Electroencephalography and Clinical Neurophysiology, 74,* 290–296.

Tiihonen, J., Hari, R., Kajola, M., Karhu, J., Ahlfors, S., & Tissari, S. (1991). Magnetoencephalographic 10-Hz rhythm from the human auditory cortex. *Neuroscience Letters, 129,* 303–305.

Tiihonen, J., Hari, R., Kajola, M., Nousiainen, U., & Vapalahti, M. (1990). Localization of epileptic foci using a large-area magnetometer and functional brain anatomy. *Annals of Neurology, 27,* 283–290.

Tiihonen, J., Hari, R., Kaukoranta, E., & M. Kajola (1989). Interaural interaction in the human auditory cortex. *Audiology, 28,* 37–48.

Tiihonen, J., Kajola, M., & Hari, R. (1989). Magnetic mu rhythm in man. *Neuroscience, 32,* 793–800.

Tiitinen, H., Sinkkonen, J., Reinikainen, K., May, P., Alho K., Lavikainen, J., & Näätänen, R. (in preparation) Effect of attention on the 40-Hz response of the human brain.

Timsit-Berthier, M., Mantanus, H., & Legros, J.J. (1983). EEG-reactivity and event-related potential approach to the study of vasopressin. In: E. Endroeczi, L. Angelucci, D. DeWied, & U. Scapagnini (Eds.), *Neuropeptides and Psychosomatic Processes* (pp. 63–71). Budapest, Hungary: Academiai Kiado.

Tomberg, C., Desmedt, J.E., Ozaki, I., Nguyen, T.H., & Chalkin, V. (1989). Mapping somatosensory evoked potentials to finger stimulation at intervals of 450 to 4000 msec and the issue of habituation when assessing early cognitive components. *Electroencephalography and Clinical Neurophysiology, 74,* 347–358.

Towe, A.L. (1973) Somatosensory cortex: Descending influences on ascending systems. In: A. Jggo (Ed.) *Somatosensory system: Handbook of Sensory Physiology, Vol. 2.* (pp. 701–718). Berlin: Springer-Verlag.

Traub, E., & Geffen, G. (1979). Phonetic and category encoding of unattended words in dichotic listening. *Memory and Cognition, 7,* 56–65.

Treisman, A.M. (1960). Contextual cues in selective listening. *Quarterly Journal of Experimental Psychology: Human Perception and Performance, 12,* 242–248.

Treisman, A.M. (1969). Strategies and models of selective attention. *Psychological Review, 76,* 282–299.

Treisman, A.M. (1982). Perceptual grouping and attention in visual search for features and for objects. *Journal of Experimental Psychology: Human Perception and Performance, 8,* 194–214.

Treisman, A.M. (1985). Preattentive processing in vision. *Computer Vision, Graphics, and Image Processing, 31,* 156–177.

Treisman, A.M. (1986a). Features and objects in visual processing. *Scientific American, 254,* 114–124.

Treisman, A.M. (1986b). Properties, parts and objects. In K. Boff, L. Kaufman, & J. Thomas (Eds.), *Handbook of perception and human performance.* (pp. 35-1–35-70) New York: Wiley.

Treisman, A.M. (1988). Features and objects: The fourteenth Bartlett memorial lecture. *The Quarterly Journal of Experimental Psychology, 40A,* 201–237.

Treisman, A.M., & Davies, A. (1973). Divided attention to ear and eye. In S. Kornblum (Ed.), *Attention and performance IV* (pp. 101–117). New York: Academic Press.

Treisman, A.M., & Geffen, G. (1967). Selective attention: Perception or response? *Quarterly Journal of Experimental Psychology, 19,* 1–18.

Treisman, A.M., & Gelade, G.A. (1980). A feature-integration theory of attention. *Cognitive Psychology, 12,* 97–136.

Treisman, A.M., & Gormican, S. (1988). Feature analysis in early vision: Evidence from search asymmetries. *Psychological Review, 95,* 15–48.

Treisman, A.M., & Riley, J. (1969). Is selective attention selective perception or selective response? *Journal of Experimental Psychology, 79,* 27–34.

Treisman, A.M., & Schmidt, H. (1982). Illusory conjunctions in the perception of objects. *Cognitive Psychology, 14,* 107–141.

Treisman, A.M., & Souther, J. (1985). Search asymmetry: A diagnostic for preattentive processing of separable features. *Journal of Experimental Psychology: General, 114,* 285–310.

Treisman, A.M., Squire, R. & Green, J. (1974). Semantic processing in dichotic listening? A replication. *Memory and Cognition, 2,* 641–646.

Treisman, A.M., Sykes, M., & Gelade, G. (1977). Selective attention and stimulus integration. In S. Dornic (Ed.), *Attention and performance VI* (pp. 333-361). Hillsdale, NJ: Lawrence Erlbaum Associates.

Tsal, Y. (1983). Movements of attention across the visual field. *Journal of Experimental Psychology: Human Perception and Performance, 9,* 523–530.

Tsang, P.S., & Wickens, C.D. (1988). The structural constraints and strategic control of resource allocation. *Human Performance, 1,* 45–72.

Tucker, D.M., & Williamson, P.A. (1984). Asymmetric neural control systems in human self-regulation. *Psychological Review, 91,* 185–215.

Tuomisto, T., Hari, R., Katila, T., Poutanen, T., & Varpula, T. (1983). Effect of stimulus repetition rate on the auditory vertex response and its magnetic counterpart. *II Nuovo Cimento, Series D,* 471–483.

Underwood, G. (1977). Contextual facilitation from attended and unattended messages. *Journal of Verbal Learning and Verbal Behavior, 16,* 99–106.

Underwood, G. (1990). Attention and awareness: Using the to-be-ignored evidence. *Behavioral and Brain Sciences, 13,* 256.

Underwood, G., & Moray, N. (1971). Shadowing and monitoring for selective attention. *Quarterly Journal of Experimental Psychology, 23,* 284–295.

Unger, S.M. (1964). Habituation of the vasoconstrictive orienting reaction. *Journal of Experimental Psychology, 67,* 11–18.

Vaughan, H.G., Jr., & Arezzo, J.C. (1988). The neural basis of event-related potentials. In T.W. Picton (Ed.), Human event-related potentials. *Handbook of Electroencephalography and Clinical Neurophysiology. Revised series,* (Vol. 3, pp. 45–96). Amsterdam: Elsevier.

Vaughan, H.G., Jr., & Ritter, W. (1970). The sources of auditory evoked responses recorded from the human scalp. *Electroencephalography and Clinical Neurophysiology, 28,* 360–367.

Vaughan, H.G., Jr., Ritter, W., & Simson, R. (1980). Topographic analysis of auditory event-related potentials. In H.H. Kornhuber & L. Deecke (Eds.), *Motivation, motor and sensory processes of the brain: Electrical potentials, behaviour and clinical use.* Progress in Brain Research, vol. 54, (pp. 279–290). Amsterdam: Elsevier.

Vaughan, H.G., Jr., Ritter, W., & Simson, R. (1983). Neurophysiological considerations in event-related potential research. In A.W.K. Gaillard & W. Ritter (Eds.), *Tutorials in ERP research: Endogeneous components* (pp. 1-7). Amsterdam: North-Holland.

Vaughn, J. (1984). *Distance of attention switch affects RT only for some stimuli.* Paper presented at Annual Meeting of Psychonomic Society, San Antonio, Texas.

Velasco, M., & Velasco, F. (1986). Subcortical correlates of the somatic, auditory and visual vertex activities in man. II. Referential EEG responses. *Electroencephalography and Clinical Neurophysiology, 63,* 62–67.

Velasco, M., Velasco, F., & Olvera, A. (1985). Subcortical correlates of the somatic, auditory and visual vertex activities in man. I. Bipolar EEG responses and electrical stimulation. *Electroencephalography and Clinical Neurophysiology, 61,* 519–529.

Velden, M. (1978). Some necessary revisions of the neuronal model concept of the orienting response. *Psychophysiology, 15,* 181–185.

Venables, P.H., & Martin, I. (1967). Skin resistance and skin potential. In P.H. Venables & I. Martin (Eds.), *A manual of psychophysiological methods* (pp. 53–102). Amsterdam: North-Holland.

Verbaten, M. (1990). Näätänen's auditory model from a visual perspective. *The Behavioral and Brain Sciences, 13,* 256–257.

Verbaten, M.N., Roelofs, J.W., Sjouw, W. & Slangen, J.L. (1986). Different effects of uncertainty and complexity on single trial visual ERPs and the SCR-OR in non-signal conditions. *Psychophysiology, 23,* 254–262.

Verleger, R. (1988). A critique of the context updating hypothesis and an alternative interpretation of P3. *Behavioral and Brain Sciences, 11,* 343–427.

Verleger, R. (1990). Top-down, fast-same, and acoustic perception. *Behavioral and Brain Sciences, 13,* 257–258.

Vinogradova, O.S. (1975). The hippocampus and the orienting reflex. In E.N. Sokolov & O.S. Vinogradova (Eds.), *The neuronal mechanisms of the orienting reflex* (pp. 128–154). Hillsdale, N.J.: Lawrence Erlbaum Associates.

Voorhis, S. van, & Hillyard, S.A. (1977). Visual evoked potentials and selective attention to points in space. *Perception and Psychophysics, 22,* 54–62.

Voorhis, S. van, Hillyard, S.A., & Näätänen, R. (1976). *Spatial Selective attention and auditory event- related potentials.* Unpublished data. University of California, San Diego, California.

Wagner, M., Alho, K., Lavikainen, J., Reinikainen, K., Teder, W., & Näätänen, R. (in press). Sequential analysis of auditory selective attention: Evidence for facilitation and inhibition of pitch discrimination. In H.-J. Heinze, G.R. Mangun, & T.F. Münte (Eds.), *Perspectives in Cognitive Neurophysiology.* Boston-Basel-Berlin: Birkhäuser.

Walker, E., & Ceci, S.J. (1983). Lateral asymmetries in electrodermal responses to nonattended stimuli: A response to Dawson and Schell. *Journal of Experimental Psychology: Human Perception and Performance, 9,* 145–147.

Walter, W.G. (1964). The convergence and interaction of visual, auditory and tactile responses in human nonspecific cortex. *Annals of the New York Academy of Science, vol 112,* (pp. 320–361). New York: The New York Academy of Sciences.

Walter, W.G., Cooper, R., Aldridge, V.J., McCallum, W.C., & Winter, A.L. (1964) Contingent negative variation. *Nature, 203,* 380–384.

Wardlaw, K.A., & Kroll, N.E.A. (1976). Automatic responses to shock-associated words in a nonattended message: A failure to replicate. *Journal of Experimental Psychology: Human Perception and Performance, 2,* 357–360.

Warr, W.B., & Guinan, Jr., J.J. (1979). Efferent innervation of the organ of Corti: Two separate systems. *Brain Research, 173,* 152–155.

Warren, R.E. (1972). Stimulus encoding and memory. *Journal of Experimental Psychology, 94,* 90–100.

Warren, R.E. (1974). Association, directionality and semantic encoding. *Journal of Experimental Psychology, 102,* 151–158.

Wastell, D.G. (1980). Temporal uncertainty and the recovery function of the auditory EP. In C. Barber (Ed.), *Evoked potentials* (pp. 491–495). Lancaster: MTP Press.

Wastell, D.G., Kleinman, D., & MacLean, A. (1982). Temporal uncertainty and the "refractoriness" of the human vertex evoked potential. *Bulletin of the Psychonomic Society, 19,* 155–158.

Weerts, T.C., & Lang, P.J. (1973). The effects of eye fixation and stimulus and response location on the contingent negative variation (CNV). *Biological Psychology, 1,* 1–19.

Weinberger, N.M. (1971). Attentive processes. In J.L. McGaugh (Ed.), *Psychobiology: Behaviour from a biological perspective* (pp. 129–198). New York: Academic Press.

Weiskrantz, L. (1986). *Blindsight: A case study and implications.* Oxford: Clarendon Press.

Weitzman, E., & Kremen, H. (1965). Auditory evoked responses during different stages of sleep in man. *Electroencephalography and Clinical Neurophysiology, 18,* 65–67.

Wickens, C.D. (1976). The effects of divided attention on human information processing in tracking. *Journal of Experimental Psychology: Human Perception and Performance, 1,* 1–13.

Wickens, C.D. (1979). Measures of workload, stress and secondary tasks. In N. Moray (Ed.), *Mental workload: its theory and measurement.* (pp. 79–99). New York: Plenum Press.

Wickens, C.D. (1980). The structure of attentional resources. In R. Nickerson (Ed.), *Attention and performance VIII.* (pp. 239–257). Hillsdale, NJ: Lawrence Erlbaum Associates.

Wickens, C.D. (1984) Processing resources in attention. In: R. Parasuraman & R. Davies (Eds.), *Varieties of attention.* (pp. 63–102). New York: Academic Press.

Wickens, C.D. (1989). Attention and skilled performance. In D. Holding (Ed.), *Human skill* (pp. 71–105). New York: Wiley.

Wickens, C.D., & Gopher, D. (1977). Control theory measures of tracking as indices of attention allocation strategies. *Human Factors, 19,* 349–365.

Wickens, C.D., Isreal, J.B., & Donchin, E. (1977). The event-related cortical potentials as an index of task workload. In: A.S. Neal & R.F. Palasek (Eds.) Proceedings of the Twenty-First Annual Meeting of the Human Factors Society. Santa Monica, California: Human Factors Society.

Wickens, C.D., & Kessel, C. (1980). The processing resource demands of failure detection in dynamic systems. *Journal of Experimental Psychology: Human Perception and Performance, 6,* 564–577.

Wickens, C.D., Kramer, A.F., Vanasse, L., & Donchin, E. (1983). The performance of concurrent tasks: A psychophysiological analysis of the reciprocity of information processing resources. *Science, 221,* 1080–1082.

Wickens, C.D., & Liu, Y. (1988). Codes and modalities in multiple resources: A success and a qualification. *Human Factors, 30,* 599–616.

Wickens, C.D., Mountford, S.J., & Schneider, W. (1981). Time-sharing efficiency: Evidence for multiple resource, task-hemispheric integrity and against a general ability. *Human Factors, 23,* 211–229.

Wickens, C.D., & Sandry, D.L. (1982). Task hemispheric integrity in dual task performance. *Acta Psychologica, 52,* 227–248.

Wiederhold, M.L. (1986). Physiology of the olivocochlear system. In R.A. Altschuler, R.P. Bobbin, & D.W. Hoffman (Eds.), *Neurobiology of hearing: The cochlea.* (pp. 349–370). New York: Raven Press.

Wijers, A.A. (1989). *Visual selective attention: An electrophysiological approach.* Academic Dissertation, University of Groningen, The Netherlands.

Wijers, A.A., Lamain, W., Slopsema, S., Mulder, G., & Mulder, L.J.M. (1989). An electrophysiological investigation of the spatial distribution of attention to colored stimuli in focused and divided attention conditions. *Biological Psychology, 29,* 213–245.

Wijers, A.A., Mulder, G., Okita, T., & Mulder, L.J.M. (1989). An ERP study on memory search and selective attention to letter size and conjunctions of letter size and color. *Psychophysiology, 26,* 529–547.

Wijers, A.A., Mulder, G., Okita, T., Mulder, L.J.M., & Scheffers, M.K. (1989). Attention to colour: An ERP-analysis of selective attention, controlled search and motor activation. *Psychophysiology, 26,* 89–109.

Wijers, A.A., Mulder, G., Otten, L., Feenstra, S., & Mulder, L.J.M. (1989). Brain potentials during selective attention, memory search and mental rotation. *Psychophysiology, 26,* 452–467.

Wijers, A.A., Okita, T., Mulder, G., Mulder, L.J.M., Lorist, M.M., Poiesz, R., & Scheffers, K.M. (1987). Visual search and spatial attention: ERPs in focused and divided attention conditions. *Biological Psychology, 25,* 33–60.

Wilkinson, R.T., & Ashby, S.M. (1974). Selective attention, contingent negative variation and the evoked potential. *Biological Psychology, 1,* 167–179.

Wilkinson, R.T., & Lee, M.V. (1972). Auditory evoked potentials and selective attention. *Electroencephalography and Clinical Neurophysiology, 33,* 411–418.

Williams, H.L., Tepas, D.I., & Morlock, H.C. (1962). Evoked responses to clicks and electroencephalographic stages of sleep in man. *Science, 138,* 685–686.

Williamson, S.J., Hoke, M., Stroink, G., & Kotani, M. (Eds.). (1989). *Advances in biomagnetism.* New York: Plenum Press.

Williamson, S.J., & Kaufman, L. (1981). Magnetic fields of the cerebral cortex. In S.N. Erné, H.D. Hahlbohm, & H. Lübbig, (Eds.), *Biomagnetism* (pp. 353–402). Berlin: Walter de Gruyter.

Williamson, S.J., & Kaufman, L. (1986). Frontiers in the new science of biomagnetism. In H. Weinberg, G. Stroink, & T. Katila (Eds.), *Biomagnetism: Applications & theory* (pp. 471–490). New York: Pergamon Press.

Williamson, S.J., Kaufman, L., & Brenner, D. (1977). Biomagnetism. In B.B. Schwartz & S. Foner (Eds.), *Superconductor applications: SQUIDs and machines* (pp. 355–402). New York: Plenum Press.

Williamson, S.J., Romani, G.L., Kaufman, L., & Modena, I. (Eds.). (1983). *Biomagnetism: An interdisciplinary approach.* Volume 66 of NATO advanced science institutes series. Series A: Life sciences. New York: Plenum Press.

Winkler, I., & Näätänen, R. (in press). Event-related brain potentials to infrequent partial omissions in series of auditory stimuli. In H.J. Heinze, G.R. Mangun, & T.F. Münte (Eds.), *Perspectives in Cognitive Neurophysiology* Boston-Basel-Berlin: Birkhäuser.

Winkler, I., Paavilainen, P., Alho, K., Reinikainen, K., Sams, M., & Näätänen, R. (1990). The effect of small variation of the frequent auditory stimulus on the event-related brain potential to the infrequent stimulus. *Psychophysiology, 27,* 228–235.

Winkler, I., Paavilainen, P., & Näätänen, R. (in press). Can echoic memory store two traces simultaneously? A study of event-related brain potentials. *Psychophysiology.*

Winkler, I., Reinikainen, K., & Näätänen, R. (1991). *Event-related brain potentials reflect traces of echoic memory in humans.* Manuscript submitted for publication.

Woldorff, M.G. (in press). Distortion of ERP averages due to overlap from temporally adjacent ERPs: Analysis and correction. *Psychophysiology.*

Woldorff, M.G., Hackley, S.A., & Hillyard, S.A. (1991). The effects of channel-selective attention on the mismatch negativity wave elicited by deviant tones. *Psychophysiology, 28,* 30–42.

Woldorff, M., Hansen, J.C., & Hillyard, S.A. (1987). Evidence for effects of selective attention in the mid-latency range of the human auditory event-related brain potential. In R. Johnson, Jr., J.W. Rohrbaugh, & R. Parasuraman (Eds.), Current trends in event-related brain potential research, (pp. 146–154). (Suppl. 40 to Electroencephalography and Clinical Neurophysiology). Amsterdam: Elsevier.

Woldorff, M.G., & Hillyard, S.A. (1991). Modulation of early auditory processing during selective listening to rapidly presented tones. *Electroencephalography and Clinical Neurophysiology, 79,* 170–191.

Wolpaw, J.R., & Penry, J.K. (1975). A temporal component of the auditory evoked response. *Electroencephalography and Clinical Neurophysiology, 39,* 609–620.

Wolpaw, J.R., & Penry, J.K. (1977). Hemispheric differences in the auditory evoked response. *Electroencephalography and Clinical Neurophysiology, 43,* 99–102.

Wolpaw, J.R., & Penry, J.K. (1978). Effects of ethanol, caffeine and placebo on the auditory evoked response. *Electroencephalography and Clinical Neurophysiology, 44,* 568–574.

Wood, C.C. (1982). Application of dipole localization to source identification of human evoked potentials. *Annals of the New York Academy of Sciences,* (Vol. 388, pp. 139–155). New York: The New York Academy of Sciences.

Wood, C.C., Cohen, D., Cuffin, B.N., Yarita, M., & Allison, T. (1985). Electrical sources in human somatosensory cortex: Identification by combined magnetic and potential recordings. *Science, 227,* 1051–1053.

Wood, C.C., & McCarthy, G. (1984). Principal component analysis of event-related potentials: Simulation studies demonstrate misallocation of variance across components. *Electroencephalography and Clinical Neurophysiology, 59,* 249–260.

Wood, C.C., McCarthy, G., Squires, N.K., Vaughan, H.G., Jr., Woods, D.L., & McCallum,

W.C. (1984). Anatomical and physiological substrates of event-related potentials. Two case studies. *Annals of the New York Academy of Sciences, (Vol. 425,* pp. 681–721). New York: The New York Academy of Sciences.

Wood, C.C., & Wolpaw, J.R. (1982). Scalp distribution of human auditory evoked potentials. II. Evidence for multiple sources and involvement of auditory cortex. *Electroencephalography & Clinical Neurophysiology, 54,* 25–38.

Woods, D.L. (1990). The physiological basis of selective attention: Implications of event-related potential studies. In J.W. Rohrbaugh, R. Parasuraman, & R. Johnson, Jr. (Eds.), *Event-related brain potentials: Basic issues and applications* (pp. 178–209). New York: Oxford University Press.

Woods, D.L., Alho, K., & Algazi, A. (1991). Brain potential signs of feature processing during auditory selective attention. *Neuroreport, 2,* 189–192.

Woods, D.L., Alho, K., & Algazi, A. (in press). Intermodal selective attention I: Effects of event-related potentials to lateralized auditory and visual stimuli. *Electroencephalography and Clinical Neurophysiology.*

Woods, D.L., & Clayworth, C.C. (1985). Click spatial position influences middle latency auditory evoked potentials (MAEPs) in humans. *Electroencephalography and Clinical Neurophysiology, 60,* 122–129.

Woods, D.L., & Clayworth, C.C. (1987). Scalp topographies dissociate N1 and Nd components during auditory selective attention. In R. Johnson, Jr., J.W. Rohrbaugh, & R. Parasuraman (Eds.), Current trends in event-related brain potential research (pp. 155–160). (Suppl. 40 to Electroencephalography and Clinical Neurophysiology). Amsterdam: Elsevier.

Woods, D.L., & Courchesne, E. (1987). Intersubject variability elucidates the cerebral generators and psychological correlates of ERPs. In R. Johnson, J.W. Rohrbaugh, & R. Parasuraman (Eds.), Current Trends in Event-Related Potential Research (pp. 293–299). (Suppl. 40 to Electroencephalography and Clinical Neurophysiology). Amsterdam: Elsevier.

Woods, D.L., & Elmasian, R. (1986). The habituation of event-related potentials to speech sounds and tones. *Electroencephalography and Clinical Neurophysiology, 65,* 447–459.

Woods, D.L., & Hillyard, S.A. (1978). Attention at the cocktail party: Brainstem evoked responses reveal no peripheral gating. In D.A. Otto (Ed.), *Multidisciplinary perspectives in event-related brain potential research* (EPA-600/9-77-043, pp. 230–233). Washington, DC: U.S. Government Printing Office.

Woods, D.L., Hillyard, S.A., Courchesne, E., & Galambos, R. (1980). Electrophysiological signs of split-second decision-making. *Science, 207,* 655–657.

Woods, D.L., Hillyard, S.A., & Hansen, J.C. (1984). Event-related brain potentials reveal similar mechanisms during selective listening and shadowing. *Journal of Experimental Psychology: Human Perception and Performance, 10,* 761–777.

Woods, D.L., & Knight, R.T. (1986). Electrophysiologic evidence of increased distractibility after dorsolateral prefrontal lesions. *Neurology, 36,* 212–216.

Woods, D.L., Knight, R.T., Scabini, D. & Clayworth, C.C. (1991). The effects of temporal and parietal lesions on event-related brain potentials during auditory selective attention. *Society for Neuroscience, Abstracts* (Vol. 17, part 1, p. 655). Abstract # 258.4. Washington: Society for Neuroscience.

Woodworth, R.S. (1938). *Experimental psychology.* New York: Holt.

Worden, F.G. (1966). Attention and auditory electrophysiology. In E. Stellar & J.M. Sprague (Eds.), *Progress in physiological psychology* (pp. 45–116). New York: Academic Press.

Wright, J.M. von (1968). Selection in immediate visual memory. *Quarterly Journal of Experimental Psychology, 20,* 62–68.

Wright, J.M. von (1970). On selection in visual immediate memory. *Acta Psychologica, 33,* 280–292.

Wright, J.M. von, Anderson, K., & Stenman, U. (1975). Generalization of conditioned GSRs in dichotic listening. In P.M.A. Rabbitt & S. Dornic (Eds.), *Attention and performance* V, (pp. 194–204). London: Academic Press.

Wurtz, R.H., Goldberg, M.E., & Robinson, D.L. (1980). Behavioral modulation of visual responses in the monkey: Stimulus selection for attention and movement. *Progress in Psychobiology and Physiological Psychology, 9,* 43–83.

Yamamoto, T., Williamson, S.J., Kaufman, L., Nicholson, C., & Llinas, R. (1988). Magnetic localization of neuronal activity in the human brain. *Proceedings of the National Academy of Sciences of the USA, 85,* 8732–8736.

Yin, T.C.T., & Mountcastle, V.B. (1977). Visual input to the visuomotor mechanisms of the monkey's parietal lobe. *Science, 197,* 1381–1383.

Yingling, C.D., & Skinner, J.E. (1977). Gating of thalamic input to cerebral cortex by nucleus reticularis thalami. In J.E. Desmedt (Ed.), *Attention, voluntary contraction and event-related cerebral potentials: Progress in clinical neurophysiology* (Vol. 1, pp. 70–96). Basel, Switzerland: Karger.

Zelnicker, T., Rattok, J., & Medem, A. (1974). Selective listening and threshold for tones appearing on a relevant and on an irrelevant input channel. *Perception and Psychophysics, 16,* 50–52.

Zimmerman, J.E. (1972). Josephson effect devices and low-frequency field sensing. *Cryogenics, 12,* 19–31.

Zimmerman, J.E., Thiene, P., & Harding, J.T. (1970). Design and optimation of stable rf-biased superconducting point-contact quantum devices, and a note on the properties of perfectly clean contacts. *Journal of Applied Physics, 41,* 1572–1580.

Zimmerman, J.T., Edrich, J., Zimmerman, J.E., & Reite, M.L. (1978). The human magnetoencephalographic averaged visual evoked field. In J.I. Martin & E.A. Calvert (Eds.), *Proceedings of the San Diego Biomedical Symposium* (pp. 217–221). New York: Academic Press.

Author Index

E

H

I

J

K

N

S

T

Y

Z

Subject Index

A

B

C

D

E

N

O

P

S

V

W